Medical Surgical Nursing I and II

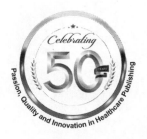

Celebrating 50

Passion, Quality and Innovation in Healthcare Publishing

Medical Surgical Nursing I and II

Second Edition

Deepak Sethi

MSc (Nursing)

Assistant Professor
Head of Department of Medical Surgical Nursing
Symbiosis International (Deemed University)
Pune, Maharashtra, India

Maj. Kirti Rani

BSc (Nursing)

Military Nursing Services (MNS)
Military Hospital (Kirkee)
Pune, Maharashtra, India

Foreword
Col. (Dr) KK Ashta

JAYPEE BROTHERS MEDICAL PUBLISHERS

The Health Sciences Publisher

New Delhi | London

Jaypee Brothers Medical Publishers (P) Ltd

Headquarters

Jaypee Brothers Medical Publishers (P) Ltd
4838/24, Ansari Road, Daryaganj
New Delhi 110 002, India
Phone: +91-11-43574357
Fax: +91-11-43574314
Email: jaypee@jaypeebrothers.com

Overseas Office

J.P. Medical Ltd
83 Victoria Street, London
SW1H 0HW (UK)
Phone: +44 20 3170 8910
Fax: +44 (0)20 3008 6180
Email: info@jpmedpub.com

Website: www.jaypeebrothers.com
Website: www.jaypeedigital.com

Inquiries for bulk sales may be solicited at: jaypee@jaypeebrothers.com

Medical Surgical Nursing I and II

First Edition: 2016
Second Edition: **2021**

ISBN 978-93-90020-97-3

Printed at Sanat Printers

Dedicated to

My Parents
Mr Sushil Kumar Sethi
and
Mrs Shashi Sethi

Foreword

This book is an enthusiastic celebration of various medical and surgical disorders. This is also a tribute to all those who have put their efforts in the past by discovering the new interventions in medicine and nursing. Medical surgical nursing is alive and well! Once considered a basic skill required of all nurses, medical surgical nursing has become increasingly complex, evolving into a vital specialty nursing practice. Medical surgical nurses must care for a growing number of healthcare consumers with complex medical needs as well as keep current with continuing developments in healthcare science, technology, and economics. They must overcome the challenges. These developments can bring to providing patient care while continuing to provide high-quality nursing care to diverse patient populations in all stages of life—from adolescents to the elderly. Specialty certification is the most important step a registered nurse can take in his/her career. It signifies a nurse's commitment to professional growth and development and, most importantly, to provide safe, effective, timely, and high-quality patient care. This book will certainly help you in pursuing certification as a medical surgical nurse. This thoroughly updated review book offers the most current content typically included in medical surgical nursing. The core content of this book reflects the best available practices that influence medical surgical nursing. It includes review topics on the foundations of nursing, legal and ethical aspects of nursing, principles of medical surgical nursing and wound care, all the medical surgical disorders and their management. **This book also offers you a free procedure manual which gives you the brief knowledge regarding advance clinical procedures such as coronary artery bypass grafting (CABG), percutaneous transluminal coronary angioplasty (PTCA), echocardiography (ECHO), cardioversion, pacemaker, central line and many more**. It also reviews the different body systems and associated diseases that certification examinations frequently cover and those medical surgical nurses commonly encounter. Whether you are a newly graduated nurse exploring the specialty of medical surgical nursing, a displaced nurse reentering the nursing profession, or a seasoned nurse wanting to update your skills and knowledge in medical surgical nursing or become certified in this prestigious specialty, I know you will find this book a valuable, addition to your library. I wish you all the best for your carrier as a Registered Nurse.

Col. (Dr) KK Ashta
Senior Advisor
Department of Medicine
Base Hospital
New Delhi, India
Assistant Professor
Armed Force Medical College (AFMC)
Pune, Maharashtra, India

Preface to the Second Edition

The complexity of the patients, increasing care demands, and increasing regulatory demands push the medical surgical nurse into new ways of thinking. In the future, the medical surgical nurse's role will continue to expand. The practice of the medical surgical nurse demands skill and expertise in a wide variety of disease states, medications, and communication techniques, as well as the ability to work with numerous members of the healthcare team. While some have interpreted this recommendation as addressing the advanced practice nurse, the intent of the recommendation was broader, including the practice of the registered nurse. When considering the practice of the medical surgical nurse, there is much that can be done in considering the full extent of practice. Often the clinical decision-making and work in care coordination by the medical surgical nurse is not fully recognized. Medical surgical nurses have long been involved in seeing the whole picture for the patient, looking beyond the patient's immediate state to the steps post-hospitalization. The medical surgical nurse has the opportunity to connect with the patient, the family, physicians, nursing staff, and the rest of the healthcare team. This provides an opportunity to make connections and carefully plan for the patients' care as they recover from their acute state to a time of rehabilitation, whether in a facility or as they return to home. In the accountable care environment, the role of the medical surgical nurse will be key in providing quality care and preventing readmissions. The practice of the medical surgical nurse is considered to be primarily in the acute care setting. The increasing complexity of patients in the home stretches the boundaries of the medical surgical nurse's practice. Nurses in long-term acute care describe their practice as that of a medical surgical nurse. Other changes within health care may continue to stretch the practice settings and opportunities for the medical surgical nurse.

This book focuses on the immediate and first aid nursing care of clients. This book includes additional chapters on medical surgical nursing, interstial lung disease, lung transplantation, etc. Significant modifications have been made in this book almost in all the chapters especially in cardiovascular disorders, respiratory disorders and immunological disorder. With these changes. I hope it will meet the most of requirement of both the students and medical surgical nursing faculty.

Deepak Sethi
Maj. Kirti Rani

Preface to the First Edition

The complexity of the patients, increasing care demands, and increasing regulatory demands push a medical surgical nurse into new ways of thinking. In the future, the medical surgical nurses' role will continue to expand. Their practice demands skill and expertise in a wide variety of disease states, medications, and communication techniques, as well as the ability to work with numerous members of the healthcare team. While some have interpreted this recommendation as addressing the advanced practice nurses, the intent of the recommendation was broader, including the practice of the registered nurses.

When considering the practice of the medical surgical nurses, there is much that can be done in considering the full extent of practice. Often the clinical decision-making and work in care coordination by the medical surgical nurses is not fully recognized. These nurses have long been involved in seeing the whole picture for the patients, looking beyond the patients' immediate state to the steps post-hospitalization. The medical surgical nurses have the opportunity to connect with the patients, the families, physicians, nursing staff, and the rest of the healthcare team. This provides an opportunity to make connections and carefully plan for the patients' care as they recover from their acute state to the time of rehabilitation, whether in a facility or as they return home. In the accountable care environment, the role of the medical surgical nurses will be the key in providing quality care and preventing readmissions. The practice of the medical surgical nurses is considered to be primarily in the acute care setting.

The increasing complexity of patients at home stretches the boundaries of the medical surgical nurses' practice. The nurses in the long-term acute care describe their practice as that of the medical surgical nurses. Other changes within health care may continue to stretch the practice settings and opportunities for the medical surgical nurses.

This book focuses on the immediate and first-aid nursing care of patients. It includes additional chapters on medical surgical nursing, interstitial lung disease, lung transplantation, etc. Significant modifications have been made in this book, almost in all the chapters, especially in Cardiovascular Disorders, Respiratory Disorders and Immunological Disorders. With these changes, I hope it will meet most of the requirements of both the students as well as the medical surgical nursing faculty.

Deepak Sethi
Maj. Kirti Rani

Acknowledgments

First and foremost, I would like to express my deepest appreciation to all those who provided me the possibility to complete this book. I would like to thank my wife **Maj. Kirti Rani** for standing beside me throughout my career and writing this book. She has been my inspiration and motivation for continuing to improve my knowledge and move my career forward. I would also like to thanks my lovely child **Kawyaa Sethi**, for always making me smile. A special gratitude I give to our final year students who gave me critiques and valuable changes as per students perceptive.

The accomplishment of this book benefits of the help and direction from my dear supervisor **Dr Sharadha Ramesh**, Director, Symbiosis College of Nursing, Pune, Maharashtra, India. I would also like to thanks **Col. (Dr) KK Ashta**, Senior Advisor, Base Hospital, New Delhi, India. He always happy and willing to help me to solve the confusions and direct me towards the final result of this book. **(Dr) Lt. Col. P Gupta**, MD (Medicine), who always gave me updates regarding the recent changes in the field of medicine and nursing. Thank you, sir.

On top of that, I would like to thanks all my colleagues of Symbiosis College of Nursing, without their encouragement, I would not finish this final work in book.

INC Syllabus

Basic BSc Nursing Year II
MEDICAL SURGICAL NURSING I
(ADULT INCLUDING GERIATRICS)

Course Description: The purpose of this course is to acquire knowledge and develop proficiency, caring for patients with medical surgical disorders in varieties of healthcare settings home.

COURSE CONTENTS

UNIT I: INTRODUCTION

- *Introduction to medical surgical nursing:* Evolution and trends of medical and surgical nursing
- Review of concepts of health and illness, disease: Concepts, causations, classification, diseases (ICD-10 or later version), acute illness, stages of illness
- Review of concepts of comprehensive nursing care in medical surgical conditions based on the nursing process
- Role of a nurse, patient and family in care of adult patients
- Role and responsibilities of a nurse in medical surgical settings:
    - Outpatient department
    - Inpatient unit
    - Intensive care unit
    - Home and community settings
- Introduction to medical surgical asepsis:
    - Inflammation and infection
    - Immunity
    - Wound healing
- Care of surgical patient (preoperative)
    - Intraoperative
    - Postoperative

UNIT II: COMMON SIGNS AND SYMPTOMS AND MANAGEMENT

- Fluid and electrolyte imbalance
- Vomiting
- Dyspnea and cough, respiratory
- Fever
- Shock
- Unconsciousness, syncope
- Pain
- Incontinence
- Edema
- Age-related problems—geriatric

UNIT III: NURSING MANAGEMENT OF PATIENTS (ADULTS INCLUDING ELDERLY) WITH RESPIRATORY PROBLEMS

- Review of anatomy and physiology of respiratory system
- *Nursing assessment:* History and physical assessment
- Etiology, pathophysiology, clinical manifestations, diagnosis, treatment modalities and medical surgical, dietetics and nursing management of adults, including elderly with:
  - Upper respiratory tract infections
  - Bronchitis
  - Asthma
  - Emphysema
  - Empyema
  - Atelectasis
  - Chronic obstructive pulmonary diseases (COPD)
  - Bronchiectasis
  - Pneumonia pulmonary tuberculosis
  - Lung abscess
  - Pleural effusion
  - Cysts and tumors
  - Chest injuries
  - Respiratory arrest and insufficiency
  - Pulmonary embolism
  - Special therapies, alternative therapies
  - Nursing procedures
  - Drugs used in treatment of respiratory disorders

UNIT IV: NURSING MANAGEMENT OF PATIENTS (ADULTS INCLUDING ELDERLY) WITH DISORDERS OF DIGESTIVE SYSTEM

- Review of anatomy and physiology of digestive system
- Nursing assessment: History and physical assessment
- Etiology, pathophysiology, clinical manifestations, diagnosis, treatment modalities and medical, surgical, dietetics and nursing management
- Disorders of:
  - *Oral cavity:* Lips, gums, tongue, salivary glands and teeth
  - *Esophagus:* Inflammation, stricture, obstruction, bleeding and tumors
  - *Stomach and duodenum:* Hiatus hernia, gastritis, peptic and duodenal ulcer bleeding, tumors, pyloric stenosis
  - *Small intestinal disorders:* Inflammation and infection, enteritis, malabsorption, obstruction, tumor and perforation
  - *Large intestinal disorders:* Colitis, inflammation and infection, obstruction and tumor and lymph hernias
  - *Appendix:* Inflammation, mass, abscess, rupture
  - *Anal and rectum:* Hemorrhoids, fissures, fistulas
  - Peritonitis/acute abdomen
  - *Pancreas:* Inflammation, cyst, abscess and tumors
  - *Liver:* Inflammation, cyst, abscess, cirrhosis, portal hypertension, hepatic failure, tumors
  - Gallbladder, inflammation, obstruction, stones and tumors
  - Special therapies, alternative therapies
  - Nursing procedures, drugs used in treatment of disorders of digestive system

UNIT V: NURSING MANAGEMENT OF PATIENTS (ADULTS INCLUDING ELDERLY) WITH BLOOD AND CARDIOVASCULAR PROBLEMS

- Review of anatomy and physiology of blood and cardiovascular system
- *Nursing assessment:* History and physical assessment
- Etiology, pathophysiology, clinical manifestations, diagnosis, treatment modalities and medical, surgical dietetics and nursing management of:
- Vascular system of:
  - Hypertension, hypotension
  - Artherosclerosis
  - Raynaud's disease
  - Aneurism and peripheral vascular disorders

Heart

- Coronary artery diseases:
  - Ischemic heart disease
  - Coronary atherosclerosis
  - Angina pectoris
  - Myocardial infarction
- Valvular disorders of the heart:
  - Congenital and acquired
  - Rheumatic heart diseases
- Endocarditis, pericarditis, myocarditis
- Cardiomyopathies
- Cardiac dysrhythmias, heart block
- Congestive cardiac failure edema, cardiogenic shock, cardiac tamponade
- Cardiac emergencies and arrest
- Cardiopulmonary resuscitation (CPR)
- Blood:
  - Anemias
  - Polycythemia
  - Bleeding disorder; clotting factor defects and platelet defects
  - Thalassemia
  - Leukopenias and agranulocytosis
  - Lymphomas
  - Myelomas
- Special therapies:
  - Blood transfusion safety checks, procedure and requirements, management of adverse transfusion reaction, records for blood transfusion
  - Management and counseling of blood donors, phlebotomy procedure, and post-donation management. Blood bank functioning and hospital transfusion committee. Biosafety and waste management in relation to blood transfusion
  - Role of a nurse in organ donation, retrieval and banking
  - Alternative therapies, nursing procedures, drugs used in treatment of blood and cardiovascular disorders

UNIT VI: NURSING MANAGEMENT OF PATIENTS (ADULTS INCLUDING ELDERLY) WITH DISORDERS OF GENITOURINARY PROBLEMS

- Review of anatomy and physiology of genitorurinary system
- Nursing assessment: History and physical assessment

- Etiology, pathophysiology, clinical manifestations diagnosis, treatment modalities and medical, surgical, dietetics and nursing management of:
  - Nephritis
  - Nephrotic syndrome
  - Nephrosis
  - Renal calculus
  - Tumors
  - Acute renal failure
  - Chronic renal failure
  - End-stage renal disease
  - Dialysis, renal transplant
  - Congenital disorders, urinary infections
  - Benign prostate hypertrophy
  - Disorders of ureter, urinary bladder and urethra—inflammation infection, stricture obstruction, tumor, prostate
- Special therapies, alternative therapies
- Nursing procedures, drugs used in the treatment of genitourinary disorders

UNIT VII: NURSING MANAGEMENT OF DISORDERS OF MALES (ADULTS INCLUDING ELDERLY) REPRODUCTIVE SYSTEM

- Review of anatomy and physiology of male reproductive system
- *Nursing assessment:* History and physical assessment
- Etiology, pathophysiology, clinical manifestation diagnosis, treatment modalities and medical, surgical dietetics and nursing management of disorders of male reproductive system
  - Congenital malformation, cryptorchidism
  - Hypospadiasis, epispadiasis
  - Infections
  - Testis and adjacent structures
  - Penis
  - *Prostate:* Inflammation, infection, hypertrophy, tumor
  - Sexual dysfunction
  - Infertility
  - Contraception
  - Breast, gynecomastia, tumor
  - Climacteric changes
- Special therapies, alternative therapies
- Nursing procedures, drugs used in treatment of disorders of male reproductive system.

UNIT VIII: NURSING MANAGEMENT OF PATIENTS (ADULTS INCLUDING ELDERLY) WITH DISORDERS OF ENDOCRINE SYSTEM

- Review of anatomy and physiology of endocrine system
- *Nursing assessment:* History and physical assessment
- Etiology, pathophysiology, diagnosis, treatment modalities and medical, surgical, dietetics and nursing management of:
  - Disorders of thyroid and parathyroid
  - Diabetes mellitus

- Diabetes insipidus
- Adrenal tumor
- Pituitary disorders
- Special therapies, alternative therapies
- Nursing procedures, drugs used in treatment of disorders of endocrine system

UNIT IX: NURSING MANAGEMENT OF PATIENTS (ADULTS INCLUDING ELDERLY) WITH DISORDERS OF INTEGUMENTARY SYSTEM

- Review of anatomy and physiology of skin and its appendages
- Nursing assessment
- History and physical assessment
- Etiology, pathophysiology, clinical manifestations, diagnosis, treatment modalities and medical, surgical, dietetics and nursing management of disorders of skin and its appendages:
  - Lesions and abrasions
  - Infection and infestations, dermatitis
  - Dermatomes, infectious and noninfectious 'inflammatory dermatoses'
  - Acne vulgaris
  - Allergies and eczema
  - Psoriasis
  - Malignant melanoma
  - Alopecia
- Special therapies, alternative therapies
- Nursing procedures, drugs used in treatment of disorders of integumentary system

UNIT X: NURSING MANAGEMENT OF PATIENTS (ADULTS INCLUDING ELDERLY) WITH MUSCULOSKELETAL PROBLEMS

- Review of anatomy and physiology of musculoskeletal system
- Nursing assessment
- History and physical assessment
- Etiology, pathophysiology, clinical manifestations, diagnosis, treatment modalities and medical, surgical, dietetics and nursing management of disorders of:
  - *Muscles, ligaments and joints:* Inflammation, infection, trauma
  - *Bones:* Inflammation, infection dislocation, fracture, tumor and trauma
  - Osteomalacia and osteoporosis
  - Arthritis
  - Congenital deformities
  - *Spinal column:* Defects and deformities, tumor, prolapsed intervertebral discs, Pott's spine
  - Paget's disease
- Amputation
- Prosthesis
- Transplant and replacement surgeries
- Rehabilitation
- Special therapies, alternative therapies
- Nursing procedures
- Drugs used in treatment of disorders of musculoskeletal system

UNIT XI: NURSING MANAGEMENT OF PATIENTS (ADULTS INCLUDING ELDERLY) WITH IMMUNOLOGICAL PROBLEMS

- Review of immune system
- *Nursing assessment:* History and physical assessment
- Etiology, pathophysiology, clinical manifestations, diagnosis, treatment modalities and medical, surgical, dietetics and nursing management of:
  - Immunodeficiency disorder
  - Primary immunodeficiency
    - Phagocyte dysfunction
    - B-cell and T-cell deficiencies
- Secondary immunodeficiency syndrome (AIDS)
- Incidence of HIV and AIDS
- Epidemiology
- Transmission–prevention of transmission
- Standard safety precautions
- Role of nurse, counseling
- Health education and home care consideration
- National AIDS Control Program—NACO, various national and international agencies
- Infection control program
- Rehabilitation
- Special therapies, alternative therapies
- Nursing procedures, drugs used in treatment of disorders of immunological system

UNIT XII: NURSING MANAGEMENT OF PATIENTS (ADULTS INCLUDING ELDERLY) WITH COMMUNICABLE DISEASE

- Overview of infectious disease, the infectious process
- *Nursing assessment:* History and physical assessment
- Epidemiology, infections, process, clinical manifestations, diagnosis, treatment, prevention and dietetics. Control and eradication of common communication diseases:
  - Tuberculosis
  - Diarrheal
  - Hepatitis A, E
  - Herpes
  - Chickenpox
  - Smallpox
  - Typhoid
  - Meningitis
  - Gas gangrene
  - Leprosy
  - Dengue
  - Plague
  - Malaria
  - Diphtheria
  - Pertussis
  - Poliomyelitis
  - Measles
  - Mumps
  - Influenza

- – Tetanus
- – Yellow fever
- – Filariasis
- – HIV, AIDS
- Reproductive tract infections
- Special infection control isolation, quarantine, immunization, infectious disease hospitals
- Special therapies, alternative therapies
- Nursing procedures, drugs used in treatment of communicable diseases

UNIT XIII: PREOPERATIVE NURSING

- Organization and physical set-up of the operation theater (OT):
  - – Classifications
  - – OT design
  - – Staffing
  - – Members of the OT team
  - – Duties and responsibilities of a nurse in an OT
- Principles of health and operating room attire
  - – Instruments
  - – Sutures and suture materials
  - – Equipment
  - – OT tables and sets for common surgical procedures
  - – Positions and draping for common surgical procedures
  - – Scrubbing procedures
  - – Gowning and gloving
  - – Preparation of OT sets
  - – Monitoring the patient during surgical procedures
- Maintenance of therapeutic environment in OT
- Standard safety measures:
  - – *Infection control:* Fumigation, disinfection and sterilization
  - – Biomedical waste
  - – Prevention of accidents and hazards in OT
- Anesthesia:
  - – Types
  - – Methods of administration
  - – Effects and stages
  - – Equipment
  - – Drugs
- Cardiopulmonary resuscitation (CPR)
- Pain management techniques
- Legal aspects

Basic BSc Nursing Year III
MEDICAL SURGICAL NURSING II
(ADULT INCLUDING GERIATRICS)

Course description: The purpose of this course is to acquire knowledge and develop proficiency in caring for patients with medical and surgical disorder in varieties of healthcare settings and at home.

COURSE CONTENTS

UNIT I: NURSING MANAGEMENT OF PATIENTS WITH DISORDER OF EAR, NOSE AND THROAT

- Review of anatomy and physiology of the ear, nose and throat
- *Nursing assessment:* History and physical assessment
- Etiology, pathophysiology, clinical manifestations, diagnosis, treatment modalities and medical and surgical nursing management of ear, nose and throat disorders:
  - *External ear:* Deformities, otalgia, foreign bodies, and tumors
  - *Middle ear:* Impacted wax, tympanic membrane perforation, otitis media, otosclerosis, mastoiditis, tumors
  - *Inner ear:* Meniere's disease, labyrinthitis, ototoxicity, tumors
  - *Upper airway infections:* Common cold, sinusitis, ethinitis, rhinitis, pharyngitis, tonsillitis and adenoiditis, peritonsilar abscess, laryngitis
- Upper respiratory airway, epistaxis
- Nasal obstruction, laryngeal obstruction, cancer of the larynx
- Cancer of the oral cavity
- Speech defects and speech therapy
- *Deafness:* Prevention, control and rehabilitation
- Hearing aids, implanted hearing devices:
  - Special therapies
  - Nursing procedures
  - Drugs used in treatment of disorders of ear, nose and throat, role of a nurse communicating with hearing impaired and muteness

UNIT II: NURSING MANAGEMENT OF PATIENTS WITH DISORDERS OF EYE

- Review of anatomy and physiology of the eye
- *Nursing assessment:* History and physical assessment
- Etiology, pathophysiology, clinical manifestations, diagnosis, treatment modalities, and medical and surgical nursing management of eye disorder
  - Refractive errors
  - *Eyelids:* Infections, tumors and deformities
  - *Conjunctiva:* Inflammation and infection, bleeding
  - *Cornea:* Inflammation and infection
  - Lens, cataract
  - Glaucoma
  - Disorder of the uveal tract
  - Ocular tumors, disorders of posterior chamber and retina, retinal and vitreous problems
  - Retinal detachment

- Ocular emergencies and their prevention
- Blindness
- National Programme for Control of Blindness
- Eye banking
- Eye prostheses and rehabilitation
- *Role of a nurse:* Communication with a visually impaired patient, eye camps
- Special therapies
- Nursing procedures
- Drugs used in the treatment of disorders of eye

UNIT III: NURSING MANAGEMENT OF PATIENTS WITH NEUROLOGICAL DISORDERS

- Review of anatomy and physiology of the neurological system
- *Nursing assessment:* History and physical and neurological assessment and Glasgow coma scale
- Etiology, pathophysiology, clinical manifestations, diagnosis, treatment modalities, and medical and surgical neurological disorders
  - Congenital malformations
  - Headache
  - Head injuries
  - Spinal injuries
  - Paraplegia
  - Hemiplegia
  - Quadriplegia
  - *Spinal cord compression:* Herniation of intervertebral disc
  - Tumors of brain and spinal cord
  - Intracranial and cerebral aneurysms abscess, neurocysticercosis
  - Movement disorders
  - Chorea
  - Seizures
  - Epilepsies
  - Cerebrovascular accidents (CVA)
  - *Cranial, spinal neuropathies:* Bell's palsy, trigeminal neuralgia
  - *Peripheral neuropathies:* Barré syndrome
  - Myasthenia gravis
  - Multiple sclerosis
  - Degenerative:
    - Delirium
    - Dementia
    - Alzheimer's disease
    - Parkinson's disease
- Management of unconscious patients and patients with stroke
- Role of a nurse in communicating with a patient having neurological deficit
- Rehabilitation of patients with neurological deficit
- Role of a nurse in long-stay facility (institutions) and at home
- Special therapies
- Nursing procedures
- Drugs used in the treatment of neurological disorders

UNIT IV: NURSING MANAGEMENT OF PATIENTS WITH DISORDERS OF FEMALE REPRODUCTIVE SYSTEM

- Review of anatomy and physiology of the female reproductive system
- *Nursing assessment:* History and physical assessment
- Breast self-examination
- Etiology, pathophysiology, clinical manifestations, diagnosis, treatment modalities, and medical and surgical nursing management of disorder of female reproductive system
    - Congenital abnormalities of female reproductive system
    - Sexuality and reproductive health
    - Sexual health assessment
    - *Menstrual disorders:* Dysmenorrheal, amenorrhea
    - Pelvic inflammatory disease
    - Ovarian and fallopian tube disorder, infections, cysts, tumors
    - *Uterine and cervical disorders:* Endometriosis, polyps, fibroids, cervical and uterine tumors
    - Uterine displacement
    - Cystocele/Urethrocele rectocele
    - *Vaginal disorders:* Infections and discharges, fistulas
    - *Diseases of breast:* Deformities, infections, cysts and tumors
    - Menopause and hormonal replacement therapy
    - Infertility
    - *Contraception:* Types methods, risk and effectiveness
    - Spacing methods
    - *Barrier methods:* Interauterine devices, hormonal, postconnectional methods, etc.
    - Terminal methods
    - Sterilization
    - Emergency contraception methods
    - *Abortion:* Natural, medical and surgical abortion; MTP Act
    - Toxic shock syndrome
    - Injuries and trauma, sexual violence
- Special therapies
- Nursing procedures
- Drugs used in the treatment of gynecological disorders
- National Family Welfare Programme

UNIT V: NURSING MANAGEMENT OF PATIENTS WITH BURNS, RECONSTRUCTIVE AND COSMETIC SURGERY

- Review of anatomy and physiology of the skin and connective tissues and various deformities
- *Nursing assessment:* History and physical assessment and assessment of burns and fluid and electrolyte loss
- Etiology, classification, pathophysiology, clinical manifestations, diagnosis, treatment modalities, and medical and surgical nursing management of burns and reconstructive and cosmetic surgery
- Types of reconstructive and cosmetic surgery; for burns, congenital deformities, injuries and cosmetic purposes
- Role of nurse
- Legal aspects
- Rehabilitation

- Special therapies
- Psychosocial aspects
- Nursing procedures
- Drugs used in the treatment of burns, reconstructive and cosmetic surgery

UNIT VI: NURSING MANAGEMENT OF PATIENTS WITH ONCOLOGICAL CONDITIONS

- Structure and characteristics of normal and cancer cells
- *Nursing assessment:* History and physical Assessment
- Prevention screening, early detection, warning signs of cancer
- Epidemiology, etiology, classification
- Pathophysiology, staging, clinical manifestations, diagnosis, treatment modalities and management of oncological conditions.
- Common malignancies of various body systems: Oral, larynx, lung, stomach and colon, liver, leukemias and lymphomas, breast, cervix, ovary, uterus, sarcoma, brain, renal, bladder, prostate, etc.
- Oncological emergencies
- Modalities of treatment:
  - Immunotherapy
  - Chemotherapy
  - Radiotherapy
  - Surgical interventions
  - Stem cell
  - Bone marrow transplant
  - Gene therapy
  - Other forms of treatment
- Psychosocial aspect of cancer
- Rehabilitation
- Palliative care; symptom and pain management, nutritional support
- Home care
- Hospice care
- Stomal therapy
- Special therapies
- Psychosocial aspects
- Nursing procedures

UNIT VII: NURSING MANAGEMENT OF PATIENTS IN EMERGENCY AND DISASTER SITUATIONS

- Concept and principles of disaster nursing
- *Causes and types of disaster:* Natural and man-made
  - Earthquakes, floods, epidemics, cyclones
  - Fire, explosion, accidents
  - Violence, terrorism: Biochemical war
- Policies related to emergency/disaster management: International, national/state, institutional
- Disaster preparedness:
- Team guidelines, protocols, equipments resources

- Coordination and involvement of community, various government departments, nongovernment organizations and international agencies
- *Role of a nurse:* Working
- Legal aspect of disaster nursing
- Impact on health and aftereffects: Post-traumatic stress disorder
- Rehabilitation; physical psychosocial, financial, relocation
- **Emergency nursing**
- Concept, priorities, principles and scope of emergency nursing
- Organization of emergency services: Physical setup, staffing, equipment and supplies, protocols, concepts of triage and role of a triage nurse
- Coordination and involvement of different departments and facilities
- *Nursing assessment:* History and physical assessment
- Etiology, pathophysiology, clinical manifestations, diagnosis, treatment modalities and medical and surgical nursing management of patient with medical and surgical emergency
- Principles of emergency management
- Common emergencies
- Respiratory emergencies
- Cardiac emergencies
- Shock and hemorrhage
- Pain
- Polytrauma, road accidents, crush injuries, wounds
- Bites
- *Poisoning:* Food, gas, drugs, and chemical poisoning
- Seizures
- *Thermal emergencies:* Heat stroke and cold injuries
- Pediatric emergencies
- Psychiatric emergencies
- Obstetric emergencies
- Violence, abuse, sexual assault
- Cardiopulmonary resuscitation
- Role of a nurse
- Medicolegal aspects
- Crisis intervention
- Communication and interpersonal relationship

UNIT VIII: NURSING CARE OF THE ELDERLY

- *Nursing assessment:* History and physical assessment
- Aging
- *Demography:* Myths and realities
- Concepts and theories of aging
- Cognitive aspects of aging
- Normal biological aging
- Age-related body system changes
- Psychosocial aspects of aging
- Medications and elderly
- Stress and coping in older adults
- Common health problems and nursing management
- Cardiovascular, respiratory, musculoskeletal

- Endocrine, genitourinary, gastrointestinal
- Neurological, skin and other sensory organs
- Psychosocial and sexual
- Abuse of elderly person
- Role of a nurse for care of elderly: Ambulation, nutritional, communicational, psychosocial and spiritual
- Role of a nurse for caregivers of elderly
- Role of a family and formal and nonformal caregivers
- Use of aids and prosthesis (hearing aids, dentures)
- Legal and ethical Issues
- Provisions and programs for elderly; privileges, community programs and health services; home and institutional care

UNIT IX: NURSING MANAGEMENT OF PATIENTS IN CRITICAL CARE UNITS

- *Nursing assessment:* History and physical assessment
- Classification
- Principles of critical care nursing
- *Organization:* Physical setup, policies, staffing norms
- Protocols, equipment and supplies
- *Special equipment:* Ventilators, cardiac monitors, defibrillators
- Resuscitation equipment
- Infection control protocols: Nursing management of critically ill patients
- Monitoring of critically ill patients
- *CPR:* Advance cardiac life support
- Treatments and procedures
- Transitional care
- Ethical and legal aspects
- Communication with patient and family
- Intensive care records
- Crisis intervention
- Death and dying—coping with them
- Drugs used in critical care unit

UNIT X: NURSING MANAGEMENT OF PATIENTS (ADULTS INCLUDING ELDERLY) WITH OCCUPATIONAL AND INDUSTRIAL DISEASES

- *Nursing assessment:* History and physical assessment
- Etiology, pathophysiology, clinical manifestations, diagnosis, treatment modalities and medical and surgical nursing management of occupational and industrial health disorders
- Role of a nurse
- Special therapies, alternative therapies
- Nursing procedures
- Drugs used in treatment of occupational and industrial disorders

- Endocrine, genitourinary, gastrointestinal
- Neurological, skin and other sensor organs
- Psychosocial and sexual
- Abuse of elderly person
- Role of nurses in care of elderly: Rehabilitation, nutritional, communication, psychosocial and palliative
- Role of nurse for care-giver of elderly
- Role of family, health related nonformal care-givers
- Use, abuse and possbilitis (like the role of nurses)
- Legal and ethical issues
- Provisions and programmes for elderly: privileges, concessions, programmes and health services, geriatric/rehabilitation care

UNIT X: NURSING MANAGEMENT OF PATIENTS IN CRITICAL CARE UNITS

- Nursing assessment: History and physical assessment
- Classification
- Principles of critical care nursing
- Organization: Physical setup, policies, staffing norms
- Protocols, equipment and supplies
- Special equipment: Ventilators, cardiac monitors, defibrillators, resuscitation equipment
- Infection control protocols, nursing management of critically ill patients
- Monitoring of critically ill patients
- CPR, haemodynamic monitoring
- Treatments and procedures
- Nutritional and...
- Ethical and legal aspects
- Communication with patient and family
- Intensive care services
- Crisis intervention
- Death and dying, coping with loss
- Drugs used in critical care unit

UNIT XI: NURSING MANAGEMENT OF PATIENTS/ADULTS, INCLUDING ELDERLY WITH OCCUPATIONAL AND INDUSTRIAL DISEASES

- Nursing assessment: History and physical assessment
- Etiology, pathophysiology, clinical manifestations, diagnosis, treatment modalities and prevention and management of occupational and industrial health disorders
- Role of nurse
- Special therapies: alternative therapies
- Nursing procedures
- Drugs used in treatment of occupational and industrial disorders

Contents

APPENDICES

Introduction

AT THE END OF THIS CHAPTER, THE STUDENTS WILL BE ABLE TO:
➤ Understand evolution and trends of medical and surgical nursing
➤ Comprehend about comprehensive nursing care
➤ Identify the role of nurse in care of adult patient
➤ Discuss inflammation and infection
➤ Discuss about immunity
➤ Discuss wound healing

EVOLUTION, ETHICS, AND TRENDS OF MEDICAL AND SURGICAL NURSING

Professional medical–surgical nurses, as direct caregivers, collaborate with different healthcare team members to provide acceptable, effective, and economical healthcare services. Medical–surgical nurses work in a variety of institutional and community settings. The role of the medical–surgical nurse depends on nursing preparation, work setting, specialized formal or informal and academic education, and clinical experiences with patients. Current treatment modalities and technologies demand distinctive data and skills. Medical–surgical nurses base clinical judgment and higher cognitive process on theory and nursing research additionally as on specific medical–surgical data.

CURRENT TRENDS IN THE NURSING PROFESSION

Moving to an all graduate, controversy continues to rage over nursing as a graduate entry profession; however, this move could be a necessity to deliver nursing care services within the 21st century. The stress on the nursing profession within the 21st century is much more complicated than those of the past. Traditionally, nursing has generally been viewed as moderate standard type profession.

Over subsequent 15 years and even on the far side, nurses can meet challenges regarding changes in human ecology, sickness patterns, lifestyle, public expectations, and information technology. Even be a growing demand for healthcare professionals with advanced nursing skills and that they will have to be compelled to develop these academic skills from a graduate knowledge domain.

SCOPE AND TRENDS IN NURSING AS A PROFESSION

Finding Your Niche in Nursing

It is not a challenging task for a new graduate nurse to step into his/her first role as a registered nurse, the responsibility of nurse to give care are:
- To ensure each client receives personal care
- To follow doctors' orders

- To ensure each patient is prepared for nursing intervention
- To monitor and record baseline data as per the need and report significant changes to the doctor.
- To ensure proper disposal of used articles, equipment, and biomedical waste segregate.
- To provide holistic care, which caters to the emotional and psychological needs as well.

Forensic Nursing

Forensic nursing is one among the latest specialty areas recognized by the American Nurses Association. It involves operating with law enforcement officers to help within the investigation of crimes such as abuse, accidental death, and assault.

They also collect evidence from the survivors of the violent crime as well as the suspect so that a case can be filed and justice can be given.

Forensic nurses work in collaboration with diverse healthcare professionals with different job responsibilities, for example, correctional nursing specialist, such as forensic clinical nurse, forensic medical specialist, forensic nurse investigator, legal nurse advisor, and nurse death investigator. The largest subspecialty of forensic nursing is sexual assault, closely followed by death investigation, forensic psychiatric nursing, and medical-legal consulting.

When sexual assault occurs, it is the responsibility of the forensic nurse to collect records and take photographs, so that the victim can be caught. This is achieved by cross-referencing the DNA sample into the criminal database system. DNA sample can be collected from the suspect and if it is match, then a legal arrest is made.

In terms of murder investigation, the forensic nurse assists the pathologist in examining the cause of death.

In order to become a forensic nurse, one has to enroll in a program offered by a university, which focuses on the criminal justice system, forensic mental health, interpersonal violence, perpetrator theory, and victimology.

Dialysis Nursing

They are registered nurses who care for patients diagnosed with chronic kidney disorders and are commonly called nephrology or dialysis nurses.

Dialysis nurses work in a hemodialysis unit and provide specific care to patients on dialysis.

Responsibilities of a dialysis nurse include:
- Assessing the patients' vital signs
- Educating the patients about their disease and its treatment modalities
- Monitoring the dialysis treatment carefully ensuring that patients are given the correct medications ordered by their physicians
- Monitoring patients' reaction to the dialysis treatment
- Reviewing the outcome of the treatment by assessing patients' conditions
- Assisting in follow-up care of the patient, for example, guiding to the transplant center and next follow-up dialysis visit.

Operating Room Nurses

The operating room nurse or perioperative nurse provides a continuity of care throughout the perioperative period. This process is dynamic and continuous and requires constant reevaluation of individual nursing practice in the operating room. They work in close collaboration with surgeons, anesthesiologists, nurse practitioners, and other allied health members.

Intensive Care Unit Nurse

Intensive care unit (ICU) nurse is one of the most demanding and challenging nursing specialties, which require specialized skill in providing immediate and long-term care to critically-ill patients. Nursing responsibilities in the ICU and emergency room will always be in great demand, but changes to the evolving healthcare system will also determine, which nursing specialties will grow at an accelerated pace.

Nurse Informaticist

A nurse specialized in the nursing informatics program effectively delivers health care with major contributions in development and utilization of healthcare technology. In other words, the nurse informatics program is a combination of nursing science and advancements in technology, which enables healthcare providers to document care and record evidence of their practice during the course of care.

Geriatric Nurse

These nursing specialties focus on geriatrics and the acute-care patient population and are expected to grow in the near future. Geriatric nursing is a growing field for nurses because of the rising disparity in the ratio of geriatric population and healthcare personnels.

Nursing Specialties in Genetics

Genetics nursing has also seen an increase in interest, as various colleges and nursing schools are now offering programs dedicated to the specialty. Advances in science and technology have contributed to the increased awareness of this specialty.

TRENDS IN MEDICAL–SURGICAL NURSING

Following are the trends in medical–surgical nursing:
1. The nursing process should be used to develop and implement the plan of care.
2. Assessment and management strategies should be developed based on a holistic approach.
3. An empathetic relationship with the client should be established.
4. Knowledge of the impact of actual or potential illness on the client's developmental, physical, social, emotional, age, spiritual, economic, vocational, and leisure status should be demonstrated.
5. The quality and effectiveness of nursing practice should be systematically evaluated.
6. Communication should be effectively done with clients, families, and other healthcare professionals.
7. There should be coordination and collaboration with clients, families, and communities.
8. The existing scientific knowledge should be applied in health care to nursing practice.
9. Clients and family members should be educated to maintain and restore health.
10. Resources should be mobilized to provide healthy environment.
11. Referrals services should be made available for patient.
12. Research findings should be applied to identify problems.
13. Standard protocols and policies should be used to increase the quality of care and quality of life for the client.
14. Leadership skills should be utilized to enhance client outcomes.
15. A mentor and role model should be there for nursing colleagues, students, and others.

ETHICS IN MEDICAL–SURGICAL NURSING

The ethics in medical–surgical nursing are as follows:
1. **Moral conflict:** It occurs when the nurse is unsure which moral principle to apply, or even what the problem is.

2. **Moral distress:** It occurs when the patient knows the right thing to do, but organizational constraints keep them away from doing it.
3. **Moral outrage:** It occurs when a patient witnesses an immoral act by another but feels powerless to do anything due to organizational constrain.
4. **Moral dilemma:** It occurs when two or more clear principles apply but, they support inconsistent courses of action.

Principles of Ethical Reasoning

The principles of ethical reasoning are as follows:
- **Confidentiality:** It means protecting patient's privacy.
- **Fidelity:** It includes implicit and explicit promises to client.
- **Autonomy:** Patients have the right to make decisions, to know procedure and complications involved, and to reject the treatment.
- **Beneficence and nonmaleficence:** Goodness, kindness, must be shown to prevent any harm to the client.

COMPREHENSIVE NURSING CARE

Comprehensive care is an approach used by nurse to provide care for the patient as a whole and fulfill all his needs. It involves the use of other health team members together, such as physician and nurse who fulfill the standard approach at all major medical concerns. Some key aspects of well-designed comprehensive care are:
- A wide range of services, such as education and counseling
- Consultation with community healthcare professionals
- Referral services
- Medical diagnosis and management
- A team of professional healthcare members
- Patient and family education programs
- School health programs
- Ongoing research that looks at and evaluates the results of all treatments and services.

ROLE OF NURSE IN CARE OF ADULT PATIENT

Adult nursing involves caring for adults from 18 years old to elder patients, both sick and well, not only in the hospital but also in the community. The role of an adult nurse is to focus on the promotion of health through education, the prevention of illness, and rehabilitation of adults.

Goals of Adult Health Nursing

The goals of adult health nursing are to:
- Determine responses to health problems, level of wellness, and needs for assistance.
- Have interventions aimed at assisting the client to meet own needs.
- Provide physical care, emotional care, teaching, guidance, and counseling.
- Prepare care plans
- Implement plans through tasks, such as preparing patients for surgeries and wound treatment
- Assist with tests, carryout routine investigations, and evaluation
- Maintain patient records
- Respond quickly to emergencies
- Monitor and record the conditions of patient
- Organize staff and workloads

- Implant teaching skills to student and junior nurses
- Make ethical decisions related to current and confidentiality.

Role of Nurse in Adult Patient Care

1. **Clinical decision maker:** To provide therapeutic care the nurse uses critical skills throughout the nursing process. Before providing any nursing care, whether it is assessing the client's condition, providing nursing care, or evaluating the outcome of the care, the nurse plans the action by deciding the best approach for each client.
2. **Protector:** As a protector the nurse helps to maintain a safe environment for the patient from possible adverse effects of diagnostic or treatment measures, such as providing accurate medicine and immunization against disease in a community-based practice.
3. **Advocate:** Adult nurse also helps patient by briefing their rights and assisting them to speak up for themselves. They help the patients to understand their right to make informed decisions about their own health and lives.
4. **Communicator:** The role of communicator is central to all other nursing roles. Nursing involves communication with clients and families, other nurses and healthcare professionals, resource persons, and the community.
5. **As a care giver:** As a caregiver, the nurse helps the patient to regain optimum health through the healing process. Adult nurses who work in the healthcare setting included those nursing approaches that assist the patient's dignity. The required nursing actions may include complete care for the completely dependent client, partial care for the partially dependent client, and supportive educative care to assist clients in their highest possible level of health.
6. **Teacher:** As a teacher, nurse must educate clients about their health and the healthcare procedures, they need to perform to restore or maintain their health. The nurse provides regular health education to patient and assesses the clients learning needs.
7. **Change agent:** The nurse acts as a change agent when she makes modifications in their own behavior.
8. **Rehabilitation:** Rehabilitation is the process by which individuals return to maximum levels of functioning after illness. Nurse helps the client to have proper follow-up with physician and to maintain their health after getting discharge from hospital.

Role and Responsibilities of a Nurse in Medical–Surgical Settings

Intensive Care Unit

Critical care nursing is a complex and challenging task done by nurse. Nursing responsibilities in the ICU and emergency room will always be in great demand, but changes to the evolving healthcare system will also determine which nursing specialties will grow at an accelerated pace.

Critical care nurses need advanced skills to care for patients who are critically ill and at high risk for life-threatening health problems, such as in the case of heart attack, stroke, shock, severe trauma, and respiratory distress. Critical care nurses provide such care in ICU, where patients can be given complex assessments and treatment.

Specific critical care nurse duties and responsibilities can include:
- Assessing a patient's condition and planning and implementing nursing care plans
- Assisting physicians in performing surgical procedures in ICU, such as lumbar puncher
- Observing and documenting patient vital signs
- Ordering lab tests
- Managing wounds and providing advanced life support
- Responding to life-saving situations, using nursing standards and protocols for treatment
- Ensuring that monitors and ventilators and other medical equipment function properly.

- Administering IV fluids and medications.
- Providing education and support to patient families.

MEDICAL–SURGICAL ASEPSIS

Inflammation

An inflammation is a defensive response of living tissue to injury. It is a protecting mechanism through which the body removes the injurious stimulant and starts the wound healing process and repair. Inflammation may be acute or chronic. Acute inflammation is for brief period and involves infiltration of neutrophils and proteins, such as albumin and globulin. Chronic inflammation is of long duration and heals very slowly and involves the infiltration of lymphocytes and macrophages.

Inflammation can either be acute or chronic and is characterized by rubor (redness), tumor (swelling), calor (heat), dolor (pain), and functio laesa (loss of function).

Acute Inflammation (Fig. 1.1)

Acute inflammation is of short duration and is characterized by redness due to increased blood flow and edema due to accumulation of fluid with in the space. These changes occur due to vascular response to inflammation.

Causes of acute inflammation

Following are the causes of acute inflammation

- Viruses, bacteria, fungi, parasites
- Physical agents such as trauma
- Chemical agents
- Hypersensitivity
- Necrosis

Cardinal signs of acute inflammation

There are five principal signs of inflammation

1. **Rubor:** It is characterized by redness and hyperemia due to dilatation of blood vessels.
2. **Tumor:** It is characterized by swelling and formation of exudate due to the migration of inflammatory cell into the affected area.

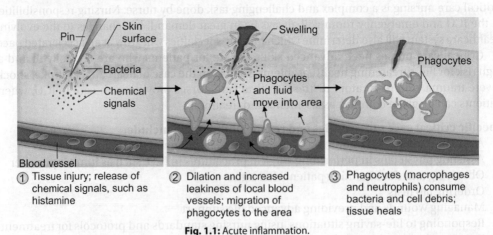

① Tissue injury; release of chemical signals, such as histamine

② Dilation and increased leakiness of local blood vessels; migration of phagocytes to the area

③ Phagocytes (macrophages and neutrophils) consume bacteria and cell debris; tissue heals

Fig. 1.1: Acute inflammation.

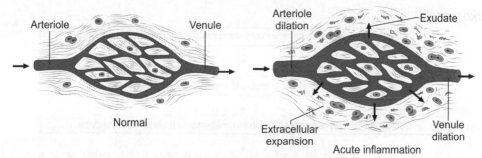

Fig. 1.2: Dilatation of blood vessels in the injured area.

3. **Color:** It is characterized by increase in temperature due to increased blood flow in the affected area resulting in circulation of warm blood in affected area.
4. **Dolor:** It is characterized by pain due to stretching and damage of tissues due to inflammatory response of bradykinin and prostaglandins.
5. **Functio laesa:** It is characterized by loss of function.

Vascular changes in acute inflammation

The vascular events occur in acute inflammation involve three main steps:
1. Changes in vessel size and blood flow
2. Increased vascular permeability
3. Formation of the fluid exudate

   1. **Changes in vessel size:** Inflammation causes dilatation of blood vessel resulting in increased flow of blood in the injured area. This dilation occurs due to release of nitric oxide, histamine, and prostaglandins **(Fig. 1.2)**.
   2. **Increased vascular permeability:** Due to increase in hydrostatic pressure and movement of plasma proteins into the extravascular space, exudates can be formed in the injured area. As a result, more and more fluid moves away from the blood vessels than is returned to them and results in exudate formation.
   3. **Formation of the cellular exudate:** Formation of exudate involves two mechanism— phagocytosis and leukocytosis. This involves the series of steps:

Phagocytosis

The process whereby cells ingest solid particles is termed phagocytosis.

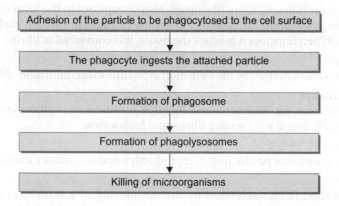

Leukocytosis

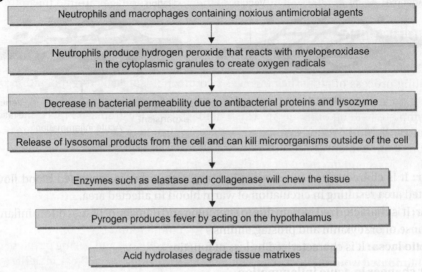

Neutrophils and macrophages containing noxious antimicrobial agents

↓

Neutrophils produce hydrogen peroxide that reacts with myeloperoxidase in the cytoplasmic granules to create oxygen radicals

↓

Decrease in bacterial permeability due to antibacterial proteins and lysozyme

↓

Release of lysosomal products from the cell and can kill microorganisms outside of the cell

↓

Enzymes such as elastase and collagenase will chew the tissue

↓

Pyrogen produces fever by acting on the hypothalamus

↓

Acid hydrolases degrade tissue matrixes

Chronic Inflammation

Chronic inflammation remains for weeks or months and characterized by the formation of granulomatous tissue and granulation tissue in the injured area. Chronic inflammation is not usually red or hot and involves the infiltration of macrophages.

Causes of chronic inflammation

The causes of chronic inflammation are as follows:

- Infections by organisms, such as bacteria and viruses
- Autoimmune diseases
- Repeated attacks of acute inflammation
- Prolonged exposure to toxins.

Granulomatous Inflammation

In chronic inflammation, the macrophages fuse together and form giant cells, called granuloma, which is a layer of macrophages surrounding a central core. Granulomas are a characteristic feature of TB, in which macrophages cannot destroy the phagocytized bacteria because the bacteria somehow prevent lysosomes from fusing with the phagocytic vesicles.

Types of exudates

Fibrinous exudate

Sometime in chronic inflammation, fibrinogen also sweeps out in the form of exudate, which is termed "fibrinogen exudate" that results in escape of larger fibrinogen molecules from the vascular system. When fibrinogen reaches the tissue, it is converted to fibrin.

Purulent exudate

Purulent exudate is characterized by the formation of pus due to accumulation of dead neutrophils.

Hemorrhagic exudate

Hemorrhagic exudates are characterized by large numbers of erythrocytes. Hemorrhagic exudates are usually mixed with serum, fibrin, and leukocytes.

Mucosal exudate

It involves excessive mucus production in reproductive and respiratory tracts.

Serous exudate

Serous inflammation is characterized by the outpouring of a translucent fluid that may accumulate on a mucosal surface of skin. Serous exudate is yellowish fluid.

Granulomatous exudate
These exudates are characterized by accumulation of macrophages around the injured area.

WOUND HEALING

Introduction

The healing process of all tissues involves two mechanisms called regeneration or repair. Regeneration is the replacement of damaged tissues by identical cells, such as liver, and repair is the complete healing of tissue, in which damaged tissue is replaced by connective tissue leaving a scar behind. Wound healing can be accomplished in one of the following two ways:
1. Healing by first intention (primary union)
2. Healing by second intention (secondary union)

Types of Wound

There are three types of wounds, which are as follows:
1. **Clean wound:** Operative incisional wounds with blunt trauma
2. **Infected wound:** Traumatic wounds containing dead tissue and having purulent drainage
3. **Contaminated wound:** Open, traumatic wounds involving a major break in sterile technique characterized by inflammation.

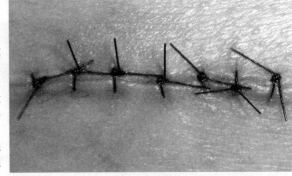

Wound Healing

Healing by first intention: Healing of a wound through primary union occurs where the wound is clean and uninfected, surgically incised, without loss of cells and edges of wound are surgically sutured **(Fig. 1.3)**.

Mechanism of wound healing through primary union (Fig. 1.4): Wound healing by primary intention follows the mentioned steps during repair.

Fig. 1.3: Sutured wound repair (healing is done by primary union).

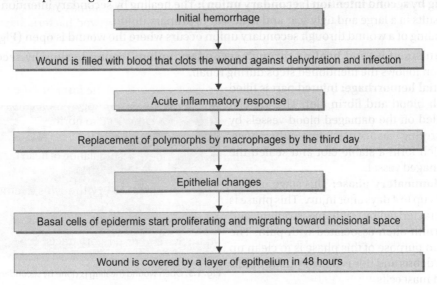

| Initial hemorrhage |
| Wound is filled with blood that clots the wound against dehydration and infection |
| Acute inflammatory response |
| Replacement of polymorphs by macrophages by the third day |
| Epithelial changes |
| Basal cells of epidermis start proliferating and migrating toward incisional space |
| Wound is covered by a layer of epithelium in 48 hours |

Contd...

Contd...

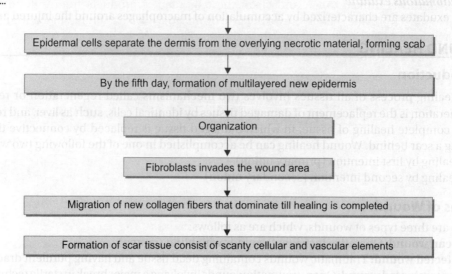

Epidermal cells separate the dermis from the overlying necrotic material, forming scab

↓

By the fifth day, formation of multilayered new epidermis

↓

Organization

↓

Fibroblasts invades the wound area

↓

Migration of new collagen fibers that dominate till healing is completed

↓

Formation of scar tissue consist of scanty cellular and vascular elements

Primary intention

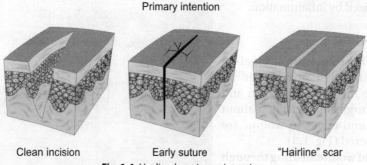

Clean incision   Early suture   "Hairline" scar

Fig. 1.4: Healing by primary intention.

Primary Wound Healing

Healing by second intention (secondary union): The healing by secondary intention is slow and results in a large and ugly scar and neat scar of primary union.

Healing of a wound through secondary union occurs where the wound is open **(Fig. 1.5)**.

Mechanism of wound healing through secondary union: Wound healing by secondary intention follows the mentioned steps during repair.

1. **Initial hemorrhage:** Injured part is filled with blood and fibrin clot. The platelet sealed off the damaged blood vessels by secreting vasoconstrictive substances, which form a stable clot and sealed the damaged vessel.

2. **Inflammatory phase:** This stage usually lasts up to 4 days after injury. This phase is characterized by erythema, swelling, and warmth often associated with pain. The main purpose of this phase is to clean up the debris and this is done by neutrophils and mast cells.

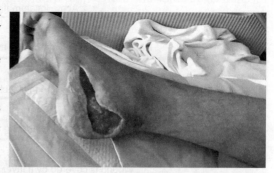

Fig. 1.5: Open wound (healing is done by secondary union).

As fibrin is broken down and clean the degradation products from injured part, macrophages provide second line of defense by phagocytized bacteria from the wound by secreting the chemotactic and growth factors.

3. **Proliferative and granulation phase:**

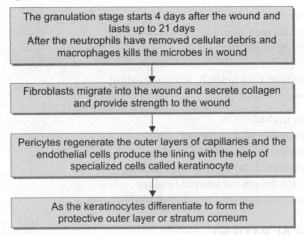

The granulation stage starts 4 days after the wound and lasts up to 21 days
After the neutrophils have removed cellular debris and macrophages kills the microbes in wound

↓

Fibroblasts migrate into the wound and secrete collagen and provide strength to the wound

↓

Pericytes regenerate the outer layers of capillaries and the endothelial cells produce the lining with the help of specialized cells called keratinocyte

↓

As the keratinocytes differentiate to form the protective outer layer or stratum corneum

4. **Wound contraction:** In primary healing, this phase is no longer active and in secondary, this is done by myofibroblasts that contract the wound to one-third to one-fourth of its original size.

5. **Remodeling or maturation phase:** This phase involves remodeling of dermal tissues to provide more tensile strength and this is done by specialized cells, fibroblast. Remodeling can take up to 2 years after wound has occurred (**Fig. 1.6**).

Complications of Wound Healing

Following are the complications of wound healing:

- Infection of wound
- Scar formation
- Incisional hernia
- Hypertrophied scars and keloid
- Excessive contraction
- Epidermal cyst
- Pigmentation

Factors influencing wound healing: Healing of wound depends on various physiological and mechanical factors, if healing is not proper and interrupted by environmental or mechanical

Secondary intension

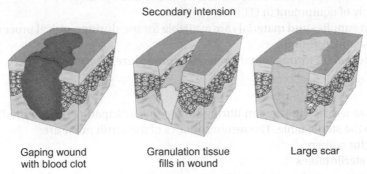

Gaping wound with blood clot

Granulation tissue fills in wound

Large scar

Fig. 1.6: Secondary wound healing.

factors, it may become poor and results in chronic inflammation and wound. Some factors are mentioned below, which can affect the wound healing process:

The local factors include:
- Infection
- Poor blood supply
- Movement of injured part
- Exposure to ionizing radiation
- Foreign bodies
- Exposure to ultraviolet rays helps in wound healing
- Type, size, and location of injury

The systemic factors include:
- Age delays the wound healing process
- Systemic infection delays the wound healing
- Uncontrolled diabetics delays the wound healing
- Nutrition deficiency delays the wound healing
- Hematologic abnormalities lead to poor wound healing

CARE OF SURGICAL PATIENT

Role of Nurse in Intraoperative Phase

The intraoperative phase extends from the time the client is admitted to the operation theater (OT) to the time of administration, performance of the surgical procedure, and until the client is transported to the recovery room.

Goals

Goals are to:
1. Promote the principle of asepsis
2. Maintain homeostasis
3. Safe administration of anesthesia

Circulating Nurse

The circulating nurse manages the OT and protects the safety and health needs of the patient by monitoring activities of members of the surgical team and checking the conditions in the operating room. Responsibilities of a circulation nurse are to:
1. Assure cleanliness in the OT
2. Guarantee the proper room temperature, humidity and lighting in OT
3. Make supply of equipment in OT
4. Ensure that supplies and materials are available for use during surgical procedures
5. Monitor aseptic technique
6. Monitor the patient throughout the operative procedure to ensure the safety.

Scrub Nurse

The scrub nurse assists the surgeon during surgery by anticipating the required instruments and setting up the sterile table. The responsibilities of the scrub nurse are:
1. Scrubbing for surgery
2. Setting up sterile tables
3. Preparing sutures and special equipment

4. Assisting the surgeon and assistant during the surgical procedure
5. Keeping track of the time the patient is under anesthesia and the time the wound is open
6. Checking equipment and materials.

Role of Nurse in Postoperative Phase

The **postoperative phase** of the surgical experience extends from the time the client is transferred to the recovery room to the time when patient transported back to the surgical unit.

Goals

Goals are:
1. Maintaining adequate body system functions
2. Restoring body homeostasis
3. Alleviating pain and discomfort
4. Preventing postoperative complications
5. Promoting adequate discharge planning and health teaching.

The mnemonic "POSTOPERATIVE" may also be helpful:
- P—Preventing complications
- O—Optimal respiratory function
- S—Support: psychosocial
- T—Tissue perfusion
- O—Observing adequate fluid intake
- P—Promoting adequate nutrition and elimination
- A—Adequate fluid and electrolyte balance
- R—Renal function maintenance
- E—Encouraging activity and mobility within limits
- T—Thorough wound care for adequate wound healing
- I—Infection control
- V—Vigilant to manifestations of anxiety
- E—Eliminating environmental hazards

Patient Assessment

Patient assessment includes:
1. Assessing skin integrity of patient
2. Verifying patient identity
3. Assessing neurologic status and level of consciousness through Glasgow Coma Scale
4. Performing cardiovascular assessment
5. Inspecting operative site

Promoting Patient Safety

When transferred to the stretcher, the patient should be covered with blankets and secured with straps above the knees and elbows. These straps anchor the blankets at the same time restrain the patient should he/she pass through a stage of excitement while recovering from anesthesia. To protect the patient from falls, side rails should be raised.
- S—Securing restraints for IV fluids and blood transfusion
- A—Assist the patient to a position appropriate
- F—Fall precaution by putting the side rails
- E—Eliminating possible sources of injuries

Postoperative Nursing Care

Care should be taken for postoperative nursing as follows:

- **Airway**
  - The airway should be kept in place until the patient is fully awake.
  - The airway is allowed to remain in place while the client is unconscious to keep the passage open and prevents the tongue from falling back.
  - Secretions should be suctioned as needed.
- **Breathing**
  - B—Bilateral lung auscultation frequently.
  - R—Rest and place the patient in a lateral position with the neck extended, if not contraindicated, and the arm supported with a pillow. This position promotes chest expansion and facilitates breathing and ventilation.
  - E—Encourage the patient to take deep breaths.
  - A—Assess and periodically evaluate the patient's orientation to name or command.
  - T—Turn the patient every 1-2 hours to facilitate breathing and ventilation.
  - H—Humidified oxygen administration.
- **Circulation**
  - Patient's vital signs should be obtained as ordered and any abnormalities should be reported.
  - Intake and output should be closely monitored.
  - Early symptoms of shock or hemorrhage, such as cold extremities and decreased urine output should be recognized.
- **Thermoregulation**
  - Hourly temperature assessment should be monitored to detect hypothermia or hyperthermia.
  - Temperature abnormalities should be reported to the physician.
  - The patient should be monitored for postanesthesia shivering.
  - A therapeutic environment should be provided with proper temperature and humidity.
- **Fluid volume**
  - Patient's skin color and turgor, mental status, and body temperature should be assessed and evaluated.
  - Fluid and electrolyte imbalances should be monitored.
  - Intake and output should be closely monitored.
  - Signs of fluid imbalances, such as decreased blood pressure, oliguria, tachycardia, tachypnea, and decreased central venous pressure should be recognized.
- **Safety**
  - Frequent dressing examination should be carried out for possible constriction.
  - The side rails should be raised to prevent the patient from falling.
  - The extremity where IV fluids are inserted should be protected.
  - Nerve damage and muscle strain should be avoided by properly supporting and padding pressure areas.
  - It must be ensured that bed wheels are locked.
- **GI function and nutrition**
  - NG tube and monitor patency and drainage should be maintained.
  - Antiemetic medications for nausea and vomiting should be provided.
  - Paralytic ileus and intestinal obstruction should be inspected for.
  - Patient should be arranged to consult with the dietitian to plan appealing, high-protein meals.

- Patient should be instructed to take multivitamins, iron, and vitamin C supplements postoperatively, if prescribed.
- Phenothiazine medications should be administered as prescribed.
- Patient should be assisted to return to normal dietary intake.
- **Comfort**
  - Behavioral and physiologic manifestations of pain should be observed and assessed.
  - Medications should be administered for pain and document its efficacy.
  - The patient should be assisted to a comfortable position.
- **Drainage**
  - There should be proper system of drainage, tubes must be connected to a specific drainage system, and presence and condition of dressings should be ensured.
- **Skin integrity**
  - The amount and type of wound drainage should be recorded.
  - Dressings should be regularly inspected and reinforced, if necessary.
  - The patient should be turned to sides every 1–2 hours.
  - The patient's good body alignment should be maintained.
  - Wound care should be proper as needed.
  - Handwashing should be performed before and after contact with the patient.
- **Assessing and managing voluntary voiding**
  - Bladder distention and urge to void should be assessed for.
  - The bedpan needs to be warmed to reduce discomfort.
  - Patient who complains of not being able to use the bedpan should be assisted.
  - Order for catheterization should be obtained before the end of the 8-hour time limit.
  - Methods should be initiated to encourage the patient to void.
  - Continue intermittent catheterization every 4–6 hours until patient can void spontaneously.
  - Safeguards should be taken to prevent the patient from falling due to orthostatic hypotension.
  - The amount of urine voided should be noted and palpated the suprapubic area for distention.

Common Signs and Symptoms

AT THE END OF THIS CHAPTER, THE STUDENTS WILL BE ABLE TO LEARN ABOUT:

The common signs and symptoms, and management of the following features:

➢ Fluid and electrolyte imbalance
➢ Vomiting
➢ Respiratory: dyspnea and cough
➢ Fever
➢ Shock
➢ Unconsciousness and syncope
➢ Pain
➢ Incontinence
➢ Edema

FLUID AND ELECTROLYTE IMBALANCE

The values of normal serum electrolyte are given in the following table.

Electrolyte	Normal value
Sodium (Na⁺)	135–145 mEq/L
Potassium (K⁺)	3.5–5.0 mEq/L
Calcium (Ca²⁺)	9.0–10.5 mg/dL
Ionized Calcium (Ca²⁺)	4.5–5.3 mg/dL
Magnesium (Mg²⁺)	1.3–2.1 mg/dL
Chloride (Cl⁻)	98–106 mEq/L
Chloride (Cl⁻)	3.0–4.5 mg/dL

SODIUM

Sodium is a major cation of extracellular fluid. The serum Na⁺ level is maintained by the sodium–potassium pump. The major function of Na⁺ is to transmit the impulse in nerve and muscle fibers and to maintain acid–base balance in order to treat acidosis and alkalosis. The normal serum Na⁺ level is 135-145 mEq/L, any deviation from the normal value will result in hyponatremia or hypernatremia.

Mechanism of Sodium Regulation

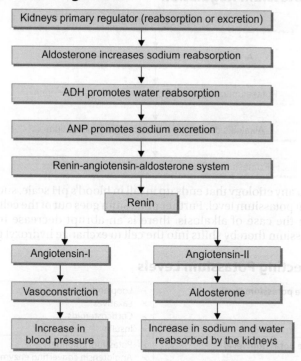

Explanation: Excessive heat and humid environment results in excessive loss of Na⁺ from body. Kidney regulates the Na⁺ excretion and absorption. Due to external changes, such as increase in temperature, aldosterone increases the absorption of Na⁺, and antidiuretic hormone (ADH) increases the reabsorption of water. At same time, renin–angiotensin–aldosterone system releases angiotensin-I and angiotensin-II. Angiotensin-I causes vasoconstriction that will increase blood pressure (BP). Angiotensin-II releases aldosterone, which increases Na⁺ and water reabsorbed by the kidneys resulting in increased BP.

Medications Affecting Sodium Levels

Drugs that decrease the sodium level	➤ Hypotonic IV solutions (D5W, 0.45% NS) ➤ Thiazide diuretics ➤ Loop diuretics ➤ Oxytocin
Drugs that increase the sodium level	➤ Hypertonic saline solutions (3% NaCl) ➤ Corticosteroids ➤ Sodium bicarbonate

POTASSIUM

Potassium could be a major cation of body fluid. The normal range of blood serum K⁺ is 3.5–5.0 mEq/L. The most important functions of K⁺ are to maintain intracellular osmolality, smooth contraction, electrical discharge conductivity, cardiac, skeletal, acid–base equilibrium, metabolism of carbohydrates, electroneutrality, and proteins. K⁺ level is regulated by sodium–potassium pump.

Mechanism of Potassium Regulation

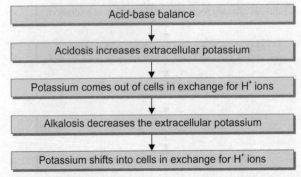

Acid-base balance
↓
Acidosis increases extracellular potassium
↓
Potassium comes out of cells in exchange for H$^+$ ions
↓
Alkalosis decreases the extracellular potassium
↓
Potassium shifts into cells in exchange for H$^+$ ions

Explanation: Due to any etiology that ends up in fall in blood's pH scale, such as acidosis leads to elevation in serum potassium level. Further potassium goes out of the cell to counterbalance the amount. Just in the case of alkalosis, there is an abrupt decrease in the extracellular potassium and potassium thereby shifts into the cell to exchange hydroxyl group ions.

Medications Affecting Potassium Levels

Drugs that decrease the potassium level	➢ Loop and thiazide diuretics ➢ Laxatives ➢ Corticosteroids ➢ Insulin
Drugs that increase the potassium level	➢ Potassium chloride ➢ Angiotensin converting enzyme inhibitors ➢ Potassium-sparing diuretics ➢ Heparin

CALCIUM

Calcium is a necessary mineral that is absorbed through gut. The normal blood serum Ca level is 9.0–10.5 mg/dL. Its major functions are the formation and maintenance of teeth and bones, internal organ and striated muscle contraction, blood coagulation, and electrical discharge transmission.

Calcium is present in serum in two forms:

1. **Bound calcium:** It is present in albumin and helps in blood coagulation.
2. **Ionized or unbound:** It covers 50% of serum calcium and helps in nerve impulses transmission and responsible for normal heart function.

Mechanism of Calcium Regulation

1. Serum calcium level increases with sunlight exposure and vitamin D.
2. The parathyroid hormone increases the serum calcium level.
3. Calcitonin (from thyroid gland) decreases the serum calcium level.

Medications Affecting Calcium Level

Drugs that decrease the calcium level	➢ Loop diuretics ➢ Citrate-buffered blood ➢ Bisphosphonates ➢ Oral phosphate supplements ➢ Magnesium antacids, laxatives ➢ Corticosteroids, calcitonin, chelating agents

Contd...

Contd...

Drugs that increase the calcium level	➢ Calcium supplements ➢ Antacids with calcium carbonate ➢ Vitamin D ➢ Parathyroid hormone ➢ Lithium ➢ Thiazide diuretics

MAGNESIUM

It is the second most abounding body fluid ion. The normal blood serum Mg^{2+} level is 1.3–2.1 mg/dL. It is useful in most of the metabolic processes, particularly energy metabolism. Its major functions are to do protein activity, bone formation, energy metabolism, sedative result on fiber bundle transmissions, having antiarrhythmic drug properties and smooth muscle relaxation.

Medications Affecting Magnesium Level

Drugs that decrease the magnesium level	➢ Loop diuretics ➢ Aminoglycosides antibiotics ➢ Corticosteroids ➢ Calcium gluconate
Drugs that increase the magnesium level	➢ Antacids ➢ Laxatives ➢ Magnesium sulfate

PHOSPHATE (PO_4^{3-})

It is a major bodily fluid ion, settled in bones, which helps in bone formation and cellular energy metabolism. Its major functions are to supply strength to bone and teeth, energy storage and transport, maintaining membrane structure and acid–base equilibrium. Parathyroid hormone lowers the phosphate by increasing urinary organ excretion and calciferol raises the phosphate level.

Medications Affecting Phosphate Level

Drugs that decrease the phosphate level	➢ Sucralfate ➢ Phosphate binders ➢ Aluminum antacids ➢ Calcium antacids ➢ Diuretics
Drugs that increase phosphate level	➢ Bisphosphonates ➢ Oral phosphate supplements ➢ IV phosphates ➢ Phosphate enema ➢ Excessive vitamin D

Intravenous Fluid Comparison

Type	Solution	Uses	Special considerations
Isotonic	Dextrose 5% in water (D5W)	➢ Fluid loss ➢ Dehydration ➢ Hypernatremia	➢ Use cautiously in renal and cardiac patients ➢ Can cause fluid overload
Isotonic	0.9% sodium chloride (Normal saline) (NaCl)	➢ Shock ➢ Hyponatremia ➢ Blood transfusions ➢ Resuscitations ➢ Fluid challengers ➢ DKA	➢ Can Lead to overload ➢ Use with caution in patients with heart failure or edema

Contd...

Contd...

Type	Solution	Uses	Special considerations
Isotonic	Lactated Ringer's (LR)	➢ Dehydration ➢ Burns ➢ Lower GI fluid loss ➢ Acute blood loss ➢ Hypovolemia due to third spacing	➢ Contains potassium, do not use with renal failure patients ➢ Do not use with liver disease, cannot metabolize lactate
Hypotonic	0.45% sodium chloride (1/2 normal saline)	➢ Water replacement ➢ DKA ➢ Gastric fluid loss from NG or vomiting	➢ Use with caution ➢ May causes cardiovascular collapse or increased intracranial pressure ➢ Do not use with liver disease, trauma, or burns
Hypertonic	Dextrose 5% in 1/2 normal saline	➢ Later in DKA treatment	➢ Use only when blood sugar falls below 250 mg/dL
Hypertonic	Dextrose 5% in normal saline	➢ Temporary treatment for shock if plasma expanders are not available ➢ Addison's crisis	➢ Do not use in cardiac or renal patients
Hypertonic	Dextrose 10% in water	➢ Water replacement ➢ Conditions where some nutrition with glucose is required	➢ Monitor blood sugar levels

VOMITING

Nausea and regurgitation often considered more of an unpleasant inconvenience than a medical problem. These are often debilitating and might cause prolonged recovery times and enhanced prices. In critically-sick patients, severe or prolonged nausea and regurgitation will result in serious complications, which may be critical.

Etiology

Nausea and vomiting are associated with a variety of medical conditions. A few have been enlisted below:

- Radiotherapy
- Chemotherapy
- Pregnancy
- Postoperative
- Motion sickness
- Drug induced
- Anxiety
- Bulimia nervosa
- Cough
- Fluid and electrolyte imbalance
- Food poisoning
- Gastrointestinal obstruction
- Increased intracranial pressure
- Infections
- Metastasis
- Peritonitis
- Tube feeding
- Uremia
- Vestibular problems

Clinical Manifestations

Nausea and emesis are basic human protecting reflexes against the absorption of poisons, likewise as responses to certain stimuli. The terms "nausea" and "emesis" are usually used along, though every phenomenon ought to be assessed individually.

Nausea is defined as a subjectively unpleasant, uneven sensation within the back of the throat or epigastrium related to achromasia or flushing, arrhythmia, and an awareness of the urge to vomit. Sweating, excess salivation, and a sensation of being cold or hot might occur.

Vomiting, or emesis, is characterized by contraction of the abdominal muscles, descent of the diaphragm, and opening of the gastric orifice, leading to forceful expulsion of abdomen contents from the mouth.

Management
Pharmacological Management

Class	Example
Antihistamines	Cyclizine, promethazine
Antimuscarinic drugs	Hyoscine
Dopamine receptor antagonists	Prochlorperazine, metoclopramide, domperidone
5HT$_3$ receptor antagonists	Granisetron, ondansetron
Neurokinin receptor antagonists	Aprepitant
Cannabinoids	Nabilone
Corticosteroids (weak antiemetic)	Dexamethasone, methylprednisolone
Benzodiazepines (no intrinsic antiemetic activity)	Lorazepam

General Management

- Positioning the patient upright while eating and for 1 hour postmeal
- Offering dry foods throughout the day
- Encouraging bland, soft, easily digestible food for main meals
- Rinsing patient's mouth after eating.

DYSPNEA

Dyspnea refers to the feeling of difficulty or discomfort in breathing. It is a subjective experience perceived and reported by an affected patient. Dyspnea on exertion may occur normally, but is considered indicative of disease when it occurs at a level of activity that is usually well tolerated.

Orthopnea is the feeling of breathlessness in the recumbent position, relieved by sitting or standing.

Paroxysmal nocturnal dyspnea is a sensation of breathlessness that awakens the patient, often after 1 or 2 hours of sleep, and is usually relieved in the upright position.

Management
Pharmacological Management

1. **β$_2$ adrenergic agonists:** albuterol and terbutaline
2. **Methylxanthines:** theophylline
3. **Muscarinic receptor antagonists:** ipratropium bromide

4. **Adrenal corticosteroids:** beclomethasone
5. **Cromolyn sodium**
6. **Leukotriene inhibitors:** montelukast sodium
7. **Monoclonal antibodies:** omalizumab

Nursing Management

Assessment

Following are the assessments of nursing management:

- The rate of respiration, easy respiration, and depth of respiration should be monitored—the common rate of respiration for adults is 10–20 breaths/min. It is necessary to require action once respirations exceed 30 breaths/min.
- It should be queried and noted whether patient has "shortness of breath" or any dyspnea— typically anxiety will cause dyspnea, thus the patient should be watched for "air hunger" that could be a sign that the cause of shortness of breath is physical.
- Hyperventilation should be check for—"sighing" with respiration should also be checked for.
- Accessory muscle use should be looked for—true respiratory problems that are physiological cause the use of accessory muscles to assist, to get air flow into the body.
- Skin color should be investigated—lack of oxygen can cause cyanosis to the lips, tongue, and fingers. Cyanosis within the mouth could be a medical emergency.
- Breathe sounds should be listened to. Crackles, wheezing, lack of breath sounds, and the other respiratory organ sounds should be checked for.
- Pulse oximetry should be checked—the patient's oxygen saturation levels should be checked upon initial assessment and on a daily basis. Normal oxygen saturation levels are between 95 and 100%.

Implementation

Implementation of nursing management should include:

- Giving respiratory medications and oxygen, per doctor's orders
- Monitoring very important signs, metastasis standing, and pulse oximetry—frequent observance of significant signs, oxygen saturation, and respiratory efforts will alert the nurse and doctor to a modification in condition
- Assisting patient to breathe slowly and keep calm
- Teaching patient to perform "pursed lip respiration"
- For acute dyspnea, helping patient to sit up straight to aid in lung expansion
- Ambulating patient as tolerated and per doctor's order three times daily
- Encouraging frequent rest periods and teaching patient to pace activity
- Consulting nutritionist for dietary modifications
- Encouraging little frequent meals to stop overloading of the diaphragm
- Place a cooler
- Encouraging the patient to "turn, cough, and deep breath" every 2 hours
- Using chest and back percussions to assist split mucosa with doctor's order

FEVER

Hyperthermia occurs once the body absorbs heat more than it will excrete. Overly elevated body temperatures are thought of medical emergency because it might lead to permanent disability and even death. Fever is one amongst the foremost common medical signs and is characterized by an elevation of body temperature higher than the normal value of 36.5–37.5°C (97.7–99.5°F) because of an increase within the temperature regulative set point.

Nursing Management

Assessment

The assessment of nursing management include:
- Assessing temperature at least every 2 hours
- Assessing BP, pulse, and respiration
- Assessing skin color and temperature
- Assessing level of consciousness
- Assessing white blood count (WBC), Hb, and Hct
- Monitoring intake and output

Implementation

Implementation of nursing management should include:
- Administering antipyretics
- Identifying and treating the underlying cause of fever
- Maintaining adequate hydration by increasing fluid intake either orally or intravenous (IV) administration.
- Performing sponge bath per the need or applying cold compress on the thigh fold, axilla, and neck to lower the temperature and avoiding sudden lowering of temperature.
- Maintaining air circulation by ensuring adequate ventilation.
- Providing measures to prevent shivering due to draught or chills and avoiding unwanted exposure of body, use of blanket, mattress, warm water bath, etc.
- Teaching the client how to prevent fatigue due to heat.
- Discussing the importance of temperature regulation and possible negative effects of cold.

SHOCK

Refer page 675 under Emergency and Disaster Nursing.

UNCONSCIOUSNESS AND SYNCOPE

Loss of consciousness is obvious in patient who is not well oriented, does not follow commands, or needs persistent stimuli to attain a state of alertness.

A person who is unconscious and unable to respond to the spoken words will typically hear what is spoken. Unconsciousness is an abnormal state resulting from disturbance of sensory perception to the extent that the patient is not aware of what is happening around him.

Levels of Unconsciousness

Alert	Normal consciousness
Automatism	Aware of surroundings, may be unable to remember actions later
Confuse	Loss of ability to speak and think in a logical coherent fashion
Delirium	Characterized by restlessness and possible violence
Stupor	Quite and uncommunicative, remains conscious but sits or lies with a glazed expression
Semi-coma	A twilight stage, patients often pass fitfully into unconsciousness
Coma	When patient is deeply unconscious

Etiology

- Head injury
- Skull fracture
- Asphyxia
- Infantile convulsions
- Fainting
- Blood loss
- Cerebrovascular accident
- Epilepsy
- Extremes of body temperature
- Cardiac arrest
- Hypothermia
- Poisonous substances and fumes
- Hypoglycemia
- Hyperglycemia
- Drug overdose

Management

Assessment of Unconscious Patients

- History
- Physical assessment

Glasgow Coma Scale

Eye opening		
	➤ Spontaneous	4
	➤ To speech	3
	➤ To pain	2
	➤ No response	1
Verbal response	➤ Oriented	5
	➤ Confusion	4
	➤ Inappropriate words	3
	➤ Incomprehensible sounds	2
	➤ No response	1
Motor response	➤ Obey commands	6
	➤ Localizes pain	5
	➤ Flexion withdrawal from pain	4
	➤ Abnormal flexion (decorticate)	3
	➤ Abnormal extension (decerebrate)	2
	➤ No response	1
	➤ Total score	15
	➤ Comatose client	8 or less
	➤ Totally unresponsive	3

Nursing Diagnosis

- Ineffective airway clearance related to altered level of consciousness
- Disturbed sensory perception related to neurologic impairment
- Risk for impaired skin integrity related to immobility
- Impaired urinary elimination related to impairment in sensing and control
- Risk for injury related to decreased level of consciousness
- Risk for impaired nutritional status
- Interrupted family process related to health crisis

Management

- Maintaining patient airway
  - Elevating the head end of the bed to 30° prevents aspiration
  - Do suctioning
  - Chest physiotherapy
  - Positioning the patient in lateral or semiprone position
  - Auscultating every 8 hours
  - Endotracheal tube insertion
- Maintaining fluid balance and managing nutritional needs
  - The hydration status should be assessed.
  - Hydration by increasing amount of liquid, or emphasizing on a liquid diet should be maintained.
- Maintaining skin integrity
  - Regular change of position should be provided.
  - Passive exercises should be performed.
  - Back massage and back care should be given to prevent development of pressure ulcers.
  - Splints or foam boots should be used to prevent foot drop.
  - Comfort devices, for example, water mattress and air cushions should be used to prevent pressure on bony prominences.
- Preventing urinary retention
  - The patient should be palpated for a full bladder.
  - An indwelling catheter should be inserted; condom catheter for male and absorbent pads for females in the case of incontinence.
  - Stimulation is induced to urinate.
- Ensuring safety of the client
  - Padded side rails, restraints should be used to prevent fall or injury.
  - The patient and attendants should be helped in verbalizing the concerns to relieve anxiety and stress.
  - The self-esteem and confidence of the patient should be enhanced by speaking positively.
- Providing sensory stimulation
  - It should be provided at proper time to avoid sensory deprivation.
  - Efforts are made to maintain the sense of daily rhythm by keeping the usual day and night patterns for activity and sleep.
  - The same schedule should be maintained each day.
  - The client should be oriented to the day, date, and time accordingly.
  - "Touch and talk" should be practiced for psychological support.
  - The client should always be addressed by name and the procedure should be explained each time.

INCONTINENCE

Urinary incontinence is an uncontrolled leakage of urine. It is a condition where inability of usually continent person to reach toilet in time to avoid unintentional loss of urine. It is caused either by the weakened or the loss of voluntary control over the urinary sphincter.

Types and Etiology

1. **Stress incontinence:** It happens during heavy lifting, exercising, laughing, forceful sneezing, and coughing that normally happens in ladies.

2. **Urge incontinence:** It is outlined as sensitive bladder leads to the urge to urinate while sleeping, drinking, or paying attention to running water.

3. **Overflow incontinence:** It happens once the bladder is not fully empty causing frequent dribble voiding.

4. **Functional incontinence:** This condition is caused by limitations in movement, thinking and communication; therefore, the patient is usually unable to manage bladder before they reach to the lavatory.

5. **Mixed incontinence:** In these two forms of incontinence that happens at the same time, usually urinary incontinence and enuresis that is usually found in girls.

6. **Anatomic or organic process abnormalities:** It is caused by anatomic or nervous system abnormalities.

7. **Temporary incontinence:** It normally happens from constipation, UTI, or side effect of treatment or medications.

8. **Bed-wetting:** Nocturnal incontinency is common in kids and normal till 5-year-old kids. This condition is the result of delayed central nervous system control of the bladder.

Management

- Monitor and record (bladder log) urine elimination and volume patterns and frequency.
- Patient should be helped in selecting and applying urine containment devices.
- A protective barrier or ointment to the perineal skin care should be applied.
- Physical examination, including inspection of the perineal skin, of the vaginal and sign of stress urinary incontinence should be performed.

Respiratory Disorders

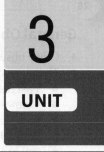

> **AT THE END OF THIS CHAPTER, THE STUDENTS WILL BE ABLE TO LEARN ABOUT NURSING MANAGEMENT OF:**
> ➤ Bronchitis
> ➤ Respiratory failure (ventilator and care of client on ventilator)
> ➤ Acute respiratory distress syndrome (ARDS)
> ➤ Asthma
> ➤ Emphysema
> ➤ Empyema
> ➤ Atelectasis
> ➤ Chronic obstructive pulmonary disease (COPD)
> ➤ Bronchiectasis
> ➤ Pneumonia pulmonary tuberculosis
> ➤ Lung abscess
> ➤ Pleural effusion
> ➤ Cysts and tumors
> ➤ Chest injuries
> ➤ Respiratory arrest and insufficiency
> ➤ Pulmonary embolism
> ➤ Edema

INTRODUCTION

The most important function of the respiratory system is to maintain the autodiffusion by providing oxygen to the body tissues and by excreting carbon dioxide. The body organs depend primarily on the central nervous system to function in an adequate manner to meet the metabolic demand of the body.

ASSESSMENT OF THE RESPIRATORY SYSTEM

Preprocedural Steps

1. Before examining the client, hands should be washed thoroughly with soap and water.
2. The procedure should be explained to the client to gain patient cooperation.
3. The client should be undressed down to the waist (in the case of male client only).
4. The client should be positioned on the examination table at a 30–45° angle, and the client should be approached from the right side.
5. The client needs to be leaned forward in order to examine the posterior side of the lung.

General Observations

- Close observation should be kept on client's respiratory status and oxygen saturation.
- The signs of respiratory distress should be noted. These include:
  - Fast respiratory rate (RR)
  - Cyanosis
  - Unusual posturing (Tripod position) to maximize air entry
  - Breathing using accessory muscles
  - Inward movement of intercostal region
- Coughing should be assessed.
- Hoarseness of voice should be assessed while speaking. It may indicate infection or malignancy.
- Abnormal breathing patterns should be observed—wheezing, crepitus, rhonchi, etc.

Physical Examination

Inspection

- The chest wall should be inspected for any scars as that would be an evidence of a previous surgery.
- The chest shape should be inspected and looked for any visible chest deformities.
- Outward and lateral curvature of the spine, which can impair respiration, should be looked for.
- "Barrel" chest movement in respiration should be assessed as it may indicate COPD and emphysema.
- Pectus excavatum, a protruding or "pigeon" chest, should be looked for.

Palpation

- The trachea is palpated in the following way:
  - The examiner/nurse stands in front of the client.
  - He/she places the right index finger in the sternal notch.
  - The lateral borders of the trachea are palpated to determine whether it is in normal position.
- The chest wall is palpated in the following way:
  - Tenderness, masses, or rib deformities are assessed.
  - The chest is palpated anteriorly and posteriorly for symmetry.
- Chest expansion is assessed in the following way:
  - The examiners hands should be placed with thumbs touching the midline and extend fingers to make contact with the lateral edges of the chest anteriorly, just below the level of the nipples.
  - The patient should be asked to take a deep breath.
  - Inference—the thumbs should be separated by approximately 5 cm or more in normal chest expansion (this technique can also be utilized posteriorly).

Auscultation

Steps for auscultation are:

1. The diaphragm of the stethoscope is used to listen to the anterior, posterior, and lateral chest during an entire inspiration and expiration at each interspace.
2. The patient should be positioned in sitting or in side-lying position and asked to breathe deeply through mouth.

3. Abnormal or adventitious sounds indicate a pathological condition. For example, eupnea, Kussmaul respiration, and hyperventilation.

DISORDERS OF RESPIRATORY SYSTEM

RESPIRATORY FAILURE

Respiratory failure is a condition in which the ability of the body to sustain respiratory drive fails or the ability of the chest wall and muscles to mechanically perform auto diffusion of gases fails to occur, as a result there is elevation of CO_2 level. It may be caused by an obstruction in the airways or by failure of the lungs to exchange gases in the alveoli.

Classification of Respiratory Failure

Respiratory failure are broadly classified into:
1. Acute respiratory failure
2. Chronic respiratory failure

Acute Respiratory Failure

Acute respiratory failure is defined as the decrease in the arterial oxygen pressure less than 50 mm Hg and increase in the arterial carbon dioxide pressure more than 50 mm Hg, with an arterial pH of less than 7.35.

It is characterized by fall in partial pressure of oxygen and fall in the ability to maintain arterial blood gases within the normal range.

Acute respiratory failure is of two types:
 I. Type 1 acute respiratory failure
 II. Type 2 acute respiratory failure
   1. **Type 1 acute respiratory failure:** Type 1 respiratory failure is characterized by hypoxia without hypercapnia, with normal partial pressure of CO_2. It is caused by a ventilation/perfusion (V/Q) mismatch.
   2. **Type 2 acute respiratory failure:** It is caused by inadequate ventilation, with poor partial pressure of both oxygen and carbon dioxide.

Chronic Respiratory Failure

It is characterized by hypoxemia and hypercapnia with a normal pH level. Chronic respiratory failure occurs over a period of months to a year.
Chronic respiratory failure may also be divided into:
1. Hypoxemic respiratory failure
2. Hypercapnia respiratory failure
   a. **Hypoxemic respiratory failure:** During any lung injury, respiratory failure occurs, and that results in poor gas exchange. It occurs due to mismatch between ventilation and perfusion and termed "hypoxemic respiratory failure," with the net result of a fall in oxygen in the blood.
   b. **Hypercapnic respiratory failure:** It occurs due to injury to respiratory muscles, which are used for breathing. The lungs of these patients are normal. This type of respiratory failure occurs in patients with neuromuscular diseases. Neuromuscular disorder results

in loss or decrease in neuromuscular function, inefficient breathing, and limitation to the flow of air into the lungs. Hypoxia and hypercapnia increase because fresh air is not brought into the alveoli.

Etiology

Brain Disorders

- **Cerebrovascular accident (CVA):** A CVA is a sudden loss of brain function resulting from a disruption of blood supply to a part of the brain.
- Brain tumors
- Narcotic tranquilizer

Chest Wall Dysfunction and Neuromuscular Factors

- Anesthetic blocking agent
- Cervical spinal cord injury
- Neuromuscular disorder
- Neuromuscular blocking agent

Obstructive Airway Disorders

- Airway inflammation
- COPD
- Hemothorax
- Foreign bodies
- Asthma
- ARDS

Interstitial Lung Diseases

- Pneumonia
- Pulmonary tuberculosis (TB)
- Pulmonary fibrosis

Pulmonary Dysfunctions Factors

- Asthma
- Emphysema
- Pneumonia
- Pneumothorax
- COPD
- Pulmonary contusion

Cardiac Dysfunctions

- Pulmonary edema
- Congestive heart failure
- Valvular disorder
- Cerebrovascular accident
- Arrhythmia

Other Dysfunctions

- Fatigue due to metabolic acidosis
- Intoxication with drugs

Traumatic Causes are as Follows

- Direct thoracic injury
- Direct brain injury

Pathophysiology

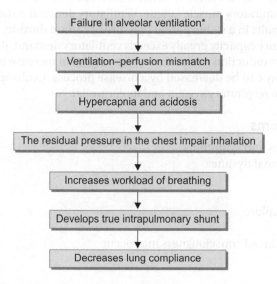

*In alveolar ventilation, nerves and muscles of respiration drive breathing.

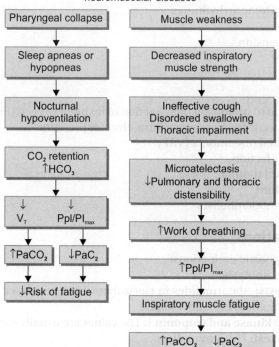

(V_T—tidal volume; PI_{max}—point of maximum impulse; $PaCO_2$—partial pressure of carbon dioxide; PaO_2—partial pressure of oxygen)

Mechanism of Pathophysiology

- Respiratory failure can occur from an abnormality in any of the components of the respiratory system, including the airways, alveoli, central nervous system, chest wall, peripheral nervous system, and respiratory muscles.
- Ventilatory capacity is the maximal spontaneous ventilation that can be maintained without development of respiratory muscle fatigue. Ventilatory demand is the spontaneous minute ventilation that results in a stable partial pressure of carbon dioxide.
- Normally, ventilatory capacity greatly exceeds ventilatory demand. Respiratory failure may result from either a reduction in ventilatory capacity or an increase in ventilatory demand. Ventilatory capacity can be decreased by a disease process involving any of the functional components of the respiratory system and its controller.

Signs and Symptoms

Following are the signs and symptoms:
- Paroxysmal nocturnal dyspnea
- Orthopnea
- Pulmonary edema
- Right ventricular failure
- Hepatomegaly
- Confusion and reduced consciousness may occur
- Restlessness
- Anxiety
- Seizures
- Polycythemia
- Cor pulmonale
- Tachycardia and cardiac arrhythmias
- Cyanosis
- Pulmonary hypertension
- Peripheral edema

Complications

- Oxygen toxicity due to prolonged high fraction of inspired oxygen (FiO_2)
- Barotrauma may occur from excessive intra-alveolar pressure
- Ventilator-associated pneumonia (VAP)
- Respiratory tract infection
- Dental or vocal cord trauma
- Gastric complications
- Deep venous thromboembolism

Diagnostic Evaluations

Following are the diagnostic evaluations:
- **Arterial blood gas analysis.**
- **Renal function tests:** Abnormalities in electrolytes, such as potassium, magnesium, and phosphate may enhance respiratory failure.
- **Serum creatinine kinase and troponin I:** The values are usually elevated.
- **Thyroid function test:** Hypothyroidism
- **Spirometry**
- **Echocardiography:** If acute respiratory failure is suspected due to cardiac cause.

- **Pulmonary function tests**
- **Electrocardiogram (ECG):** It helps to evaluate a cardiovascular cause.
- **Right heart catheterization**
- **Pulmonary capillary wedge pressure:** It may be helpful in distinguishing cardiogenic from no cardiogenic edema.

Management of Acute Respiratory Failure

Management of acute respiratory failure depends on the cause and its severity. The *principle* of management of acute respiratory failure includes:
- Treating the cause
- Providing optimum oxygen
- Carrying out chest physiotherapy
- Maintaining a patient airway
- Providing adequate ventilation.

The main goal of treating respiratory failure is:
- To get oxygen to lungs and organs and remove the carbon dioxide from body
- To promote effective airway clearance effective gas exchange
- To promote comfort
- To prevent complication of immobility
- To monitor and document
- To correct hypoxemia and hypercapnia

Medical Management

- Antibiotics for pneumonia
- Bronchodilators
- Diuretics
- Mucolytic
- Chest physical therapy
- Intravenous (IV) fluids to maintain fluid and electrolytes
- Intubation and mechanical ventilation

Nursing Management

The *general nursing care* for patients with acute respiratory failure are as follows:
- **Anxiety reduction:** Restlessness, fear, and uneasiness should be minimized.
- **Calming technique:** Anxiety should be reduced in client with acute distress.
- **Hemodynamic regulation:** Heart rate, preload, and afterload should be maintained.
- **Circulatory care:** *Mechanical assist devices should be used for* temporary support of the circulation.
- **Nutrition management:** Balanced dietary intake of foods and fluids should be provided.
- **Security enhancement:** Patient's sense of physical and psychological safety should be assessed.
- **Coping enhancement:** A patient should be assisted to adapt to perceived stressors and changes that interfere with meeting life demands and roles.
- **Exercise therapy:** Active or passive body movement should be performed to maintain or restore flexibility.
- **Pain management**
- **Respiratory monitoring:** Airway patency and adequate gas exchange should be maintained.
- **Oxygen therapy:** Administration of oxygen and monitoring of its effectiveness should be taken care of.

- **Active listening:** It is necessary to actively listen and give attention to patient's verbal and nonverbal messages.
- **Cough enhancement:** It includes promotion of deep inhalation by the patient with subsequent generation of high intrathoracic pressures and compression of underlying lung parenchyma for the forceful expulsion of air.
- **Decision-making support:** Information and support should be provided to a person who is making a decision regarding health care.
- **Skin surveillance:** Skin and mucous membrane integrity should be maintained.
- **Pressure management:** Pressure to body parts should be minimized and pressure ulcers should be prevented.
- **Fluid and electrolyte management:** Fluid and electrolyte balance and prevention of complications should be promoted.
- **Cerebral perfusion promotion:** Adequate perfusion and limitation of complications should be promoted for a patient experiencing or at risk for inadequate cerebral perfusion.
- **Infection protection:** Prevention and early detection of infection and maintenance of patient's hygiene should be taken care of.
- **Infection control:** The acquisition and transmission of infectious agents should be minimized.
- **Energy management:** Energy use should be regulated to prevent fatigue.
- **Exercise promotion:** Regular physical exercise should be encouraged to maintain fitness and health.

Nursing Care Plan

Nursing Assessment

- The increased work of breathing and changes in breathing pattern or pulmonary edema should be assessed.
- Breathing sound should be assessed.
- Sign of hypoxemia and hypercapnia should be assessed.
- The arterial blood gas (ABG) should be analyzed.
- Hemodynamic status should be determined.
- Cyanosis of the oral mucosa, lips, and nail beds and skin should be assessed.
- Assess for cold, clammy skin, and asymmetrical chest movement, which indicates pneumothorax,
- Percussion may reveal hyperresonance. If acute respiratory failure results from atelectasis or pneumonia, percussion usually produces a dull or flat sound.
- Auscultation may reveal adventitious breath sounds as wheezing and rhonchi.

Nursing Diagnosis

- Impaired gas exchange related to airway obstruction
- Ineffective airway clearance related to increase secretion
- Acute pain related to inflammatory process and dyspnea
- Anxiety related to pain dyspnea.

Nursing Interventions

- **Improving gas exchange:**
  - Oxygen should be administered to maintain partial pressure.
  - Fluid balance should be monitored by intake and output measurement.
  - Body weight should be assessed daily.

- Measures should be provided to prevent to atelectasis and promote chest expansion.
- Steam inhalation should be done to remove chest secretions.
- Head level should be elevated 30°.
- Adequacy of alveolar ventilation should be monitored.
- **Maintaining airway clearance**
  - Medication should be administered to increase alveolar function and chest movement.
  - Chest physiotherapy should be performed to remove mucus and secretions.
  - Suctioning should be performed as required to assist with removal of secretions.
- **Relieving pain**
  - Patient should be monitored for sign of discomfort and pain.
  - The head of patient should be elevated to encourage maximum lung expansion.
  - Prescribed morphine should be given and pain relieving sign should be monitored.
- **Reducing anxiety**
  - It is advised to speak calmly and slowly.
  - Diagnostic procedure should be explained.

CARE OF PATIENT ON MECHANICAL VENTILATOR

Mechanical ventilation is one of the main components of supportive therapy for critically-ill patients in critical care unit and is often lifesaving. But it may result in a number of lung injuries, known as ventilator-induced lung injury.

Basics of Mechanical Ventilation

A breath cycle is classified into four phases:
1. Initiation of inspiration or a switch from expiration to inspiration
2. Inspiration
3. A switch from inspiration to expiration
4. Expiration

Phase Variables

These four phases are controlled by phase variables, which include trigger, limit, and cycle variables and can be manually manipulated on the ventilator.

Trigger Variables

A ventilator can be triggered automatically or manually by the machine itself. There are four common trigger variables: time, flow, pressure, and volume.
- With **time triggering**, mechanical inspiration is initiated at a regular preset time interval, which is determined by the preset RR. Time triggering is also called machine triggering.
- A client's breathing efforts cause changes in pressure, flow, or volume within the ventilator circuit.
- When inspiration starts, there is decrease in the baseline gas flow during exhalation, it is called **flow triggering**. It is supposed to reduce the work of breathing compared with pressure triggering.
- If the ventilator is initiated by delivering inspiratory flow by a drop in baseline pressure resulting from a patient's inspiratory effort during exhalation, it is known as **pressure triggering**.
- **Volume triggering** is when during exhalation, a decrease in volume to a certain extent within the ventilator circuit activates inspiration.

After selecting a trigger variable, the operator has to set up a sensitivity setting that evaluates the extent of change in flow or pressure, or the amount of a client's effort that is required to activate the ventilator. In order to reduce the work load of breathing and avoid patient–ventilator mismatch, it is important to adjust settings to meet the requirements of individual clients.

Limit Variables

- When the maximum tidal volume (TV or V_T) that can be delivered to a client during inspiration is preset, it is called **volume-controlled ventilation**.
- If the maximum pressure rise during inspiration is predetermined, it is referred to as **pressure-controlled ventilation**. With pressure-support ventilation, inspiration is limited by the preset level of pressure support.
- The **flow limit** involves setting the maximum flow that can be delivered by the ventilator. Setting a flow limit may cause patient–ventilator mismatch, if a client's inspiratory flow demand exceeds the preset flow limit.

Cycle Variables

Inspiration can be terminated by a predefined pressure, flow, volume, or time variable.

- With **pressure-cycled ventilation**, inspiration is ended once the peak inspiration pressure achieved the targeted pressure.
- In **flow-cycled ventilation**, the inspiratory flow ceases when its flow rate is dropped to the predetermined percentage of peak inspiratory flow rate. Flow cycle criteria vary with different kinds of ventilators and are determined by a patient's clinical status.
- With **volume-cycled ventilation**, inspiration is terminated once the preset volume is delivered.
- In **time-cycled ventilation**, the cycling between inspiration and expiration spontaneously works at a regular preset time interval.

Breath Types

Following are the types of breathing:

- When the mandatory breath is initiated by the client, it is termed **assisted breath**. If spontaneous breaths are assisted or through the ventilator, such as the pressure support mode, they are termed "assisted breaths."
  - There are volume-controlled and pressure-controlled mandatory breaths. With **volume-controlled ventilation**, the inspiration of mandatory and assisted breaths is limited by the preset volume.
  - For **pressure-controlled ventilation**, mandatory and assisted breaths are restricted by the preset inspiratory pressure. Volume and flow are variable and affected by the preset pressure, respiratory resistance, chest wall, lung compliance, and inspiratory time.
  - During spontaneous breathing, the client controls his/her own tidal volumes and terminates his/her own inspiration. Both volume and pressure variable depend on the client's inspiratory effort, lung compliance, and respiratory resistance.
  - Pressure support is commonly indicated for clients with spontaneous breaths to overcome the resistance developed by the ventilator circuit, reduce the work load of breathing, and improve a patient's comfort.
  - With volume-controlled ventilation, the mandatory breath is time triggered, time cycled, and volume limited; the assisted breath is patient triggered, limited, and cycled by the same mechanisms as the mandatory breath.
  - Pressure-support ventilation is patient triggered, pressure limited, and usually flow cycled.

Ventilator-induced Lung Injury

Ventilator-induced lung injury is of four types—barotrauma, volutrauma, atelectrauma, and biotrauma.

1. **Barotrauma** is characterized by extra-alveolar air. It is induced by high airway pressure or over ventilation that damages the alveolar tissue and leads to alveolar rupture.

2. **Volutrauma** is caused by over ventilation that results in alveolar over distension, which may manifest itself as pulmonary edema.

3. **Atelectrauma** occurs with repeated recruiting and derecruitments of ventilator. Ventilation with low positive end-expiratory pressure (PEEP) increases the chances of atelectrauma in patients with heterogeneous damage of lung parenchyma, such as ARDS.

4. **Biotrauma** results from the production, activation, and release of both local and systemic inflammatory mediators secondary to lung parenchymal damage caused by volutrauma, barotrauma, and atelectrauma.

Nursing Care of Ventilated Patient

The top 10 essentials of nursing care for ventilator patients are as follows:

Review Communications

Review communications include the following:

- Communication among care providers promotes optimal outcomes and better recovery. For mechanically ventilated clients, care providers may include primary care physicians, pulmonary specialists, hospitalists, respiratory therapists, and nurses.

- To make sure nurse is aware of other team members' communications about the patient's condition, find out the approach of therapy for his/her patient. The reasons behind to keep a patient in ventilation are to improve oxygenation or give sedation if required or reverse respiratory muscle fatigue.

General Instructions to Check Ventilator Settings and Modes

General instructions include:

- Assessing vital signs, checking oxygen saturation, inspecting for breath sounds, and noting changes from previous findings.

- Assessing the patient's pain and anxiety levels.

- Going through the client's order and obtaining information about the ventilator.

- Familiarizing self with ventilator alarms and the actions to take when an alarm sounds.

- Locating suction equipment and being ready with all.

- Being ready with bag-valve mask, which should be available for every client with an artificial airway.

- Ventilators that generally display ordered settings and patient parameters.

- Checking the following settings-RR, FiO_2, Tidal volume (TV or V_T), Peak inspiratory pressure (PIP).

- Finding out which ventilation mode or method patient is receiving and checking the ventilator itself or the respiratory flow sheet.

- Providing adjuvant therapy to some patients, such as positive PEEP. With PEEP, a small amount of continuous pressure is added to the airway to increase therapeutic effectiveness.

- Finally, determining whether a capnography monitor is recording the patient's partial pressure of exhaled carbon dioxide.

- ***Suction*** appropriately. General suctioning recommendations include the following:
  - Suction only as needed—not according to a schedule.
  - The client should be hyperoxygenated before and after suctioning to help prevent oxygen desaturation.
  - Normal saline solution should not be used into the endotracheal (ET) tube in an attempt to promote secretion removal.
  - Suctioning pressure should be limited to the lowest level that needed to remove secretions.
  - Suction should be for the shortest duration, if possible.
  - If client has an ET tube, tube slippage into the right main-stem bronchus should be checked.
  - Complications of tracheostomy tubes should be assessed, such as tube dislodgment, bleeding, and infection by assessing the tube insertion site, breath sounds, vital signs, and PIP trends.
  - If client has a tracheostomy, routine cleaning and care should be performed according to facility policies and procedures.

Assess Pain and Sedation Needs

- Even though patient cannot verbally express his/her needs, nurse will need to assess client's pain level using a pain scale.
- It should be kept in mind that a client's acknowledgment of pain means pain is present and must be treated.
- Two scales can be used to assess sedation level are the Richmond Agitation–Sedation Scale and the Ramsay Sedation Scale.

Prevent Infection

VAP is a major complication of mechanical ventilation. VAP prevention "bundle" includes:
- Keeping the head of the bed elevated 30–45° at all times
- Regularly assessing vital signs and arterial blood gas values
- Providing peptic ulcer disease prophylaxis, as with a histamine-2 blocker
- Providing deep vein thrombosis prophylaxis, as with an intermittent compression device
- Performing oral care with chlorhexidine daily to prevent oral infection
- Extubating the client as quickly as possible
- Performing range-of-motion exercises daily to increase blood circulation
- Client's turning and positioning to prevent the effects of muscle disuse
- Having the client sit up and move or walk when possible to improve gas exchange
- Providing appropriate nutrition to prevent a catabolic state
- Keeping bacteria out of oral secretions and thus reducing VAP risk
- Avoid changing the ventilator circuit or tubing unnecessarily
- Brushing the patient's teeth at least twice a day and providing oral moisturizers every 2–4 hours.

Prevent Hemodynamic Instability

The following points are how to prevent hemodynamic instability:
- The client's blood pressure (BP) should be regularly assessed every 2–4 hours, especially after ventilator settings are changed or adjusted.

- Mechanical ventilation causes thoracic-cavity pressure to rise on inspiration, which creates pressure on blood vessels and may minimize the blood flow to the heart; as a result, BP may drop.
- IV fluids should be administered to maintain hemodynamic stability or a drug, such as dopamine or norepinephrine should also be administered, if ordered.
- High levels of inspiratory pressure with pressure support ventilation (PSV) and PEEP increase the risk of barotrauma and pneumothorax. To detect these complications, breath sounds and oxygenation status need to be assessed often.

Manage the Airway

The following points are about managing the airway:
- The cuff on the ET tube provides airway occlusion. Proper cuff inflation ensures that the client receives the proper ventilator parameters.
- Air must never be added to the cuff without using the proper technique.
- Following hospital policy, the cuff should be inflated and measured for proper inflation pressure using the minimal leak technique or minimal occlusive volume.
- When performing mouth care, suctioning oral secretions and brushing the patient's teeth, gums, and tongue at least twice a day should be done.

Meet the Patient's Nutritional Needs

If patient cannot swallow normally, they need an alternative nutrition route, preferably, NG tube feeding. They should have feeding tubes with liquid nutrition provided through the gut.

Educate the Patient and Family

Seeing a loved one attached to a mechanical ventilator is frightening. To ease distress in the patient and family, they should be taught why mechanical ventilation is needed by emphasizing the positive outcomes it can provide.

Wean the Patient from the Ventilator Appropriately

Weaning methods are as follows:
- ❖ Weaning method is indicated when patients are able to take more breaths on their own efforts.
- ❖ Some clients may need weeks for gradually reduced ventilator assistance before they can be extubated others cannot be weaned at all.
- ❖ Factors that affect weaning include underlying disease processes, such as COPD or peripheral vascular disease, medications used to treat anxiety and pain, and nutritional status of client.

Weaning Criteria	Guide
1. Adequate oxygenation	PaO_2/FiO_2 ratio >200 or FiO_2 ≤40 and SpO_2 ≥90% and/or PaO_2 ≥60 Peep ≤8 cmH_2O
2. Adequate ventilation	PH ≥7.30 RR ≤35 bpm VE ≤15 lpm Inspiratory effort by patient
3. Hemodynamic stability	HR ≤140 bpm SBP 90–80 mm Hg No or minimal vasopressors or inotropes*
4. Appropriate LOC	No continuous sedation infusion No neuromuscular blocking agents
5. Afebrile	Temp >36°C and <38°C
6. Adequate hemoglobin	Hb ≥70 and/or no evidence of hemorrhage

*Dopamine <5 µg/kg/min

The spontaneous breathing trial will be terminated if any of the following termination criteria occur.

	Termination criteria
1.	SpO_2 <90 % with ↑ FiO_2 ≥.50
2.	RR >35 bpm
3.	RSBI >80
4.	Blood pressure ↑ 20 mm Hg
5.	HR ↑ 20 bpm
6.	New arrhythmia's
7.	↑ WOB
8.	Patient agitation or anxiety

Other Care Essentials

Other care essentials are as follows:

Care of the airway

- It is very essential that all cares and procedures are carried out with maintaining a patent airway.
- It should be ensured that the ET tube is held securely in position.
- The placement of the ET tube should be checked by listening to equal bilateral breath sounds.
- The cuff pressure of the ET tube should be checked and adjusted.
- The client's facial expression, color, respiratory effort, and vital signs should be observed.

Ventilation

- It must be ensured that the ventilation tubing is not blocked.
- Ventilator circuits are changed weekly.
- The type of humidification and when the filters and ventilation tubing were last changed should be checked.
- The ventilator should be checked regularly and documented the settings.
- Whether the ventilator and the cardiac monitor are plugged into emergency power supply should be ensured.
- The alarm parameters should be looked at and reset, if necessary.
- Indications for an actively humidified circuit include:
  - Minute volume more than 10 L
  - Chest trauma with pulmonary contusion
  - Airway burns
  - Hypothermia
  - Pulmonary hemorrhage
  - Consultant order
  - Severe asthma
  - Severe sputum.

Suction of an artificial airway

- To maintain a patent airway
- To prevent effects of retained secretions
- To promote improved gas exchange
- Suction the oropharynx to remove potentially infected secretions
- Tracheal suctioning should be attended 2–3 hours
- To obtain tracheal aspirate specimens
- It is important to oxygenate before and after suctioning.

Monitor
- The level of any invasive monitoring transducers should be assessed.
- The alarm parameters should be assessed and reset if needed.
- The client's vital signs should be documented hourly.
- A manual BP should be assessed and documented.

Oral care
- The goal of oral care is to promote hygiene and prevent infection and dryness of mouth.
- A soft toothbrush can be used for oral hygiene and a small amount of toothpaste can help to give freshness.
- Diluted sodium bicarbonate can be used to remove resistant coating on the tongue.
- The lips should be kept moisturized to stop them becoming sore and cracked.

Eye care
- The unconscious, sedated, or paralyzed clients are at risk of developing eye infection due to dryness that may result in ulceration, perforation, and scarring of the cornea.
- Sedation and muscle relaxants may cause inadequate closure of the eye, lack of random eye movements, and a loss of the blink reflex, which may further contribute in eye infection.
- Fluid imbalances and increased permeability can promote conjunctival edema.
- Regular eye care using saline soaked gauze to clean the eye after every 2 hours will prevent eye complication due to dryness.

Gastrointestinal tract (GIT)
- Intubated clients must need an NG tube for gastric decompression or nutritional support.
- Bowel sounds and the turgor of the abdomen should be assessed regularly.
- Clients who have poor nutritional status are prone to infection, weight loss fluid and electrolyte imbalance, intestinal fluid retention, pressure ulcers, and delayed wound healing.
- Diarrhea, dehydration, and fluid overload should be monitored regularly.
- Elevating the head of the bed to 30–45° is effective in reducing the risk of aspiration.

Genital/urinary tract
- Urinalysis should be performed twice a day.
- Regular catheter care should be given.
- The catheter should be secured to the leg carefully.
- Hourly urine monitoring is carried out.

Repositioning and pressure area care
- Client's hygiene should be maintained especially for the skin to prevent pressure ulcer.
- The patient's position should be changed regularly to prevent bed ulcers.
  - Routine turning and positioning assist in the mobilization of secretions.
  - The head of the bed should be elevated if the patient's condition allows to help prevent aspiration and improve oxygenation.
  - If the patient has any signs of developing pressure areas, he/she should be nursed on an air mattress.
  - It prevents the development of pressure areas.
  - If the patient has leg splints on them, it should not be bandaged and the skin integrity should be checked with each turn.
  - It improves oxygenation and can encourage weaning from the ventilator.
  - The ET tube should be secure and safeguarded.
  - The skin should be kept dry and inspected for pressure ulcers.

- The ET tube should be repositioned at alternate sides of the mouth to prevent developing of pressure areas.
- The NG tube should be secured in such a way as to minimize pressure on the nares and changed at least daily.

Complications of Mechanical Ventilation

Mechanical ventilation has been associated with complications, such as VAP, cardiovascular compromise, gastrointestinal disturbances, renal impairment, asymmetric chest movement, pneumothorax.

Complications can be categorized as under:

1. *Associated with patient's response to mechanical ventilation:*

A. **Decreased cardiac output**
   - **Cause:** Venous return to the right atrium impeded by the dramatically increased intrathoracic pressures during inspiration from positive pressure ventilation.
   - **Symptoms:**
     ◆ Increased heart rate
     ◆ Decreased BP
     ◆ Perfusion to vital organs
     ◆ Decreased central venous pressure (CVP)
     ◆ Cool clammy skin.
   - **Treatment:** Fluid administration

B. **Barotrauma**
   - **Etiology:** Damage to pulmonary system due to alveolar rupture from excessive airway pressures.
   - **Symptoms:** Pneumothorax or subcutaneous emphysema.

C. **Nosocomial pneumonia**
   - **Cause:** Invasive procedure in critically-ill patients becomes colonized with pathological bacteria within 24 hours.
   - **Treatment:** Aimed at prevention by:
     ◆ Frequent handwashing
     ◆ Decreasing the risk of aspiration
     ◆ Using of sterile technique
     ◆ Maintaining closed system setup on ventilator circuitry
     ◆ Ensuring adequate nutrition
     ◆ Avoiding neutralization of gastric contents with antacids.

D. **Positive water balance**
   - **Syndrome of inappropriate antidiuretic hormone (ADH):** Due to vagal stimulation, receptors in right atrium observe a decrease in venous return and finally cause hypovolemia, resulting in a release of ADH and lead to retention of sodium and water. This fluid overload is evidenced by decreased urine specific gravity, dilutional hyponatremia, increased heart rate, and BP.

E. **Decreased renal perfusion:** It can be managed by low-dose dopamine therapy.

F. **Increased intracranial pressure:** It reduces PEEP.

G. **Hepatic congestion:** It reduces PEEP.

2. *Other complications related to endotracheal intubation*

A. **Sinusitis and nasal injury:** It can be prevented by avoiding nasal intubations; cushion nares from tube and tape and administering antibiotics.

B. **Tracheoesophageal fistula:** It can be prevented by inflating the cuff with minimal amount of air and monitoring of cuff pressures.

C. **Mucosal lesions:** It can be prevented by inflating cuff with minimal amount of air and regular monitoring of cuff pressure.

D. **Laryngeal or tracheal stenosis:** It can be prevented by inflating cuff with minimal amount of air and regular monitoring of cuff pressure and suction area above cuff frequently.

3. *Other common potential:* Aspiration, GI bleeding, inappropriate ventilation dysrhythmias, or vagal reactions during or after suctioning and incorrect PEEP setting.

Nursing Care Plan for the Ventilated Patient

Nursing Assessment

Critical care nurses can identify subtle changes in a patient's clinical status and initiate appropriate nursing interventions rapidly and effectively. This includes the following (Table 3.1):

	Assessment parameters	Relevant numerical data
A. Airway	Is the airway patent and secure? ➢ Listen to air movement ➢ Observe rise and fall of chest ➢ Check tube is secure and length is correct	
B. Breathing	Is the patient breathing? ➢ Observe chest rise and fall ➢ Observe patient color	SpO_2, tidal volume, respiratory rate
C. Circulation	Does the patient have adequate circulation? Check for a pulse Assess strength of pulse Observe patient color	Heart rate and rhythm, arterial blood pressure
D. Disability	What is the patient's level of consciousness?	
E. Exposure	What Is the patient's surrounding environment? Is the patient's dignity preserved	

TABLE 3.1: Primary survey.

Goals

- Patient will have effective breathing pattern.
- Patient's nutritional status will be well maintained.
- Patient will have adequate gas exchange.
- Possibility of pulmonary infection should be avoided.
- Patient will not develop problems related to immobility.

Nursing Diagnosis and the Related Nursing Interventions

1. Ineffective breathing pattern related to secretions

Interventions:

- Changes in RR and depth and observation for dyspnea and use of accessory muscles should be assessed.
- Tube misplacement should be observed.

- Accidental extubation should be prevented by taping tube securely.
- Thorax should be inspected for symmetry of movement.
- Tidal volume and vital capacity should be measured.
- Pain should be assessed.
- Head of the bed 60–90° should be elevated.
- Ventilator settings should be maintained as ordered.

2. Impaired gas exchange related to alveolar–capillary membrane changes

Interventions:

- ABGs should be monitored.
- Skin color and capillary refill should be observed.
- Complete blood count (CBC) should be monitored.
- Oxygen should be administered as ordered.
- It is necessary to observe for tube obstruction, suction prn, and ensure adequate humidification.

3. Poor nutritional status less than body requirement related to nil per oral (NPO) status

Interventions:

- Total parenteral nutrition, lipids, or enteral feedings should be provided.
- Nutrition consultation should be obtained.
- Lymphocytes and albumin should be monitored.

4. Risk for pulmonary infection related to poor tissue integrity

Interventions:

- Airway should be assessed and secured regularly and ventilator tubing should be supported.
- Good oral care should be provided.
- Proper handwashing with antimicrobial for 30 seconds before and after patient should be done.

ACUTE RESPIRATORY DISTRESS SYNDROME

It is the clinical condition that is characterized by a sudden and progressive pulmonary edema, increased bilateral infiltrates on chest X-ray, and the absence of an elevated atrial pressure.

Etiology

- Aspiration
- Drug ingestion
- Prolong inhalation of high concentrations oxygen
- Smoking
- Fat embolism
- Systemic sepsis
- Shock

Signs and Symptoms

- Increase pulse rates
- Low partial pressure of oxygen
- Dyspnea

- Restlessness
- Poor mental status
- Tachycardia
- Acute breathlessness
- Tachypnea
- Hypotension

Complications

- Dysrhythmias
- Infection
- Decreased cardiac output
- Multiorgan failure
- Renal failure
- Stress ulcer

Pathophysiology

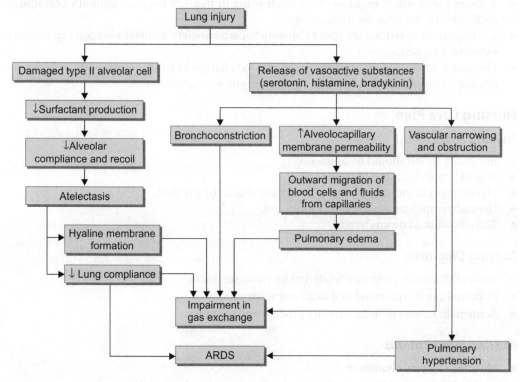

Diagnostic Evaluations

- Echocardiography
- ABG
- Computed tomography (CT) scan of thorax
- Chest X-ray
- Sputum culture
- Pulmonary artery catheterization

Management

The primary focus in the management of ARDS includes:
- Identification and treatment of the underlying condition
- Providing supportive therapy, such as intubation and mechanical ventilation
- Supplementation of oxygen as required

Medical Management

- IV fluids are given to provide nutrition and prevent dehydration.
- Antibiotic therapy is provided for infection.
- Antianxiety to reduce the anxiety
- Diuretics to eliminate fluid from lungs
- Antibiotics for the infection

Nursing Management

General Measure
- A patient with ARDS requires close monitoring in the ICU because patient's conditions could quickly become life threatening.
- It is important to reduce the client's anxiety because anxiety increases oxygen expenditure by preventing rest.
- The nurse must closely monitor the client for change in oxygenation with a change in position. The patient should be elevated to improve oxygenation.

Nursing Care Plan

Nursing Assessment

- Breathing sound should be assessed.
- Sign of hypoxemia should be assessed.
- The changes in increased work of breathing should be notified.
- Hemodynamic status should be monitored.
- The ABG should be analyzed.

Nursing Diagnosis

- Ineffective airway clearance related to increase secretion.
- Impaired gas exchange related to airway obstruction.
- Acute pain related to inflammatory process and dyspnea.

Nursing interventions

- **Maintain airway clearance**
  - Medication should be administered to increase alveolar function.
  - IV fluids should be administered.
  - Chest physiotherapy should be performed to remove mucus.
  - Patient should be suctioned as needed.
- **Relieving pain**
  - Client should kept under watch for any sign of discomfort and pain.
  - The client's head should be elevated.
  - Prescribed morphine should be administered for pain.

- **Reducing anxiety**
  - Dyspnea is corrected and physical discomfort is relieved.
  - It is advised to speak calmly and slowly.
  - Diagnostic procedure should be explained well.

PULMONARY HYPERTENSION

Pulmonary hypertension is an increase of BP in the pulmonary blood vessels together known as the lung vasculature, resulting in shortness of breath, dizziness, fainting, and leg swelling.

Types of Pulmonary Hypertension

Types of pulmonary hypertension are as follows:
1. **Idiopathic or primary pulmonary hypertension:** When an underlying cause for high BP in the lungs cannot be found, the condition is called idiopathic pulmonary hypertension.
2. **Secondary pulmonary hypertension:** Pulmonary hypertension that is caused due to medical conditions is called secondary pulmonary hypertension. Secondary pulmonary hypertension can be caused due to—
   - Blood clots in the respiratory blood vessels
   - COPD
   - Scleroderma
   - Congenital heart disease
   - Sickle cell anemia
   - Chronic liver disease
   - Sleep apnea
   - HIV/AIDS

Other Types of Pulmonary Hypertension

The World Health Organization divides pulmonary hypertension into five groups:
1. **Group 1 pulmonary arterial hypertension:** Group 1 PAH has no known cause or inherited or caused by drugs or toxins.
2. **Group 2 pulmonary hypertension:** Group 2 includes pulmonary hypertension with left heart disease, such as mitral valve disease.
3. **Group 3 pulmonary hypertension:** Group 3 pulmonary hypertension includes disorders associated with lung diseases, such as COPD.
4. **Group 4 pulmonary hypertension**: Group 4 includes pulmonary hypertension caused by blood clots in the lungs or blood clotting disorders.
5. **Group 5 pulmonary hypertension:** Group 5 includes pulmonary hypertension caused by blood disorders.

Etiology

Etiologies are as follows:
- Drugs, such as dexfenfluramine and phentermine
- Liver diseases
- Aortic valve disease and left heart failure
- Thromboembolic disease
- Low-oxygen conditions
- Obesity and sleep apnea
- Genetic predisposition

Pathophysiology

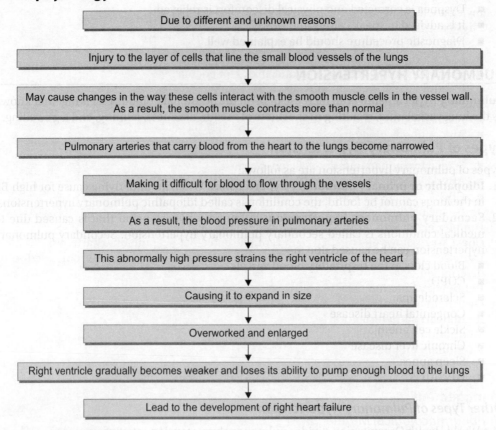

Due to different and unknown reasons

↓

Injury to the layer of cells that line the small blood vessels of the lungs

↓

May cause changes in the way these cells interact with the smooth muscle cells in the vessel wall. As a result, the smooth muscle contracts more than normal

↓

Pulmonary arteries that carry blood from the heart to the lungs become narrowed

↓

Making it difficult for blood to flow through the vessels

↓

As a result, the blood pressure in pulmonary arteries

↓

This abnormally high pressure strains the right ventricle of the heart

↓

Causing it to expand in size

↓

Overworked and enlarged

↓

Right ventricle gradually becomes weaker and loses its ability to pump enough blood to the lungs

↓

Lead to the development of right heart failure

Signs and Symptoms

Following are the signs and symptoms:
- Fatigue
- Dizziness
- Bluish lips or skin
- Fainting spells
- Chest pain
- Irregular heart beat (palpitations or strong, throbbing sensation)
- Tachycardia
- Swelling in the ankles, abdomen, or legs
- Progressive shortness of breath

Complications

- **Right-sided heart failure:** Enlargement of right ventricle that will result in thickening of septum walls and expanding the chamber of the right ventricle to increase the amount of blood it can hold. But this thickening and enlarging work only for a period and finally the right ventricle fails from the extra pressure.
- **Blood clots:** A number of small clots block the veins and travel to the lungs, resulting in pulmonary hypertension.
- **Arrhythmias:** These can lead to palpitations, dizziness, or fainting.
- **Bleeding:** Pulmonary hypertension can lead to bleeding into the lungs and hemoptysis.

Diagnostic Evaluations

Following are the diagnostic evaluations:

- **Physical examination includes:**
  - Auscultating abnormal heart sounds
  - Examining the jugular vein for engorgement
  - Examining the abdomen, legs, and ankles for edema
  - Examining nail beds for cyanosis.
- **Blood tests include:**
  - Liver and kidney function test
  - Autoantibody blood tests
  - Thyroid-stimulating hormone
  - Screen for human immunodeficiency virus
  - Arterial blood gases
  - CBC
  - B-type natriuretic peptide, for heart failure
- **Doppler echocardiogram** to rule out heart problem.
- **Chest X-ray** shows an enlarged right ventricle and enlarged pulmonary arteries.
- Exercise tolerance level and blood oxygen saturation level during exercise need to be determined.
- **Pulmonary function tests**
- **Overnight oximetry,** for sleep apnea
- **Right heart catheterization**
- **Ventilation perfusion scan (V/Q scan)**
- **Pulmonary angiogram**
- **Chest CT scan**

Management

Nonpharmacological Management

- **Oxygen therapy:** It replaces the low oxygen in blood.
- **Nutrition:** Nutritious diet that is low in fat, cholesterol, and sodium and rich in high fiber.
- It is advised to quit smoking.
- Physical activities and exercise should be performed.

Pharmacological Management

- **Anticoagulants,** such as warfarin sodium
- **Vasodilators and calcium channel blockers**
- **Prostaglandins** help prevent blood clots formation
- **Diuretics:** frusemide, spironolactone
- **Potassium** supplement
- **Inotropic agents** (such as digoxin)
- **Phosphodiesterase type 5 inhibitors, such as sildenafil to** relax pulmonary smooth muscle cells.

Surgical Management

Surgical managements are as follows:

a. **Atrial septostomy:** It is a surgical procedure that creates a communication between the right and left atria and relieves pressure on the right side.

b. **Pulmonary thromboendarterectomy:** It is the surgically removal of clot to improve blood flow in pulmonary circulation.

c. **Lung transplantation**
d. **Heart transplantation**

Nursing Care Plan

Nursing Assessment

- Breathing sound should be assessed.
- Sign of hypoxemia should be assessed.
- The changes in increased work of breathing should be notified.
- Hemodynamic status should be monitored.
- The ABG should be analyzed.

Nursing Diagnosis

- Ineffective airway clearance related to increase secretion.
- Impaired gas exchange related to airway obstruction.
- Acute pain related to inflammatory process and dyspnea.

Nursing Intervention

- **Improving gas exchange includes:**
  - Administering oxygen
  - Monitoring fluid balance by intake and output
  - Elevating head level 30°
  - Administering antibiotic, cardiac medication, and diuretics as prescribed by physician.
- **Maintaining airway clearance includes:**
  - Administering medication to increase alveolar function
  - Performing chest physiotherapy to remove mucus
  - Administering IV fluids
  - Suction to remove secretions
- **Relieving pain includes:**
  - Monitoring the client for discomfort and pain
  - Positioning the head elevated
  - Administering prescribed morphine pain relief
- **Reducing anxiety includes:**
  - Correcting dyspnea and relive physical discomfort
  - Speaking in a calm and slow manner
  - Explaining diagnostic procedure

COR PULMONALE

Cor pulmonale refers to the hypertrophy of heart chambers and impaired function of the right ventricle, which results from pulmonary hypertension that is caused by COPD or any other respiratory-associated condition.

Etiology

- Blood clots in the lungs
- COPD
- Lung tissue damages
- Sleep apnea

- Cystic fibrosis
- Congestive heart failure (CHF)

Pathophysiology

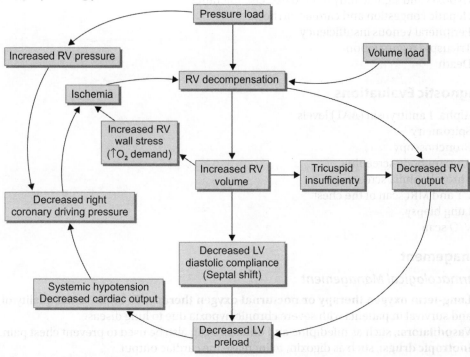

Signs and Symptoms

- Tachypnea
- Fatigue
- Ankle swelling
- Exertional dyspnea
- Worsening cough
- Angina
- Exertional syncope
- Labored respiratory effort
- Crackles and wheeze in the chest
- Systolic bruits
- Distended neck veins
- Murmur
- Hepatic congestion
- Cyanosis
- Split second heart sound
- Systolic ejection murmur
- Hemoptysis
- Hoarseness of voice
- Diastolic pulmonary regurgitation
- Hepatomegaly
- Ascites

Complications

- Exertional syncope
- Peripheral edema
- Hypoxia and significantly limited exercise tolerance
- Hepatic congestion and cardiac cirrhosis
- Peripheral venous insufficiency
- Tricuspid regurgitation
- Death

Diagnostic Evaluations

- Alpha-1 antitrypsin (AAT) levels
- Spirometry
- Bronchoscopy
- Autoantibody screening
- Thrombophilia screening
- CT and MRI scan of the chest
- Lung biopsy
- V/Q scan

Management

Pharmacological Management

- **Long-term oxygen therapy or nocturnal oxygen therapy:** To improve the quality of life and survival in patients with severe chronic hypoxia due to lung disease.
- **Vasodilators:**, such as nifedipine and diltiazem can also be used to prevent chest pain.
- **Inotropic drugs:**, such as digoxin, to increase the cardiac output
- **Bronchodilators:**, such as theophylline
- **Diuretics:**, such as furosemide and bumetanide can be used in management of associated peripheral edema.
- **Anticoagulation:** It is used where patients have venous thromboembolism as the underlying cause of their cor pulmonale.
- **Transplantation of lung and heart**.

Nursing Care Plan

1. Impaired gas exchange related to fluid in the alveoli

Interventions:

- Auscultation of breath sounds every 4 hours
- Monitoring ABG
- Maintaining Fowler's position
- Administering oxygen
- Encouraging to turn cough and deep breath
- Intubation and mechanical ventilation

2. Fluid volume excess related to reduced cardiac output and Na and water retention

Interventions:

- Monitor intake output chart
- Provide Fowler's position
- Ensure frequent oral care
- Perform daily weighing

- Assess jugular vein distension
- Fluid restriction
- Ensure diet modification, i.e., 2–4 g salt diet.

3. Decreased cardiac output related to heart failure and dysrhythmias

Interventions:

- Monitor vital signs every hour
- Administer oxygen
- Monitor hourly urine output
- Auscultate lung and heart sounds every 2 hours
- Assessing changes in mental status
- Provide small and frequent meals

4. Decreased peripheral tissue perfusion related to reduced cardiac output

Interventions:

- Monitor peripheral pulses
- Assess color and temperature of skin
- Keep extremities warm
- Assess for thrombophlebitis
- Perform active or passive range of motion (ROM)

5. High risk for impaired skin integrity related to reduced peripheral tissue perfusion

Intervention:

- Changing position every 2 hours
- Provide pressure mattress
- Provide heel protectors

6. High risk for digitalis toxicity related to impaired excretion

Interventions:

- Assess for hypokalemia and heart block
- Assess the serum digitalis levels and potassium

BRONCHITIS

Bronchitis is defined as inflammation of the bronchial tubes, which results in excessive secretions of mucus, leading to tissue swelling that can narrow or close off bronchial lumen.

Etiology

- **Acute bronchitis** is caused by viruses, such as influenza, respiratory virus it last longer for days to 1 week and can be managed by antimicrobial drugs.
- **Chronic bronchitis** is a cough with mucus for at least 3 months in each of 2 consecutive years. It may results in permanent damage to lungs.

Risk Factors

Risk factors include the following:

- **Cigarette smoke:** People who smoke or who live with a smoker are at higher risk of both acute bronchitis and chronic bronchitis.
- **Low immunity:** Older adults, infants, and young children have greater vulnerability to infection.

Pathophysiology

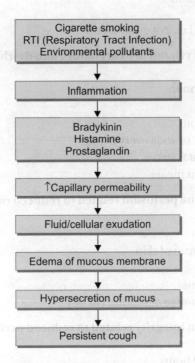

Signs and Symptoms

For either acute bronchitis or chronic bronchitis, signs and symptoms may include:

- Cough
- Production of mucus
- Tiredness
- Slight fever and chills
- Chest discomfort

Complications

- Chronic bronchitis
- Asthma
- TB
- Sinusitis
- Breathlessness
- Respiratory failure
- Pneumonia
- Bronchiectasis
- Cor pulmonale
- Pneumothorax
- Emphysema
- Polycythemia
- COPD
- High mortality rate

Diagnostic Evaluations

- **Chest X-ray:** A chest X-ray can help determine pneumonia or another condition that may explain cough.
- **Sputum culture:** This test checks for the presence of bacteria in sputum produced when cough.
- **Pulmonary function test**

Management

The goal of treatment for bronchitis is to relieve symptoms and ease breathing. In most cases, acute bronchitis requires only self-care treatments, such as:

- Getting more rest
- Taking over-the-counter pain medications
- Drinking fluids
- Breathing in warm, moist air

Medical Management

- **Antibiotics:** Such as fluoroquinolones
- **Cough medicine:** Such as expectorants and mucolytic
- **Steroids:** Such as prednisone and methylprednisolone to reduce the inflammatory reaction.
- Bronchodilators
- **Phosphodiesterase-4 (PDE4) inhibitors** are a class of anti-inflammatory agents for exacerbations of COPD.

Nursing Care Plan

Nursing Diagnosis and Interventions

1. Impaired gas exchange related to altered oxygen supply

Interventions:

- Respirations should be assessed.
- Signs of hypoxemia should be assessed.
- Life-threatening problems should be assessed.
- Lung sounds should be auscultated.
- Vital signs should be monitored.
- Changes in orientation and behavior should be assessed.
- Skin color for cyanosis should be assessed.
- Supplemental oxygen should be provided.
- ABG should be monitored.
- The patient should be placed on continuous pulse oximetry.
- The patient for intubation should be prepared.

2. Ineffective airway clearance related to tracheobronchial obstruction

Interventions:

- Airway for patency should be assessed.
- Respiratory should be assessed.
- Supplemental oxygen should be administered.
- Mouth, neck, and position of trachea should be inspected.
- Lungs should be auscultated.
- Changes in vital signs should be assessed.
- Patient with head of bed 45° should be positioned.

- Mental status changes should be assessed.
- Arterial blood gases should be monitored.
- Patient should be assisted with coughing and deep breathing techniques.
- Placement of endotracheal should be prepared.
- Placement of the artificial airway should be confirmed.

3. Poor nutritional status less than body requirement related to NPO status

Interventions:
- Total parenteral nutrition, lipids, or enteral feedings should be provided.
- Nutrition consult should be obtained.
- Lymphocytes and albumin should be monitored.

4. Risk for pulmonary infection related to poor tissue integrity

Interventions:
- Airway and support ventilator tubing should be regularly assessed and secured.
- Good oral care should be provided.
- Proper handwashing with antimicrobial for 30 seconds before and after patient should be done.

CHRONIC OBSTRUCTIVE PULMONARY DISEASES

COPD is a condition of chronic dyspnea with expiratory airflow limitation that is characterized by airway inflammation, mucous plugging, and narrowed airway.

The term "COPD" includes chronic bronchitis and emphysema and asthma.

Asthma: It is characterized by reversible inflammation and constriction of bronchial smooth muscle, hypersecretion of mucus, hyperventilation, and mucosal edema.

Chronic bronchitis: Bronchitis is defined as inflammation of the bronchial tubes, which results in excessive secretions of mucus, leading to tissue swelling that can narrow or close off bronchial lumen **(Fig. 3.1)**.

Emphysema: It is the most severe form of COPD characterized by damages and destruction of alveolar walls **(Fig. 3.2)**.

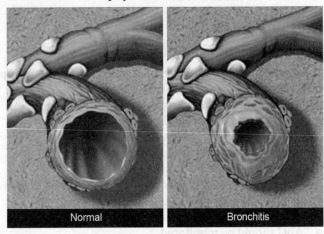

Normal   Bronchitis

Fig. 3.1: Abnormal bronchus in bronchitis.

Etiology

Primary causes:
- **Smoking:** Smoking damages the cilia in the lungs, which normally help clear away mucus and secretions. This creates blockage in the airways that further causes inflammation and irritation in the lungs.
- **AAT deficiency:** These are susceptible to irritants in the environment cause symptoms of COPD.

- **Air pollution:** It also plays a role in the development of COPD.
- **Environmental factors:** COPD does occur in individuals who have never smoked. Although the role of air pollution of COPD is quite common.
- **Hereditary:** AAT deficiency is the genetic risk factor that leads to COPD.
- Occupational chemicals and dusts
- Breathing in secondhand smoker
- Aging

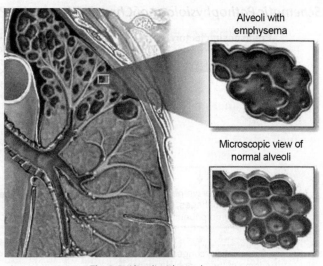

Alveoli with emphysema

Microscopic view of normal alveoli

Fig. 3.2: Alveoli with emphysema.

Pathophysiology

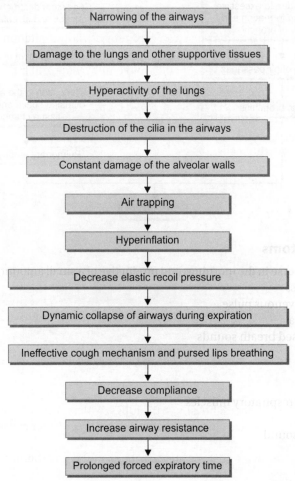

Narrowing of the airways

↓

Damage to the lungs and other supportive tissues

↓

Hyperactivity of the lungs

↓

Destruction of the cilia in the airways

↓

Constant damage of the alveolar walls

↓

Air trapping

↓

Hyperinflation

↓

Decrease elastic recoil pressure

↓

Dynamic collapse of airways during expiration

↓

Ineffective cough mechanism and pursed lips breathing

↓

Decrease compliance

↓

Increase airway resistance

↓

Prolonged forced expiratory time

Schematic Pathophysiology of Chronic Obstructive Pulmonary Diseases

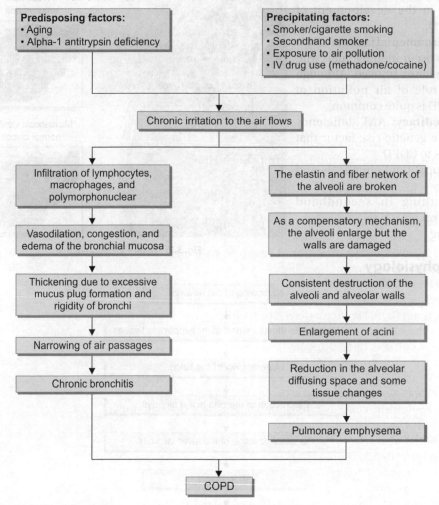

Predisposing factors:
- Aging
- Alpha-1 antitrypsin deficiency

Precipitating factors:
- Smoker/cigarette smoking
- Secondhand smoker
- Exposure to air pollution
- IV drug use (methadone/cocaine)

Chronic irritation to the air flows

Infiltration of lymphocytes, macrophages, and polymorphonuclear

The elastin and fiber network of the alveoli are broken

Vasodilation, congestion, and edema of the bronchial mucosa

As a compensatory mechanism, the alveoli enlarge but the walls are damaged

Thickening due to excessive mucus plug formation and rigidity of bronchi

Consistent destruction of the alveoli and alveolar walls

Narrowing of air passages

Enlargement of acini

Chronic bronchitis

Reduction in the alveolar diffusing space and some tissue changes

Pulmonary emphysema

COPD

Signs and Symptoms

- Cough, usually worse in the mornings and productive of a small amount of colorless sputum
- Acute chest illness
- Elevated jugular venous pulse
- Peripheral edema
- Diffusely decreased breath sounds
- Breathlessness
- Wheezing
- Tachypnea
- Use of accessory respiratory muscles
- Cyanosis
- Coarse crackles sound
- Barrel chest
- Hyperresonance
- Prolonged expiration

Characteristics

Chronic bronchitis	Emphysema
➢ Patients may become obese ➢ Frequent cough and expectoration are typical ➢ Coarse bronchi and wheezing may be heard on auscultation ➢ Patients may have signs of right heart failure	➢ Patients may be very thin with a barrel chest ➢ Patients typically have little or no cough or expectoration ➢ Breathing may be assisted by pursed lips and use of accessory respiratory muscles; patients may adopt the tripod sitting position ➢ The chest may be hyper resonant, and wheezing may be heard ➢ Heart sounds are very distant

Diagnostic Evaluations

Following are the diagnostic evaluations:

- **Chest X-ray:** It may indicate hyperinflation of lungs.
- **Pulmonary function tests**
- **Arterial blood gas analysis:** It may reveal acidosis and mild respiratory alkalosis secondary to hyperventilation.
- **The forced expiratory volume over 1 second (FEV$_1$):** Reduced FEV$_1$ is an indication of reversibility in response to therapy.
- **Total lung capacity, functional residual capacity, and residual volume:** It may be increased, indicating air trapping.
- **D$_L$ CO test:** It is used to assess diffusion in lungs.
- **Bronchogram:** It can show cylindrical dilation of bronchi.
- **Lung scan:** COPD is characterized by a mismatch of perfusion and ventilation.
- **Blood chemistry:** AAT is measured to verify deficiency and diagnosis of primary emphysema.
- **Sputum culture:** It identifies pathogen.
- **Cytologic examination:** It helps to rule out malignancy or allergic disorder.
- **ECG**
- **Exercise ECG and stress test**
- **CBC:** It shows increased hemoglobin and increased eosinophils.

Complication

Following is the list of complications:

- **Pneumothorax:** Air filled in the lungs
- **Cor pulmonale**
- **Giant bullae:** Empty spaces, called bullae, develop in the lungs
- **Recurring infections**

Management

An effective COPD plan includes **four components**:

1. Assess and monitor disease
2. Reduce risk factor
3. Manage stable COPD
4. Manage exacerbations

The **goals** of effective COPD management are to:

- Prevent progression
- Relieve symptoms
- Prevent and treat complications
- Prevent and treat exacerbations
- Improve exercise tolerance
- Improve health status
- Reduce mortality

Component 1: Assess and monitor disease

- Measurement of arterial blood gas tensions should be considered.

Component 2: Reduce risk factors

- Reduction of total exposure to tobacco smoke, occupational dusts and chemicals, and indoor and outdoor air pollution are important goals to prevent the onset and progression of COPD.

Component 3: Manage stable COPD

- For patients with COPD, health education can play a role in improving ability to cope with illness.
- Bronchodilator medications are central to the symptomatic management of COPD.
- Beta 2-agonists, anticholinergics, theophylline, and a combination can be used as bronchodilator.
- Inhaled glucocorticosteroids should only be prescribed for symptomatic patients with COPD.
- The long-term administration of oxygen to patients with chronic respiratory failure has been shown to increase survival.

Component 4: Manage exacerbations

- Inhaled bronchodilators and glucocorticosteroids are effective for treatments for acute exacerbations of COPD.
- Noninvasive positive pressure ventilation in acute exacerbations improves blood gases and pH.
- AAT deficiency treatment reduces the neutrophil elastase burden.

Management of Sputum Viscosity and Secretion Clearance

Mucolytic agents reduce sputum viscosity and improve secretion clearance.

Other managements are:

- **Stop smoking**
- **Bronchodilators**
- **Steroid aerosol sprays**
- **Antibiotics**
- **Rehabilitation techniques**
- **Oxygen**
- **Lung transplant**

Pharmacological Therapy

Pharmacological therapy includes:

- Short-acting beta 2-agonist bronchodilators
- Long-acting beta 2-agonist bronchodilators
- Respiratory anticholinergics
- Phosphodiesterase-4 inhibitors
- Inhaled corticosteroids
- Oral corticosteroids
- Beta 2-agonist and anticholinergic combinations
- Beta 2-agonist and corticosteroid combinations.

Nursing Care Plan

Nursing Diagnosis

1. Ineffective airway clearance related to bronchospasm

Interventions:

- Auscultating breath sounds
- Assessing RR

- Keeping environmental pollution to a minimum
- Encouraging abdominal breathing exercises
- Observing characteristics of cough
- Noting inspiratory/expiratory ratio
- Elevating head of bed
- Increasing fluid intake to 3,000 mL/day

2. Impaired gas exchange related to altered oxygen supply

Interventions:

- Assessing RR and depth
- Elevating head of bed
- Suctioning when indicated
- Auscultating breath sounds
- Assessing routinely monitoring of skin and mucous membrane color
- Monitoring vital signs and cardiac rhythm
- Monitoring level of consciousness
- Evaluating level of activity tolerance

3. Nutrition: imbalanced, less than body requirements related to dyspnea and sputum production.

Interventions:

- Assessing dietary habits and recent food intake
- Auscultating bowel sounds
- Evaluating weight and body size
- Avoiding gas-producing foods and carbonated beverages
- Avoiding very hot or very cold foods
- Giving frequent oral care
- Encouraging a rest period
- Administering supplemental oxygen during meals as indicated.

4. Risk for infection related to inadequate primary defense

Interventions:

- Monitoring temperature
- Observing color, character, and odor of sputum
- Recommending rinsing mouth with water and spitting
- Demonstrating and assist patient in disposal of tissues and sputum
- Encouraging balance between activity and rest
- Discussing need for adequate nutritional intake
- Monitoring visitors and providing masks as indicated
- Administering antimicrobials as indicated.

5. Knowledge deficit related to lack of information

Interventions:

- Providing a detailed plan of care
- Discussing importance of medical follow-up
- Providing information and encourage participation in support groups
- Instructing asthmatic patient in use of peak flow meter
- Reviewing the harmful effects of smoking
- Stressing need for routine influenza and pneumococcal vaccinations
- Stressing importance of oral care and dental hygiene
- Instructing rationale for breathing exercises and coughing effectively
- Discussing importance of avoiding people with active respiratory infections

- Reviewing oxygen requirements and dosage
- Discussing respiratory medications, side effects, and adverse reactions.

ASTHMA

Asthma is a condition in which the airways become narrow and swell and produce extra mucus and characterized by airway hyperresponsiveness, hyperventilation, and mucosal edema.

Etiology

Etiologies are as follows:
- Airborne allergens, such as pollen and dust
- Respiratory infections
- Physical activity
- Cold air
- Air pollutants
- Certain medications
- Strong emotions and stress
- Menstrual cycle

Risk Factors

A number of factors are thought to increase chances of developing asthma, including:
- History of asthma
- Overweight
- Smokers
- Exposure to exhaust fumes
- History of allergic condition and allergic rhinitis
- Second-hand smoke
- Smoking during pregnancy
- Exposure to occupational hazards

Pathophysiology

Stage 1: Bronchoconstriction

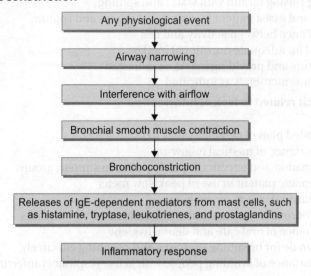

Stage 2: Airway Edema

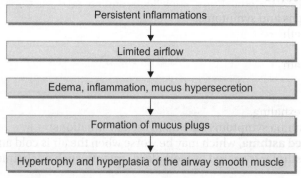

Persistent inflammations

↓

Limited airflow

↓

Edema, inflammation, mucus hypersecretion

↓

Formation of mucus plugs

↓

Hypertrophy and hyperplasia of the airway smooth muscle

Stage 3: Airway Hyperresponsiveness

It include inflammation, dysfunctional neuroregulation, and structural changes in respiratory tree.

Stage 4: Airway Remodeling

In some persons who have asthma, airflow limitation may be only partially reversible. Permanent structural changes can occur in the airway. These are associated with a progressive loss of lung function.

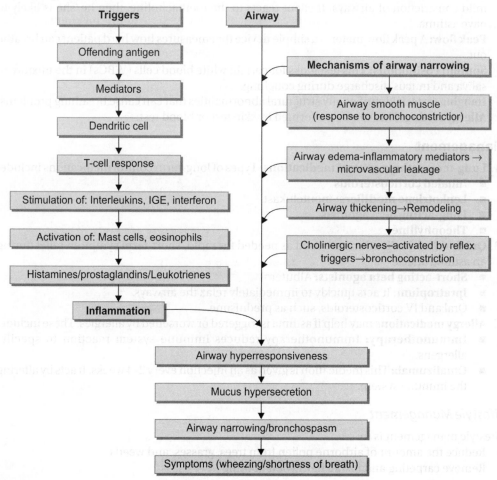

Triggers

Offending antigen

↓

Mediators

↓

Dendritic cell

↓

T-cell response

↓

Stimulation of: Interleukins, IGE, interferon

↓

Activation of: Mast cells, eosinophils

↓

Histamines/prostaglandins/Leukotrienes

↓

Inflammation

Airway

Mechanisms of airway narrowing

Airway smooth muscle
(response to bronchoconstrictior)

Airway edema-inflammatory mediators →
microvascular leakage

Airway thickening→Remodeling

Cholinergic nerves–activated by reflex
triggers→bronchoconstriction

Airway hyperresponsiveness

↓

Mucus hypersecretion

↓

Airway narrowing/bronchospasm

↓

Symptoms (wheezing/shortness of breath)

Signs and Symptoms

Following are the signs and symptoms:
- Shortness of breath
- Chest tightness
- Shortness of breath
- Coughing
- Wheezing
- Whistling when exhaling.

For some people, asthma symptoms flare up in certain situations:
- **Exercise-induced asthma,** which may be worse when the air is cold and dry.
- **Occupational asthma,** triggered by workplace irritants, such as chemical fumes, gases, or dust.
- **Allergy-induced asthma,** triggered by particular allergens, such as pet dander, cockroaches, or pollen.

Diagnostic Evaluations

Following are the diagnostic evaluations:
- **Spirometry:** This test estimates how much air can exhale after a deep breath.
- **Methacholine challenge:** Methacholine triggers the asthma when inhaled and will cause mild constriction of airways. If client reacts to the methacholine, then he/she is likely to have asthma.
- **Peak flow:** A peak flow meter is a simple device that measures how hard patient can breathe out.
- **Sputum eosinophils:** This test looks for certain white blood cells (WBCs) in the mixture of saliva and mucus discharge during coughing.
- **Imaging tests:** It identifies any structural abnormalities that can cause breathing problems.
- **Allergy testing:** This can be performed by skin test or blood test.

Management

A. **Long-term asthma control medications:** Types of long-term control medications include:
   - **Inhaled corticosteroids**
   - **Leukotriene modifiers:** montelukast
   - **Long-acting beta agonists**
   - **Theophylline**
B. **Quick-relief medications** are used as needed for rapid, short-term symptom relief during an asthma attack.
   - **Short-acting beta agonists:** Albuterol
   - **Ipratropium:** It acts quickly to immediately relax the airways.
   - Oral and IV corticosteroids, such as prednisone.
C. **Allergy medications** may help if asthma is triggered or worsened by allergies. These include:
   - **Immunotherapy:** Immunotherapy reduces immune system reaction to specific allergens.
   - **Omalizumab:** This medication is given as an injection every 2–4 weeks. It acts by altering the immune system.

Lifestyle Management

Lifestyle management is to:
- Reduce the amount of airborne pollen from trees, grasses, and weeds
- Remove carpeting and install hardwood flooring

- Dehumidify the room
- Prevent spores
- Clean home at least once a week
- Cover nose and mouth

Nursing Care Plan

Nursing Diagnosis

1. Ineffective airway clearance related to tracheobronchial obstruction

Interventions:
- Assessing airway for patency
- Inspecting the mouth and neck for potential obstruction
- Auscultating lungs
- Assessing respiratory quality, rate, and depth
- Monitoring arterial blood gases
- Administering supplemental oxygen
- Positioning patient with head of bed 45°
- Assessing for mental status changes
- Assessing changes in vital signs
- Helping patient with coughing and deep breathing techniques
- Always being ready with artificial airway

2. Impaired gas exchange related to altered oxygen supply

Interventions:
- Assessing respirations
- Assessing for signs of hypoxemia
- Monitoring vital signs
- Assessing for life-threatening problems
- Auscultating lung sounds
- Providing supplemental oxygen
- Assessing for changes in level of consciousness
- Monitoring ABGs
- Continuous pulse oximetry
- Assessing skin color for cyanosis
- Preparing the patient for intubation

PNEUMONIA

Pneumonia is an inflammation the lung parenchyma characterized by inflammatory process associated with increased in interstitial, alveoli fluid fever, chest tightness, and a lack of air space.

Etiology and Risk Factors

The main cause of pneumonia is the
- *Streptococcus pneumoniae*, influenza, *Staphylococcus aureus* bacteria.
- Rhinoviruses, coronaviruses, and influenza virus
- Fungal agents, such as *Histoplasma capsulatum*
- Parasites, such as *Toxoplasma gondii.*

The major risk factors of pneumonia include:

- Advanced age
- Smoking
- Upper respiratory infections
- Tracheal intubation
- Bedridden patient
- Immunosuppressive therapy
- Diabetes
- Expose to air pollution
- Alcoholism
- Malnutrition
- Dehydration

Other Risk Factors

Other risk factors include:

- Previous stroke
- Age
- Weakened immune system
- Drug abuse
- Certain medical conditions

Types of Pneumonia

Pneumonia according to site:

- **Segmental pneumonia:** It involves one or more segments of the lungs.
- **Lobar pneumonia:** It involves one or more entire lobes.
- **Bilateral pneumonia:** It involves lobes in both the lungs.

Pneumonia according to location:

- Bronchopneumonia
- Interstitial pneumonia
- Alveolar pneumonia
- Narcotizing pneumonia.

Pneumonia according to organism:

- Pneumococcal pneumonia
- *Staphylococcus pneumonia*
- *Haemophilus* influenzae pneumonia
- Gram-negative bacterial pneumonia
- Legionnaires disease
- *Mycoplasma pneumoniae*
- Viral pneumonia
- Fungal pneumoconiosis
- Parasitic pneumonia

Other type of pneumonia:

- **Aspiration pneumonia:** It occurs due to aspiration of foreign particles, gastric content or food.
- **Hypostatic pneumonia:** It is caused by lack of mobility.
- **VAP:** It is defined as pneumonia occurring in a patient within 48 hours or more after intubation with an endotracheal tube.

Pathophysiology

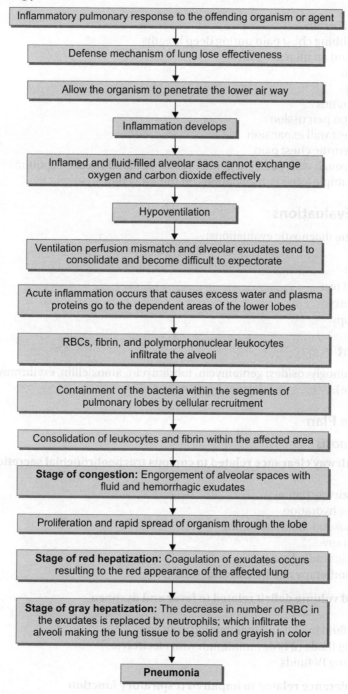

| Inflammatory pulmonary response to the offending organism or agent |
| Defense mechanism of lung lose effectiveness |
| Allow the organism to penetrate the lower air way |
| Inflammation develops |
| Inflamed and fluid-filled alveolar sacs cannot exchange oxygen and carbon dioxide effectively |
| Hypoventilation |
| Ventilation perfusion mismatch and alveolar exudates tend to consolidate and become difficult to expectorate |
| Acute inflammation occurs that causes excess water and plasma proteins go to the dependent areas of the lower lobes |
| RBCs, fibrin, and polymorphonuclear leukocytes infiltrate the alveoli |
| Containment of the bacteria within the segments of pulmonary lobes by cellular recruitment |
| Consolidation of leukocytes and fibrin within the affected area |
| **Stage of congestion:** Engorgement of alveolar spaces with fluid and hemorrhagic exudates |
| Proliferation and rapid spread of organism through the lobe |
| **Stage of red hepatization:** Coagulation of exudates occurs resulting to the red appearance of the affected lung |
| **Stage of gray hepatization:** The decrease in number of RBC in the exudates is replaced by neutrophils; which infiltrate the alveoli making the lung tissue to be solid and grayish in color |
| **Pneumonia** |

Signs and Symptoms

Following are the signs and symptoms:

- Productive cough
- Hyperthermia

- Headache
- Fatigue
- Shortness of breath
- Sharp or stabbing chest pain during deep breaths
- Confusion and an increased RR
- Malnutrition
- Hemoptysis
- Crackling sounds
- Dull sound on percussion
- Unequal chest wall expansion
- Stabbing pleuritic chest pain
- Productive cough with purulent golden yellow or blood streaked sputum
- Single or multiple lobar consolidations on the X-ray film.

Diagnostic Evaluations

Following are the diagnostic evaluations:
- Chest CT
- Sputum test
- Pleural fluid test
- Pulse oximetry
- Bronchoscopy

Management

Antibiotics (aminoglycosides: gentamycin, tobramycin, amoxicillin, erythromycin, penicillin, and tetracycline).

Nursing Care Plan

Nursing Diagnosis

1. Ineffective airway clearance related to copious tracheobronchial secretions
Interventions:
- Improving airway patency
- Encouraging hydration
- Providing nasotracheal suctioning
- Oxygen therapy
- Providing humidified air
- Chest physiotherapy and incentive spirometry

2. Risk for fluid volume deficit related to fever and dyspnea
Interventions:
- Promoting fluid intake and maintaining nutrition
- Encouraging fluids (2 L/day minimum with electrolytes)
- Administering IV fluids

3. Activity intolerance related to impaired respiratory function
Interventions:
- Promoting activity tolerance
- Encouraging patient to have rest
- Providing comfortable position (e.g., semi-Fowler's)
- Changing position

4. Knowledge deficit about treatment regimen and preventive measures

Interventions:

- Informing patient
- Instructing on management of symptoms
- Explaining treatments using appropriate language
- Repeating instructions and explanations as needed

Monitoring and Preventing Complications

Monitoring and preventing complications include:

- Assessing for signs and symptoms of shock and respiratory failure
- Administering IV fluids
- Assessing for atelectasis and pleural effusion
- Assisting with thoracentesis
- Monitoring for superinfection

Health Education

Health education should be:

- Instructing client to continue taking antibiotics until complete
- Advising client to increase activities gradually after fever subsides
- Advising client that fatigue and weakness may occur
- Encouraging breathing exercises
- Encouraging follow-up
- Encouraging client to avoid fatigue
- Encouraging adequate nutrition and rest
- Recommending influenza vaccine

BRONCHIECTASIS

Bronchiectasis is a condition characterized by destruction, loosening of integrity, and permanently enlargement of bronchial wall.

Etiology

- Cystic fibrosis
- HIV
- Recurrent aspiration of fluid into the lungs
- Inhalation of a foreign object into the lungs
- Inhalation of harmful chemicals

Types

Following are the types:

1. **Cylindrical bronchiectasis:** Bronchi are enlarged and cylindrical.
2. **Varicose bronchiectasis:** Bronchi are irregular with areas of dilatation.
3. **Saccular:** Dilated bronchi form clusters of cysts.

Signs and Symptoms

Following are the signs and symptoms:

- Mucus-producing cough
- Hypophysis

- Foul breath
- Wheezing chest
- Recurring lung infections

Diagnostic Evaluations

Following are the diagnostic evaluations:
- Chest X-ray
- CT scan
- Blood tests
- Mucus swab culture
- ABG analysis
- Lung function tests

Management

Medications:
- Antibiotics are used to treat acute lung infections
- Bronchodilators
- Corticosteroids
- Mucolytic
- Vaccination against flu and pneumococcus

Physiotherapy and exercise: Chest physiotherapy and postural drainage

Prevention

The Ministry of Health recommends the following measures to help prevent bronchiectasis in children:
- Not smoking during pregnancy
- Immunization against measles and whooping cough
- Exclusive breastfeeding
- Making sure homes are warm and dry
- Eating a healthy balanced diet
- Early detection and treatment of chest infections

Nursing Care Plan

1. Ineffective airway clearance related to copious tracheobronchial secretions
Interventions:
- Improving airway patency
- Encouraging hydration
- Providing nasotracheal suctioning
- Oxygen therapy
- Provide humidified air
- Chest physiotherapy and incentive spirometry

2. Risk for fluid volume deficit related to fever and dyspnea
Interventions:
- Promoting fluid intake and maintaining nutrition
- Encouraging fluids (2 L/day minimum with electrolytes)
- Administering IV fluids

3. Activity intolerance related to impaired respiratory function
Interventions:
- Promoting activity tolerance
- Encouraging patient to have rest
- Providing comfortable position (e.g., semi-Fowler's)
- Changing position frequently

4. Knowledge deficit about treatment regimen and preventive measures
Interventions:
- Informing patient
- Instructing on management of symptoms
- Explaining treatments using appropriate language
- Repeating instructions and explanations as needed.

INTERSTITIAL LUNG DISEASE

Interstitial lung disease describes a large group of disorders, most of which cause progressive scarring of lung tissue, which affects the ability to breathe and decrease the partial pressure of oxygen.

Types of Interstitial Lung Disease

Following are the types of interstitial lung disease:
- **Interstitial pneumonia:** Caused by *Mycoplasma pneumoniae*
- **Idiopathic pulmonary fibrosis:** Its cause is unknown
- **Hypersensitivity pneumonitis:** Caused by ongoing inhalation of dust
- **Cryptogenic organizing pneumonia:** Pneumonia-like interstitial lung disease but without an infection present
- **Acute interstitial pneumonitis:** A sudden, severe interstitial lung disease often requires life support
- **Desquamative interstitial pneumonitis:** Caused by smoking
- **Sarcoidosis:** Characterized by swollen lymph nodes
- **Asbestosis:** Caused by asbestos exposure
- **Nonspecific interstitial pneumonitis:** Due to autoimmune conditions
- **Silicosis:** Silicosis is a condition caused by inhaling too much silica over a long period
- **Pneumoconiosis:** Caused by inhaling coal dust

Etiology

- **Occupational and environmental factors:** Long-term exposure to a number of toxins and pollutants can damage the lungs. These may include:
  - Silica dust
  - Asbestos fibers
  - Grain dust
  - Bird and animal droppings
- **Radiation treatments:** The severity of the damage depends on:
  - How much of the lung was exposed to radiation?
  - The total amount of radiation administered
  - Whether chemotherapy also was used
  - The presence of underlying lung disease.

- **Medications:**
  - **Chemotherapy drugs:** Methotrexate and cyclophosphamide
  - **Antibiotics:** Nitrofurantoin and sulfasalazine.
- **Medical conditions:** Lung damage can also result from:
  - Systemic lupus erythematosus
  - Sarcoidosis
  - Rheumatoid arthritis
  - Scleroderma

Risk Factors

Risk factors include:

a. Age
b. Exposure to occupational and environmental toxins
c. Smoking
d. Radiation and chemotherapy
e. Oxygen

Pathophysiology

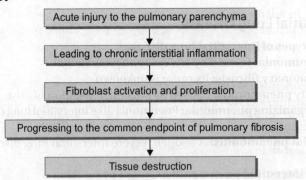

Acute injury to the pulmonary parenchyma

↓

Leading to chronic interstitial inflammation

↓

Fibroblast activation and proliferation

↓

Progressing to the common endpoint of pulmonary fibrosis

↓

Tissue destruction

Signs and Symptoms

Following are the signs and symptoms:

- Shortness of breath
- Cyanosis
- Clubbing (a painless enlargement of the fingertips)
- Cardiomyopathy
- Weight loss
- Anorexia
- Dry cough
- Cachexia
- Fatigue

Diagnostic Evaluations

Following are the diagnostic evaluations:

- Medical history and physical examination
- Blood tests
- Chest X-ray

- Pulmonary function testing
- Bronchoscopy
- Video-assisted thoracoscopic surgery
- Lung biopsy
- CT
- High-resolution CT scan
- Open lung biopsy (thoracotomy)

Management

Following is the list of management:
- **Inhaled oxygen**
- **Antibiotics:** Azithromycin and levofloxacin
- **Vaccines:** Influenza vaccine and pneumococcal pneumonia vaccine
- **Corticosteroids:** Prednisone and methylprednisolone
- **Immune-suppressing drug:** Azathioprine or cyclophosphamide
- **Smoking cessation**

Surgical Management

Lung transplant: In advanced interstitial lung disease causing severe impairment, a lung transplant may be the best option. Most people undergoing lung transplant for interstitial lung disease make large gains in quality of life and their ability to exercise.

Contraindications
Following are the contradictions:
- Current or recurring infection
- Metastatic cancer
- Severe cardiac disorder
- Noncompliance with treatment regimen

Risks of the Procedure
The risks of the procedure are as follows:
- Hemorrhage
- Septicemia
- Blockage of the blood vessels
- Blockage of the airways
- Severe pulmonary edema
- Blood clots

Requirements for Potential Recipients
While a transplant center is free to set its own criteria for transplant candidates, certain requirements are generally agreed upon, which are as follows:
- End-stage lung disease
- Age
- Acceptable psychological profile
- Financially able to pay for expense
- Has exhausted other available therapies without success
- No other chronic medical conditions
- No current infections or recent cancer
- No HIV or hepatitis

- Within an acceptable weight range
- Has social support system
- Able to comply with post-transplant regimen
- No alcohol, smoking, or drug abuse

Medical tests for potential transplant
- **Blood typing:** The recipient's blood type must match the donor.
- **Tissue typing:** The lung tissue would also match as closely as possible between the donor.
- **Chest X-ray:** It is done to verify the size of the lungs and the chest cavity.
- **Pulmonary function tests**
- **V/Q scan**
- **ECG**
- **CT scan**
- Bone mineral density scan
- Cardiac stress test
- Cardiac catheterization
- Echocardiogram

Types of lung transplant
Types of lung transplant are as follows:
A. **Lobe: One lob is transplanted**
B. **Single lung:** Transplantation of a single healthy lung.
C. **Heart lung:** Some respiratory patients may also have severe cardiac disease, which would necessitate a heart transplant.

Procedure
- **Procedure should be as follows:**
  - Before operating on the recipient, the transplant surgeon inspects the donor lung(s) for signs of damage or disease.
  - If the lung or lungs are approved, then the recipient is connected to an IV line and various monitoring equipment, including pulse oximetry.
  - The patient will be given general anesthesia, and a machine will breathe for him/her.
  - It takes about 1 hour for the preoperative preparation of the patient.
  - A single-lung transplant takes about 4–8 hours, while a double-lung transplant takes about 6–12 hours to complete.
  - A history of prior chest surgery may complicate the procedure and require additional time.
- **Single lung:**
  - The process starts out after the donor lung has been inspected.
  - The decision to accept the donor lung for the patient has been made.
  - An incision is generally made from under the shoulder blade around the chest, ending near the sternum.
  - An alternate method involves an incision under the breastbone.
  - In the case of a singular lung transplant, the lung is collapsed, the blood vessels in the lung tied off, and the lung removed at the bronchial tube.
  - The donor lung is placed, the blood vessels reattached, and the lung reinflated. To make sure the lung is satisfactory and to clear any remaining blood and mucus in the new lung, a bronchoscopy will be performed.
  - When the surgeons are satisfied with the performance of the lung, the chest incision will be closed.

- **Double lung**
  - A double-lung transplant, also known as a bilateral transplant, can be executed sequentially or simultaneously. Sequential is more common. This is effectively like having two separate single-lung transplants done.
  - The transplantation process starts after the donor lungs are inspected and the decision to transplant has been made.
  - An incision is then made from under the patient's armpit, around to the sternum, and then back toward the other armpit; this is known as a clamshell incision.
  - In the case of a sequential transplant, the recipient's lung with the poorest lung functions is collapsed, the blood vessels tied off and cut at the corresponding bronchi.
  - The new lung is then placed and the blood vessels reattached. To make sure that the lung is satisfactory before transplanting the other, a bronchoscopy is performed.
  - When the surgeons are satisfied with the performance of the new lung, surgery on the second lung will proceed.
  - In 10–20% of double-lung transplants, the patient is hooked up to a heart-lung machine that pumps blood for the body and supplies fresh oxygen.

Signs of rejection:
- Fever
- Flu-like symptoms
- Dyspnea
- Increase or decrease in body weight
- Worsening pulmonary test results
- Increased chest pain.

Prevention of rejection

The antirejection medications most commonly used include:
- Cyclosporine
- Tacrolimus
- Azathioprine
- Mycophenolat
- Prednisone

Complications

- Pulmonary hypertension
- Right-sided heart failure
- Respiratory failure

SILICOSIS

Silicosis is a chronic lung disease caused by breathing in tiny bits of silica dust. When people inhale silica dust, they inhale tiny particles of silica that has crystallized and cause fluid buildup and scar tissue in the lungs, which cuts down effects of the ability to breathe.

Classification of Silicosis

There are three types of silicosis:
1. **Chronic silicosis:** It is the most common type of silicosis, which usually occurs after 10 or more years of exposure to crystalline silica at low levels.
2. **Accelerated silicosis:** It occurs 5–10 years after exposure and is caused by exposure to higher levels of crystalline silica.
3. **Acute silicosis:** It can occur after only weeks or months of exposure to very high levels of crystalline silica.

Etiology and Risk factors

Following are etiology and risk factors:
- Mining
- Quarrying
- Abrasive blasting
- Masonry work
- Stone cutting
- Highway and bridge construction
- Building construction
- Sand and gravel screening
- Rock crushing
- Concrete finishing
- Drywall finishing
- Rock drilling

Pathophysiology

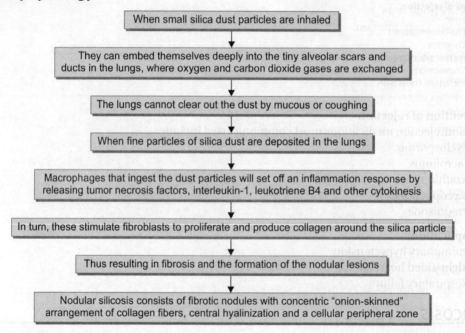

When small silica dust particles are inhaled

↓

They can embed themselves deeply into the tiny alveolar scars and ducts in the lungs, where oxygen and carbon dioxide gases are exchanged

↓

The lungs cannot clear out the dust by mucous or coughing

↓

When fine particles of silica dust are deposited in the lungs

↓

Macrophages that ingest the dust particles will set off an inflammation response by releasing tumor necrosis factors, interleukin-1, leukotriene B4 and other cytokinesis

↓

In turn, these stimulate fibroblasts to proliferate and produce collagen around the silica particle

↓

Thus resulting in fibrosis and the formation of the nodular lesions

↓

Nodular silicosis consists of fibrotic nodules with concentric "onion-skinned" arrangement of collagen fibers, central hyalinization and a cellular peripheral zone

Signs and Symptoms

Following are the signs and symptoms:
- Dyspnea
- Coughing
- Fatigue
- Tachypnea
- Anorexia
- Chest pain
- Fever

Diagnostic Test

Diagnostic tests include:
- Chest X-ray
- Chest CT scan
- Pulmonary function tests
- Purified protein derivative skin test (for TB)
- Serologic tests for connective tissue diseases

Treatment

Following are the types of treatment:
- Stopping further exposure to silica
- Antibiotics for bacterial lung infection
- TB prophylaxis
- Prolonged antituberculosis (multidrug regimen)
- Chest physiotherapy
- Oxygen administration
- Bronchodilators
- Lung transplantation

Complications

Following are the complications:
- Connective tissue disease
- Lung cancer
- Progressive massive fibrosis
- Respiratory failure
- TB

ASBESTOSIS

Asbestosis is a chronic inflammatory and fibrotic medical condition affecting the parenchymal tissue of the lungs caused by the inhalation and retention of asbestos fibers.

Etiology

Tiny asbestos fibers—they can get stuck deep inside lungs.

Symptoms of Asbestosis

Following are the symptoms of asbestosis:
- Dry inspiratory crackles
- Clubbing of the fingers
- Misshapen nails
- Shortness of breath
- A persistent, dry cough
- Loss of appetite with weight loss
- Chest tightness or pain
- Coughing
- Chest pain

- Blood in the sputum
- Swelling in the neck or face
- Difficulty swallowing
- Loss of appetite
- Weight loss

Pathophysiology

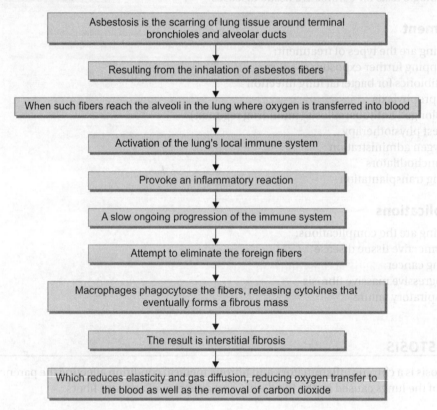

Asbestosis is the scarring of lung tissue around terminal bronchioles and alveolar ducts

↓

Resulting from the inhalation of asbestos fibers

↓

When such fibers reach the alveoli in the lung where oxygen is transferred into blood

↓

Activation of the lung's local immune system

↓

Provoke an inflammatory reaction

↓

A slow ongoing progression of the immune system

↓

Attempt to eliminate the foreign fibers

↓

Macrophages phagocytose the fibers, releasing cytokines that eventually forms a fibrous mass

↓

The result is interstitial fibrosis

↓

Which reduces elasticity and gas diffusion, reducing oxygen transfer to the blood as well as the removal of carbon dioxide

Diagnosis

- Complete physical examination
- Chest X-ray
- Lung function tests
- A **lung biopsy**

Treatment

- Oxygen therapy to relieve shortness of breath
- Respiratory physiotherapy to remove secretions from the lungs
- Medications to thin secretions and relieve pain.

COAL WORKERS' PNEUMOCONIOSIS

Coal worker's pneumoconiosis can be defined as the accumulation of coal dust in the lungs and the tissue's reaction to its presence.

Pathophysiology

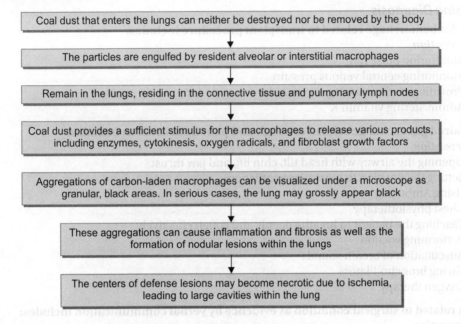

Coal dust that enters the lungs can neither be destroyed nor be removed by the body

↓

The particles are engulfed by resident alveolar or interstitial macrophages

↓

Remain in the lungs, residing in the connective tissue and pulmonary lymph nodes

↓

Coal dust provides a sufficient stimulus for the macrophages to release various products, including enzymes, cytokinesis, oxygen radicals, and fibroblast growth factors

↓

Aggregations of carbon-laden macrophages can be visualized under a microscope as granular, black areas. In serious cases, the lung may grossly appear black

↓

These aggregations can cause inflammation and fibrosis as well as the formation of nodular lesions within the lungs

↓

The centers of defense lesions may become necrotic due to ischemia, leading to large cavities within the lung

Clinical Signs and Symptoms

Following are the clinical signs and symptoms:

- Chronic cough
- Fever
- Expectoration
- Dyspnea

Diagnostic Evaluations

Following are the diagnostic evaluations:

- History of exposure
- Lung function test
- Radiography
- Pulmonary function tests

Management

Management includes: Corticosteroids, pulmonary lavage, and lung transplant.

Prevention and Control

Following are the steps to be taken for prevention and control:

- Preplacement and periodic medical examination of workers
- Use of protective equipment by the workers
- Use of dust suppression measure
- Exhaust ventilation

Nursing Care Plan

Nursing Diagnosis

Risk for hemorrhage related to transplant procedure includes:
Intervention
- Monitoring pulse rate
- Monitoring central venous pressure
- Providing sterile dressing on wound
- Administering vitamin K

Impaired gas exchange related to cough and pain from incision includes:
Intervention
- Opening the airway with head tilt, chin lift, and jaw thrust
- Setting the position to maximize ventilation
- Using Ambu bag
- Chest physiotherapy
- Teaching the patient to breathe deeply and cough effectively
- Performing suction
- Auscultation of breath sounds
- Giving bronchodilators
- Oxygen therapy

Pain related to surgical condition as evidence by verbal communication includes:
Intervention
- Assessing the intensity of pain
- Teaching the patient about pain management
- Securing the chest tube to restrict movement
- Assessing pain reduction measures
- Providing analgesics as indicated

RESTRICTIVE LUNG DISEASES

"Restrictive lung disease is a chronic disorder that causes a decrease in the ability to expand the lung and sometimes makes it harder to get enough oxygen to meet the body's needs."

Types

Types of restrictive lung disease are as follows:
  I. Interstitial pulmonary fibrosis or interstitial lung disease
 II. Extrapulmonary restrictive lung disease

Etiology

- **Intrinsic**
  - Radiation fibrosis
  - Certain drugs
  - Hypersensitivity pneumonitis
  - Acute ARDS
  - Infant ARDS
- **Extrinsic**
  - Neuromuscular diseases
  - Nonmuscular diseases
  - Pleural thickening

Pathophysiology

In cases of intrinsic lung disease

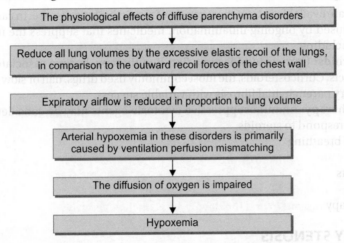

The physiological effects of diffuse parenchyma disorders

Reduce all lung volumes by the excessive elastic recoil of the lungs, in comparison to the outward recoil forces of the chest wall

Expiratory airflow is reduced in proportion to lung volume

Arterial hypoxemia in these disorders is primarily caused by ventilation perfusion mismatching

The diffusion of oxygen is impaired

Hypoxemia

In cases of extrinsic disorders

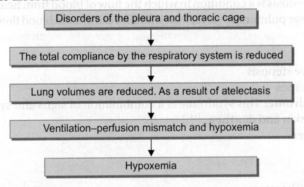

Disorders of the pleura and thoracic cage

The total compliance by the respiratory system is reduced

Lung volumes are reduced. As a result of atelectasis

Ventilation–perfusion mismatch and hypoxemia

Hypoxemia

Signs and Symptoms

Symptoms of restrictive lung disease include:

- Cough
- Shortness of breath
- Wheezing and chest pain
- Difficulty in inhaling and exhaling
- Wheezing and noisy breathing
- Coughing up blood

Diagnostic Evaluations

- Physical examination
- Pulmonary function tests
- Chest X-ray
- CT scans
- Bronchoscopy
- Pulse oximetry
- Lung biopsy

Management

Medical Management

Few medicines are available to treat most causes of restrictive lung disease. In cases of restrictive lung disease caused by ongoing inflammation, medicines that suppress the immune system may be used, including:

- **Corticosteroids:** Corticosteroids are a first-line therapy, but are associated with myriad adverse effects. Corticosteroids, the most commonly used drugs, halt or slow the progression of pulmonary parenchymal fibrosis with variable success.
- **Cytotoxic therapy:** Immunosuppressive cytotoxic agents may be considered for patients who do not respond to steroids.
- Mechanical breathing
- Inhalers
- Expectorants
- Antibiotics
- Chemotherapy

PULMONARY STENOSIS

Pulmonary valve stenosis is a condition in which the flow of blood from heart to lungs is slowed by a deformity or near pulmonary valve, which finally restricts the blood flow to pulmonary tree.

Etiology

- Pulmonary valve stenosis
- Heart abnormalities
- **Carcinoid syndrome:** This syndrome is a combination of signs and symptoms, including flushing of the skin and diarrhea.
- **Rheumatic fever**

Risk Factors

Following are the risk factors:
- Carcinoid syndrome
- Rheumatic fever
- Noonan's syndrome

Signs and Symptoms

Following are the signs and symptoms:
- Heart murmur
- Shortness of breath
- Chest pain
- Palpitations
- Loss of consciousness
- Fatigue

Diagnostic Evaluations

- **ECG:** An ECG records the electrical activity of heart each time it contracts. During this procedure, patches with wires are placed on chest, wrists, and ankles. The electrodes measure electrical activity, which is recorded on paper. This test helps determine whether the muscular wall of right ventricle is thickened (ventricular hypertrophy).

- **Echocardiography:** Echocardiograms use high-pitched sound waves to produce an image of the heart. Sound waves bounce off the heart and produce moving images that can be viewed on a video screen. This test is useful for checking the structure of the pulmonary valve, the location, and severity of the narrowing and the function of the right ventricle of the heart.
- **Other imaging tests:** Magnetic resonance imaging and CT scans are sometimes used to confirm the diagnosis of pulmonary valve stenosis.
- **Cardiac catheterization:** During this procedure, doctor inserts a thin, flexible tube into an artery or vein in groin and weaves it up to the heart or blood vessels. A dye is injected through the catheter to make blood vessels visible on X-ray pictures. Doctors also use cardiac catheterization to measure the BP in the heart chambers and blood vessels.

Management

Medical Management

A physician may prescribe medications that make it easier for blood to flow through the heart's chambers. **Examples of medications** prescribed may include:
- Prostaglandins to improve blood flow
- Blood thinners to reduce clotting
- Antiarrhythmic that prevents irregular heart rhythms

Surgical Management

Balloon valvuloplasty

This technique, which tends to be the first choice for treatment, uses cardiac catheterization to treat pulmonary valve stenosis. During this procedure, doctor threads a small tube through a vein in leg and up to heart. An uninflated balloon is placed through the opening of the narrowed pulmonary valve and then inflates the balloon, opening up the narrowed pulmonary valve and increasing the area available for blood flow. The balloon is then removed.

Open-heart surgery

- Balloon valvuloplasty cannot be used for cases of pulmonary stenosis that occur above the pulmonary valve (supravalvular) or below the valve (subvalvular). Open-heart surgery is required for these types of stenosis and occasionally for valvular stenosis.
- During the surgery, doctor repairs the pulmonary artery or the valve to allow blood to pass through more easily. In certain cases, doctor may replace the pulmonary valve with an artificial valve.
- Some people with pulmonary stenosis have other congenital heart defects, and these may be repaired at the time of surgery. As with balloon valvuloplasty, there is a slight risk of bleeding, infection, or blood clots associated with the surgery.

Nursing Care Plan

Nursing Diagnosis

- Ineffective airway clearance related to bronchoconstriction, increased mucus production, ineffective cough, possible bronchopulmonary infection.
- Risk for infection related to compromise pulmonary function, retained secretions, and compromised defense mechanism.
- Impaired gas exchange related to chronic pulmonary obstruction due to destruction of alveolar capillary membrane.

- Imbalanced nutritional status less than body requirements related to increased work of breathing, air swallowing, and drug effects with resultant wasting of respiratory and skeletal muscles.
- Activity intolerance related to compromised pulmonary function, resulting in the shortness of breath and fatigue.
- Ineffective coping related to the stress of living with chronic disease, loss of independence, depression, and anxiety disorder.

Nursing Interventions

Improving airway clearance

- All pulmonary irritants, particularly cigarette smoking, should be eliminated.
- Cessation of smoking usually results in less pulmonary irritation, sputum production, and cough.
- Patient's room should be kept as dust free as possible.
- Moisture should be added to indoor environment.
- Bronchodilators should be administered to control bronchospasm and assist with raising sputum.
- Side effects—tremulousness, tachycardia, cardiac dysrhythmias, central nervous system stimulation, and hypertension—should be assessed.
- The chest should be auscultated after administration of aerosol bronchodilator to assess for improvement of aeration and reduction of adventitious breath sounds.
- Whether patient has reduction in dyspnea need to be observed.
- Serum theophylline level should be monitored, as ordered, to ensure therapeutic level and prevent toxicity.
- Postural drainage position should be used to aid in clearance of secretions, because mucopurulent secretions are responsible for airway obstruction.
- The patient should be encouraged to take high liquid fluids.
- Inhalation nebulized water should be provided to humidify bronchial tree and liquefy sputum.

Controlling infection

- It is necessary to recognize early manifestations of respiratory infection-increased dyspnea, fatigue, and change in color, amount and character of sputum, nervousness, irritability, and low-grade fever.
- Sputum for smear and culture should be obtained.
- Prescribed antimicrobial tree should be administered to clear the airway.
- The patients should be advised to live in proper ventilated room.
- The patients should be advised to take medicine regularly as advised by doctor.
- The patients should be advised to live in hygienic place, that is, free from dust.

Improving gas exchange

- It is necessary to watch for restlessness, aggressiveness, anxiety, or confusion; central cyanosis and shortness of breath at rest, which frequently is caused by acute respiratory insufficiency and may signal respiratory failure.
- Low-flow oxygen therapy should be given as ordered to correct hypoxemia in a controlled manner and minimize carbon dioxide retention.
- It is advised to be prepared to assist with intubation and mechanical ventilation if acute respiratory failure and rapid carbon dioxide retention occurs.
- The patients should be advised to live in ventilated room and contact with fresh air daily.
- The patients should be advised to do breathing exercise as advised by doctors.

Improving nutrition

- Nutritional history, height, and anthropometric measurements should be considered.
- Frequent small meal should be encouraged if patient is dyspneic, even small increase in abdominal contents may press on diaphragm and impede breathing.
- Food that causes abdominal discomfort should be avoided.
- Supplemental oxygen therapy should be given while patient is eating to relieve dyspnea, as directed.
- Body weight should be monitored regularly.

Increased activity tolerance

- The patient should be encouraged for daily exercise and benefits of walking, bicycling, and swimming should be discussed.
- The patient should be encouraged to carry out regular exercise program to increase physical endurances.
- The patient should be trained in energy conservation techniques.
- The patients as well as the family should be educated about the benefits of exercise.

Enhancing coping

- It is necessary to understand the constant shortness of breath and fatigue make the patient irritable, anxious, and depressed, with feeling of helplessness/hopelessness.
- The patient should be assessed for reactive behavior (anger, depression, and acceptance).
- The patient's self-image should be strengthened.
- The patient should be allowed to express feelings, and the mechanisms of dental and repression should be retained.
- The patient should be always supported by spouse/family members.

PULMONARY EMBOLISM

- Pulmonary embolism refers to the obstruction of one or more pulmonary arteries, by a thrombus that originates somewhere in the venous system or in the right heart. It may be associated with trauma, surgery, pregnancy CCF, advanced age (above 60 years), and immobility.
- Pulmonary embolism is defined as an obstruction of one or more pulmonary arteries of the lungs are blocked, or thrombus that originates somewhere in the venous system or right side of the heart.

Etiology

- Venous stasis
- Hypercoagulation
- Damage to the endothelium of blood vessels

Risk Factors

- Prolonged immobilization
- Concurrent phlebitis heart failure
- Heart failure and strokes
- Malignancy
- Advancing age and estrogen therapy
- Oral contraceptives
- Obesity

Pathophysiology

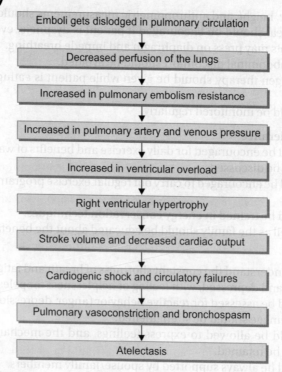

Emboli gets dislodged in pulmonary circulation

↓

Decreased perfusion of the lungs

↓

Increased in pulmonary embolism resistance

↓

Increased in pulmonary artery and venous pressure

↓

Increased in ventricular overload

↓

Right ventricular hypertrophy

↓

Stroke volume and decreased cardiac output

↓

Cardiogenic shock and circulatory failures

↓

Pulmonary vasoconstriction and bronchospasm

↓

Atelectasis

Clinical Manifestation

- Rapid onset of dyspnea at rest, pleuritic chest pain cough and syncope, delirium, apprehension, tachypnea, diaphoresis, and hemoptysis.
- Chest pain with apprehension and a sense of impending doom occurs when most of the pulmonary artery is obstructed.
- Tachycardia, rales, fever, hypotension, cyanosis, heart gallop, and loud pulmonic component of S2.
- Calf and thigh pain, edema, erythema, tenderness, or palpable cord.

Diagnostic Evaluations

- History taking
- Assess for signs and symptoms blood study
- Thrombotic imaging: V/Q scan or single photo emission computerized
- Pulmonary angiography
- D-Dimer assay for low intermediate probability of pulmonary embolism
- ABG levels—decreased PaO_2 usually found due to perfusion abnormality of lung
- Chest X-ray—normal or possible wedge-shaped infiltrate.

Management

Medical Management

It is focused on anticoagulant to reduce the size of thrombus and maintain the cardiopulmonary stability.

1. **Anticoagulant:** It begins with heparin 5,000 IU and warfarin, 2.5 mg/day, as maintained dose regulation upon prothrombin time.

2. **Thrombolytic therapy:** Cytokines resolve the thrombus or emboli quickly and restore normal hemodynamic therapy to reducing pulmonary hypertension improving pulmonary perfusion, oxygenation, and cardiac output.
3. Also to improve patients respiratory and vascular status.
   - Oxygenation therapy to correct hypoxia
   - Venous stasis is reduced by using elastic stoking
   - Elevating leg for increase venous flow
   - Hypotension relaxed with fluids
   - Chest pain and apprehension one treated with analgesics.

Surgical Management

When anticoagulation is contraindicated or patient has recurrent embolization or develops serious complication from drug therapy.
- **Interruption of vena cava:** It reduces channel size to prevent lower extremity from reaching lungs and accomplished by:
  - Ligation, placation, or clipping of the inferior vena cava
  - Placement of transversely inserted intraluminal filter inferior vena cava to prevent migration of emboli
- **Embolectomy**

Nursing Care Plan

Assessment

- The signs and symptoms of pulmonary embolism should be assessed.
- The vital signs of patient especially respiration should be assessed.
- The chest pain intensity should be assessed.
- Edema and fever should be assessed.
- The hypotension and cyanosis of the patient should be assessed.

Nursing Diagnosis

- Ineffective breathing pattern related to increase in alveolar dead airspace and possible changes in lung mechanics from embolism.
- Ineffective tissue perfusion (pulmonary) related to decreased blood circulation.
- Acute pain (pleuritic) related to congestion, possible pleural effusion, and lung infraction.
- Anxiety related to dyspnea to altered hemodynamic factors and anticoagulant therapy.

Nursing Interventions

Improving the breathing

- Hypoxia, dyspnea, headache, restlessness, apprehension, pallor, cyanosis, and behavioral changes should be assessed.
- Vital signs, ECG, oximetry, and ABG levels for adequacy of oxygenation should be monitored.
- Patient's response to IV fluids/vasopressor should be monitored.
- Oxygen therapy that is used to relieve hypoxia should be monitored.
- Prepare patient for assisted ventilation who doest not respond to supplemental oxygen. Hypoxia is due to abnormalities of V/Q mismatch.

Improving tissue perfusion

- Shock-decreasing BP, tachycardia, cool, and clammy skin should be closely monitored.
- Prescribed medication given to preserve right-sided heart filling pressure and increase BP should be monitored.

- Patient should be maintained on bed rest during acute phase to reduce oxygen demand and risk of bleeding.
- Urinary output should be monitored hourly due to assess reduce renal perfusion.
- Anti-embolism compression stocking should provide a compression of 30–40 mm Hg.

Relieving pain

- Patient should be watched for sign of discomfort and pain.
- Whether pain worsens with deep breathing and coughing for friction rub should be ascertained.
- Morphine should be given, as prescribed, and monitored for pain relief.
- Signs of hypoxia should be monitored, thoroughly when anxiety, restlessness, and agitation of new onset are noted.

Relieving anxiety

- Dyspnea should be corrected and physical discomfort should be relieved.
- Diagnostic procedure and the role should be explained and any misconception should be corrected.
- The patient's concerns should be listened to; attentive listing relieves anxiety and reduces emotional distress.
- It is advised to speak calmly and slowly.

Complications

- Bleeding as a result of treatment
- Respiratory failure
- Pulmonary hypertension

Health Education

Health education should be:

- Advising patient for possible need to continue taking anticoagulant therapy for 6 weeks up to an indefinite period.
- Teaching about the sign of bleeding, especially of gum, nose, bruising, blood in urine and stool.
- Instructing patient to tell dentist about taking anticoagulant therapy.
- Warning against inactivity for prolonged periods or sitting with legs crossed to prevent reoccurrence.
- Warning against support activity that may cause trauma or injury to legs and predispose to thrombus.
- Encouraging to wear medic alert bracelet and identifying as an anticoagulant user.

Prevention

Preventing clots in the deep veins in legs (deep vein thrombosis) will help prevent pulmonary embolism. For this reason, most hospitals are aggressive about taking measures to prevent blood clots:

- **Anticoagulants:** Anticoagulants are given to people at risk of clots before and after an operation as well as to people admitted to the hospital with a heart attack, stroke, or complications of cancer.
- **Graduated compression stockings:** Compression stockings steadily squeeze your legs, helping veins and leg muscles move blood more efficiently. They offer a safe, simple, and inexpensive way to keep blood from stagnating after general surgery.
- **Pneumatic compression:** This treatment uses thigh-high or calf-high cuffs that automatically inflate with air and deflate every few minutes to massage and squeeze the veins in legs and improve blood flow.

- **Physical activity:** Moving as soon as possible after surgery can help prevent pulmonary embolism and hasten recovery overall. This is one of the main reasons nurse may push to get up, even on your day of surgery, and walk despite pain at the site of your surgical incision.

PNEUMOTHORAX, HEMOTHORAX, AND PYOTHORAX

Pneumothorax

Air in the pleural space due to trauma.. Pneumothorax is the presence of air in the pleural space that prohibits complete lung expansion.

"Pneumothorax is an abnormal collection of air or gas in the pleural space separating the lung from the chest wall which may interfere with normal breathing."

The lung expansion occurs when the pleural lining of the chest wall and the visceral lining of the lung maintain negative pressure in the pleural space. When the continuity of this system is lost, the lung collapses, resulting in a pneumothorax.

Classification of Pneumothorax

a. **Spontaneous pneumothorax:** Sudden onset of air in the pleural space with deflation of the affected lung in the absence of trauma.

b. **Open pneumothorax:** It implies an opening in the chest wall large enough to allow air to pass freely in and out of thoracic cavity with each attempted respiration.

c. **Tension pneumothorax:** Buildup of air under pressure in the pleural space resulting in interference with filling of both the heart and lungs.

Etiology

Primary spontaneous: The exact cause of primary spontaneous pneumothorax is unknown.

Risk Factors

- Male
- Smoking
- Family history

In children, additional causes include:

- Measles
- Echinococcosis
- Inhalation of a foreign body
- Congenital malformations
- Marfan's syndrome
- Homocystinuria
- Ehlers-Danlos syndrome
- AAT deficiency (which leads to emphysema)

Pathophysiology

- When there is a large hole in the chest wall, the patient will have a steal in the ventilation of other lung.
- A portion of the tidal volume will move back and forth through the hole in the chest wall, rather than the trachea as it normally does.

- Spontaneous pneumothorax is usually due to rupture of a subpleural bleb.
  - May occur secondary to chronic respiratory disease or idiopathically.
  - May occur in healthy people, particularly in thin, white males and those with family history of pneumothorax.

Signs and Symptoms

- Hyperresonance (tympany) to percussion on, diminished breath sounds on affected side.
- Tracheal deviation away from affected side of tension pneumothorax.
- Clinical picture of open or tension pneumothorax is one of air hunger, agitation, hypotension, and cyanosis.
- Mild-to-moderate dyspnea and chest discomfort may be present with spontaneous pneumothorax.
- Tachypnea
- Asymmetrical chest expansion

Diagnostic Evaluations

- **Chest X-ray:** Chest X-ray of left-sided pneumothorax. The left thoracic cavity is partly filled with air occupying the pleural space. The mediastinum is shifted to the opposite side.
- **CT:** CT can be useful in particular situations. In some lung diseases, especially emphysema, it is possible for abnormal lung areas, such as bullae (large air-filled sacs) to have the same appearance as a pneumothorax on chest X-ray, and it may not be safe to apply any treatment before the distinction is made and before the exact location and size of the pneumothorax is determined.
- **Ultrasound:** Ultrasound is commonly used in the evaluation of people who have sustained physical trauma. It may be more sensitive than chest X-rays in the identification of pneumothorax after blunt trauma to the chest.

Management

Non-pharmacological management

- **Conservative:** Oxygen given at a high flow rate may accelerate resorption as much as fourfold.
- **Aspiration:** By aspiration is equally effective as the insertion of a chest tube. This involves the administration of local anesthetic and inserting a needle connected to a three-way tap, up to 2.5 L of air (in adults) are removed. If there has been significant reduction in the size of the pneumothorax on subsequent X-ray, the remainder of the treatment can be conservative.
- **Chest tube:** A chest tube (or intercostal drain) is the most definitive initial treatment of a pneumothorax. These are typically inserted in an area under the axilla called the "safe triangle," where damage to internal organs can be avoided, this is delineated by a horizontal line at the level of the nipple and two muscles of the chest wall (latissimus dorsi and pectoralis major). Local anesthetic is applied. Two types of tubes may be used. In spontaneous pneumothorax, small-bore (smaller than 14 F, 4.7 mm diameter) tubes may be inserted by the Seldinger technique, and larger tubes do not have an advantage. In traumatic pneumothorax, larger tubes (28 F, 9.3 mm) are used.

Surgical Management

Pleurodesis and surgery

- Pleurodesis is a procedure that permanently obliterates the pleural space and attaches the lung to the chest wall.

- Thoracotomy (surgical opening of the chest), with identification of any source of air leakage and stapling of blebs.
- Pleurectomy (stripping of the pleural lining) of the outer pleural layer and pleural abrasion (scraping of the pleura) of the inner layer.

Hemothorax

"A **Hemothorax** is a condition that results from blood accumulating in the pleural cavity."

Etiology

Following are the etiologies:
- Penetrating trauma
- Blunt trauma
- Broken ribs
- Shearing forces
- Violent compression of the lungs.

Pathophysiology

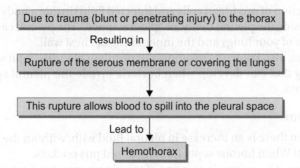

Signs and Symptoms

- Tachypnea
- Dyspnea
- Cyanosis
- Decreased or absent breath sounds on affected side
- Tracheal deviation to unaffected side
- Dull resonance on percussion
- Unequal chest rise
- Tachycardia
- Hypotension
- Pale, cool, clammy skin
- Possibly subcutaneous emphysema
- Narrowing pulse pressure

Diagnostic Evaluations

- Chest X-ray
- CT scan
- Pleural fluid analysis
- Thoracentesis

Management

Thoracostomy: A hemothorax is managed by removing the source of bleeding and by draining the blood already in the thoracic cavity. Blood in the cavity can be removed by inserting a drain (chest tube) in a procedure called a tube thoracostomy.

Thrombolytic agents have been used to break up clot in tubes or when the clot becomes organized in the pleural space; however, this is risky as it can lead to increased bleeding and the need for reoperation.

Complications

- Collapsed lung, leading to respiratory failure
- Death
- Fibrosis or scarring of the pleural membranes
- Infection of the pleural fluid (empyema)
- Pneumothorax
- Shock

Pyothorax or Empyema

Empyema is a collection of pus (dead cells and infected fluid) inside a body cavity. Usually, this term refers to pus inside the pleural cavity, or "pleural space." The pleural cavity is the thin space between the surface of your lungs and the inner lining of chest wall.

Pleural empyema, also known as pyothorax or purulent pleuritis, is an accumulation of pus in the pleural cavity that can develop when bacteria invade the pleural space, usually in the context of pneumonia.

Stages of Pyothorax

1. **Exudative:** When there is an increase in pleural fluid with/without the presence of pus.
2. **Fibrin purulent:** When fibrous septa form localized pus pockets.
3. **Organizing stage:** When there is scarring of the pleura membranes with possible inability of the lung to expand.

Etiology and Risk Factors

- It is the complication of the other medical conditions.
- Bacteria and fungi
- Lung infections
- After surgery of lung
- COPD
- Lung cancer
- Procedure, such as thoracentesis

Types

1. **Simple empyema:** Simple empyema is seen early in the course of the illness. In simple empyema, pus is present, but it is free flowing. Treatment at the simple stage is best, because the pleural cavity can easily be drained.
2. **Complex empyema:** In complex empyema, the inflammation is more severe. The longer the patient have empyema that is left untreated, the greater the chance that it will develop complex empyema.
    - In cases of severe inflammation, body forms lots of scar tissue in the pleural space. Formation of scar tissue causes the cavity to become divided into multiple, smaller cavities. This is called loculation, which creates complications, because infected areas

that have been walled off can be difficult to drain. Complete drainage of pus from the pleural cavity is essential for treatment.

Signs and Symptoms

Following are the signs and symptoms:
- Fever
- Cough
- Shortness of breath
- **Pleurisy:** Pleurisy is chest pain that occurs when you breathe and is caused by inflammation.
- The shortness of breath experienced by patients with empyema occurs when the lungs cannot fully expand.
- Fatigue
- Loss of appetite
- Weight loss
- The most severe signs of empyema are associated with sepsis (the presence of bacteria in the blood).
- Signs of sepsis include high fever, chills, rapid breathing, a fast heart rate, and low BP. Sepsis is life threatening and requires emergency treatment.

Diagnostic Evaluations

Diagnosis of empyema begins with a complete medical history and physical examination. Tests that are useful for diagnosing empyema include:

a. **Blood tests, such as:**
- Blood cultures (to identify what bacterium or organism is causing the infection)
- C-reactive protein (elevated levels are seen in inflammatory conditions)
- WBC count (elevated levels in inflammatory and infectious conditions).

b. **X-ray** (to diagnose pneumonia, lung abscess document fluid accumulation).

c. **Thoracentesis** (aspiration of pleural fluid for microscopic examination and testing).

d. **Thoracic ultrasound** (use of sound waves to tell if loculations are present).

e. **CAT scan** of the chest (use of computerized X-ray analysis to evaluate the lungs and pleural space).

Treatment Options for Empyema

- Empyema is treated with IV antibiotics, such as cephalosporins, metronidazole, and penicillins with beta-lactamase (ampicillin/sulbactam). Clindamycin can be used for patients who are allergic to penicillin.
- Fluids lost, due to lack of appetite and fever, are replaced, and medications, such as acetaminophen.
- **Pleural fluid drainage:** A chest tube is used to drain pus from the pleural space and allow the lungs to expand normally.

PLEURAL EFFUSION

Pleural effusion is a collection of fluid in the pleural space and is rarely a primary disease process but is usually occurred secondary to other disease. Normally small amount of fluid is present in the pleural space (5–15 mL), which acts as lubricant that allows the pleural surfaces to move without friction. Pleural effusion may be a complication of heart failure, TB, pneumonia, pulmonary infection, connective tissue disease, pulmonary embolus, and neoplastic tumors. A pleural effusion is an abnormal amount of fluid around the lungs. A pleural effusion is a buildup of fluid between the layers of tissue that line the lungs and chest cavity.

Etiology

- Congestive heart failure
- Pneumonia
- Liver disease (cirrhosis)
- End-stage renal disease

Signs and Symptoms

- Shortness of breath
- Chest pain, especially on breathing in deeply (pleurisy or pleuritic pain)
- Fever
- Cough

Diagnostic Evaluations

- Physical examination
- Chest X-ray film
- CT scan
- Kidney and liver function blood tests
- Pleural fluid analysis (examining the fluid under a microscope to look for bacteria, amount of protein, and presence of cancer cells)
- Thoracentesis (a sample of fluid is removed with a needle inserted between the ribs)
- Ultrasound of the chest and heart

Management

Medical and Surgical Management

Medical and surgical management includes:
- Thoracocentesis is done to remove the fluid, collect a specimen, and relieve dyspnea
- Drug therapy—analgesics, antibiotic, corticosteroid therapy.

For malignant effusion
- Chest tube drainage, radiation and chemotherapy, surgical pleurectomy, pleuroperitoneal shunt.
- Pleurodesis: Production of adhesions between the parietal and visceral pleura accomplished by tube thoracostomy.

Nursing Care Plan

Assessment

- The history of previous pulmonary conditions should be obtained.
- Patient should be assessed for dyspnea and tachypnea.
- Auscultation and percussion for lung abnormalities should be done.

Nursing Diagnosis

- Ineffective airway breathing pattern related to collection of fluid after space
- Pain related to pleuritic fluid in lungs
- Disturbed sleep pattern related to the pain and dyspnea
- Anxiety related to the disease process.

Nursing Interventions

Ineffective airway breathing pattern related to collection of fluid in the air space:
Intervention
- Instituting treatment to solve the underlying cause ordered
- Assisting with thoracocentesis if indicated
- Maintaining chest diseases
- Providing care after pleurodesis
- Monitoring for excessive pain from the sclerosing agent, which may cause hypoventilation
- Administering prescribed analgesic
- Administering oxygen to prevent hypoxemia and dyspnea
- Observing patient's breathing pattern

Pain related to pleuritic fluid in lungs:
Intervention
- Assessing the pain intensity
- Providing breathing exercises
- Providing analgesics to relieve the pain.

Disturbed sleep pattern related to the pain and dyspnea:
Intervention
- Assessing the sleeping hours of the patient
- Providing oxygen administration
- Providing analgesics to patient
- Providing cool and calm environment
- Providing side line position to patient to increase the lung capacity.

Complications

- Infection that turns into an abscess, called an empyema, which will need to be drained with a chest tube.
- Pneumothorax (air in the chest cavity) after thoracentesis
- Cancer
- Pulmonary embolism
- Lung damage

TUBERCULOSIS

"Tuberculosis is an infectious bacterial disease caused by *Mycobacterium tuberculosis*, which most commonly affects the lungs." It is transmitted from person to person via droplets from the throat and lungs of people with the active respiratory disease.

Etiology

- *Mycobacterium tuberculosis*
- Immunocompromised person
- Chemical industries

Risk Factor

- Aging
- Alcoholism
- Crowded living conditions
- Diseases that weaken the immune system

- Healthcare workers
- HIV infection
- Homelessness
- Low socioeconomic status
- Malnutrition, migration from a country with a high number of cases
- Nursing homes
- Unhealthy immune system

Types

1. **Pulmonary TB:** If a TB infection does become active, it most commonly involves the lungs (in about 90% of cases). Symptoms may include chest pain and a prolonged cough producing sputum.
2. **Extrapulmonary TB:** In 15–20% of active cases, the infection spreads outside the lungs, causing other kinds of TB. These are collectively denoted as "extrapulmonary TB," which occurs more commonly in immunosuppressed persons and young children.
3. **Active TB:** Active TB means the bacteria are active in the body. The immune system is unable to stop these bacteria from causing illness. People with active TB in their lungs can pass the bacteria on to anyone they come into close contact with. When a person with active TB coughs, sneezes, or spits, people nearby may breathe in the TB bacteria and become infected.
4. **Inactive TB:** Inactive TB infection is also called latent TB. If a person has latent TB, it means their body has been able to successfully fight the bacteria and stop them from causing illness. People who have latent TB do not feel sick, do not have symptoms and cannot spread TB.

Pathophysiology

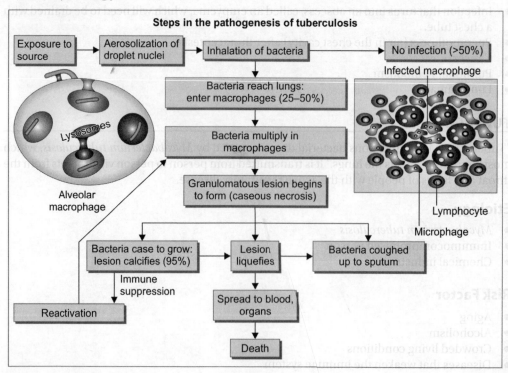

Signs and Symptoms

- A cough lasting for more than 2–3 weeks
- Chest pain
- Chills
- Discolored or bloody sputum
- Fatigue
- Loss of appetite
- Night sweats
- Pain with breathing
- Severe headache
- Shortness of breath
- Slight fever
- Tiredness or weakness
- Weight loss

Diagnostic Evaluations

- **Injection of protein:** By injecting a protein found in TB bacteria into the skin of an arm. If the skin reacts by swelling, then the person is probably infected with TB.
- **X-ray:** Diagnosis of TB in the lungs may be made using an X-ray.
- **Sputum test:** Sample of sputum is test in laboratory to diagnose the TB.
- **Bacteria:** A culture of TB bacteria can also be grown in a laboratory. However, this requires specialized and costly equipment and can take 6–8 weeks to produce a result.

Management

Medical Management

The five basic or "first-line" TB drugs are:
- Isoniazid
- Rifampicin
- Pyrazinamide
- Ethambutol
- Streptomycin

Surgical Management

If medications are NOT effective, there are three surgical treatments for pulmonary TB:
- Pneumothorax, in which air is introduced into the chest to collapse the lung
- Thoracoplasty, in which one or more ribs are removed
- Removal of a diseased lung

Nursing Care plan

The goal of management is:
- To control the inflammatory process
- To relieve symptoms
- To correct metabolic and nutritional problems and promote healing
- To achieve the previous health status

Nursing Assessment

- Promoting airway clearance
- Advocating adherence to treatment regimen

- Promoting activity and adequate nutrition
- Preventing spreading of TB infection

Nursing Diagnosis

- Ineffective airway clearance related to increased sputum
- Risk for of infection related to lower resistance of others who are around people
- Ineffective breathing pattern related to inflammation
- Hyperthermia related to the infection process
- Fluid volume deficit related to fatigue due to lack of fluid intake
- Activity intolerance related to fatigue
- Imbalanced nutrition, less than body requirements related to decreased appetite
- Ineffective management and therapeutic regimen related to lack of knowledge about the disease process
- Impaired gas exchange related to alveoli function decline.

Interventions

- **Ineffective airway clearance:**
  - Auscultating lungs for wheezing, decreased breath sounds, and coarse sounds
  - Using universal precautions if secretions are purulent even before culture reports
  - Assessing cough for effectiveness and productivity
  - Noting the amount, color, odor, and consistency of sputum
  - Sending sputum specimens for culture as prescribed
  - Instituting appropriate isolation precautions if cultures are positive
  - Using humidity to help loosen sputum
  - Administering medications and noting effectiveness and side effects
  - Teaching effective deep breathing and coughing techniques.
- **Risk for infection:**
  - Monitoring sputum for changes indicating infection
  - Monitoring vital signs
  - Teaching patient and family the purpose and techniques for infection control, such as handwashing, patient covering mouth when coughs, maintaining isolation if necessary
  - Teaching patient the purpose, importance, and how to take medications as prescribed consistently over the long-term therapy.
- **Deficient knowledge:**
  - Determining who will be the learner, patient, or family
  - Assessing ability to learn
  - Identifying any existing misconceptions about the material to learn
  - Assisting the learner to integrate the information into daily life
  - Giving clear thorough explanations and demonstrations.
- **Activity intolerance:**
  - Assessing patient's level of mobility
  - Observing and documenting response to activity
  - Assessing emotional response to change in physical status
  - Anticipating patient's needs to accommodate
  - Teaching energy conservation techniques
  - Referring to community resources as needed.
- **Ineffective therapeutic regimen management:**
  - Assessing prior efforts to follow regimen
  - Assessing patient's perceptions of their health problem

■ Assessing other factors that may affect success in a negative way
■ Informing patient of the benefits of conforming with the regimen
■ Concentrating on the behaviors that will make the most difference to the therapeutic effect
■ Family and support system in teachings and explanations

Health Education

Health education should be:
● Explaining about the disease condition causes and risk factors.
● Using universal precautions if secretions are purulent even before culture reports
● Assessing cough for effectiveness and productivity
● Noting the amount, color, odor, and consistency of sputum
● Sending sputum specimens for culture as prescribed or prn
● Instituting appropriate isolation precautions if cultures are positive
● Using humidity to help loosen sputum
● Administering medications and noting effectiveness and side effects
● Assessing patient's perceptions of their health problem
● Assessing other factors that may affect success in a negative way
● Informing patient of the benefits of conforming with the regimen
● Concentrating on the behaviors that will make the most difference to the therapeutic effect.

Complications

Complications are as follows:
● Miliary TB
● Pleural effusion
● Emphysema
● TB pneumonia

CHEST INJURIES

Chest injuries (or **thoracic trauma**) are a serious injury of the chest. Thoracic trauma is a common cause of significant disability and mortality, the leading cause of death from physical trauma after head and spinal cord injury. Blunt thoracic injuries are the primary or a contributing cause of about a quarter of all trauma-related deaths.

Classification

Chest trauma can be classified as:
  a. Blunt injuries
  b. Crush injuries
  c. Penetrating injuries.

  a. **Blunt trauma:** Mode of injury important where there has been massive deformity of a car or a history of a fall of 5 m or more major intrathoracic injuries should always be suspected. The physical nature of chest wall allows for considerable elastic recoil, especially in young patients, and therefore, the degree of injury within chest may need to be judged initially by deformity to car rather than appearance of patient.
  b. **Penetrating injuries**
    ■ These result in parenchymal damage related to track of missile or stabbing implement and velocity.
    ■ More solid structures (e.g., heart and major vessels) suffer greater injury where high-velocity missiles are penetrating weapon.

- Most lethal complication is hemorrhage
- It is often associated with abdominal trauma.
c. **Crush injury**
    - It occurs where elastic limits of chest and its contents have been exceeded.
    - Patients usually have AP deformity.
    - Majority have flail chests with multiple fractures, pneumothorax, or hemothorax.
    - Most have pulmonary contusion
    - Injuries of heart, aorta, diaphragm, liver, kidney, and spleen are common.

Specific types of chest trauma include:
a. **Injuries to the chest wall:**
    - Rib fractures
    - Flail chest
    - Sternal fractures
b. **Pulmonary injury (injury to the lung) and injuries involving the pleural space**
    - Pulmonary contusion
    - Pulmonary laceration
    - Pneumothorax
    - Hemothorax
    - Hemopneumothorax
c. **Injury to the airways**
    - Tracheobronchial tear
d. **Cardiac injury**
    - Pericardial tamponade

Signs and Symptoms

Following are the signs and symptoms:
- Air hunger, use of accessory muscles, tracheal deviation, cyanosis, or distended neck veins (evidence of tension pneumothorax or tamponade)
- Tracheal deviation (evidence of tension pneumothorax)
- Major defects in the chest (sucking chest wounds)
- Unilaterally diminished breath sounds or hyperresonance to percussion (evidence of closed pneumothorax or tension pneumothorax).
- Decreased heart sounds (pericardial tamponade)
- Location of foreign bodies
- Location of entry and exit wounds

Diagnostic Evaluations

Following are the diagnostic evaluations:
a. **Chest X-ray:**
    - CXR is most useful screening investigation
    - Subcutaneous air, foreign bodies, bony fractures, widening of mediastinum, and atelectasis should be looked for.
    - Inspiratory and expiratory films for checking for pneumothorax.
b. **CT scan**
    - It is valuable tool.
    - It aids in diagnosis and precise location of numerous lesions.
    - Contrast is useful particularly when looking for mediastinal hemorrhage and periaortic hematomas.

c. **Echocardiography:** Cardiac wall motion abnormalities and valve function and presence of pericardial fluid or blood.

d. **ECG:** Most common abnormality in thoracic trauma are S-T and T wave changes and findings indicative of bundle branch block.

e. **Angiography:** Remains the gold standard for defining thoracic vascular injuries.

f. **Bronchoscopy:** Indications include evaluation of airway injury, hemoptysis, segmental or lobar collapse, and removal of aspirated foreign bodies.

Management

Immediate Management

- Patent airway, oxygenation, and ventilation should be assured
- Following should be excluded or treated:
  - Pneumothorax
  - Hemothorax
  - Cardiac tamponade
- Extrathoracic injuries should be assessed for
- Stomach should be decompressed.
- Pain relief should be provided.
- Endotracheal intubation and ventilation should be reconsidered. In particular, gross obesity, significant preexisting lung disease, severe pulmonary contusion or aspiration, and need for surgery for thoracic or extrathoracic injuries should be taken into account.

General Management

a. **Monitoring**

Following are danger signs requiring full reassessment:
  - Respiratory rate >20/min
  - Heart rate >100/min
  - Systolic BP <100 mm Hg
  - Reduced breath sounds on affected side
  - PaO_2 <9 kPa on room air
  - $PaCO_2$ >8 kPa
  - Increased size of pneumothorax, hemothorax or increased width of mediastinum on CXR.

Deterioration in any of these signs must be followed by a search for evidence of blood loss, tension pneumothorax, head injury, sepsis, or fat embolism. Chest drains should be checked for patency.

- **Chest drains:** Indications for insertion of chest drains in stable patients:
  - Pneumothorax >10% in nonventilated patient (i.e., >1 intercostal space)
  - Hemothorax >500 mL (i.e., above neck of seventh rib)
  - Surgical emphysema
- **Antibiotics:**
  - Use of prophylactic antibiotics controversial. Some recommend them for patients treated conservatively in whom a chest drain is inserted.
  - Cefuroxime and metronidazole for patients with perforated viscous (in addition to exploration and drainage).
- **Mechanical ventilation:**
  - Most centers use packed cell volume (PCV) or PSV to reduce incidence of barotraumas.
  - PCV and PSV also provide some compensation for air leaks.

- **Analgesia:**
  - IV opioids in frequent small doses or by continuous infusion
  - Entonox inhalation during physiotherapy
  - Intercostal nerve block
  - Multiple individual nerve blocks
  - Single large volume (e.g., 20 mL .5% bupivacaine) into 1 intercostal space. It spreads to block nerves above and below.
  - Intrapleural bupivacaine via intercostal catheters using intermittent injections or continuous infusions.
  - NSAIDs: Fully resuscitated patients with normal renal function.

Postoperative intensive care
- Following tracheobronchial, lung, or diaphragmatic repair high inflation pressures should be avoided.
- Tracheal suction must be minimal where there is a tracheobronchial suture line.
- Fluid overload should be avoided.
- Gastric distension should be prevented.

RIB FRACTURE

Rib fracture includes the following:
- Fractures of the first and second ribs may be more likely to be associated with head and facial injuries than other rib fractures. The middle ribs are the ones most commonly fractured.
- Fractures usually occur from direct blows or from indirect crushing injuries. The weakest part of a rib is just anterior to its angle, but a fracture can occur anywhere. The most commonly fractured ribs are the 7th and 10th.
- A lower rib fracture has the complication of potentially injuring the diaphragm, which could result in a diaphragmatic hernia. Rib fractures are usually quite painful because the ribs have to move to allow for breathing. Even a small crack can inflame a tendon and cripple an arm.
- When several ribs are broken in several places, a flail chest results, and the detached bone sections will move separately from the rest of the chest.
- A rib fracture is a breaking or fracture in one or more of the bones making up the rib cage. The first rib is rarely fractured because of its protected position behind the clavicle. If it is broken, serious damage can occur to the brachial plexus of nerves and the subclavian vessels.

Etiology

Etiologies are as follows:
- Rib fractures can occur without direct trauma and have been reported after sustained coughing.
- Various sports, for example, rowing and golf, often in elite athletes. They can also occur as a consequence of diseases, such as cancer or infections.
- Fragility fractures of ribs can occur due to diseased bone structure, for example, osteoporosis and metastatic deposits.

Signs and Symptoms

Following are the signs and symptoms:
- Pain when breathing or with movement
- A portion of the chest wall moving separately from the rest of the chest (flail chest).
- A grating sound with breathing or movement.
- The mechanism of injury would indicate substantial force to the ribs.

Treatment

Following are the types of treatments:

- There is no specific treatment for rib fractures, but various supportive measures can be taken. In simple rib fractures, pain can lead to reduced movement and cough suppression; this can contribute to the formation of secondary chest infection.
- Adequate analgesia can avoid pain.
- It is a potentially life-threatening injury and will often require a period of assisted ventilation.
- Acute innovations RibLoc is a titanium U-shaped plate that is sized to match rib thickness and uses screws that fixate to anterior and posterior of plate and provide fixation without needing bone purchase for screws and without risking damage to the neurovascular bundle. These plates can be contoured to match the rib segment being plated and come in various lengths.
- Judet and/or sanchez plates/struts are a metal plate with strips that bend around the rib and then are further secured with sutures.
- Synthes MatrixRIB fixation system has two options: A precontoured metal plate that uses screws to secure the plate to the rib and an intramedullary splint, which is tunneled into the rib and secured with a set screw.
- Anterior locking plates are metal plates that have holes for screws throughout the plate. The plate is positioned over the rib and screwed into the bone at the desired position. The plates may be bent to match the contour of the rib section.

FLAIL CHEST

A flail chest is a life-threatening medical condition that occurs when a segment of the rib cage breaks under extreme stress and becomes detached from the rest of the chest wall. It occurs when multiple adjacent ribs are broken in multiple places, separating a segment, so a part of the chest wall moves independently.

Characteristic

Following are the characteristics:

- During normal inspiration, the diaphragm contracts and intercostal muscles push the rib cage out. Pressure in the thorax decreases below atmospheric pressure, and air rushes in through the trachea. However, a flail segment will not resist the decreased pressure and will appear to push in while the rest of the rib cage expands.
- During normal expiration, the diaphragm and intercostal muscles relax, allowing the abdominal organs to push air upward and out of the thorax. However, a flail segment will also be pushed out while the rest of the rib cage contracts.

Etiology

Etiologies are as follows:

- This typically occurs when three or more adjacent ribs are fractured in two or more places, allowing that segment of the thoracic wall to displace and move independently of the rest of the chest wall.
- Flail chest can also occur when ribs are fractured proximally in conjunction with disarticulation of costal cartilages distally.
- For the condition to occur, generally there must be a significant force applied over a large surface of the thorax to create the multiple anterior and posterior rib fractures.
- Rollover and crushing injuries most commonly break ribs at only one point—for flail chest to occur a significant impact is required, breaking the ribs in two or more place.

Signs and Symptoms

- Pain
- Puncher of pleural sac
- Pneumothorax

Management

Treatment of the flail chest initially follows the principles of advanced trauma life support. Further treatment includes:

- Good analgesia, including intercostal blocks, avoiding narcotic analgesics as much as possible. This allows much better ventilation, with improved tidal volume, and increased blood oxygenation.
- Positive pressure ventilation, meticulously adjusting the ventilator settings to avoid pulmonary barotrauma.
- Chest tubes as required.
- Adjustment of position to make the patient most comfortable and provide relief of pain.
- Aggressive pulmonary toilet

Surgical fixation: It can help in significantly reducing the duration of ventilatory support and in conserving the pulmonary function.

A patient may be intubated with a double-lumen tracheal tube. In a double-lumen endotracheal tube, each lumen may be connected to a different ventilator. Usually one side of the chest is affected more than the other, so each lung may require drastically different pressures and flows to adequately ventilate.

STERNAL FRACTURE

A sternal fracture is a fracture of the sternum located in the center of the chest. The injury that experience significant blunt chest trauma may occur in vehicle accidents, when the still moving chest strikes a steering wheel or dashboard or is injured by a seat belt. Sternal fractures may also occur as a fracture, in people who have weakened bone in their sternum, due to another disease process.

Etiology

Etiologies are as follows:

- Vehicle collisions are the usual cause of sternal fracture. The injury is estimated to occur in about 3% of auto accidents.
- The chest of a driver who is not wearing a seat belt may strike the steering wheel, and the shoulder component of a seat belt may injure the chest if it is worn without the lap component.

Signs and Symptoms

Following are the signs and symptoms:

- Crepitus (a crunching sound made when broken bone ends rub together)
- Pain
- Tenderness
- Bruising
- Swelling over the fracture site
- Palpation

Diagnostic Evaluations

Following are the diagnostic evaluations:

- X-rays of the chest are taken in people with chest trauma and symptoms of sternal fractures.
- CT scanning
- ECG and radionucleotide abnormalities (abnormal test results indicating cardiac dysfunction.

Treatment

Following are the two types of treatment:

1. Tracheal intubation
2. Mechanical ventilation

PULMONARY CONTUSION

Contusion is a bruise of the lung, caused by chest trauma. As a result of damage to capillaries, blood and other fluids accumulate in the lung tissue. The excess fluid interferes with gas exchange, potentially leading to inadequate oxygen levels hypoxia.

Pulmonary contusion: It is not only usually caused directly by blunt trauma but can also result from explosion injuries or a shock wave associated with penetrating trauma.

Etiology

Etiologies are as follows:

- Motor vehicle accidents are the most common cause of pulmonary contusion.
- Chest strikes the inside of the car
- Falls
- Assaults
- Sports injuries
- Explosions

Pathophysiology

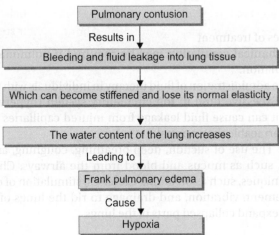

Pulmonary contusion

Results in ↓

Bleeding and fluid leakage into lung tissue

↓

Which can become stiffened and lose its normal elasticity

↓

The water content of the lung increases

Leading to ↓

Frank pulmonary edema

Cause ↓

Hypoxia

Signs and Symptoms

Following are the signs and symptoms:

- Dyspnea (painful breathing or difficulty breathing)
- Rapid breathing
- Rapid heart rate

- Rales (an abnormal crackling sound in the chest accompanying breathing)
- Bronchorrhea (the production of watery sputum)
- Wheezing and coughing are other signs
- Coughing up blood or bloody sputum
- Cardiac output (the volume of blood pumped by the heart
- Hypotension (low BP)
- Tender or painful

Diagnostic Evaluations

Following are the diagnostic evaluations:

- **X-ray:** A chest X-ray showing right-sided pulmonary contusion associated with rib fractures and subcutaneous emphysema
- **CT:** A chest CT scan reveals pulmonary contusions, pneumothorax, and pseudocysts. CT (CT scanning) is a more sensitive test for pulmonary contusion, and it can identify abdominal, chest, or other injuries that accompany the contusion. CT scans also help differentiate between contusion and pulmonary hematoma.
- **Ultrasound:** An ultrasound image showing early pulmonary contusion, at this moment, is not visible on radiography.

Prevention

Following are the preventative measures:

- Airbags in combination with seat belts can protect vehicle occupants by preventing the chest from striking the interior of the vehicle during a collision.
- Child restraints, such as car seats protect children in vehicle collisions from pulmonary contusion.
- Equipment exists for use in some sports to prevent chest and lung injury, for example, in softball the catcher is equipped with a chest.
- Protective garments can also prevent pulmonary contusion in explosions.

Treatment

Following are the types of treatment

- **Ventilation:** Mechanical ventilation may be required if pulmonary contusion causes inadequate oxygenation.
- **Fluid therapy:** The administration of fluid therapy in individuals with pulmonary contusion is controversial. Excessive fluid in the circulatory system (hypervolemia) can worsen hypoxia because it can cause fluid leakage from injured capillaries (pulmonary edema), which are more permeable than normal.
- **Supportive care:** The use of suction, deep breathing, coughing, and other methods to remove material, such as mucus and blood from the airways. Chest physical therapy makes use of techniques, such as breathing exercises, stimulation of coughing, suctioning, percussion, movement, vibration, and drainage to rid the lungs of secretions, increase oxygenation, and expand collapsed parts of the lungs.

Complications

Complications are as follows:

- Pneumonia
- Acute ARDS
- Pulmonary edema
- Acute ARDS

PULMONARY LACERATION

Pulmonary laceration: In which lung tissue is torn or cut, differs from pulmonary contusion in that the former involves disruption of the macroscopic architecture of the lung.

Pulmonary hematoma: When lacerations fill with blood, the result is pulmonary hematoma, a collection of blood within the lung tissue.

Etiology: Pulmonary laceration is a common result of:
- Penetrating trauma
- Blunt trauma
- Broken ribs
- Shearing forces
- Violent compression of the lungs

Classification

Classification of lacerations is as follows:
- **Type 1 lacerations:** These occur in the mid lung area, the air-filled lung bursts as a result of sudden compression of the chest. Also called compression-rupture lacerations, type 1 are the most common type and usually occur in a central location of the lung. They tend to be large, ranging in size from 2 to 8 cm.
- **Type 2 lacerations:** These result when the lower chest is suddenly compressed and the lower lung is suddenly moved across the vertebral bodies. These are also called compression –shear, tend to occur near the spine, and have an elongated shape. Type 2 lacerations usually occur in younger people with more flexible chests.
- **Type 3 laceration:** These are caused by punctures from fractured ribs and occur in the area near the chest wall underlying the broken rib. Also called rib penetration lacerations, type 3 lacerations tend to be small and accompanied by pneumothorax.
- **Type 4 lacerations:** These are also called adhesion tears, which occur in cases where a pleuropulmonary adhesion had formed prior to the injury, in which the chest wall is suddenly fractured or pushed inward.

Pathophysiology

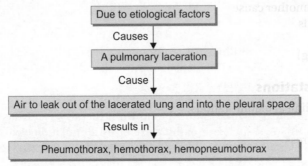

Due to etiological factors

Causes ↓

A pulmonary laceration

Cause ↓

Air to leak out of the lacerated lung and into the pleural space

Results in ↓

Pneumothorax, hemothorax, hemopneumothorax

Diagnostic Evaluations
- **X-ray:** A chest X-ray of a right-sided pulmonary contusion associated with flail chest and subcutaneous emphysema. Contusion may mask pulmonary laceration on chest X-ray.
- **CT scanning:** On a CT scan, pulmonary lacerations show up in a contused area of the lung typically appearing as cavities filled with air or fluid that usually have a round or ovoid shape due to the lung's elasticity.
- **Thoracoscopy** may be used in both diagnosis and treatment of pulmonary laceration.

Management

Following are the managements:

- As with other chest injuries, such as pulmonary contusion, hemothorax, and pneumothorax, pulmonary laceration can often be treated with just supplemental oxygen, ventilation, and drainage of fluids from the chest cavity.
- A thoracostomy tube can be used to remove blood and air from the chest cavity. About 5% of the cases require surgery, called thoracotomy.

Surgical Treatment

Surgical treatments are as follows:

- **Lobectomy:** In which a lobe of the lung is removed
- **Pneumonectomy:** In which an entire lung is removed.

Complications

Complications are as follows:

- Pulmonary abscess.
- Bronchopleural fistula (a fistula between the pleural space and the bronchial tree).
- **Air embolism:** In which air enters the bloodstream, is potentially fatal, especially when it occurs on the left side of the heart.

TRACHEOBRONCHIAL INJURY

Tracheobronchial injury (TBI) is damage to the tracheobronchial tree (the airway structure involving the trachea and bronchi). It can result from blunt or penetrating trauma to the neck or chest, inhalation of harmful fumes or smoke, or aspiration of liquids or objects.

Etiology

Etiologies are as follows:

- Falls from height
- Motor vehicle accidents
- Explosions are another cause
- Gunshot wounds
- Knife wounds
- Edema (swelling)

Clinical Manifestations

Following are the clinical manifestations:

- Dyspnea
- Respiratory distress
- Coughing
- Hemoptysis
- Stridor (an abnormal, high-pitched breath sound indicating obstruction of the upper airway can also occur)
- Necrosis (death of the tissue)
- Scar formation
- Stenosis
- Due to inhalation of foreign body aspiration
- Medical procedures are uncommon

Diagnostic Evaluation

Following are the diagnostic evaluations:
- **Chest X-ray** is the initial imaging technique used to diagnose TBI. X-rays may also show accompanying injuries and signs, such as fractures and subcutaneous emphysema.
- **CT scanning** detects results of blunt trauma. It is a replacement of bronchoscopy.

Prevention: Vehicle occupants who wear seat belts have a lower incidence of TBI after a motor vehicle accident.

Treatment

Following are the types of treatment:
- **Endotracheal tube:** It may be used to bypass a disruption in the airway.
- **Tracheotomy:** An incision can be made in the trachea (tracheotomy).
- **Mechanical ventilation:** Such as PEEP and ventilation at higher than normal pressures may be helpful in maintaining adequate oxygenation.

Complications

Complications are as follows:
- Bronchial stenosis
- Pneumonia
- Bronchiectasis.

MULTIPLE CHOICE QUESTIONS

1. **Most patients with COPD have a history of:**
   A. Cigarette smoking
   B. Excessive alcohol consumption
   C. Seasonal allergies
   D. Injection drug use

2. **Untreated obstructive sleep apnea may result in all of the following, *except*:**
   A. Excessive daytime sleepiness
   B. Sexual dysfunction
   C. COPD
   D. Increased risk for cardiovascular disease

3. **Low birth weight is linked to increased risk of developing:**
   A. Seasonal allergies
   B. Sinusitis
   C. Childhood asthma
   D. Bronchitis

4. **A history of smoking, abnormal permanent enlargement of the alveoli, cough, and dyspnea suggest:**
   A. Asthma
   B. Emphysema
   C. Chronic bronchitis
   D. Obstructive sleep apnea

5. **All of the following increase the risk of developing lung cancer, *except*:**
   A. Smoking
   B. Exposure to radon or asbestos
   C. Exposure to coal products or radioactive substances, such as uranium
   D. History of seasonal allergies

6. **Which of the following statement about lymphangioleiomyomatosis not true?**
   A. It is a rare lung disease that affects many more women than men
   B. It involves the growth of smooth muscle cells in the lungs, pulmonary blood vessels, lymphatics, and pleurae
   C. It is of unknown etiology
   D. It is considered a neoplastic disease

7. **Treatment for influenza generally includes all of the following, *except*:**
   A. Ampicillin and tetracycline
   B. Rest and ample fluids
   C. Oseltamivir and zanamivir
   D. Over-the-counter medications to relive fever, myalgias, and headache

8. **Pneumonia may be caused by any of the following, *except*:**
   A. Bee sting   B. Bacteria
   C. Viruses   D. Mycoplasmas

9. **The most common causes of pneumonia in children under age 5 are:**
   A. Fungi   B. Viruses
   C. Bacteria   D. Mycoplasmas

10. **Concern about the possibility of pandemic TB has been fueled by a rise in all of the following, *except*:**
    A. H1N1
    B. The number of reported cases in the United States
    C. MDR TB and XDR TB
    D. AIDS

11. **Occupational exposure to asbestos is associated with increased risk of developing:**
    A. AIDS   B. Mesothelioma
    C. Cystic fibrosis   D. Aspiration pneumonia

12. **Actions to prevent acute bronchitis may include all of the following, *except*:**
    A. Frequent handwashing
    B. Annual flu shot
    C. Wearing a protective mask while using paint or solvents
    D. Taking high doses of vitamin C

13. **All of the following are true about histoplasmosis, *except*:**
    A. Symptoms appear suddenly and are moderate to severe
    B. It is caused by inhaling the spores of a fungus that arise from soil
    C. Many cases are asymptomatic
    D. Symptoms arise within 24 hours of exposure

14. **Workers who handle unprocessed cotton are at risk of developing:**
    A. Coccidioidomycosis   B. Byssinosis
    C. Pertussis   D. Sarcoidosis

15. **All of the following statements about pulmonary sarcoidosis are true, *except*:**
    A. It causes dyspnea, dry cough, and chest pain
    B. African-Americans and Scandinavians are disproportionately affected
    C. It is treated with antiviral agents
    D. Many cases resolve without intervention

16. **Cystic fibrosis patients suffer pulmonary infections of all of the following pathogens, *except*:**
    A. *Pseudomonas aeruginosa*   B. *Haemophilus influenzae*
    C. *Staphylococcus aureus*   D. *Candida albicans*

17. **All of the following are true about acute respiratory distress syndrome (ARDS), *except*:**
    A. It generally arises in persons with serious comorbidities
    B. It may be life threatening
    C. It is a common complication of anesthesia
    D. Some patients with ARDS suffer permanent lung damage

18. Hantavirus pulmonary syndrome arises from contact with any of the following, *except*:

A. Infected rodents

B. Infected rodent urine or droppings

C. Infected rodent saliva

D. Infected people

19. Symptoms of pertussis include all of the following, *except*:

A. Runny nose and mild fever

B. Severe coughing

C. Choking in infants

D. Rash

20. Silicosis is a disorder characterized by all of the following, *except*:

A. Dyspnea

B. Severe cough, tachypnea, and weakness

C. Fever, night sweats, and chest pain

D. Paralysis of the lower extremities

Answers

1. A	2. C	3. C	4. B	5. D	6. D	7. A	8. A	9. B	10. A
11. B	12. D	13. A	14. B	15. C	16. D	17. C	18. D	19. D	20. D

Gastrointestinal Disorder

AT THE END OF THIS CHAPTER, THE STUDENTS WILL BE ABLE TO LEARN ABOUT NURSING MANAGEMENT OF PATIENT WITH:
➢ Gastroesophageal reflux disease
➢ Hiatal hernia
➢ Peptic ulcer
➢ Appendicitis
➢ Hemorrhoids
➢ Ulcerative colitis
➢ Crohn's disease
➢ Gastrointestinal (GI) bleeding
➢ Portal hypertension
➢ Liver cirrhosis
➢ Cholelithiasis
➢ Cholecystitis
➢ Irritable bowel syndrome
➢ Esophageal varices
➢ Pancreatitis
➢ Abdominal hernia
➢ Hepatitis

REVIEW OF ANATOMY AND PHYSIOLOGY

Introduction to the Gastrointestinal System

The **gastrointestinal tract** (GIT) consists of a hollow muscular tube starting from the oral cavity, where food enters the mouth, continuing through the pharynx, esophagus, stomach, and intestines to the rectum and anus, where food is expelled. There are various **accessory organs** that assist the tract by secreting enzymes to help break down food into its component nutrients. Thus, the salivary glands, liver, pancreas, and gallbladder have important functions in the **digestive system**. Food is propelled along the length of the GIT by peristaltic movements of the oral cavity.

The oral cavity or mouth is responsible for the intake of food. It is lined by a stratified squamous oral mucosa with keratin covering those areas subject to significant abrasion, such as the tongue, hard palate, and roof of the mouth. Mastication refers to the mechanical breakdown of food by chewing and chopping actions of the teeth. The tongue, a strong muscular organ, manipulates the food bolus to come in contact with the teeth. It is also the sensing organ of the mouth for touch, temperature, and taste using its specialized sensors known as papillae.

In salivation refers to the mixing of the oral cavity contents with salivary gland secretions. The mucin (a glycoprotein) in saliva acts as a lubricant. The oral cavity also plays a limited role in the digestion of carbohydrates. The enzyme serum amylase, a component of saliva, starts the process of digestion of complex carbohydrates. The final function of the oral cavity is the absorption of small molecules, such as glucose and water, across the mucosa. From the mouth, food passes through the pharynx and esophagus via the action of swallowing.

Gastrointestinal Assessment

Components may include in GI assessment are as follows:
- Chief complaints, such as change in appetite, weight gain or loss, dysphagia, intolerance to certain foods, nausea and vomiting, change in bowel habits, and abdominal pain
- Present health status
- Past health history
- Current lifestyle
- Psychosocial status
- Family history
- Physical assessment
  - **Appetite:**
    - Any changes in appetite should be queried.
    - A loss of taste sensation
  - **Weight loss or gain:**
    - Any change in weight should be documented.
    - If weight loss or gain is rapid, further investigation should be done.
    - Weight loss may also be associated with illness, while weight gain may be attributed to fluid retention or a mass.
  - **Dysphagia or odynophagia:** People with dysphagia have difficulty swallowing and may also experience pain while swallowing—any difficulty swallowing that may indicate cerebral palsy or Parkinson's disease should be queried.
  - **Intolerance to food:**
    - Any intolerance to food should be asked for.
    - Symptoms of intolerance to a particular food might include stomach discomfort, gas, bloating, burping, flatulence, abdominal pain, and diarrhea.
  - **Nausea and vomiting:** The frequency of these symptoms should be determined. Nausea and vomiting may also indicate food poisoning.
  - **Changes in bowel habits:**
    - The frequency, color, and consistency of bowel should be assessed.
    - Black, tarry stools may indicate an upper GI bleed.
    - Bright red blood in the stools may indicate hemorrhoids.

Physical Examination

During physical assessment of GI system, at least one of the following four basic techniques inspection, auscultation, percussion, and palpation should be used. Inspection is first, as it is noninvasive. Auscultation is performed after inspection; the abdomen should be auscultated before percussion or palpation to prevent production of false bowel sounds.
- **Inspection:** During inspection the following should be carefully watched: bulges, masses, hernias, ascites, enlarged veins, pulsations or movements, and inability to lie flat.
- **Auscultation**
  - Auscultation from right lower quadrant should be started. If bowel sounds are not heard, a total of 5 minutes should be listened to.
  - Bowel sounds echo during the movement of food in the intestines. It is normal to hear high-pitched clicking and gurgling sounds approximately every 5–15 seconds.

- **Percussion**
  - Percussion is used to evaluate tenderness that gives an idea about GI problems. During percussion, the area for tenderness should be assessed and the client should be monitored for signs of discomfort.
  - During percussion, general tympany, liver span, and splenic dullness should be examined for.
  - Dullness is usually heard over solid organs or masses, such as the liver, spleen, or full bladder.
- **Palpation**
  - During light palpation, the skin should be pressed about 1/2–3/4 inch with the pads of fingers. During deep palpation, finger pads should be used to compress the skin about 1.5–2 inches.
  - Palpation lightly at first then deeply will give clue about any muscle guarding, rigidity, and masses.
  - Palpation allows you to assess for texture, tenderness, temperature, moisture, pulsations, masses, and internal organs.

GASTROINTESTINAL DISORDERS

GASTROESOPHAGEAL REFLUX DISEASE

Gastroesophageal reflux occurs when stomach contents flow back up into the esophagus due to weak or relaxes esophageal sphincter and characterized by heartburn, burning feeling in the mid-chest.

Etiology

- Obesity
- Pregnancy
- Certain medications, such as nonsteroidal antiinflammatory drugs (NSAIDs)
- Smoking
- Use of spicy foods
- Sudden fall of sleep after meal
- Congenital weakness of esophageal sphincter

Signs and Symptoms

- Dry, chronic cough
- Wheezing
- Asthma
- Nausea
- Vomiting
- Sore throat
- Hoarseness
- Dysphagia
- Pain in the chest
- Dental erosion
- Foul breath

Pathophysiology

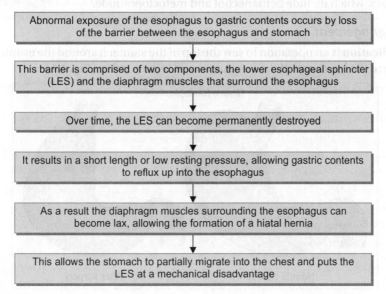

Abnormal exposure of the esophagus to gastric contents occurs by loss of the barrier between the esophagus and stomach

↓

This barrier is comprised of two components, the lower esophageal sphincter (LES) and the diaphragm muscles that surround the esophagus

↓

Over time, the LES can become permanently destroyed

↓

It results in a short length or low resting pressure, allowing gastric contents to reflux up into the esophagus

↓

As a result the diaphragm muscles surrounding the esophagus can become lax, allowing the formation of a hiatal hernia

↓

This allows the stomach to partially migrate into the chest and puts the LES at a mechanical disadvantage

Diagnostic Evaluation

- **Barium meal:** An X-ray, during the procedure, the person will stand or sit in front of an X-ray machine and drink barium. Barium coats the esophagus, stomach, and small intestine so the radiologist can see these organs' shapes more clearly on X-rays.
- **Endoscopy:** This procedure involves using an endoscope, a small, flexible tube with a light, to see the upper GIT.
- **Esophageal pH monitoring:** The most accurate test to detect acid reflux, esophageal pH monitoring measures the amount of liquid or acid in the esophagus. A gastroenterologist will pass a thin tube, called a nasogastric (NG) probe, through the person's nose or mouth to the stomach. The gastroenterologist will then pull the tube back into the esophagus, where it will be taped to the person's cheek and remain in place for 24 hours. The end of the tube in the esophagus has a small probe to measure when and how much liquid or acid comes up into the esophagus.
- **Esophageal manometry:** Esophageal manometry measures muscle contractions in the esophagus.

Management

Lifestyle Changes

- Loss of weight
- Wearing loose-fitting
- Remaining upright for 3 hours after meals
- Raising the head of the bed
- Avoiding smoking

Medical Management

- Antacids, magnesium hydroxide and aluminum hydroxides
- H₂ blockers, such as cimetidine

- Proton pump inhibitors include omeprazole
- Prokinetics, which include bethanechol and metoclopramide.

Surgical Management

1. **Fundoplication** is an operation to sew the top of the stomach around the esophagus to add pressure to the lower end of the esophagus and reduce reflux **(Fig. 4.1)**.

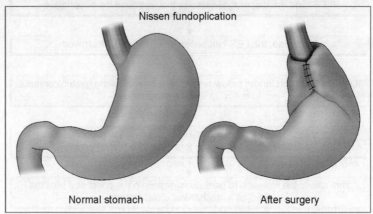

Fig. 4.1: Fundoplication.

2. **Endoscopic techniques,** such as endoscopic sewing and radiofrequency, endoscopic sewing use small stitches to tighten the sphincter muscle. Radiofrequency creates heat lesions that help tighten the sphincter muscle.

Nursing Management

1. Make a diet for the patient
2. To reduce intraabdominal pressure, encourage the patient to sleep in reverse Trendelenburg's position
3. Encourage the client to avoid lying down immediately after meals
4. Monitor the client's response to therapy and compliance with treatment
5. Monitor his intake and output and vital signs
6. Monitor for complication of the disease and of surgery
7. Discuss the recommended dietary changes
8. Instruct the client to avoid situations or activities that increase intraabdominal pressure
9. Encourage the patient compliance with his drug regimen
10. Avoid spicy foods and beverages
11. Encourage client to eat small and frequent meals
12. Encourage relaxation techniques
13. Explain diagnostic test

HIATAL HERNIA

A hiatal hernia occurs when part of stomach pushes upward through diaphragm. The stomach can push up through this opening and cause a hiatal hernia **(Fig. 4.2)**.

Etiology

- Injury to the area
- Born with an unusually large hiatus
- Persistent and intense pressure on the surrounding muscles

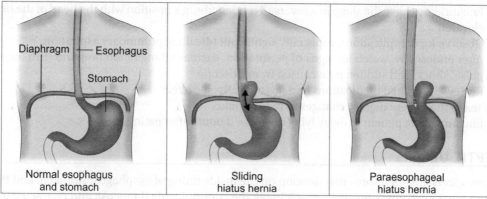

Fig. 4.2: Types of hernia.

Signs and Symptoms

- Most small hiatal hernias cause no signs or symptoms
- Heartburn
- Belching
- Difficulty swallowing
- Fatigue

Diagnostic Evaluation

- **Barium meal:** An X-ray, during the procedure, the person will stand or sit in front of an X-ray machine and drink barium. Barium coats the esophagus, stomach, and small intestine so the radiologist can see these organs' shapes more clearly on X-rays.
- **Endoscopy:** This procedure involves using an endoscope, a small, flexible tube with a light, to see the upper GIT.
- **Esophageal pH monitoring:** The most accurate test to detect acid reflux, esophageal pH monitoring measures the amount of liquid or acid in the esophagus. A gastroenterologist will pass a thin tube, called an NG probe, through the person's nose or mouth to the stomach. The gastroenterologist will then pull the tube back into the esophagus, where it will be taped to the person's cheek and remain in place for 24 hours. The end of the tube in the esophagus has a small probe to measure when and how much liquid or acid comes up into the esophagus.
- **Esophageal manometry:** Esophageal manometry measures muscle contractions in the esophagus.

Management

- Antacids that neutralize stomach acid are magnesium hydroxide and aluminum hydroxides.
- H_2-receptor blockers, cimetidine, famotidine, and ranitidine
- Proton pump inhibitors block acid production

Surgical Management

Fundoplication is an operation to sew the top of the stomach around the esophagus to add pressure to the lower end of the esophagus and reduce reflux.

Nursing Management

- Prepare the client for diagnostic tests
- Administer prescribed antacids

- Encourage to have the sleep in a reverse Trendelenburg's position with the head of the bed elevated
- Observe for complications, especially significant bleeding, pulmonary aspiration.
- After endoscopy, watch for signs of perforation, such as falling blood pressure (BP), rapid pulse, shock, and sudden pain caused by endoscope.
- Review prescribed medications and possible adverse effect
- Teach the patient dietary changes to reduce reflux
- Encourage the patient to delay lying down for 2 hours after eating.

PEPTIC ULCERS

Peptic ulcers are open sores that develop on the inside lining of esophagus, stomach, and the upper portion of small intestine, which break the continuity of GI mucosa and characterized by abdominal pain **(Fig. 4.3)**.

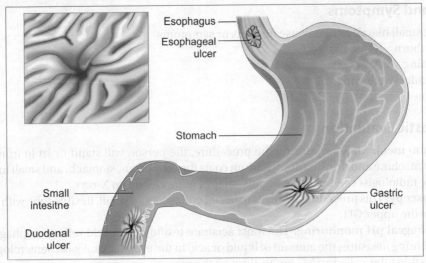

Fig. 4.3: Peptic ulcer.

Classification of Peptic Ulcer

1. **According to area affected**
   - Duodenal ulcer
   - Esophageal ulcer
   - Gastric ulcer
   - Meckel's diverticulum.
2. **Modified Johnson classification**
   - **Type I:** Ulcer along the body of the stomach, most often along the lesser curve
   - **Type II:** Ulcer in the body in combination with duodenal ulcers
   - **Type III:** In the pyloric channel within 3 cm of pylorus
   - **Type IV:** Proximal gastroesophageal ulcer
   - **Type V:** Can occur throughout the stomach

Etiology

- *Helicobacter pylori*
- Obesity
- Pregnancy

- Certain medications, such as NSAIDs
- Smoking
- **Alcohol:** Ulcers are more common in people who have cirrhosis of the liver.
- **Stress:** Emotional stress increases ulcer pain
- Use of spicy foods
- Sudden fall of sleep after meal
- **Acid and pepsin:** The stomach's inability to defend itself against the powerful digestive fluids, acid and pepsin, contributes to ulcer formation.
- Congenital weakness of esophageal sphincter

Characteristics	Gastric ulcer	Duodenal ulcer
Incidence	**Age** = 50 years or above Male:Female = 1:1 15% of peptic ulcers are gastric	**Age** = 30–60 years Male:Female = 2–3:1 80% of peptic ulcers are duodenal
Definition	Ulcers that occur in the stomach are called gastric ulcers	The duodenum ulcer refers to the upper region of the small intestine
Causes	*Helicobacter pylori* infection or consumption of nonsteroidal antiinflammatory drugs (NSAIDs)	Excess stomach acid *H. pylori* bacteria
Signs and symptoms	Gastric ulcers cause stomach pain immediate and 1–2 h after eating	Duodenal ulcers cause pain 3–4 h later
	Gastric ulcers cause hematemesis or vomiting of blood	Duodenal ulcers cause melena or blood in the stool
	It is located in epigastric area (area between belly button and rib cage)	Pain below the ribs and just below the breastbone
	Gastric ulcers cause an aching, burning	Duodenal ulcers cause an aching, burning, hunger-like pain in the upper–middle portion of the abdomen
	Vomiting is common	Vomiting is uncommon
	Normal and hyposecretion of HCl	Hypersecretion of HCl
	No telltale sign of a duodenal ulcer is pain that occurs during the middle of the night	Telltale sign of a duodenal ulcer is pain that occurs during the middle of the night
	This pain tends to develop or worsen when the stomach is full	This pain tends to develop or worsen when the stomach is relatively empty
Malignancy possibility	Rare	Occasionally
Risk factors	Alcohol, smoking, cirrhosis, stress	Use of NSAIDs, gastritis, alcohol, smoking
Diet	A gastric ulcer has a special diet	Duodenal ulcers do not

Signs and Symptoms

- Pain is the most common symptom and worsens when stomach is empty
- Temporarily relieved by eating certain foods that buffer stomach acid or by antacids
- Disappear and then return for a few days or weeks
- Hemoptysis
- Melena
- Nausea or vomiting
- Unexplained weight loss
- Anorexia

Pathophysiology

Duodenal ulcer:

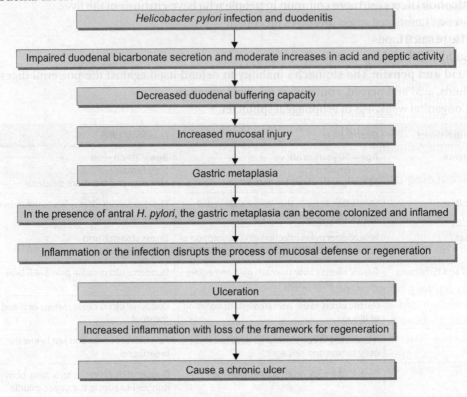

Helicobacter pylori infection and duodenitis

↓

Impaired duodenal bicarbonate secretion and moderate increases in acid and peptic activity

↓

Decreased duodenal buffering capacity

↓

Increased mucosal injury

↓

Gastric metaplasia

↓

In the presence of antral *H. pylori*, the gastric metaplasia can become colonized and inflamed

↓

Inflammation or the infection disrupts the process of mucosal defense or regeneration

↓

Ulceration

↓

Increased inflammation with loss of the framework for regeneration

↓

Cause a chronic ulcer

Gastric ulcer:

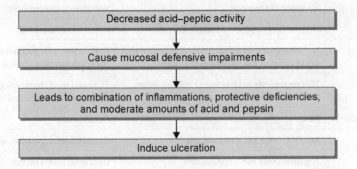

Decreased acid–peptic activity

↓

Cause mucosal defensive impairments

↓

Leads to combination of inflammations, protective deficiencies, and moderate amounts of acid and pepsin

↓

Induce ulceration

Complications

- **GI bleeding:** Melena or hemoptysis
- GI infection and perforation

Diagnostic Evaluation

- **Blood tests:** The body produces antibodies against *H. pylori* in an attempt to fight the bacteria.
- **Breath tests:** Breath tests measure carbon dioxide in exhaled breath. Patients are given a substance called urea with carbon to drink. Bacteria break down this urea and the carbon is

absorbed into the blood stream and lungs and exhaled in the breath. By collecting the breath, physician can measure this carbon and determine whether *H. pylori* are present or absent.
- **Tissue tests:** A rapid urease test detects the bacteria's enzyme urease.

Management

Lifestyle Changes
- Loss of weight
- Wearing loose-fitting
- Remaining upright for 3 hours after meals
- Raising the head of the bed
- Avoiding smoking

Pharmacological Management
- Antacids, magnesium hydroxide, aluminum hydroxides
- H_2 blockers, such as cimetidine
- Proton pump inhibitors include omeprazole
- Prokinetics, which include bethanechol and metoclopramide
- **Sucralfate and misoprostol:** Sucralfate coats the ulcer surface and promotes healing.

Helicobacter pylori Treatment
The treatment of *H. pylori* includes the following:
- **Antibiotics:** Tetracycline, amoxicillin, metronidazole, clarithromycin, and levofloxacin (Levaquin) to eradicate *H. pylori*.
- Probiotic supplement
- **Vitamin C:** 500–1,000 mg one to three times daily

Surgical Management

Vagotomy: A vagotomy is a surgical procedure that involves resection of the vagus nerve, it reduces acid secretion.

Types of Vagotomy
- **Truncal vagotomy:** It involves division of the anterior and posterior vagal trunks close to the abdominal esophagus and just below the diaphragm.
- **Selective vagotomy:** It is one operative means of reducing gastric acid output.
- **High selective vagotomy:** A vagotomy for peptic ulceration is to reduce parietal cell acid output.
- **Antrectomy:** In this surgery, the lower part of the stomach is removed. This section of the stomach produces a hormone that stimulates the stomach to secrete digestive juices **(Fig. 4.4)**.
- **Billroth I (gastroduodenostomy):** Removal of lower portion of the antrum of the stomach as well as a small portion of duodenum and pylorus. The remaining segment is anastomosed to the duodenum **(Fig. 4.5)**.
- **Billroth II (gastrojejunostomy):** Removal of lower portion of the antrum of the stomach as well as a small portion of duodenum and pylorus. The remaining segment is anastomosed to the jejunum.
- **Pyloroplasty:** This surgery enlarges the opening to the duodenum and small intestine, which enables stomach contents to pass more freely out of the stomach.
- **Gastrectomy:** Gastrectomy is surgery to remove part or all of the stomach.
  - **Partial gastrectomy:** Removing part of the stomach is called partial gastrectomy.
  - **Complete gastrectomy:** Removing the complete stomach is called gastrectomy.

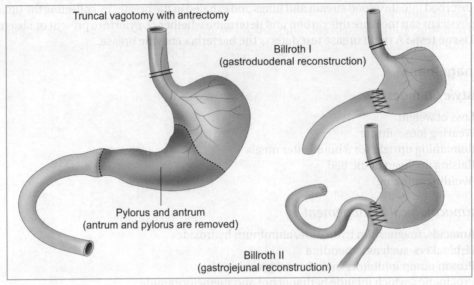

Fig. 4.4: Antrectomy.

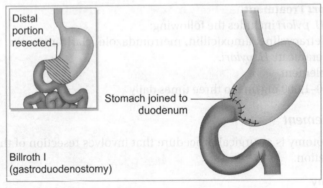

Fig. 4.5: Billroth I.

Nutritional Management

- Encouraging to have foods containing flavonoids, such as apples, which may inhibit the growth of *bacteria*.
- Eating antioxidant-rich foods
- Eating foods high in B vitamins and calcium, such as almonds
- Avoiding spicy foods
- Using healthy oils, such as olive oil or vegetable oil
- Reducing or eliminating *trans*-fatty acids
- Avoiding beverages that may irritate the stomach lining
- Drinking six to eight glasses of filtered water daily
- Exercising at least 30 minutes daily, 5 days a week
- Reducing stress by performing exercise daily

Complications

- **Gastrointestinal bleeding**
- **Perforation**

- **Gastric outlet obstruction**
- **Gastric cancer**
- **Dumping syndrome:** It occurs after gastrojejunostomy because ingested food rapidly enter the jejunum without proper mixing and without the duodenum digestive process.

Nursing Care Plan

1. Acute pain related to irritation of the mucosa and muscle spasms

Interventions:

- Administering pain killers and antacids as ordered
- Instructing to avoid spicy foods
- Encouraging clients to avoid caffeine and alcohol
- Encouraging clients to have small and frequent meals
- Instructing patient to stop smoking

2. Anxiety related to the nature of the disease and long-term management

Interventions:

- Encouraging clients to express their problems and fears
- Explaining the reasons for the dietary restrictions and to reduce or stop smoking
- Assisting clients to identify situations that cause anxiety
- Teaching stress management strategies.

3. Imbalanced nutrition, less than body requirements related to pain

Interventions:

- Encouraging to eat foods and drinks that do not irritate
- Instructing to avoid spicy foods
- Encouraging clients to avoid caffeine and alcohol
- Encouraging clients to have small and frequent meals
- Encouraging to eat food in a relaxed environment

APPENDICITIS

Appendicitis is an inflammation of the appendix. The inflamed appendix gradually swells and fills with pus.

Etiology

An obstruction: Stool can block the opening of the cavity that runs the length of appendix.

Signs and Symptoms

- Pain usually occurs at **McBurney's point** over the right side of the abdomen that is one-third of the distance from the anterior superior iliac spine to the umbilicus **(Fig. 4.6)**.
- Tenderness
- Pain that worsens during coughing (Dunphy's sign)
- Nausea

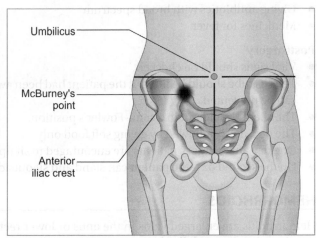

Fig. 4.6: Location of McBurney's point.

- Vomiting
- Anorexia
- Low-grade fever
- Constipation
- Inability to pass gas
- Diarrhea
- Ascites

Diagnostic Evaluation

- **Physical examination:** A gentle pressure on the painful area. When the pressure is suddenly released, appendicitis pain will often feel worse, signaling that the adjacent peritoneum is inflamed
- Complete blood count (CBC)
- Urinalysis
- Abdominal X-ray, computerized tomography (CT) scan

Complications

- Ruptured appendix
- Peritonitis

Management

Laparoscopic appendectomy
- Lifestyle and home remedies
  - Strenuous activity should be avoided
  - Abdomen should be supported when coughing
  - It is advised not to wear tight clothes, such as tight belt

Nursing Management

Intraoperative Phase
- Installation of NG tube to decompress
- Catheters to control urine production
- Rehydration
- Giving antibiotics with broad spectrum
- Medicines for fever

Postsurgery
- Vital signs should be checked.
- The NG tube should be lifted; if the patient had been aware of that aspiration of gastric fluid can be prevented.
- The client should put in a semi-Fowler's position.
- The next day is followed by giving soft food only.
- One day after surgery patients are encouraged to sit up in bed.
- On the second day, the patient can stand and sit outside the room.

HEMORRHOIDS

Hemorrhoids are enlarged veins in the anus or lower rectum, which compromises the blood supply to the anus and distal rectum.

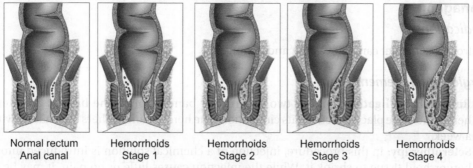

| Normal rectum Anal canal | Hemorrhoids Stage 1 | Hemorrhoids Stage 2 | Hemorrhoids Stage 3 | Hemorrhoids Stage 4 |

Fig. 4.7: Types of hemorrhoids.

Etiology

- Constipation
- Diarrhea
- Lack of exercise
- Low-fiber diets
- Increased intra-abdominal pressure
- Genetics
- Aging
- Obesity
- Prolonged sitting
- Chronic cough
- Pregnancy

Types

1. **External hemorrhoids:** These appear on the outside of the anus, especially around the anal opening.
2. **Prolapsed hemorrhoids:** When it becomes bulky due to clogging of the veins with blood they begin to sag and consequently protrude from the anus.
3. **Bleeding hemorrhoids** These are also a more severe form or stage of internal hemorrhoids characterized by profuse bleeding **(Fig. 4.7)**.

Pathophysiology

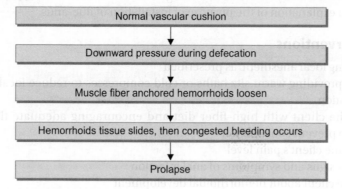

Normal vascular cushion

↓

Downward pressure during defecation

↓

Muscle fiber anchored hemorrhoids loosen

↓

Hemorrhoids tissue slides, then congested bleeding occurs

↓

Prolapse

Diagnostic Evaluation

- Examination of anal canal and rectum for abnormalities
- Visual inspection of anal canal and rectum

Management

Medications

Hydrocortisone that can relieve pain and itching.

Surgical Management

- **Rubber band ligation:** One or two tiny rubber bands around the base of an internal hemorrhoid are placed to cut off its circulation. The hemorrhoid withers and falls off within a week.
- **Sclerotherapy:** In this procedure, injection of a chemical solution is introduced into the hemorrhoid tissue to shrink it. While the injection causes little or no pain, it may be less effective than rubber band ligation.
- **Coagulation:** Coagulation techniques use laser or infrared light or heat. They cause small, bleeding, internal hemorrhoids to harden and shrivel.
- **Hemorrhoidectomy:** During a hemorrhoidectomy, removal of excessive tissue that causes bleeding.
- **Hemorrhoid stapling:** It blocks the blood flow to hemorrhoidal tissue and makes it necrotized.

Nursing Management

Preoperative care
- Giving soak seat
- Giving lubricant during defecation would
- Giving a diet low in residual
- Instructing the patient to avoid prolonged standing or sitting
- Observing patient's complaints
- Providing an explanation of the emergence of pain and explain briefly
- Giving the patient suppository

Postoperative care
- Giving the patient a pleasant sleeping position
- Changing the bandage every morning according to aseptic techniques
- Exercising as early as possible
- Observing the rectal area if there is bleeding
- Providing an explanation of the purpose of installation of flue-anus.

Nursing Interventions

- Administering local anesthetic as prescribed
- As needed, providing warm sitz baths or cold compresses to reduce local pain, swelling, and information
- Providing the client with high-fiber diet and encouraging adequate fluid intake and exercising to prevent constipation
- Monitoring the client's pain level
- Checking for signs and symptoms of anal infection
- Teaching the client about hemorrhoidal development
- Encouraging the client to eat high-fiber diet to promote regular bowel movement
- Emphasizing the need for good anal hygiene
- Encouraging the use of medicated astringent pads and toilet paper without dyes or perfumes.

GASTROINTESTINAL BLEEDING

Gastrointestinal bleeding or **GI hemorrhage** is a form of hemorrhage in the GIT, from the pharynx to the rectum. The degree of bleeding can range from nearly undetectable to acute or massive, life-threatening bleeding.

Etiology

- Peptic ulcers: *H. pylori*
- Overuse of NSAIDs
- Esophageal varices
- **Mallory-Weiss tears:** These tears in the lining of the esophagus usually result from vomiting
- Gastritis
- Esophagitis
- Gastroesophageal reflux disease (GERD)
- Benign tumors and cancer
- Diverticular disease
- Colitis
- Hemorrhoids

Types of Gastrointestinal Bleeding

- **Upper GI bleeding:** Bleeding in the esophagus, stomach, or the beginning of small intestine.
- **Lower GI bleeding:** Bleeding in the small intestine, large intestine, rectum, or anus.
- **Frank bleeding:** Active bleeding that can be easily seen. For example, vomiting blood.
- **Occult bleeding:** Slow bleeding that cannot be seen easily. Tests may be needed to find occult bleeding.
- **Acute GI bleeding:** Blood loss that is new or sudden and lasts only for a short time.
- **Chronic GI bleeding:** Blood loss that has been going on for a long time, or that comes back often.

Signs of bleeding in the upper digestive tract include

- Bright red blood in vomit
- Vomit that looks, such as coffee grounds
- Black or tarry stool
- Dark blood mixed with stool
- Stool mixed or coated with bright red blood

Signs of bleeding in the lower digestive tract include:

- Black or tarry stool
- Dark blood mixed with stool
- Stool mixed or coated with bright red blood
- Weakness
- Dizziness or faintness
- Shortness of breath
- Crampy abdominal pain
- Diarrhea
- Paleness

Signs and symptoms of losing too much blood may include:

- Chest pain
- Palpitation
- Extreme tiredness

- Dizziness or fainting
- Pale skin
- Dry mouth
- Feeling confused or short of breath

Diagnostic Evaluation

- *Endoscopy*
- *Enteroscopy*
  - **Push enteroscopy:** A long endoscope is used to examine the upper portion of the small intestine.
  - **Double-balloon enteroscopy:** Balloons are mounted on the endoscope to help the endoscope move through the entire small intestine.
  - **Capsule endoscopy:** The person swallows a capsule containing a tiny camera. The camera transmits images to a video monitor as the capsule passes through the digestive tract. This procedure is designed to examine the small intestine.
- *Barium X-rays*
- *Radionuclide scanning*
- *Angiography*

Management

Pharmacological Management

There are many medicines that may be given to treat bleeding, which include:
- **Antibiotics**
- **Antiemetic**
- **Antiulcer medicine**
- **Pain medicine:** Caregivers may give you medicine to take away or decrease your pain.

Nursing Care Plan

Nursing Diagnosis

1. Nutrition: Imbalanced, less than body requirements related to inadequate diet

Interventions:
- Measuring dietary intake by calorie count
- Weighing as indicated
- Restricting intake of caffeine
- Suggesting soft foods, avoiding roughage
- Providing NG tube feedings
- Encouraging client to have small and frequent diet
- Avoiding spicy foods
- Encouraging client to eat all meals, including supplementary feedings unless contraindicated
- Giving small, frequent meals
- Encouraging frequent mouth care
- Promoting undisturbed rest periods, especially before meals
- Avoiding smoking
- Referring to dietitian to provide diet high in calories and simple carbohydrates, low in fat

2. Skin integrity, risk for impaired related to altered circulation

Interventions:
- Inspecting pressure points for pressure ulcers
- Recommending elevating lower extremities

- Keeping linens dry and free of wrinkles
- Suggesting clipping fingernails short and providing mittens, gloves, if indicated
- Using calamine lotion and providing baking soda baths
- Using alternating pressure mattress
- Providing perineal care following urination and bowel movement
- Using emollient lotions
- Assisting with active and passive range of motion (ROM) exercises.

3. Risk for injury related to internal bleeding

Interventions:

- Closely assessing for signs and symptoms of GI bleeding
- Observing the presence of petechiae and ecchymosis
- Monitoring vital signs
- Encouraging the use of soft toothbrush, electric razor, avoiding straining for stool, vigorous nose blowing
- Using small needles for injections
- Advising to avoid aspiring-containing products
- Taking supplemental vitamins: vitamins K, D, and C
- Administering stool softeners
- Noting changes in mental status
- Avoiding rectal temperature and be gentle with GI tube insertions
- Assisting with insertion and maintenance of GI tube
- Providing gastric lavage

IRRITABLE BOWEL SYNDROME

Irritable bowel syndrome (IBS) is a common disorder that affects large intestine, characterized by cramping, bloating gas, diarrhea, constipation, and abdominal pain.

Etiology and Risk Factors

- Carbonated beverages and some fruits and vegetables may lead to bloating
- Stress
- Hormones
- More women than men are diagnosed with this condition
- Having a family history of IBS

Pathophysiology

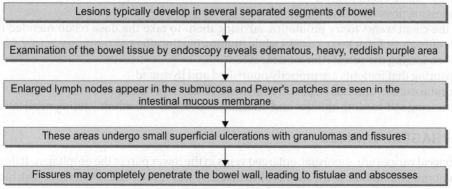

Lesions typically develop in several separated segments of bowel

↓

Examination of the bowel tissue by endoscopy reveals edematous, heavy, reddish purple area

↓

Enlarged lymph nodes appear in the submucosa and Peyer's patches are seen in the intestinal mucous membrane

↓

These areas undergo small superficial ulcerations with granulomas and fissures

↓

Fissures may completely penetrate the bowel wall, leading to fistulae and abscesses

Contd...

Contd...

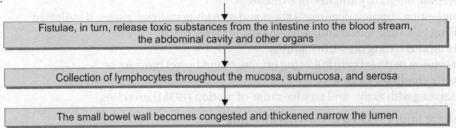

Fistulae, in turn, release toxic substances from the intestine into the blood stream, the abdominal cavity and other organs

Collection of lymphocytes throughout the mucosa, submucosa, and serosa

The small bowel wall becomes congested and thickened narrow the lumen

Signs and Symptoms

- Abdominal pain
- A bloated feeling
- Gas
- Diarrhea or constipation
- Mucus in the stool

Diagnostic Evaluation

- Flexible sigmoidoscopy
- Colonoscopy
- CT
- Lactose intolerance tests
- Blood tests

Management

- **Fiber supplements:** Such as psyllium or methylcellulose
- **Antidiarrheal medications:** Such as loperamide
- Elimination of high-gas foods
- **Anticholinergic medications:** To relieve bowel spasms
- **Antidepressant medications:** Such as tricyclic antidepressant or a selective serotonin reuptake inhibitor.

Nursing Management

- Changing in bowel habit
- Providing information about self-help, physical activity, diet, and symptom-targeted medication
- Encouraging client to relax
- Assessing physical activity levels
- If the client wants to try probiotics, advising them to take the dose recommended by the manufacturer for at least 4 weeks while monitoring the effect
- Discouraging the use of *Aloe vera* for IBS
- Ensuring that patients are properly nourished and hydrated
- Administration and management of alternative forms of nutrition
- Assessing self-feeding abilities and assisting as needed, and administering medications.

ESOPHAGEAL VARICES

Esophageal varices are abnormal, enlarged veins in the lower part of the esophagus. It develops when normal blood flow to the liver is obstructed by scar tissue. The vessels may leak blood or even rupture, causing life-threatening bleeding.

Etiology

- Prehepatic cause
  - Portal vein thrombosis
  - Portal vein obstruction
  - Increased portal blood flow
  - Increased splenic flow
- Intrahepatic cause
  - Cirrhosis
  - Idiopathic portal hypertension
  - Acute hepatitis
  - Schistosomiasis
  - Congenital hepatic fibrosis
- Posthepatic cause
  - Compression
  - Budd–Chiari syndrome

Signs and Symptoms

- Hemoptysis
- Black, tarry, or bloody stools
- Shock
- Jaundice
- Spider veins
- Palmar erythema
- Shrunken testicles
- Swollen spleen
- Ascites

Diagnostic Evaluation

- Endoscopic examination
- Imaging tests: Both CT and MRI scans
- Capsule endoscopy
- CBC
- Clotting, including International Normalized Ratio (INR)
- Renal function
- Liver function tests (LFTs).

Management

- **Beta blocker**
- **Band ligation:** Using an endoscope, the varices are wrapped with each other with an elastic band, which essentially "strangles" the veins so they cannot bleed.
- **Transjugular intrahepatic portosystemic shunt (PSS) (TIPS):** The shunt is a small tube that is placed between the portal vein and the hepatic vein, which carries blood from liver back to heart. By providing an additional path for blood, the shunt reduces pressure in the portal vein and often stops bleeding from esophageal varices.
- **Sengstaken–Blakemore tube:** It is inserted through the mouth and into the stomach. The gastric balloon is inflated with air and the gastric balloon in then pulled up against the esophagogastric junction, compressing submucosal varices. The Sengstaken tube also contains an esophageal balloon, which is only rarely required when the gastric balloon does not work **(Fig. 4.8)**.

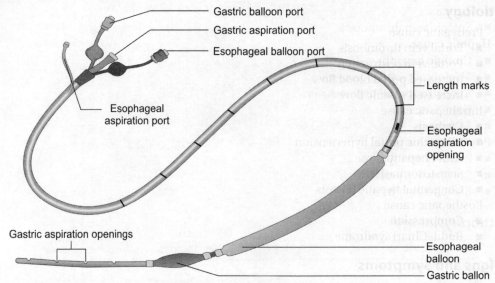

Fig. 4.8: Sengstaken-Blakemore tube.

Nursing Care Plan

Nursing Diagnosis

- Risk for bleeding related to obstruction in blood flow
- **Imbalanced nutrition:** Less than body requirements related to vomiting and jaundice.

Nursing Interventions
- Providing ongoing assessment
  - Ecchymosis, epistaxis, petechiae, and bleeding gums should be assessed for.
  - Level of consciousness should be monitored.
  - The client should be monitored during blood transfusion administration if prescribed.
  - Small-gauge needles should be used, and pressure or cold should be applied for bleeding.
  - The procedure should be explained to the client to reduce fear and enhance cooperation with insertion and maintenance of the esophageal tamponade tube.
  - The client should be monitored closely to prevent accidental removal or displacement of the tube with resultant airway obstruction.
- Administering prescribed vasopressin and vitamin K
  - Stool softeners should be administered.
  - It is required to assist with insertion and maintenance of GI tube.
  - Gastric lavage with room temperature and cool saline solution or water as indicated should be provided.

PORTAL HYPERTENSION

Portal hypertension refers to abnormally high pressure in the hepatic portal vein more than 10 mm Hg.

Etiology

- **Prehepatic cause**
  - Congenital atresia
  - Portal-vein thrombosis

- Tumors
- Splenic vein thrombosis
- **Hepatic cause**
  - Chronic hepatitis
  - Myeloproliferative diseases
  - Idiopathic portal hypertension
  - Granulomata
  - Toxins
- **Posthepatic cause**
  - Budd–Chiari syndrome
  - Constrictive pericarditis
  - Right heart failure

Pathophysiology

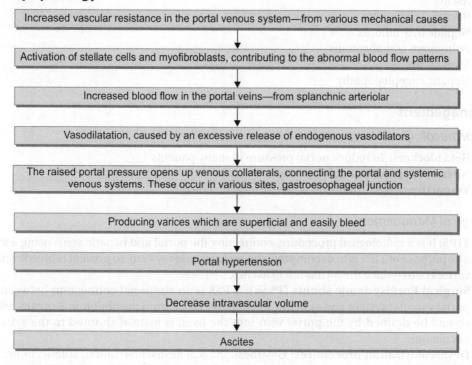

Increased vascular resistance in the portal venous system—from various mechanical causes

↓

Activation of stellate cells and myofibroblasts, contributing to the abnormal blood flow patterns

↓

Increased blood flow in the portal veins—from splanchnic arteriolar

↓

Vasodilatation, caused by an excessive release of endogenous vasodilators

↓

The raised portal pressure opens up venous collaterals, connecting the portal and systemic venous systems. These occur in various sites, gastroesophageal junction

↓

Producing varices which are superficial and easily bleed

↓

Portal hypertension

↓

Decrease intravascular volume

↓

Ascites

Signs and Symptoms

- Dilated veins
- Splenomegaly
- Ascites
- Jaundice
- Confusion
- Enlarged or small liver
- Gynecomastia
- Testicular atrophy
- Spider veins
- Palmar erythema

Diagnostic Evaluation

- Blood tests
- Abdominal ultrasound
- Doppler ultrasound
- CT scan
- Endoscopy
- Hepatic venous pressure gradient
- Liver biopsy
- Vascular imaging
- Hepatic venography

Complications

- Esophageal varices
- Ascites
- Bacterial peritonitis
- Hepatic hydrothorax
- Pulmonary complications
- Liver failure
- Hepatic encephalopathy

Management

Pharmacological Management

- **Beta blockers:** To reduce portal pressure in many patients
- **Nitrates:** To reduce portal pressure
- **Vasoactive drugs:** To control acute variceal bleeding

Surgical Management

- **TIPS:** It is a radiological procedure, connecting the portal and hepatic veins using a stent. The purpose of TIPS is to decompress the portal venous system, to prevent rebleeding from varices or to reduce the formation of ascites.
- **Surgical Portosystemic shunts (PSSs):** A PSS is an abnormal connection between the portal vascular system and systemic circulation. Blood from the abdominal organs, which should be drained by the portal vein into the liver, is instead shunted to the systemic circulation.
- **Devascularization procedures:** Gastroesophageal devascularization, splenectomy, and esophageal transaction.

Nursing Care Plan

Nursing Diagnosis

- Risk for infection related to ascites
- Risk for imbalanced fluid volume related to vomiting and edema
- Activity intolerance related to weakness

Nursing Interventions

- Administering medications, as ordered
- Assisting the healthcare provider with paracentesis

- Measuring and record abdominal girth and body weight daily
- Encouraging the client to elevate the lower extremities
- Administering salt-poor albumin, which temporarily elevates the serum albumin level
- Giving small, frequent meals
- Restricting intake of caffeine
- Measuring dietary intake by calorie count
- Weighing as indicated
- Encouraging patient to eat, explaining reasons for the types of diet
- Encouraging patient to eat all meals, including supplementary feedings unless contraindicated
- Promoting undisturbed rest periods, especially before meals
- Measuring intake and output chart
- Monitoring BP and respiratory status
- **Auscultating lungs**
  - Cardiac dysrhythmias should be monitored.
  - Degree of peripheral edema should be assessed.
  - Soft foods should be suggested, avoiding roughage, if indicated.
  - Frequent mouth care, especially before meals, should be encouraged.
  - Abdominal girth should be measured.
  - Bed rest should be encouraged when ascites is present.
  - Sodium and fluids should be restricted as indicated.
  - Salt-free albumin, plasma expanders should be administered.
- Diuretics should be administered

CHOLELITHIASIS

It refers to the presence of stones in gallbladder. A gallstone is a crystalline concretion formed within the gallbladder by accretion of bile components. These calculi are formed in the gallbladder and may obstruct the flow of bile **(Fig. 4.9)**.

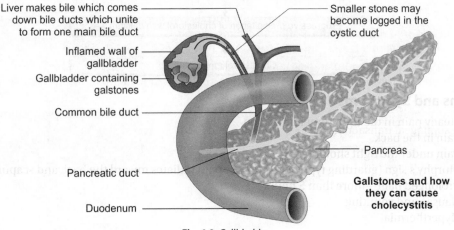

Fig. 4.9: Gallbladder.

Types of Gallstones

- **Cholesterol stones:** Yellow to dark green
- **Pigment stones:** Pigment stones are small and dark
- **Mixed stones:** Contain 20–80% cholesterol

Etiology

- **Gender:** Women are twice as likely as men
- **Family history**
- **Obesity**
- **Diet:** Diets high in fat and cholesterol
- **Age:** People older than age 60 are more likely to develop gallstones than younger people
- **Hypolipidemic drugs**
- **Hyperglycemia**

Pathophysiology

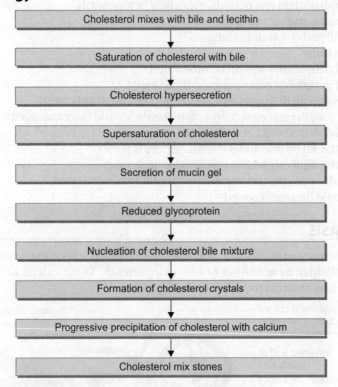

Cholesterol mixes with bile and lecithin

↓

Saturation of cholesterol with bile

↓

Cholesterol hypersecretion

↓

Supersaturation of cholesterol

↓

Secretion of mucin gel

↓

Reduced glycoprotein

↓

Nucleation of cholesterol bile mixture

↓

Formation of cholesterol crystals

↓

Progressive precipitation of cholesterol with calcium

↓

Cholesterol mix stones

Signs and Symptoms

- Steady pain in the right upper abdomen
- Pain in the back
- Pain under the right shoulder
- Murphy's sign (guarding type of respiratory pain radiates toward the back and scapula)
- Prolonged pain—more than 5 hours
- Nausea and vomiting
- Hyperthermia
- Jaundice
- Clay-colored stool

Diagnostic Evaluation

- CT scans
- Cholescintigraphy scan

- **Endoscopic retrograde cholangiopancreatography (ERCP):** ERCP is used to locate and remove stones in the bile ducts. The physician inserts an endoscope—a long, flexible, lighted tube with a camera—down the throat and through the stomach and into the small intestine. The physician guides the endoscope and injects a special dye that helps the bile ducts appear better on the monitor. The endoscope helps the physician locate the affected bile duct and the gallstone.
- **Blood tests**

Management

Pharmacological Management

- Opioid analgesic
- Antispasmodic
- Antiemetic
- Bile acid therapy
- Chenodeoxycholic acid to reduce the cholesterol stone
- Anticholelithiotic agents

Surgical Management

- **Extracorporeal shock wave lithotripsy:** It is a noninvasive procedure used as an ambulatory treatment. A machine called lithotripter generates a powerful shock to shatter the gallstones **(Fig. 4.10).**

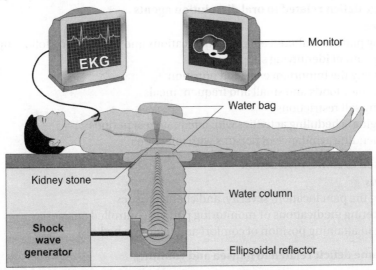

Fig. 4.10: Extracorporeal shock wave lithotripsy.

- **Percutaneous transhepatic biliary catheter insertion:** Insertion of a percutaneous transhepatic biliary catheter under fluoroscopic guidance. This procedure will decompress obstructed extrahepatic ducts, so that the bile can flow.

Other surgical interventions are:
- Cholecystectomy
- Laparoscopic laser cholecystectomy
- Cholecystotomy
- Choledochotomy
- Choledocholithotomy (incision of common bile duct and removal of gallstones).

Nonsurgical Treatment

- **Oral dissolution therapy:** Drugs made from bile acid are used to dissolve gallstones, for example, ursodiol and chenodiol.
- **Contact dissolution therapy:** This experimental procedure involves injecting a drug directly into the gallbladder to dissolve cholesterol stones. The drug—methyl *tert*-butyl ether—can dissolve some stones in 1–3 days.

Nursing Care Plan

Nursing Diagnosis

1. Risk for injury related to medication during retrograde endoscopy for stone removal

Interventions

- Assessing signs and symptoms of GI bleeding
- Noting changes in mentation and level of consciousness
- Observing the presence of petechiae, ecchymosis
- Monitoring vital signs
- Using small needles for injections
- Applying pressure to small bleeding
- Avoiding rectal temperature
- Encouraging the use of soft toothbrush, electric razor, avoiding straining for stool
- Recommending avoidance of aspirin-containing products.

2. Knowledge deficit related to oral dissolution agents

Interventions

- Informing patient of altered effects of medications and encouraging follow-up
- Assisting patient identifying support person
- Emphasizing the importance of good nutrition
- Avoiding spicy foods and small and frequent meals
- Discussing salt restrictions
- Encouraging scheduling activities with adequate rest periods
- Recommending avoidance of persons with infections

3. Pain related to stone obstruction

Interventions

- Assessing the pain location, severity, and characteristics
- Administering medications or monitoring patient-controlled analgesia
- Assisting in attaining position of comfort and maintain bed rest

4. Fluid volume deficit related to nausea and vomiting

Interventions

- Administering fluids and electrolytes as ordered
- Administering antiemetic as ordered
- Maintaining NG decompression
- Beginning food and fluids as tolerated by the client

5. Activity intolerance related to fatigue, general discomfort

Interventions

- Encouraging alternating periods of rests and ambulation
- Maintaining some periods of rest
- Encouraging and assisting with gradually increasing periods of exercise.

6. Imbalanced nutrition less than body requirement related to pain

Interventions

- Encouraging a diet that is low in residue fiber and fat and high in calories
- Monitoring weight daily
- Providing small frequent meals
- Planning a meal per preference of client and as ordered
- Preparing the patient for element diet
- Restarting oral fluid intake gradually

7. Ineffective coping related to feeling of rejection

Interventions

- Assessing the level of fear and note nonverbal communication
- Asking the client usual coping pattern
- Assuring client a close monitoring
- Allowing client to verbalize fear of dying
- Providing diversional materials

CHOLECYSTITIS

Cholecystitis is inflammation of the gallbladder.

Etiology

- Gallstones
- Tumor
- Bile duct blockage

Risk Factors

- **Gender:** Women are twice as likely as men
- **Family history**
- **Obesity**
- **Diet:** Diets high in fat and cholesterol
- **Age:** People older than age 60 are more likely to develop gallstones than younger people
- **Hypolipidemic drugs**
- **Hyperglycemia**

Signs and Symptoms

- Steady pain in the right upper abdomen
- Pain in the back
- Pain under the right shoulder
- Murphy's sign (guarding type of respiratory pain radiates toward the back and scapula)
- Prolonged pain more than 5 hours
- Nausea and vomiting
- Hyperthermia
- Jaundice
- Clay-colored stool

Complications

- Enlarged gallbladder
- Perforation in gallbladder
- Gangrene

Diagnostic Evaluation

- **Blood tests:** CBC
- **Imaging tests:** Imaging tests, such as abdominal ultrasound or a CT scan
- **Hepatobiliary iminodiacetic acid (HIDA):** A HIDA scan tracks the production and flow of bile from liver to small intestine and shows if bile is blocked or not.

Management

- **Antibiotics:** To treat the infection
- **Analgesics:** To help control pain until the inflammation in gallbladder is relieved.

Surgical Interventions

- Cholecystectomy
- Laparoscopic laser cholecystectomy
- Cholecystectomy
- Choledochotomy
- Choledocholithotomy

Nursing Care Plan

Nursing Assessment

- Obtaining history
- Assessing mental status
- Perform abdominal examination for ascites
- Assessing the client's bowel elimination pattern
- Assessing the client's abdomen for bowel sounds
- Assessing hemorrhage
- Monitoring for temperature and white blood cell (WBC) counts.

Nursing Diagnosis

- Pain related to stone obstruction
- Risk for injury related to medication during retrograde endoscopy for stone removal
- Fluid volume deficit related to nausea and vomiting
- Activity intolerance related to fatigue, general discomfort
- Imbalanced nutrition less than body requirement related to pain
- Ineffective coping related to feeling of rejection
- Knowledge deficit related to oral dissolution agents
- Anxiety-related inflammatory disease of gallbladder

1. Risk for injury related to medication during retrograde endoscopy for stone removal

Interventions

- Assessing for signs and symptoms of GI bleeding
- Noting changes in mentation and level of consciousness
- Observing the presence of petechiae, ecchymosis
- Monitoring vital signs
- Using small needles for injections
- Applying pressure to small bleeding
- Avoiding rectal temperature
- Encouraging the use of soft toothbrush, electric razor and avoiding straining for stool
- Recommending avoidance of aspirin-containing products

2. Knowledge deficit related to oral dissolution agents

Interventions
- Informing patient of altered effects of medications and encouraging follow-up
- Assisting patient identifying support person
- Emphasizing the importance of good nutrition
- Avoiding spicy foods and small and frequent meals
- Discussing salt restrictions
- Encouraging scheduling activities with adequate rest periods
- Recommending avoidance of persons with infections

3. Pain related to stone obstruction

Interventions
- Assessing the pain location, severity, and characteristics
- Administering medications or monitoring patient-controlled analgesia
- Assisting in attaining position of comfort and maintaining bed rest

4. Fluid volume deficit related to nausea and vomiting

Interventions
- Administering fluids and electrolytes as ordered
- Administering antiemetic as ordered
- Maintaining NG decompression
- Beginning food and fluids as tolerated by the client

5. Activity intolerance related to fatigue, general discomfort

Interventions
- Encouraging alternating periods of rests and ambulation
- Maintaining some periods of rest
- Encouraging and assist with gradually increasing periods of exercise.

6. Imbalanced nutrition less than body requirement related to pain

Interventions
- Encouraging a diet that is low in residue fiber and fat and high in calories
- Monitoring weight daily
- Providing small frequent meals
- Planning a meal per preference of client and as ordered
- Preparing the patient for element diet
- Restarting oral fluid intake gradually

7. Ineffective coping related to feeling of rejection

Interventions
- Assessing the level of fear and noting nonverbal communication
- Asking the client about usual coping pattern
- Assuring client a close monitoring
- Allowing client to verbalize fear of dying
- Providing diversional materials

Complications

- **Acute cholangitis:** Acute cholecystitis is a condition indicated by a sudden attack of pain in the upper abdomen that lasts more than 12 hours.
- **Acute biliary pancreatitis**
- **Gallstone ileus**

- **Obstructive jaundice or cholestasis**
- **Gallbladder cancer**

LIVER CIRRHOSIS

In cirrhosis of the liver, progressive scarring and fibrosis of the liver cause scar tissue to replace normal liver tissue, which alters the normal architectural structure of liver, which is characterized by scar, distorted, hardened, and lumpy liver surface with nodules.

Etiology and Types

- **Chronic alcoholism:** The amount of alcohol intake is broken down and acts as a toxin, leading to inflammation results in scarring of liver tissue.
- **Autoimmune hepatitis:** This disease appears to be caused by the immune system and inflammatory responses.
- **Inherited or genetic disorder**
- **Bile ducts obstruction:** It happens due to blockage in bile duct flow which damages liver tissue.
- **Drugs and toxin:** Prolonged exposure to drugs and environmental toxins can lead to hepatic cell damage.
- **Chronic hepatitis C:** The hepatitis C virus is a liver infection that is spread by contact with an infected person's blood.
- **Nonalcoholic fatty liver disease:** In this, fat builds up in the liver and eventually causes cirrhosis.

Pathophysiology

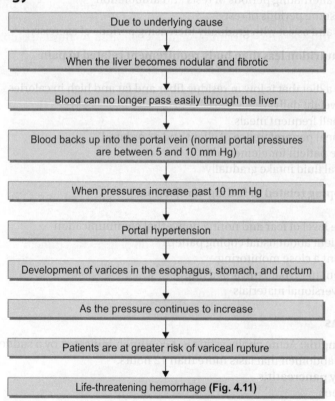

Due to underlying cause

↓

When the liver becomes nodular and fibrotic

↓

Blood can no longer pass easily through the liver

↓

Blood backs up into the portal vein (normal portal pressures are between 5 and 10 mm Hg)

↓

When pressures increase past 10 mm Hg

↓

Portal hypertension

↓

Development of varices in the esophagus, stomach, and rectum

↓

As the pressure continues to increase

↓

Patients are at greater risk of variceal rupture

↓

Life-threatening hemorrhage **(Fig. 4.11)**

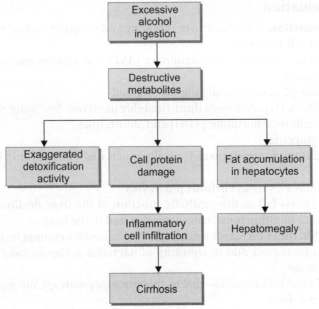

Fig. 4.11: Pathophysiology of cirrhosis.

Signs and Symptoms

- **Spider angiomata:** Vascular lesions consisting of a central arteriole surrounded by many smaller vessels
- **Palmar erythema:** Exaggerations of normal speckled mottling of the palm
- **Nail changes**
- **Muehrcke's lines:** Paired horizontal bands separated by normal color resulting from hypoalbuminemia
- **Terry's nails:** Proximal two-thirds of the nail plate appears white
- **Clubbing:** Angle between the nail plate and proximal nail fold >180°
- **Hypertrophic osteoarthropathy:** Chronic proliferative periostitis of the long bones that can cause considerable pain
- **Dupuytren's contracture:** Thickening and shortening of palmar fascia that leads to flexion deformities of the fingers
- **Gynecomastia**
- **Hypogonadism**
- **Enlarged liver size**
- **Splenomegaly**
- **Ascites**
- **Fetor hepaticus:** Musty odor in breath as a result of increased dimethyl sulfide
- **Jaundice**
- **Asterixis:** Bilateral asynchronous flapping of outstretched, dorsiflexed hands seen in patients with hepatic encephalopathy
- Lack of energy
- Weight loss or sudden weight gain
- Bruises
    - Itchy skin
    - Edema
    - A brownish or orange tint to the urine

Diagnostic Evaluation

- **Physical examination:** A cirrhotic liver is bumpy and irregular instead of smooth
- **Blood tests:** Liver function tests
- Aminotransferases—Aspartate transaminase (AST) and alanine transaminase (ALT) are moderately elevated
  - **Alkaline phosphatase:** Usually slightly elevated
  - **Serum sodium:** Hyponatremia due to inability to excrete free water resulting from high levels of antidiuretic hormone (ADH) and aldosterone.
  - Thrombocytopenia
  - **Gamma-glutamyl transferase:** Typically much higher in chronic liver disease from alcohol.
  - **Bilirubin:** May elevate as cirrhosis progresses
  - **Albumin:** Levels fall as the synthetic function of the liver declines with worsening cirrhosis since albumin is exclusively synthesized in the liver.
  - **Prothrombin time:** Increases since the liver synthesizes clotting factors
  - **Globulins:** Increased due to shunting of bacterial antigens away from the liver to lymphoid tissue
  - Leukopenia and neutropenia—due to splenomegaly with splenic margination
  - Coagulation defects
  - Immunoglobulin levels
- **CT**
- **Endoscopy**
- **Ultrasound**
- **Biopsy.**

Management

The goal of treatment includes:
- Treating the cause of cirrhosis, to prevent further liver damage
- Avoiding substances that may further damage the liver, especially alcohol
- Preventing and treating the symptoms and complications of cirrhosis.

1. **Supportive treatment**
   - Eating a nutritious
   - Avoiding alcohol and other substances.
2. **Medical management**
   - **Diuretics**—for edema
   - **Oral antibiotics** may be prescribed to prevent infection
   - **Beta blocker** or nitrate for portal hypertension
   - **Lactulose**—for cleansing the bowel
   - Interferon.
3. **Surgical management**
   - **Liver transplantation.**
     Prevention of cirrhosis of the liver:
   - It is advised not to abuse alcohol
   - It is better to avoid high-risk sexual behavior.
   - It is necessary to get vaccinated against hepatitis B
   - It is also advised to eat a well-balanced, low-fat diet and take vitamins.
   - It is better to avoid NSAIDs.
   - The patient should be immunized with cirrhosis against infection with hepatitis A and B.

Complications

- Edema and ascites
- Bruising and bleeding
- Portal hypertension
- Esophageal varices
- Splenomegaly
- Jaundice
- Hepatic encephalopathy
- Insulin resistance and type 2 diabetes
- **Liver cancer**

Nursing Care Plan

Nursing Diagnosis

1. Nutrition: imbalanced, less than body requirements related to vomiting secondary to jaundice

Interventions

- Measuring dietary intake by calorie count
- Weighing as indicated
- Assisting and encouraging patient to eat and explain reasons for the types of diet
- Encouraging patient to eat all meals and supplementary feedings
- Encouraging a diet that is low in residue fiber and fat and high in calories
- Monitoring weight daily
- Providing small frequent meals
- Planning a meal per preference of client and as ordered
- Preparing the patient for element diet
- Restarting oral fluid intake gradually
- Recommending and providing small, frequent meals
- Providing salt substitutes; if allowed, avoiding those containing ammonium
- Restricting intake of caffeine, gas-producing or spicy and excessively hot or cold foods
- Suggesting soft foods, avoiding roughage, if indicated
- Encouraging frequent mouth care, especially before meals.

2. Fluid volume excess related to excess sodium and fluid intake

Interventions

- Measuring intake and output chart
- Monitoring BP respiratory status
- Auscultating lungs
- Assisting the healthcare provider with paracentesis
- Measuring and record abdominal girth and body weight daily
- Encouraging the client to elevate the lower extremities
- Administering salt-poor albumin, which temporarily elevates the serum albumin level
- Giving small, frequent meals
- Restricting intake of caffeine
- Measuring dietary intake by calorie count
- Weighing as indicated
- Encouraging patient to eat, explaining reasons for the types of diet
- Measuring abdominal girth

- Encouraging bed rest when ascites is present
- Providing frequent mouth care
- Restricting sodium and fluids as indicated
- Administering salt-free albumin and plasma expanders as indicated

3. Impaired skin integrity related to altered metabolic state and edema

Interventions

- Inspecting skin surfaces and pressure points regularly
- Gently massaging bony prominences
- Encouraging and assisting with repositioning
- Recommending elevating lower extremities
- Suggesting clipping fingernails short
- Encouraging and provide perineal care
- Using alternating pressure mattress
- Applying calamine lotion and providing baking soda baths.

4. Ineffective breathing pattern related to ascites

Interventions

- Monitoring respiratory rate, depth, and effort
- Keeping head of bed elevated
- Encouraging frequent repositioning
- Monitoring temperature
- Monitoring serial arterial blood gases (ABGs), pulse oximetry
- Providing supplemental O_2 as indicated.

5. Risk for injury related to abnormal blood profile

Interventions

- Assessing for signs and symptoms of GI bleeding
- Observing the presence of petechiae, ecchymosis
- Monitoring pulse, BP
- Avoiding rectal temperature
- Encouraging the use of soft toothbrush, electric razor
- Using small needles for injections
- Recommending avoidance of aspirin-containing products
- Administering s tool softeners
- Providing gastric lavage
- Assisting with insertion of GI or esophageal

6. Risk for acute confusion related to liver encephalopathy

Interventions

- Observing changes in behavior and mentation
- Reviewing current medication regimen
- Evaluating sleep and resting schedule
- Reporting deterioration of ability
- Reorienting to time, place, and person
- Maintaining a pleasant, quiet environment
- Providing continuity of care
- Assessing potential for violent behavior
- Maintaining bed rest

- Identifying and providing safety needs
- Investigating temperature elevations
- Monitoring for signs of infection
- Eliminating or restrict protein in diet

7. Disturbed body image and self-esteem related to biophysical changes

Interventions

- Discussing situation and encouraging verbalization of fears and concerns
- Supporting and encouraging patient provide care with a positive, friendly attitude
- Encouraging family to verbalize feelings
- Referring to support services, for example, counselors, psychiatric resources, social service, clergy, and/or alcohol treatment program.

8. Knowledge deficit related to lack of exposure, information misinterpretation

Interventions

- Reviewing disease process and prognosis and future expectations
- Stressing importance of avoiding alcohol
- Giving information about community services
- Inform the client about adverse drug effects
- Assisting client identifying support person
- Emphasizing the importance of good nutrition
- Recommending avoidance of high-protein, salty foods, onions, and strong cheeses
- Providing written dietary instructions
- Discussing sodium and salt substitute restrictions
- Encouraging scheduling activities
- Promoting diversional activities
- Recommending avoidance of persons with infections, especially upper respiratory tract infection
- Identifying environmental dangers

PANCREATITIS

Pancreatitis is an inflammation and potential necrosis of the pancreas. It may be acute or chronic.

Types

1. **Acute pancreatitis:** It ranges from a mild self-limiting disorder to a severe, rapidly fatal disease. It is very sudden and characterized by edema and inflammation confined to the pancreas.
2. **Chronic pancreatitis:** Chronic pancreatitis is an inflammatory disorder characterized by progressive anatomic and functional destruction of the pancreas. It occurs over many years and has multiple causes and painful symptoms.

Etiology

- Certain drugs, antiinflammatory drugs (NSAIDs), and antibiotics
- Infection with mumps, hepatitis virus, rubella
- Pancreatic cancer
- High levels of triglycerides
- Hereditary diseases
- Injury to the abdomen

Pathophysiology

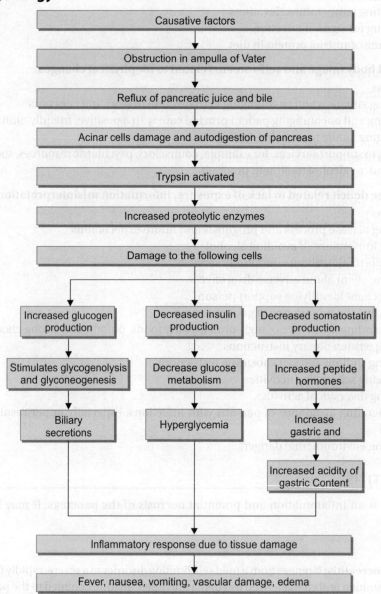

```
                    Causative factors
                           ↓
              Obstruction in ampulla of Vater
                           ↓
            Reflux of pancreatic juice and bile
                           ↓
        Acinar cells damage and autodigestion of pancreas
                           ↓
                   Trypsin activated
                           ↓
             Increased proteolytic enzymes
                           ↓
             Damage to the following cells
```

Increased glucogen production	Decreased insulin production	Decreased somatostatin production
Stimulates glycogenolysis and glyconeogenesis	Decrease glucose metabolism	Increased peptide hormones
Biliary secretions	Hyperglycemia	Increase gastric and
		Increased acidity of gastric Content

```
          Inflammatory response due to tissue damage
                           ↓
      Fever, nausea, vomiting, vascular damage, edema
```

Signs and Symptoms

Acute Pancreatitis

- Severe abdominal pain
- Abdominal tenderness and back pain
- Abdominal distention
- Nausea and vomiting
- Abdominal guarding
- Ecchymosis (bruising) in the flank
- Fever, jaundice, mental confusion

- Hypotension
- Acute renal failure
- Respiratory distress
- Myocardial depression

Chronic Pancreatitis

- Severe upper abdominal and back pain
- Nausea and vomiting
- Weight loss
- Malabsorption
- **Steatorrhea:** The stools become frequent, frothy, and foul-smelling
- Dependence on opioids

Diagnostic Evaluation

- **History of abdominal pain**
- **Physical examination**
- **Diagnostic findings:**
  - Serum amylase and lipase levels are used in making the diagnosis of acute pancreatitis
  - Urinary amylase levels also become elevated
  - The white blood cell count is usually elevated
  - Hematocrit and hemoglobin levels
  - Hypocalcemia
  - The stools of patients with pancreatic disease are often bulky, pale, and foul-smelling
  - Glucose tolerance test
  - X-ray studies
  - Ultrasonography
  - Contrast-enhanced CT scans and MRI
  - Peritoneal fluid examination

Management

Medical Management

Management of the patient with acute pancreatitis is directed toward relieving symptoms and preventing or treating complications.

- Acute pancreatitis may require patient to be admitted to the hospital.
- Nil per orally is maintain to allow the pancreas to rest and stabilize.
- Intravenous fluids and nutrition
- NG suction may be used to relieve nausea and vomiting.

Intensive care

- Correction of fluid and blood loss and low albumin levels to maintain fluid volume
- Prevent renal failure
- Insulin may be required if significant hyperglycemia occurs
- Intubation and mechanical ventilation if required
- Monitor in the intensive care unit
- Antibiotic agents

Pharmacological Management

- **Analgesics:** Morphine
- Antiemetic agents

- Histamine-2 (H2) antagonists
- Antibiotics
- Enzyme supplements, such as pancrelipase
- Probiotic supplement
- Multivitamin daily
- Omega-3 fatty acids

Nutrition and supplements
- Eliminate all suspected food allergens
- Eat foods high in B-vitamins and iron
- Eat antioxidant foods
- Avoid refined foods, such as white breads, pastas, and sugar
- Eat less red meat and more lean meats
- Use healthy oils for cooking
- Eliminate trans-fatty acids
- Avoid coffee and other stimulants, alcohol, and tobacco
- Drink six to eight glasses of filtered water daily
- Exercise moderately daily

Surgical Management

Surgery is required to:
- Remove damaged and infected tissue
- Drain an abscess
- Maintain pancreatic duct patency
- Relief pain in chronic pancreatitis.
    - **Endoscopic retrograde cholangiopancreatography:** In ERCP, a specialist inserts a tube-like instrument through the mouth and down into the duodenum to access the pancreatic and biliary ducts and the gallstones are removed.
    - **Biliary drainage:** Placement of biliary drains (for external drainage) and stents (indwelling tubes) in the pancreatic duct through endoscopy has been performed to reestablish drainage of the pancreas.
    - **Diagnostic laparotomy**
    - **Pancreaticojejunostomy**
    - **Whipple resection (pancreaticoduodenectomy)**
    - **Pancreatectomy:** Total removal or excision of the pancreas
    - **Autotransplantation**
    - **Sphincterotomy**

Nursing Care Plan

Nursing Diagnosis

1. Acute pain related to disease process

Interventions
- Administering opioid analgesics as ordered to control pain
- Assisting patient to a comfortable position
- Maintaining nil per os (NPO) status
- Maintaining patency of NG suction
- Providing frequent oral hygiene and care
- Administering antacids as ordered
- Reporting increase in severity of pain

2. Nutrition: imbalanced, less than body requirements related to vomiting secondary to jaundice

Interventions
- Measuring dietary intake by calorie count
- Weighing as indicated
- Assisting and encouraging patient to eat and explaining reasons for the types of diet
- Encouraging patient to eat all meals and supplementary feedings
- Encouraging a diet that is low in residue fiber and fat and high in calories
- Monitoring weight daily
- Providing small frequent meals
- Planning a meal per preference of client and as ordered
- Preparing the patient for element diet
- Restarting oral fluid intake gradually
- Recommending and providing small, frequent meals
- Providing salt substitutes, if allowed, avoiding those containing ammonium
- Restricting intake of caffeine, gas-producing or spicy and excessively hot or cold foods
- Suggesting soft foods, avoiding roughage if indicated
- Encouraging frequent mouth care, especially before meals

3. Risk for fluid and electrolyte imbalance related to vomiting, self-restricted intake

Interventions
- Monitoring and recording vital signs, skin color, and temperature
- Monitoring intake and output and weight daily
- Evaluating hemoglobin, hematocrit, albumin, calcium, potassium, and sodium levels
- Observing and measuring abdominal girth

4. Ineffective breathing pattern related to severe pain and pulmonary complications.

Interventions
- Assessing respiratory rate and rhythm
- Positioning in upright or semi-Fowler's position
- Administering oxygen supplementation
- Reporting signs of respiratory distress
- Instructing patient in coughing and deep breathing

5. Imbalanced nutrition: Less than body requirements related to malabsorption, and glucose intolerance

Interventions
- Assessing nutritional status
- Administering pancreatic enzyme
- Administering antacids or H_2-receptor antagonists
- Monitoring intake and output and daily weight
- Assessing for GI discomfort with meals and character of stools
- Monitoring blood glucose levels
- Identifying foods that aggravate symptoms and teach low-fat diet

Complications

- Shock
- Hypocalcemia

- High blood glucose
- Dehydration
- Respiratory complications
- Hemorrhagic Pancreatitis
- Pancreatic pseudocysts

INTESTINAL OBSTRUCTION

Intestinal obstruction is an interruption in the normal flow of intestinal contents along the intestinal tract. The obstruction may occur in small intestine or colon and can be partial or complete, may be mechanical or may be paralytic, may/may not comprise the vascular supply.

Etiology

- Inflammation of intestine
- Neoplasms or adhesions of intestine
- Hernia of intestine
- Paralytic ileus

Risk Factors

Mechanical factors: A physical block to passage of intestinal contents without disturbing blood supply of bowel, which includes the following two factors:

1. **Extrinsic**
2. **Intrinsic.**

Extrinsic

- **Adhesions:** These fibrous bands of scar tissue can become looped over a portion of the bowel. The loops can twist and obstruct the bowl by external pressure.
- **Hernia:** An incarcerated hernia may/may not cause obstruction. A strangulated hernia is always obstructed because the bowel cannot function when its blood supply is cut off.
- **Volvulus:** Volvulus is a twisting of the bowel.

Intrinsic

Hematoma, tumor, stricture, or stenosis.

Non-mechanical factor

- **Neurologic factors:** Neurogenic factors are responsible for a dynamic obstruction, also called paralytic ileus, caused by lack of peristaltic activity.
- **Vascular factor:** When the blood supply to any part of the body is interrupted, the part ceases to function and pain occurs.

Other Causes Include

- Spinal cord injuries
- Vertebral fractures
- Postoperatively after any abdominal surgery
- GIT surgery
- Strangulation
- Peritonitis, pneumonia
- Wound dehiscence

Signs and Symptoms

- Crampy pain that is wave like and colicky in character
- The patient may pass blood and mucus but no fecal matter and no flatus
- Crampy, lower abdominal pain
- Fecal vomiting
- Shock
- Constipation
- Vomiting
- Obstruction
- Abdominal distension

Pathophysiology

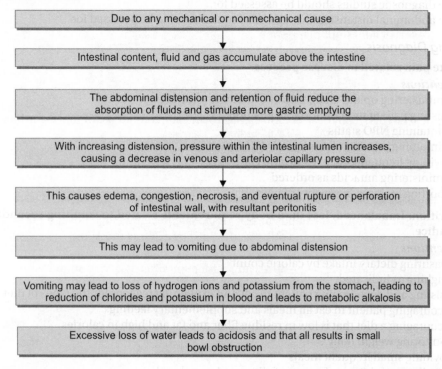

Due to any mechanical or nonmechanical cause

↓

Intestinal content, fluid and gas accumulate above the intestine

↓

The abdominal distension and retention of fluid reduce the absorption of fluids and stimulate more gastric emptying

↓

With increasing distension, pressure within the intestinal lumen increases, causing a decrease in venous and arteriolar capillary pressure

↓

This causes edema, congestion, necrosis, and eventual rupture or perforation of intestinal wall, with resultant peritonitis

↓

This may lead to vomiting due to abdominal distension

↓

Vomiting may lead to loss of hydrogen ions and potassium from the stomach, leading to reduction of chlorides and potassium in blood and leads to metabolic alkalosis

↓

Excessive loss of water leads to acidosis and that all results in small bowl obstruction

Diagnostic Evaluation

- **X-ray studies**
- **Lab studies:** Complete blood cell count electrolytes, and blood urea nitrogen
- **Hematocrit**

Surgical Management

- **Strictureplasty:** In this, the narrowed area of intestine is widened without removing any portion of the small intestine. The surgeon makes a lengthwise incision along the narrowed area and then sews it up crosswise.
- **Small bowel resection:** In this, a segment of the small intestine is removed and the two ends of healthy intestine are joined together.
- **Large bowel resection:** In this, the diseased portion of the colon is removed and the healthy intestine on either side of the removed area is sewn together.

- **Colectomy and proctocolectomy:** If the colon must be removed entirely, but the rectum is unaffected by the disease, a colectomy will be performed. Once the colon is taken out, the ileum will be joined to the rectum. This allows the person to continue to pass stool through the anus. If the rectum is affected and must be removed along with the colon, the surgeon will perform a proctocolectomy with end ileostomy.
- **Total proctocolectomy:** In this surgery, the colon and rectum are removed and the anus is closed.

Nursing Care Plan

Assessment

- The signs and symptoms of abdominal pain should be assessed.
- The history of prolonged constipation should be taken.
- The diagnostic studies should be assessed for.
- The abdominal distension through bowel sounds should be assessed for.

Nursing Diagnosis

1. Acute pain related to disease process

Interventions

- Administering opioid analgesics as ordered to control pain
- Assisting patient to a comfortable position
- Maintaining NPO status
- Maintaining patency of nasogastric (NG) suction
- Providing frequent oral hygiene and care
- Administering antacids as ordered
- Reporting increase in severity of pain

2. Nutrition: Imbalanced, less than body requirements related to vomiting secondary to jaundice

Interventions

- Measuring dietary intake by calorie count
- Weighing as indicated
- Assisting and encouraging patient to eat and explaining reasons for the types of diet
- Encouraging patient to eat all meals and supplementary feedings
- Encouraging a diet that is low in residue fiber and fat and high in calories
- Monitoring weight daily
- Providing small frequent meals
- Planning a meal per preference of client and as ordered
- Preparing the patient for element diet
- Restarting oral fluid intake gradually
- Recommending and providing small, frequent meals
- Providing salt substitutes, if allowed, avoiding those containing ammonium
- Restricting intake of caffeine, gas-producing or spicy and excessively hot or cold foods
- Suggesting soft foods, avoiding roughage, if indicated
- Encouraging frequent mouth care, especially before meals.

3. Ineffective breathing pattern related to abdominal distension, interfering with normal lung expansion

Interventions

- Keeping the patient in Fowler's position to promote ventilation
- Providing oxygenation to the patient
- Monitoring ABG level for oxygenation to decompress

4. Risk for fluid and electrolyte imbalance related to vomiting, self-restricted intake

Interventions

- Monitoring and recording vital signs, skin color, and temperature
- Monitoring intake and output and weight daily
- Evaluating hemoglobin, hematocrit, albumin, calcium, potassium, and sodium levels
- Observe and measure abdominal girth

5. Diarrhea related to obstruction

Interventions

- Collecting stool sample for test for occult blood if occur
- Maintaining adequate fluid balance
- Recording and amount of consistency of stools
- Maintaining NG tube as prescribed to decompress bowel.

Nonsurgical Treatment

- Introducing colonoscope for the removal of polyps and dilated strictures
- Correction of fluid and electrolyte imbalances with normal saline or Ringer's solution with potassium as required
- NG suction to decompress bowel
- Treatment of shock and peritonitis
- Topical negative pressure (TNP) therapy is the application of negative pressure across a wound to aid wound healing. The pressure is thought to aid the drainage of excess fluid, reduce infection rates and increase localized blood flow.
- Analgesics and sedative
- Ambulation for the patients with paralytic ileus

Complications

- Dehydration due loss of water, sodium, and chloride
- Peritonitis
- Shock due to lass of electrolyte and dehydration
- Death due to shock

CROHN'S DISEASE

Crohn's disease is a chronic idiopathic inflammatory disease that can affect any part of GI system commonly the small intestine and large intestines that is characterized by ulceration, swelling and scarring of the part of intestine.

Etiology

- Idiopathic
- Family history of inflammatory bowel disease
- Immune system disorders
- Genetics

Types

- Crohn's colitis is inflammation that is confined to the colon.
- Crohn's enteritis refers to inflammation confined to the small intestine.
- Crohn's terminal ileitis is inflammation that affects only the very end of the small intestine (terminal ileum).

- Crohn's enterocolitis and ileocolitis are the terms to describe inflammation that involve both the small intestine and the colon.

Pathophysiology

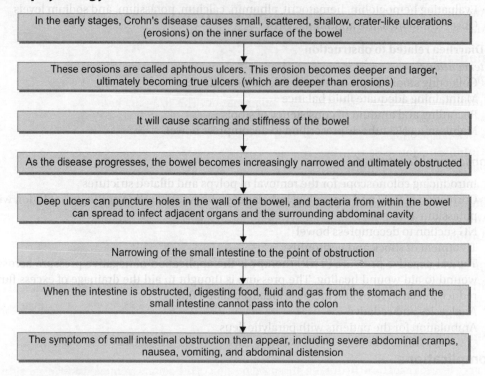

In the early stages, Crohn's disease causes small, scattered, shallow, crater-like ulcerations (erosions) on the inner surface of the bowel

↓

These erosions are called aphthous ulcers. This erosion becomes deeper and larger, ultimately becoming true ulcers (which are deeper than erosions)

↓

It will cause scarring and stiffness of the bowel

↓

As the disease progresses, the bowel becomes increasingly narrowed and ultimately obstructed

↓

Deep ulcers can puncture holes in the wall of the bowel, and bacteria from within the bowel can spread to infect adjacent organs and the surrounding abdominal cavity

↓

Narrowing of the small intestine to the point of obstruction

↓

When the intestine is obstructed, digesting food, fluid and gas from the stomach and the small intestine cannot pass into the colon

↓

The symptoms of small intestinal obstruction then appear, including severe abdominal cramps, nausea, vomiting, and abdominal distension

Signs and Symptoms

- Swelling of the tissue of the anal sphincter colon that controls defecation
- Ulcers and fissures within the anal sphincter
- Anal fistulae between the anus or rectum
- Perirectal abscesses

Diagnostic Evaluation

- **Laboratory blood tests:** CBC
- **Colonoscopy**
- **Computerized axial tomography**
- **Video capsule endoscopy (VCE): VCE** has also been added to the list of tests for diagnosing Crohn's disease. For VCE, a capsule containing a miniature video camera is swallowed. As the capsule travels through the small intestine, it sends video images of the lining of the small intestine to a receiver carried on a belt at the waist. The images are downloaded and then reviewed on a computer.
- **Stool test**
- Barium enema

Complications

- Bowel strictures
- Nutritional deficiencies

- Growth retardation
- Delayed puberty
- Formation of fistulas
- Loss of weight
- Anemia
- Massive intestinal bleeding

Management
Medical Management

- **Immunosuppressant**—to reduce the inflammation. This drugs includes
  - Azathioprine
  - Cyclosporine
- **Aminosalicylates:** Balsalazine
- **Corticosteroids:** Prednisolone
- **Corticosteroids (rectal):** Hydrocortisone
- **Immune modifiers:** 6-mercaptourine
- **Monoclonal antibodies:** Infliximab reduces inflammation
- **Antibiotics:** Metronidazole

Surgical Management

- **Strictureplasty:** In this, the narrowed area of intestine is widened without removing any portion of the small intestine. The surgeon makes a lengthwise incision along the narrowed area and then sews it up crosswise.
- **Small bowel resection:** In this, a segment of the small intestine is removed and the two ends of healthy intestine are joined together.
- **Large bowel resection:** In this, the diseased portion of the colon is removed and the healthy intestine on either side of the removed area is sewn together.
- **Colectomy and proctocolectomy:** If the colon must be removed entirely, but the rectum is unaffected by the disease, a colectomy will be performed. Once the colon is taken out, the ileum will be joined to the rectum. This allows the person to continue to pass stool through the anus.

  If the rectum is affected and must be removed along with the colon, the surgeon will perform a proctocolectomy with end ileostomy.
- **Total proctocolectomy:** In this surgery, the colon and rectum are removed and the anus is closed.

  Dietary recommendations are to
  - Eat regularly, not to skip meals
  - Have small, frequent meals that are best
  - Avoid spicy foods
  - Recommend high-potassium foods

Nursing Care Plan

The goal of nursing management is:
- To control the inflammatory process
- To relieve symptoms
- To correct metabolic and nutritional problems and promote healing
- To achieve the previous health status

Nursing Diagnosis

- Diarrhea related to inflamed intestinal mucosa
- Chronic pain related inflammatory disease of small intestine
- Imbalanced nutrition less than body requirement related to pain
- Deficit fluid volume related to diarrhea
- Ineffective coping related to feeling of rejection

1. Diarrhea related to inflamed intestinal mucosa

Interventions

- Antidiarrheal medications
- Monitoring the number and consistency of stools
- Perineal care
- Reporting reduction in frequency of stools, return to more normal stool consistency
- Identifying and avoiding contributing factors
- Promoting bed rest and providing bedside commode

2. Deficit fluid volume related to diarrhea

Interventions

- Monitoring intake and output chart
- Providing fluids as prescribed
- Monitoring electrolytes and acid-base balance because diarrhea can lead to metabolic acidosis
- Watching for cardiac dysrhythmias and muscular weakness

3. Acute pain related to disease process

Interventions

- Administering opioid analgesics as ordered to control pain
- Assisting patient to a comfortable position
- Maintaining NPO status
- Maintaining patency of NG suction
- Providing frequent oral hygiene and care
- Administering antacids as ordered
- Reporting increase in severity of pain

4. Nutrition: Imbalanced, less than body requirements related to vomiting secondary to jaundice

Interventions

- Measuring dietary intake by calorie count
- Weighing as indicated
- Assisting and encouraging patient to eat and explain reasons for the types of diet
- Encouraging patient to eat all meals and supplementary feedings
- Encouraging a diet that is low in residue fiber and fat and high in calories
- Monitoring weight daily
- Providing small frequent meals
- Planning a meal per preference of client and as ordered
- Preparing the patient for element diet
- Restarting oral fluid intake gradually

- Recommending and providing small, frequent meals
- Providing salt substitutes, if allowed, avoiding those containing ammonium
- Restricting intake of caffeine, gas-producing or spicy and excessively hot or cold foods
- Suggesting soft foods, avoiding roughage, if indicated
- Encouraging frequent mouth care, especially before meals

5. Ineffective coping related to feeling of rejection
Interventions

- Offering understanding concern and encouragement
- Facilitating supportive psychological counseling if appropriate
- Encouraging the patients usual support people to be involved in management of disease
- Encouraging health promoting behavior

Health Education

- Comprehensive education should be provided about anatomy and physiology of GI system.
- Client should be instructed about all prescribed medications, including the purpose, dosage, and adverse effects.
- The client should be encouraged to participate in stress reducing activities.
- Nutrition and dietary considerations need to be discussed.
- Regular follow-up should be encouraged and signs of complications should be reported.
- The importance of adequate hydration and nutrition monitoring weight should be explained.
- If the client is on medications, instruction should be given regarding the dose, when and how to take the drug.
- Regular follow-up should be encouraged and signs of complications should be reported.

ABDOMINAL HERNIA

An abdominal hernia occurs when there is a tear in the inner lining of the abdominal wall causing a bulge in the abdominal wall where the organs protrude.

Etiology and Risk Factors

- A chronic cough
- Obesity
- Straining
- Pregnancy
- Straining to lift heavy objects
- Persistent sneezing
- Prolonged seating or standing

Signs and Symptoms

The main sign of an abdominal hernia is a bulge or swelling appearing on a part of abdomen.

Types of Abdominal Hernia

The following are different types of abdominal hernia:

1. **Inguinal hernia:** When a male's testicles descend into the scrotum, this causes a naturally weakened area in the wall of the abdomen, called the internal ring.
2. **Epigastric hernia:** This type of hernia occurs as a result of a weakness in the muscles of the upper middle abdomen, above the navel.
3. **Indirect inguinal hernia:** An indirect inguinal hernia is the most common type of inguinal hernia. It occurs at the internal ring in the groin area. The intestine drops down into the internal ring and can extend down into the scrotum in men or to the outer folds of the vagina in women.
4. **Direct inguinal hernia:** Less common than an indirect inguinal hernia, a direct inguinal hernia occurs near the internal ring instead of within it.
5. **Femoral hernia:** Femoral hernias occur just below the inguinal ligament, when abdominal contents pass into the weak area at the posterior wall of the femoral canal.
6. **Incisional hernia:** An incisional hernia occurs when the defect is the result of an incompletely healed surgical wound.
7. **Diaphragmatic hernia:** Higher in the abdomen, diaphragmatic hernia results when part of the stomach or intestine protrudes into the chest cavity through a defect in the diaphragm.
8. **Umbilical hernia:** It involves protrusion of intra-abdominal contents through a weakness at the site of passage of the umbilical cord through the abdominal wall.

Diagnostic Evaluations

- Taking history
- Physical examination
- Examining the bulge or swelling
- Ultrasound scan
- X-ray
- CT scan

Management

Nonsurgical Treatment

1. **Trusses**

   There are two kinds of trusses for hernias, the spring truss and the umbilical truss. The spring truss is worn around the waist and acts as a support, while the umbilical truss is worn around the midsection. Trusses also come in different sizes and are usually worn under briefs.

2. **Hernia belts**

   Hernia belts are lightweight and made so that movement is not restricted while you are recovering. These belts were designed to be worn over briefs, are made with adjustable straps and are lined with foam for extra comfort. The foam compression pads provide gradual pressure and support to the weakened muscles.

3. **Bindings**

   Abdominal bindings are made of elastic and provide uniform compression and support of the abdominal muscles. They can be fastened around the waist.

4. **Hernia briefs**

   Hernia briefs look like regular briefs except they are made with spandex and foam pads for extra support and are designed to provide rupture relief.

Surgical treatment: Surgery of hernia can be performed through various approaches:

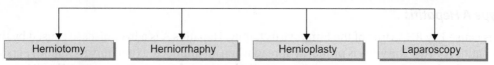

1. **Herniotomy** (removal of the hernial sac only)
2. **Herniorrhaphy** (herniotomy plus repair of the posterior wall of the inguinal canal)
3. **Hernioplasty** (reinforcement of the posterior inguinal canal wall with a synthetic mesh).

HEPATITIS

Hepatitis is a viral infection of the liver associated with a broad spectrum of nonsymptom-producing infection through icteric hepatitis to hepatic necrosis.

Viral hepatitis is a systemic, viral infection in which necrosis and inflammation of liver cells produce a characteristics cluster of clinical, biochemical, and cellular changes. There are five definite types of viral hepatitis have been identified, hepatitis A, B, C, D, and E. Hepatitis A and E are similar in mode of transmission, whereas hepatitis B, C, and D share many characteristics.

Pathophysiology

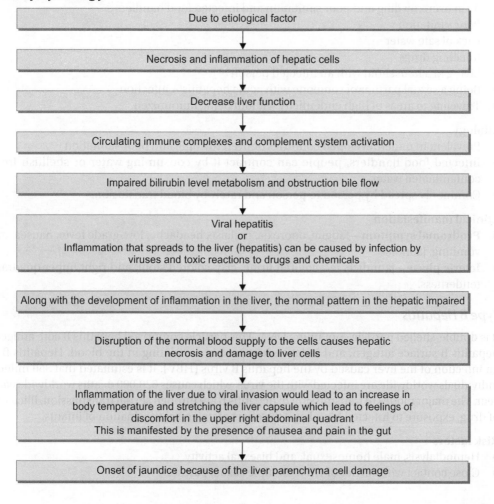

Types of Hepatitis

Type A Hepatitis

It is caused by RNA virus of the Enterovirus family. Hepatitis A is a liver disease caused by the hepatitis A virus. The virus is primarily spread when an uninfected (and unvaccinated) person ingests food or water that is contaminated with the feces of an infected person. The disease is closely associated with a lack of safe water, inadequate sanitation, and poor personal hygiene. Unlike hepatitis B and C, hepatitis A infection does not cause chronic liver disease and is rarely fatal, but it can cause debilitating symptoms and fulminant hepatitis (acute liver failure), which is associated with high mortality. Hepatitis A occurs sporadically and in epidemics worldwide, with a tendency for cyclic recurrences. Every year there are an estimated 1.4 million cases of hepatitis A worldwide.

Modes of transmission
- This is primarily fecal–oral, usually through ingestion of food or liquid contaminated with virus.
- The virus has been found in the stool of infected patient.
- Children acquire the infection at school by poor hygiene, hand-to-mouth contact.

Risk factors
- As in overcrowding and poor sanitation and infected food handlers
- Poor sanitation
- Lack of safe water
- Injecting drugs
- Living in a household with an infected person
- Being a sexual partner of someone with acute hepatitis A infection
- Traveling to areas of high endemicity without being immunized.

Etiology
- Prevalent in underdeveloped countries or overcrowding and poor sanitation
- Infected food handlers, people can contract it by consuming water or shellfish from contaminated water
- Commonly spread by person to person and rarely by blood transfusion.

Clinical manifestation
- **Prodromal symptom**—fatigue, anorexia, malaise, headache, low-grade fever, nausea and vomiting, jaundice
- **Icteric phase**—jaundice, tea-colored urine, clay-colored stool, and right upper quadrant tenderness.

Type B Hepatitis

It is double-shelled particle containing DNA. This particle comprised hepatitis B core antigen, hepatitis B surface antigen, and independent protein circulating in the blood. Hepatitis B is an infection of the liver caused by the hepatitis B virus (HBV). It is estimated that 350 million individuals worldwide are infected with the virus, which causes 620,000 deaths worldwide each year. The major modes of transmission of hepatitis B are through sexual transmission, illicit use of drug, exposure to infected blood and the effect of universal vaccination of infants.

Risk factors
- Hemodialysis, male homosexual, and bisexual activity
- Close contact with carrier of HBV, multiple sexual partner

- Receipt of blood or blood products, recent history of sexual transmitted disease
- Frequent exposure to blood or blood products

Modes of transmission
- It is primarily through blood and oral route through saliva or through breastfeeding.
- Sexual activity through blood—semen, saliva or vagina secretions
- Gay men are high at risk
- Multiple sexual partners.

Clinical manifestation
- One week to 2 months of prodromal symptoms appear.
- Extrahepatic manifestation may include photophobia, arthritis, urticaria, maculopapular eruptions, skin rashes, and vacuities.
- Jaundice in icteric phase.
- In rare cases, it may progress to fulminant hepatitis of hepatic failure.
- It may become chronic active or chronic persistent hepatitis.

Type C Hepatitis

It was formerly called non-A, non-B hepatitis, an RNA virus.

Risk factors
- Receipt of blood product, health care, and safety workers after needle stick injury
- Children born to women infected with hepatitis C virus
- Past treatment with chronic hemodialysis, sex with infected partners, history of STD
- Unprotected sex

Modes of transmission
- In most cases through blood or blood product, as through blood transfusion
- IV drugs users and renal dialysis patients, sexual intercourse
- Through piercing, and tattooing and ink

Clinical manifestation
Similar to those associated with HBV but usually less severe. Symptom usually occurs 6–7 weeks after transfusion, but may be attributed to another viral infection and not diagnosed as hepatitis.

Type D Hepatitis (Delta Hepatitis)

Hepatitis D virus is a defective RNA agent that appears to replicate only with the HBV. It requires HBsAg to replicate, occurs along with HBV, or may superinfect a chronic HBV carrier. It cannot outlast a hepatitis B infection and may be acute or chronic. Hepatitis D or delta hepatitis is caused by the hepatitis delta virus (HDV), a defective RNA virus.

Risk factors
- Chronic HBV carriers are at risk for infection with HDV.
- Individuals, who are not infected with HBV and have not been immunized against HBV, are at risk of infection with HBV with simultaneous or subsequent infection with HDV.
- Since HDV absolutely requires the support of a hepadnavirus for its own replication, inoculation with HDV in the absence of HBV will not cause hepatitis D. Alone, the viral genome indeed replicates in a helper-independent manner, but virus particles are not released.

Modes of transmission

Transmission is similar to that of HBV:

- Blood-borne and sexual
- Percutaneous (injecting drug use)
- Permucosal (sexual)
- Perinatal

Clinical manifestation

It is similar to HBV but more severe.

With superinfection of chronic HBV carriers, it causes sudden worsening of condition and rapid progression of cirrhosis.

Type E Hepatitis

A single identified no enveloped single strand RNA virus.

Modes of transmission

The hepatitis E virus is transmitted mainly through the fecal–oral route due to fecal contamination of drinking water. Other transmission routes have been identified, which include:

- Food-borne transmission from ingestion of products derived from infected animals
- Zoonotic transmission from animals to humans
- Transfusion of infected blood products
- Vertical transmission from a pregnant woman to her fetus.

Although humans are considered the natural host for the hepatitis E virus, antibodies to the hepatitis E virus or closely related viruses have been detected in primates and several other animal species.

Hepatitis E is a water-borne disease, and contaminated water or food supplies have been implicated in major outbreaks. The ingestion of raw or uncooked shellfish has also been identified as the source of sporadic cases in endemic areas.

The risk factors for hepatitis E are related to poor sanitation in large areas of the world and shedding of the hepatitis E virus in feces.

Signs and Symptom

- Jaundice (yellow discoloration of the skin and sclera of the eyes, dark urine and pale stools)
- Anorexia
- Hepatomegaly
- Abdominal pain and tenderness
- Nausea and vomiting
- Fever

Diagnostic Evaluation

- Elevated serum transferase levels AST, ALT of all form of hepatitis.
- Radioimmunoassay that reveal immunoglobulin M antibodies to hepatitis virus in the acute phase of HAV.
- Radioimmunoassay to include HBsAg, anti-HBc, anti-HBsAg detected in various stages of HBV.
- Hepatitis C antibody may not be detected for 3–6 months after onset of HCV illness, antibody test used for screening purpose.
- Polymerase chain reaction test to confirm viral activity in HIV illness

- Anti-delta antibodies of ABsAg for HDV or detection of IgM in acute disease and IgG in chronic disease
- Hepatitis E antigen
- Liver biopsy to detect chronic active disease, progression, and response to therapy.

Hepatitis B infection is diagnosed with blood tests. These tests can detect pieces of the virus in the blood (antigens), antibodies against the virus, and viral DNA (viral load). Blood tests for HBV are often done when routine blood work shows abnormal liver function tests or in patients who are at an increased risk for exposure. If a patient has had a large amount of vomiting or has not been able to take in liquids, blood electrolytes may also be checked to ensure that the patient's blood chemistry is in balance.

- X-rays and other diagnostic images are needed only in very unusual circumstances.
- **CT scan or ultrasound:** These diagnostic imaging tests are used to detect the extent of liver damage and may also detect cancer of the liver caused by chronic hepatitis B.
- **Liver biopsy:** This involves removal of a tiny piece of the liver. It is usually done by inserting a long needle into the liver and withdrawing the tissue. The tissue is examined under a microscope to detect changes in the liver. A biopsy may be done to detect the extent of liver damage or to evaluate how well a treatment is working.

Self-Care at Home

The goals of self-care are to relieve symptoms and prevent worsening of the disease.

- Plenty of fluids should be consumed to prevent dehydration. Although, broth, sports drinks, gelatin, frozen ice treats, and fruit juices may be better because they also provide calories.
- It is necessary to consult with physician before taking any medications, even those that are over-the-counter. Some medications depend on the liver, and liver damage may impair the body's ability to metabolize these drugs. If you are on prescription medications, check with your physician to see if the doses should be adjusted or if the medication should be temporarily discontinued.
- Alcohol needs to be avoided until your healthcare practitioner allows it. Individuals with chronic HBV should avoid alcohol for the rest of their lives.
- It is advised to eat a diet that provides adequate nutrition. Take it easy. It may take some time for your energy level to return to normal.
- Prolonged, vigorous exercise should be avoided until symptoms start to improve.
- It is necessary to ask healthcare practitioner for advice if your condition worsens or new symptoms appear.
- Any activity that may spread the infection to other people (sexual intercourse, sharing needles, etc.) should be avoided.

Management

- Rest according to patient level of fatigue
- Therapeutic measures to control dyspeptic symptom and malaise.
- Hospitalization for protracted nausea and vomiting
- Small, frequent feeding of high calories, low-fat diet, and proteins are restricted when liver cannot metabolize protein by products
- Vitamin K injected subcutaneous (SC) if prothrombin time (PT) is prolonged
- IV fluids and electrolyte replacement is indicated
- Antiemetic drugs are administered
- After jaundice has cleared gradual increase in physical activity

Active immunization: A hepatitis B vaccine prepared from plasma of humans chronically infected with HBV is used only rarely and in patient who are immunodeficient or allergic to recombinant yeast derived vaccines. It provides active immunity. The need for booster doses may be revisited if reports of hepatitis B increase prevalence of carrier state develops, indicating the protection is declining. Vaccines are administered IM in three doses, the second and third dose 1 and 6 months after the first dose. The third dose is very important in provide long immunity. It should be administered in deltoid muscle in adults. Antibody response may be measured by anti-HBs levels 1–3 months after completing the basic course of vaccine.

Passive immunity: Hepatitis B immune globulin provides passive immunity to hepatitis B and is indicated for people exposed to HBV who have never had hepatitis B and have never received hepatitis B vaccine.

Indication: Inadvertent exposure to HBAg-positive blood through percutaneous or transmural routes, sexual contact with people positive for HBAg, perinatal exposure. Hepatitis B immune globulin (HBIG), which provides passive immunity, is prepared from plasma selected from high titers of anti-HBs. Both active and passive immunization are recommended for people exposed to hepatitis B through sexual contact or through percutaneous routes.

Pharmacological Intervention

Hepatitis B medications: All of the following medications described that are used to treat chronic hepatitis B are antiviral medications. They reduce the ability of the virus to reproduce in the body and give the liver a chance to heal it. These drugs are not a cure for hepatitis B, but they do reduce the damage caused by the virus.

- Pegylated interferon alfa-2b
  - Pegylated interferon is used alone or in combination with other medications.
  - Pegylated interferon slows the replication of the virus and boosts the body's immune system to fight the infection.
  - It works best in people who have relatively low levels of HBV DNA (low viral load).
  - Pegylated interferon usually is not given to people whose liver damage has progressed to cirrhosis, because it can make the liver damage worse.
  - Treatment is often given for 48 weeks, which is shorter than for other medications, but pegylated interferon requires regular shots (injections) while other medications are taken orally.
  - Pegylated interferon has unpleasant side effects in many people. The side effects are similar to having the flu. For many people, side effects are so severe that they cannot continue taking the medication.
  - Liver function tests and HBV DNA tests are used to check how well the treatment is working.
  - Interferon appears to stop the liver damage in up to 40% of people although relapse is possible.
- **Nucleoside/nucleotide analogs (NAs):** NAs are compounds that mimic normal building blocks for DNA. When the virus tries to use the analogs, it is unable to make new viral particles. For example, adefovir (Hepsera), entecavir (Baraclude), lamivudine (Epivir-HBV, Heptovir, Heptodin), telbivudine (Tyzeka), and tenofovir (Viread).
  - NAs reduce the amount of virus in the body. Between 20% and 90% of patients may have levels reduced so far that they become undetectable. Obviously, this is a broad range. The higher success rates are achieved in patients who do not have "hepatitis B

e-antigen" (HBeAg). HBeAg is detected by a blood test and indicates that the virus is actively multiplying.

- Side effects are less common than with pegylated interferon. NAs have been associated with changes in body fat distribution, reduced blood cell counts, and increased levels of lactic acid in the blood. Rarely, NAs are associated with a severe flare of hepatitis that can be serious or fatal.
- HBV may become resistant to NAs over time.
- NAs do not cure the infection. Relapse is possible even in patients who have had a good response to treatment.

Dietary Management of Viral or Drug-induced Hepatitis

- Small frequent meals should be recommended.
- Intake of 20,000–3,000 kcal/day should be provided during acute illness.
- High-protein, high-calorie diet may be beneficial, so patient should not be forced to take food and be restricted to fat intake.
- Fluid balance should be carefully monitored.
- Patient should be instructed to abstain from alcohol during acute illness and for 6 months after recovery.
- Patient should be advised to avoid substances (medication, herbs, drugs, and toxins), which may affect liver function.

Preventive Measures

Hepatitis A

- Washing hands with soap after going to the toilet
- Consuming only food that has just been cooked
- Drinking only commercially bottled water, or boiled water if you unsure of local sanitation
- Eating only fruits that you can peel if you are somewhere where sanitation is unreliable
- Eating only raw vegetables if you are sure they have been cleaned/disinfected thoroughly
- Getting a vaccine for hepatitis A if you travel to places where hepatitis may be endemic.

Hepatitis B

- Telling the partner if you are a carrier or try to find out whether he/she is a carrier
- Practicing safe sex
- Using only clean syringes that have not been used by anyone else
- Avoid sharing toothbrushes, razors, or manicure instruments
- Having a hepatitis B series of shots if you are at risk
- Allow only well-sterilized skin perforating equipment (tattoo, acupuncture, etc.).

Hepatitis C

- If anybody is infected, he/she must not share his/her toothbrush, razor, and manicure equipment.
- If anybody is infected, he/she should cover his/her open wounds.
- It is advised not to share needles, toothbrushes, or manicure equipment.
- If the skin is to be pierced, equipment should be well sterilized (tattoo, etc.).
- The consumption of alcohol should be avoided.
- Drug equipment must not be shared.

Hepatitis D

Same guidelines should be followed as for hepatitis B. Only a person who is infected with hepatitis B can become infected with hepatitis D.

Hepatitis E

- Maintaining quality standards for public water supplies
- Establishing proper disposal systems to eliminate sanitary waste
- Maintaining hygienic practices, such as handwashing with safe water, particularly before handling food.
- Avoiding drinking water or ice of unknown purity.
- Avoiding eating uncooked shellfish, and uncooked fruits or vegetables that are not peeled or that are prepared by people living in or traveling in highly endemic countries.

NONVIRAL HEPATITIS

Certain chemicals have toxic effects on the liver and produce acute liver cell necrosis or toxic hepatitis when inhaled, injected parenterally or are taken by mouth. The chemicals most commonly implicated in this disease are carbon tetrachloride, phosphorus, chloroform, and gold compounds. These substances are true hepatotoxins.

Toxic Hepatitis

It resembles the viral hepatitis. Obtaining the history of exposure to hepatotoxic chemicals, medications, or other toxic agents assists in early treatment and removal of causative agent.

Symptoms: Anorexia, nausea, and vomiting are usual symptoms; jaundice and hepatomegaly are noted in physical assessment, fever.

Treatment: Therapy is to maintain fluid and electrolyte balance, blood replacement, comfort and supportive measures.

Drug-induced Hepatitis

This liver disease is most common cause of acute liver failure.

Symptoms: Chills, fever, rash, pruritus, arthralgia, anorexia, and nausea. Later may produce symptom jaundice, dark urine, or enlarged or tender liver.

Treatment: The use of medication should be stopped, a short course of high-dose corticosteroids may be used in patients with severe hypersensitivity reactions. Liver transplantation is an option for drug-induced hepatitis, but outcomes may not be as successful as with other causes of liver failure.

Fulminant Hepatitis

Acute liver failure or fulminant hepatitis is a rare, but potentially fatal disease. Fulminant liver failure is acute necrosis of liver cell without preexisting liver disease, resulting inability of liver to perform its many functions.

Etiology: Viral hepatitis is common cause. Poisons, chemicals, such as acetaminophen, tetracycline, isoniazid, methyldopa, may cause liver disease.

- Ischemia and hypoxia because of hepatic vascular occlusion, hypovolemic shock, acute circulatory failure, septic shock, and heat stroke.
- Other cause includes hepatic vein obstruction, acute fatty liver of pregnancy, autoimmune hepatitis, partial hepatectomy, complication of liver transplantation.
- Progression of hepatocellular injury and necrosis with development of encephalopathy.

Clinical Features

- Malaise, anorexia, nausea, vomiting, fatigue, jaundice, urine is tea colored and frothy when shaken
- Purities caused by bile salts deposited in skin
- Steatorrhea and diarrhea because of decrease of fat absorption, peripheral edema as fluid move from intravascular to interstitial spaces, secondary to hypoproteinemia.
- Ascites from hypoproteinmia or portal hypertension
- Easy bruising, petechiae, overt bleeding because of clotting deficiency
- Altered level of consciousness (LOC), ranging from irritability and confusion to stupor, somnolence and coma
- Change in tendon reflexes—initially hyperactive become flaccid, tremor.
- Breath odor of acetone and portal systemic encephalopathy, also known as hepatic coma
- Cerebral edema as cause of death because of brain stem herniation.

Diagnostic Evaluation

- Prolonged PT, decreased platelets count
- Elevated ammonia, amino acid levels
- Hypoglycemia or hyperglycemia

Management

- Oral or rectal administration of lactulose to minimize formation of ammonia and other nitrogenous byproducts in bowel.
- Rectal administration of neomycin to suppress urea-splitting enteric bacteria in the bowel and decrease ammonia formation.
- Low molecular weight or albumin followed by potassium sparing diuretic (spironolactone) to enhance fluid shift from interstitial back to intravascular spaces.
- Pancreatic enzymes, if diarrhea and steatorrhea.

Complications

- Encephalopathy and cerebral edema
- Sepsis
- Gastrointestinal bleeding
- Renal failure
- Hemodynamic complications.

Nursing Care Plan

Nursing Assessment

- Assess for systemic and liver related symptom.
- Obtain history, such as IV drug use, sexual activity, ingestion of possible contaminated food or water to assess for any mode of transmission of virus.
- Assess size and shape of liver to detect enlargement or characteristics of cirrhosis.
- Obtain vital history, including temperature.

Nursing Diagnosis

- Imbalanced nutrition less than body requirement related to effects of liver dysfunction
- Deficient fluid volume related to nausea and vomiting

- Activity intolerance related to anorexia and liver dysfunction
- Deficient knowledge related to transmission

1. Imbalanced nutrition less than body requirement related to effects of liver dysfunction
Interventions
- Encouraging frequent small feedings of high-calorie, low-fat diet
- Encouraging eating meal in sitting position to decrease pressure in liver
- Encouraging taking pleasing meal in the environment with noxious stimuli
- Administering antiemetic drug to patient

2. Deficient fluid volume related to nausea and vomiting
Interventions
- Providing frequent oral fluid as tolerated
- Administering IV fluids for patient with inability to maintain oral fluids
- Monitoring intake and output

3. Activity intolerance related to anorexia and liver dysfunction
Interventions
- Promoting periods of rest during symptom-producing phase
- Promoting comfort by administering the analgesic to patient
- Providing emotional support and diversional activities when recovery is prolonged
- Encouraging gradual resumption of activities and mild exercise during convalescent period.

4. Knowledge deficit regarding transmission of disease related to lack of exposure of health services and information
Interventions
- Encouraging specific protection for close contacts immune globin and hepatitis B immune globin, followed by HBV vaccine series
- Explaining precautions to patient and family about transmission and prevention of transmission to others.
- Good handwashing and maintaining hygiene
- Avoidance of sexual activity
- Avoidance of sharing needles and toothbrushes to prevent blood or body fluid contact.

MULTIPLE CHOICE QUESTIONS

1. **Persons with celiac disease cannot tolerate:**
   A. Gluten
   B. Lactose
   C. Peanuts
   D. Eggs

2. **GERD is a risk factor for the development of:**
   A. Celiac disease
   B. Biliary atresia
   C. Barrett's esophagus
   D. Inguinal hernia

3. **Risk factors for hepatitis A include all of the following, *except*:**
   A. Men who have sex with men
   B. Illegal drug users
   C. Overweight
   D. Persons who visit developing countries

4. **Interferon is prescribed for the treatment of:**
   A. Hepatitis A
   B. Chronic hepatitis B
   C. GERD
   D. Diverticulitis

5. **Persons of Jewish heritage are disproportionately affected by:**
   A. Barrett's esophagus
   B. Diverticulosis
   C. Appendicitis
   D. Crohn's disease

6. **Which of the following conditions usually is asymptomatic?**
   A. Diverticulitis
   B. Crohn's disease
   C. Inflammatory bowel disease
   D. Diverticulosis

7. **Bowel diversion surgery may be indicated for all of the following conditions, *except*:**
   A. Gastroparesis
   B. Cancer
   C. Inflammatory bowel disease
   D. Bowel obstruction

8. **The most frequent cause of abdominal adhesions is:**
   A. Abdominal surgery
   B. Gastroenteritis
   C. Hepatitis A
   D. Hepatitis B

9. **The most frequent cause of emergency abdominal surgery is:**
   A. Inflammatory bowel disease
   B. Appendicitis
   C. Viral gastroenteritis
   D. Barrett's esophagus

10. **Abdominal pain associated with appendicitis is generally described as:**
    A. Near the diaphragm
    B. Relieved by eating
    C. Near or around the umbilicus and in the right lower quadrant of the abdomen
    D. Worse in the morning

11. **Physical examination of a patient with acute appendicitis may reveal all of the following, *except*:**
    A. Guarding
    B. Rectal bleeding
    C. Rebound tenderness
    D. Rovsing's sign

12. **Symptoms of ulcerative colitis may include abdominal pain, rectal bleeding, diarrhea, and all of the following, *except*:**
    A. Anemia
    B. Weight loss
    C. Joint pain
    D. Bradycardia

13. **Peptic ulcers may be caused by all of the following, *except*:**
    A. Emotional stress and eating spicy foods
    B. Bacterial infection with *Helicobacter pylori*
    C. Long-term use of nonsteroidal anti-inflammatory agents (NSAIDs)
    D. Malignant tumors in the stomach or pancreas

14. **All of the following are symptoms of peptic ulcer, *except*:**
    A. Pain is relieved by eating
    B. Pain is unrelenting and quickly worsens
    C. Pain is relieved by antacids
    D. Pain occurs at night when the stomach is empty

15. **Which of the following symptoms is not associated with dyspepsia?**
    A. Feeling overly full after a normal meal
    B. Mild to severe epigastric pain
    C. Black tarry stools
    D. Epigastric burning sensations

16. **In the United States, the most common causes of hepatitis C are:**
    A. Wilson disease, cystic fibrosis, and glycogen storage diseases
    B. Alpha-1 antitrypsin deficiency and hemochromatosis
    C. Chronic hepatitis B and D
    D. Excessive alcohol consumption, hepatitis C, and obesity

17. Food-borne illness associated with eating raw and undercooked eggs is generally attributable to:
   A. *Campylobacter jejuni*
   B. *Listeria monocytogenes*
   C. *Salmonella* enteritidis
   D. *Clostridium botulinum*

18. About 80% of gallstones are composed of:
   A. Calcium
   B. Bile
   C. Bilirubin
   D. Hardened cholesterol

19. Persons at risk for gallstones include all of the following, *except*:
   A. Adults age 60 and older
   B. Pregnant women or women using hormone replacement therapy or oral contraceptives
   C. Native Americans and Mexican Americans
   D. People with rheumatoid or osteoarthritis

20. Disorders that increase risk for chronic pancreatitis include all of the following, *except*:
   A. Cystic fibrosis
   B. Hypercalcemia
   C. Excessive alcohol consumption
   D. Hyperthyroidism

Answers

1. A 2. C 3. C 4. B 5. D 6. D 7. A 8. A 9. B 10. C
11. D 12. D 13. A 14. B 15. C 16. D 17. C 18. D 19. D 20. D

Cardiovascular Disorders

REVIEW OF ANATOMY AND PHYSIOLOGY OF HEART

The heart is a muscular organ about the size of a closed fist that functions as the body's circulatory pump. It takes in deoxygenated blood through the veins and delivers it to the lungs for oxygenation before pumping it into the various arteries (which provide oxygen and nutrients to body tissues by transporting the blood throughout the body). The heart is located in the thoracic cavity medial to the lungs and posterior to the sternum **(Fig. 5.1)**.

Structure of the Heart Wall

The heart wall is made up of three layers: epicardium, myocardium, and endocardium.

1. **Epicardium:** The epicardium is the outermost layer of the heart wall and is just another name for the visceral layer of the pericardium. Thus, the epicardium is a thin layer of serous membrane that helps to lubricate and protect the outside of the heart. Below the epicardium is the second, thicker layer of the heart wall: the myocardium.

2. **Myocardium:** The myocardium is the muscular middle layer of the heart wall that contains the **cardiac muscle tissue**. Myocardium makes up the majority of the thickness and mass of the heart wall and is the part of the heart responsible for pumping blood. Below the myocardium is the thin endocardium layer.

3. **Endocardium:** Endocardium is the simple squamous endothelium layer that lines the inside of the heart. The endocardium is very smooth and is responsible for keeping blood from sticking to the inside of the heart and forming potentially deadly blood clots.

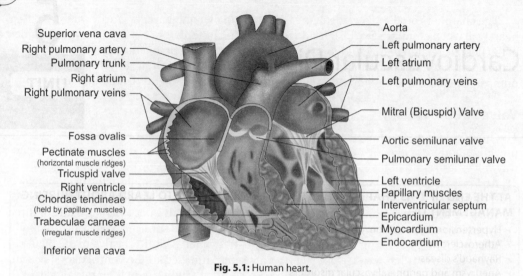

Superior vena cava
Right pulmonary artery
Pulmonary trunk
Right atrium
Right pulmonary veins

Fossa ovalis
Pectinate muscles
(horizontal muscle ridges)
Tricuspid valve
Right ventricle
Chordae tendineae
(held by papillary muscles)
Trabeculae carneae
(irregular muscle ridges)
Inferior vena cava

Aorta
Left pulmonary artery
Left atrium
Left pulmonary veins

Mitral (Bicuspid) Valve

Aortic semilunar valve
Pulmonary semilunar valve

Left ventricle
Papillary muscles
Interventricular septum
Epicardium
Myocardium
Endocardium

Fig. 5.1: Human heart.

The thickness of the heart wall varies in different parts of the heart. The atria of the heart have a very thin myocardium because they do not need to pump blood very far—only to the nearby ventricles. The ventricles, on the other hand, have a very thick myocardium to pump blood to the lungs or throughout the entire body. The right side of the heart has less myocardium in its walls than the left side because the left side has to pump blood through the entire body, while the right side only has to pump to the lungs **(Fig. 5.2)**.

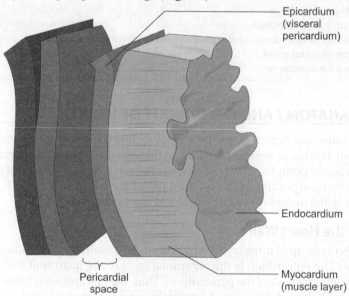

Epicardium
(visceral
pericardium)

Endocardium

Pericardial
space

Myocardium
(muscle layer)

Fig. 5.2: Layers of heart.

Chambers of the Heart

The heart contains four chambers—the right atrium, left atrium, right ventricle, and left ventricle. The atria are smaller than the ventricles and have thinner, less muscular walls than the ventricles. The atria act as receiving chambers for blood, so they are connected to the veins that carry blood to the heart. The ventricles are the larger, stronger pumping chambers that send blood out of the heart. The ventricles are connected to the arteries that carry blood away from the heart.

The chambers on the right side of the heart are smaller and have less myocardium in their heart wall when compared to the left side of the heart. This difference in size between the sides of the heart is related to their functions and the size of the two circulatory loops. The right side of the heart maintains pulmonary circulation to the nearby lungs, while the left side of the heart pumps blood all the way to the extremities of the body in the systemic circulatory loop.

Valves of the Heart

The heart functions by pumping blood both to the lungs and to the systems of the body. To prevent blood from flowing backward or "regurgitating" back into the heart, a system of one-way valves is present in the heart. The heart valves can be broken down into two types:

1. **Atrioventricular (AV) valves:** The AV valves are located in the middle of the heart between the atria and ventricles and only allow blood to flow from the atria into the ventricles. The AV valve on the right side of the heart is called the **tricuspid valve** because it is made of three cusps (flaps) that separate to allow blood to pass through and connect to block regurgitation of blood. The AV valve on the left side of the heart is called the **mitral valve** or the bicuspid valve because it has two cusps. The AV valves are attached to the ventricular side with tough strings called **chordae tendineae**. The chordae tendineae pull on the AV valves to keep them from folding backward and allowing blood to regurgitate past them. During the contraction of the ventricles, the AV valves look like domed parachutes with the chordae tendineae acting as the ropes holding the parachutes taut.
2. **Semilunar valves:** The semilunar valves, so named for the crescent moon shape of their cusps, are located between the ventricles and the arteries that carry blood away from the heart. The semilunar valve on the right side of the heart is the **pulmonary valve**, so named because it prevents the backflow of blood from the pulmonary trunk into the right ventricle. The semilunar valve on the left side of the heart is the **aortic valve**, named for the fact that it prevents the **aorta** from regurgitating blood back into the left ventricle. The semilunar valves are smaller than the AV valves and do not have chordae tendineae to hold them in place. Instead, the cusps of the semilunar valves are cup shaped to catch regurgitating blood and use the blood's pressure to snap shut.

CARDIOVASCULAR ASSESSMENT

An intensive and focused cardiovascular assessment indicates a potential cardiovascular problem.
1. **Past health history:** The past health history should collect relevant history of previous health history of hypertension, elevated blood cholesterol heart murmurs, congenital heart disease, rheumatic fever or unexplained joint pains, and cardiac surgeries.
2. **Current lifestyle and psychosocial status:** Current lifestyle and psychosocial issues include:
   - **Nutrition:** Dietary pattern should be determined. Body weight and any recent weight gain or weight loss should be assessed.
   - **Smoking:** Any smoking habits should be informed.
   - **Alcohol:** The quantity of alcohol the patient normally consumes daily should be recorded.
   - **Exercise:** Activity level and exercise regimen should be considered.
   - **Drugs:** Medication history should be queried.
3. **Family history:** Any history of hypertension, obesity, diabetes, coronary artery disease (CAD), or sudden death should be queried.
4. **Assessment of chest pain:** The following characteristics of pain should be informed:
   - Quality of pain: Is it punching, squeezing, throbbing, or chest heaviness?
   - Radiation of pain: If pain radiates toward left side, left arm, left jaw, or left scapula should be queried.
   - Severity: On a scale of 1–10.

- It should be queried about what worsens the pain, such as cold, emotional stress, or sexual activity.
5. **Orthopnea:** Orthopnea is the inability to breathe when in a lying position. Whether the client feels the same during sleep should be asked.
6. **Cough:** History of consistent cough, frequency, timing, or severity should be queried.
7. **Edema, cyanosis, and pallor:** Whether any swelling or skin color changes should be enquired—whether it is cyanosis or pallor.
8. **Physical examination:**
   - **Inspection:** When inspecting the neck vessels, abnormalities in jugular venous pulse should be looked for. Central venous pressure and the cardiac output (CO) are estimated.
   - **Auscultation:** The carotid arteries should be auscultated. The presence of a bruit, which is a blowing or swishing sound, indicating turbulent blood flow should be assessed for. blood pressure (BP) should be auscultated for.
   - **Palpation:** Palpation allows you to assess the neck for tenderness, abnormal temperature, excessive moisture, pulsations, or abnormal masses. The carotid arteries are to be palpated in order to feel the contour and amplitude of the pulse. Also the peripheral arteries, such as brachial, radial, femoral, and popliteal should be palpated.
9. **Heart sounds:** The heart sounds and murmurs should be auscultated.
   - S1 is accelerated during exercise, anemia, hyperthyroidism, and mitral stenosis, while it is diminished in first-degree heart block. S1 split is most audible in tricuspid area.
   - Splitting of S2 sound can occur during pulmonic stenosis, left bundle branch block, atrial septal defect, and right ventricular failure.
   - S3 is produced by the rapid filling of the ventricle and is normal in pregnancy and in children.
   - S4 is typically heard in late diastole before S1 due to decreased ventricular compliance.

DISORDERS OF CARDIOVASCULAR SYSTEM

CORONARY ARTERY DISEASE

CAD is characterized by atherosclerosis in the coronary arteries, which results in progressively narrowing of the coronary artery lumen and minimizes myocardial blood flow. The plaque becomes thick, calcified, and solid causing obstruction in coronary blood flow **(Fig. 5.3)**.

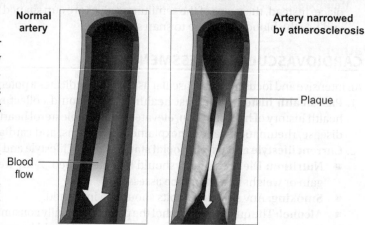

Fig. 5.3: Fatty streak formation in coronary artery.

Etiology and Risk Factors

- **Nonmodifiable major risk factors are as follows:**
  1. **Heredity:** Children whose parents had heart disease, hypertension, and diabetes are at higher risk of CAD.
  2. **Advance age:** People older than 40 are at greater risk.
  3. **Gender:** Men are at higher risk for heart attacks at younger ages. However, the risk for women increases significantly at menopause.

- **Modifiable major risk factors are as follows:**
  1. **Cigarette and smoking:** Both active and passive smoking have been strongly implicated as a risk factor in the development of CAD.
  2. **Hypertension:** High BP increases the workload of cardiac muscles by increasing stroke volume, enlarging and weakening the left ventricle muscles, hence increase the chances of CAD.
  3. **Elevated serum cholesterol level:** The risk of CAD increases as blood cholesterol level increases.
  4. **Physical inactivity:** Those who exercise reduce their risk of CAD.
  5. **Obesity:** Obesity elevates serum cholesterol and triglyceride levels.
  6. **Diabetes:** Patients with diabetes have a two- to eight-fold higher prevalence, incidence and mortality.

Contributing Factors

- **Response to stress:** Stress is associated with elevated BP; hence, it contributes to CAD.
- **Inflammatory responses:**

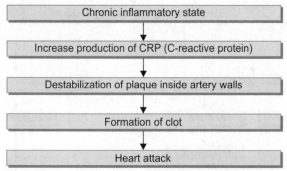

- **Menopause:** The incidence of coronary heart disease (CHD) increases among women after menopause.

Pathophysiology

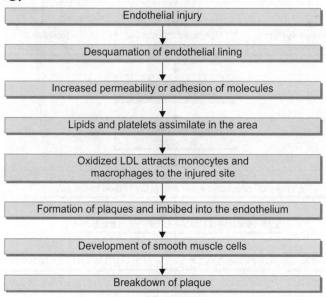

Contd...

Contd...

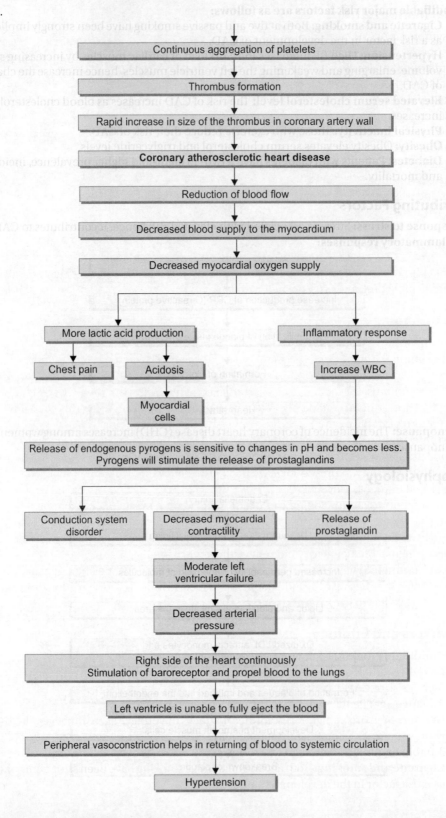

Continuous aggregation of platelets

↓

Thrombus formation

↓

Rapid increase in size of the thrombus in coronary artery wall

↓

Coronary atherosclerotic heart disease

↓

Reduction of blood flow

↓

Decreased blood supply to the myocardium

↓

Decreased myocardial oxygen supply

More lactic acid production | Inflammatory response

Chest pain | Acidosis | Increase WBC

Myocardial cells

Release of endogenous pyrogens is sensitive to changes in pH and becomes less. Pyrogens will stimulate the release of prostaglandins

Conduction system disorder | Decreased myocardial contractility | Release of prostaglandin

Moderate left ventricular failure

↓

Decreased arterial pressure

↓

Right side of the heart continuously Stimulation of baroreceptor and propel blood to the lungs

↓

Left ventricle is unable to fully eject the blood

↓

Peripheral vasoconstriction helps in returning of blood to systemic circulation

↓

Hypertension

Clinical Manifestations

Other symptoms of CAD include:

- Dyspnea
- Palpitations
- Weakness
- Nausea
- Discomfort, pressure and pain in the chest, left arm
- Discomfort radiating to the back, jaw, throat, or left arm
- Choking feeling
- Sweating
- Nausea, vomiting
- Extreme weakness
- Arrhythmias

ANGINA PECTORIS

Angina is pain in the chest that occurs during activity or rest, after having heavy meals, or at other predictable time and is associated with CAD.

Types of Angina

Types of angina are as follows:

1. **Stable angina:** Angina pectoris is said to be stable when its pattern of frequency, intensity, does not change over a period of several weeks. Sublingual nitroglycerin is required to relieve symptoms. It occurs during exertional activity.
2. **Accelerating angina:** Angina pectoris is said to be accelerating when there is a change in the pattern of stable angina.
3. **Unstable angina:** Unstable angina occurs during rest or during minimal activity. Unstable angina usually is related to the rupture of an atherosclerotic plaque and the abrupt narrowing of a coronary artery, representing a medical emergency and will not be relieved by rest or sublingual nitroglycerine.
4. **Variant angina:** Variant angina can occur while resting or sleeping. It can be relieved by taking sublingual nitroglycerine.
5. **Microvascular angina:** Microvascular angina can be more severe and last longer than other types of angina. Medicine may not relieve this type of angina.
6. **Decubitus angina:** It is a type of chest pain occurs in lying down position. It usually occurs at night. It occurs because the fluid in the body is redistributed in this position due to gravity and the heart has to work harder.

Risk Factors and Etiology

- **Nonmodifiable major risk factors are as follows:**
  1. **Heredity:** Children whose parents had heart disease, hypertension and diabetes are at higher risk of CAD.
  2. **Advance age:** People older than 40 are at greater risk.
  3. **Gender:** Men are at higher risk for heart attacks at younger ages. However, the risk for women increases significantly at menopause.
- **Modifiable major risk factors are as follows:**
  1. **Cigarette and smoking:** Both active and passive smoking have been strongly implicated as a risk factor in the development of CAD.

2. **Hypertension:** High BP increases the workload of cardiac muscles by increasing stroke volume, enlarging and weakening the left ventricle muscles, hence increase the chances of CAD.

3. **Elevated serum cholesterol level:** The risk of CAD increases as blood cholesterol level increases.

4. **Physical inactivity:** Those who exercise reduce their risk of CAD.

5. **Obesity:** Obesity elevates serum cholesterol and triglyceride levels, high BP, and diabetes so contributes to CAD.

6. **Diabetes:** Patients with diabetes have a two- to eight-fold higher prevalence, incidence and mortality.

Pathophysiology

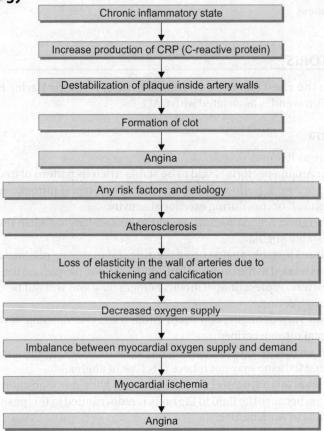

Chronic inflammatory state

↓

Increase production of CRP (C-reactive protein)

↓

Destabilization of plaque inside artery walls

↓

Formation of clot

↓

Angina

Any risk factors and etiology

↓

Atherosclerosis

↓

Loss of elasticity in the wall of arteries due to thickening and calcification

↓

Decreased oxygen supply

↓

Imbalance between myocardial oxygen supply and demand

↓

Myocardial ischemia

↓

Angina

Diagnostic Evaluation

History

The history should include:

- Any current symptoms
- An inventory of cardiac risk factors
- Family history
- Character and location of pain

Physical Examination

- Evaluation should include measurements of BP and the ankle-brachial index.

- Examination of the carotid arteries
- Examination of the chest wall, neck, and shoulders
- Cardiac auscultation
- Assessment of the abdominal aorta for an aneurysm
- Palpation of all peripheral pulses

Diagnostic and Imaging Studies

- Electrocardiography (further elaborated in this chapter).
- Chest radiograph.
- Cardiac computed tomography (CT) angiography
- **Echocardiography:** Echocardiography is recommended for patients with stable angina and physical findings suggesting valvular heart disease.
- **Laboratory studies:** Routine laboratory measurements recommended as a part of the initial evaluation of patients with CAD should include determination of fasting glucose and fasting lipid levels, C-reactive protein (CRP).
- **Stress testing:** Stress testing is another method for determining the presence of flow-limiting, functionally significant CAD. It can be done by two ways—treadmill or pharmacological method. During exercise, a higher rate pressure product and therefore greater cardiovascular workload can be obtained. The most common pharmacologic agent used for nonexercise stress testing is dobutamine.

Contraindications to Exercise Stress Testing

Absolute contraindications
❖ Acute MI within 2 days
❖ Symptomatic or severe aortic stenosis
❖ Acute aortic dissection
❖ Acute myocarditis or pericarditis
❖ Decompensated heart failure
❖ Cardiac arrhythmias
❖ Unstable angina
❖ Acute pulmonary embolus

- Coronary arteriography or catheterization (explained further with **Percutaneous Transluminal Coronary Angioplasty**).

Treatment and Management

Once a cardiac catheterization has been performed, the four most common therapeutic options are:
- Lifestyle modification
- Pharmacological therapy
- Surgical management
  - Percutaneous coronary intervention
  - Coronary artery bypass graft (CABG)

Nonpharmacological Therapy

Lifestyle modification
- Quit smoking
- Regular exercise
- Weight control

Pharmacological Therapy

- **Antiplatelet agents:** Aspirin
- **Antianginal agents:** Beta blockers, calcium channel blockers, and nitrates are the mainstays of antianginal therapy.

Surgical Management: Revascularization

The primary revascularization options are percutaneous coronary intervention (PCI) and coronary artery bypass grafting (CABG) surgery.

Percutaneous Transluminal Coronary Angioplasty

It is performed to open blocked coronary arteries caused by CAD to restore arterial blood flow to the heart tissue without open-heart surgery. It involves the following steps:

- A special catheter is inserted into the coronary artery with a small balloon at the tip.
- Once the catheter is placed into the coronary artery, the balloon is then inflated.
- The inflation of the balloon compresses the plaque and improves blood flow.
- Fluoroscope is used to find the location of blockages in the coronary arteries.
- A small sample of cardiac tissue can also be taken for further examination for any abnormality.
- Intravascular ultrasound waves are used to visualize and measure the size of the clot.
- Atherectomy is also done during same time to break the hard plaque.
- Atherectomy is used when the plaque is calcified and hardened. It is done with the help of a laser, which opens the artery by "vaporizing" the plaque **(Figs. 5.4A and B)**.

Coronary Artery bypass Graft Surgery

- CABG surgery is a procedure used to treat CAD.
- A graft of blood vessel from femoral vein is used to treat the blocked arteries.

Risks of the Procedure

Possible risks associated with CABG surgery include **(Fig. 5.5)**:

- Hemorrhage
- Coagulopathy

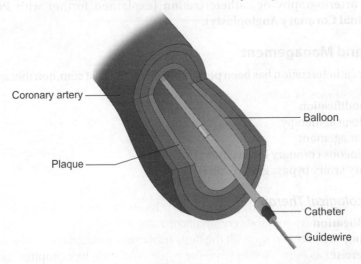

Inflation of balloon inside a coronary artery

Coronary artery

Balloon

Plaque

Catheter

Guidewire

Fig. 5.4A

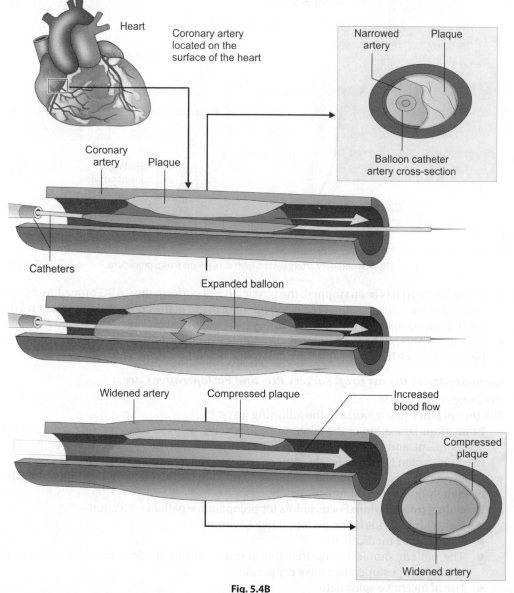

Fig. 5.4B
Figs. 5.4A and B: Percutaneous transluminal coronary angioplasty (PTCA).

- Sepsis
- Pneumonia
- Respiratory problem
- Cardiac dysrhythmias.

Procedure

- CABG is a very delicate procedure so the heart has to be stopped during the procedure, in order to sew the grafts onto the very small coronary arteries.
- The blood can be pumped through the body by a cardiopulmonary bypass machine.
- Once the blood has been diverted into the bypass machine for pumping, the heart will be stopped by injecting it with a cold solution.

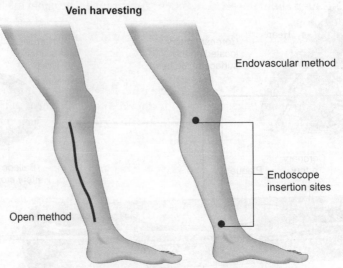

Fig. 5.5: Coronary artery bypass graft surgery-on-pump procedure.

- When the heart has been stopped, the physician will perform the CABG procedure by tying one end of a section of vein over a small opening made in the aorta, and the other end over a tiny opening made in the coronary artery just below the blockage.
- Once the CABG has been completed, the blood circulating through the bypass machine will be allowed back into heart and the tubes to the machine will be removed.

Coronary Artery Bypass Graft Surgery Pre- and Postoperative Care

The Preoperative Phase

The preoperative phase works in the following ways:

- **Education:** Education of the client prior to surgery helps in recovery, increases patient's contentment, and decreases postoperative complications. Appropriate timing of preoperative preparation is helpful for the patient's information retention.
- **Assessment:** It is important for the nurse to provide the information regarding procedure in a timely manner to minimize anxiety.
- **Providing information:** Focus points for preoperative patient education—
  - Sights and sounds in the perioperative environment
  - Preoperative medications
  - The patient should be assured that a nurse will be in close proximity during the immediate postoperative recovery period.
  - Use of incentive spirometer
  - Insertion of monitoring lines
  - Length of the operation
  - Client should be informed that an ET will probably be in place postoperatively, resulting in a temporary inability to speak
  - The client should be assured that the ET will be removed.
  - Expectations related to postoperative phase
  - Pain control
  - Communication with client during the intraoperative period is helpful to minimize anxiety
  - Pulmonary care is an important part of the postoperative care for the client after CABG surgery.
  - Teaching coughing exercise
  - Early mobilization is effective in improving postoperative pulmonary complications

- Teaching them about the expected client appearance. The client may appear pale, cool, and edematous.
- The nurse should also discuss equipment that will be connected to the client.

The Intraoperative Phase

The intraoperative phase should be as follows:
- Insertion of an intravenous (IV) catheter, an arterial line, and a pulmonary artery catheter.
- After the insertion of the invasive lines, anesthesia will be administered.
- After the patient is anesthetized, there will be a head-to-toe surgical preparation.
- Insert urinary catheter after anesthesia.
- Heparin is administered to promote anticoagulation.
- The client may receive protamine to reverse the heparin at the end of the operation.

The Postoperative Phase

- It is essential for the nurse to assess for the possible complications so that appropriate interventions can be started immediately.
- The operating room nurse and the anesthesiologist report the patient's condition to the receiving nurse.
- A history of smoking, chronic obstructive pulmonary disease (COPD), steroid use, gastro-esophageal reflux disease (GERD), heart failure, and poor nutrition may increase postoperative pulmonary complications.
- Routine postoperative care to promote oxygenation and ventilation involves prevention and treatment of atelectasis and pulmonary infection.
- Nurse should be conscious about atelectasis. Atelectasis can be related to cardiopulmonary bypass, surfactant inhibition, and stimulation of the inflammatory response.

Postoperative management includes:
- Accurate and frequent physical assessment
- Arterial blood gas analysis
- Continuous pulse oximetry
- Intubation and incentive spirometry
- Early mobilization
- Control of pain and shivering
- Pain control is usually achieved with IV narcotics
- The nurse must assess the client for early extubation
- Physical assessment must be done with laboratory analysis of arterial blood gases
- During the weaning process, the nurse should assess the client's respiratory and heart rates.

Postoperative management of hemodynamics: Transfer of the client from the operating room to the recovery room can create hemodynamic instability.
- The client should be assessed for cardiac dysfunction and hemodynamic instability.
- The receiving nurse must monitor heart rhythm and rate, preload, afterload, contractility, and myocardial compliance to achieve this outcome.
- BP must be maintained.
- The nurse must monitor right atrial pressure and pulmonary capillary wedge pressure.
- Fluid volume must be replaced with a colloid solution unless the hematocrit is low and then volume may be replaced with packed red blood cells.
- Dopamine or dobutamine can be used if BP and cardiac output (CO) are low.
- Trendelenburg position can relief hypotension, especially in the early postoperative phase.
- Nitroprusside is administered to lower the BP to the ordered parameter. Nitroglycerine, a nitrate, may also be used to cause vasodilation and lower the BP.
- The nurse must rewarm the patient after surgery if hypothermia persists.
- Rewarming may be accomplished by the use of warm blankets, warm humidified oxygen.

Postoperative management of hemorrhage:
- Clients who are on anticoagulants and antiplatelet drugs before surgery are at a risk of postoperative bleeding; therefore sites for bleeding, such as the chest wall, and chest tube must be assessed.
- Administration of heparin can all contribute to postoperative bleeding.
- The nurse should be aware that heparin can be stored in adipose tissue and some clients may have an increase in bleeding 4 hours postoperatively.
- IV infusion of aprotinin intraoperatively should be done to minimize the risk of postoperative bleeding.
- The nurse should monitor the client for signs of bleeding from the chest tubes and the surgical sites.
- Hemoglobin and hematocrit should be monitored at regular intervals during the postoperative period.
- Protamine sulfate can be used to reverse the effects of heparin.
- Blood products, such as fresh frozen plasma and platelets may also be ordered.

Postoperative neurologic management:
- Stroke can be a complication of an embolic event during or after surgery.
- Pupils should be assessed initially.
- A motor and sensory assessment should also be performed.
- Before the extubation, client should follow commands and have equal movement and strength of the extremities.
- The nurse should do neurologic assessment in the postoperative period.
- The nurse should provide needed comfort but not give false hope.
- A positive result is a good indication that an intraoperative stroke can be ruled out.

Postoperative renal management:
- Renal insufficiency may be related to advanced age, hypertension, and diabetes.
- The nurse must monitor the urinary output at least hourly during the early postoperative period.
- The urine should be assessed for color and characteristics as well as for amount.
- One indicator of effective CO is adequate renal perfusion as evidenced by urinary output of at least.
- The client's potassium level should be monitored at least every 4–6 hours for the first 24 hours.
- Diuresis is likely in the postoperative period when renal function is adequate, as the fluids mobilize from the interstitial to the intravascular space.
- IV potassium replacement should be administered if needed.

Postoperative gastrointestinal management:
- Some risk factors for gastrointestinal (GI) dysfunction include age over 70, a history of GI disease, and a history of alcohol misuse and smoking.
- The nurse should monitor the client for bowel sounds and abdominal distention.
- If the gastroepiploic artery is used as a conduit for bypass, this may also increase the risk of GI dysfunction.
- When the NG tube is removed, the client will be started on a clear liquid diet.
- The intubated patient will have an NG tube to low intermittent suction.
- Placement and patency should be assessed as well as amount, color, and characteristics of the drainage.
- The presence of bowel sounds prior to extubation should be assessed.
- Anesthetic agents and analgesics can also contribute to GI dysfunction.
- The nurse should administer antiemetic agents.

Postoperative pain management:
- Manipulation of the chest cavity, positioning on the operating room table and length of time of the surgery, use of retractors during surgery, and electrocautery may all contribute to postoperative pain.
- The nurse should evaluate the effectiveness of pain management interventions regularly.
- Nurses must do pain assessment.
- Poorly controlled pain can stimulate the sympathetic nervous system that results in cardiovascular problems.
- Pain control management is essential for comfort, hemodynamic stability, and prevention of pulmonary complications.
- Analgesics, relaxation techniques, and proper positioning are used for pain control.
- Keeping serum levels of opioid analgesics in the therapeutic range.
- Teaching the patient to splint the incision when coughing and moving minimize pain.

Postoperative management of infection:
- Risk factors for infection include diabetes, malnutrition, chronic diseases, and patients requiring emergent surgery or prolonged surgery.
- Regular dressings should be done.
- Control of blood glucose level may help with prevention of infection.
- Corticosteroids can be used postoperatively.
- Regular assessment for local and systemic infection must be done.
- Postoperative antibiotics should be administered.
- Clients need to be taught how to slowly discontinue the medication after discharge per physician orders.

Additional postoperative management:
- This intensive monitoring and postoperative discomfort can interfere with the patient's need for sleep; intervention must be done to enhance sound sleep.
- Hospital routines should be maintained and too many visits should be avoided to minimize the sleep deprivation problem.
- A balance should be there between the need for rest and sleep.
- Therapeutic touch postoperatively and giving reassurance to patient are important.

Nursing Care Plan

1. **Acute pain related to an imbalance of oxygen supply to myocardial demands.**
   Interventions
   - Assessing pain location, duration, radiation
   - Reviewing the history of previous activities that provoke chest pain
   - Creating a 12-lead electrocardiogram (ECG)
   - Administering oxygen therapy, if necessary
   - Giving analgesics as ordered
   - Maintaining a rest period
   - Checking vital signs
2. **Decreased CO related to poor myocardial contraction.**
   Interventions
   - Maintaining bed rest
   - Elevating head at 30°
   - Assessing and monitoring vital signs
   - Monitoring and recording ECG

3. **Anxiety related to the needs of the body is threatened.**
   Interventions
   - Assessing signs and verbal expressions of anxiety
   - Taking action to reduce anxiety by creating a calm environment
   - Encouraging patients to express feelings
   - Accompanying patient during periods of high anxiety
   - Providing an explanation of procedures and treatment
   - Referring to the spiritual adviser if necessary

4. **Activity intolerance related to conduction problem as evidenced by tachycardia.**
   Interventions
   - Checking the vital signs of the patient
   - Checking for the activity level of the patient
   - Providing small activity
   - Involving in activities of daily living
   - Avoiding staining activity

CARDIOMYOPATHY

Cardiomyopathy is weakening of the heart muscle which is characterized by cardiomegaly, heart failure, endocarditis, or other heart problems.

Causes and Types

There are three types of cardiomyopathy:

1. Dilated
2. Restrictive
3. Hypertrophic

1. **Dilated cardiomyopathy** is a condition characterized by week heart muscles and hypertrophy of chambers.

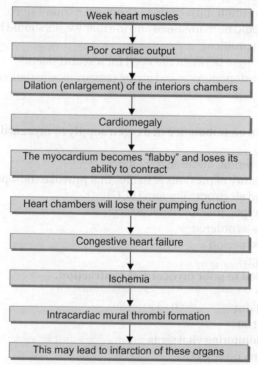

Week heart muscles

↓

Poor cardiac output

↓

Dilation (enlargement) of the interiors chambers

↓

Cardiomegaly

↓

The myocardium becomes "flabby" and loses its ability to contract

↓

Heart chambers will lose their pumping function

↓

Congestive heart failure

↓

Ischemia

↓

Intracardiac mural thrombi formation

↓

This may lead to infarction of these organs

2. **Hypertrophic cardiomyopathy** is a condition in which the heart muscle becomes thick.

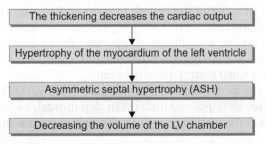

3. **Restrictive cardiomyopathy** is a group of disorders. Restrictive cardiomyopathy can either be idiopathic or can be caused by diseases that deposit abnormal substances within the myocardium. The classic example is amyloidosis, whereby the abnormal amyloid protein accumulates within the myocardium resulting in stiffness.

Clinical Manifestation

- Breathlessness
- Fatigue
- Pounding or fluttering heartbeat
- Dizziness
- Swelling of the legs, ankles, and feet
- Bloating of the abdomen
- Chest pain
- Palpitations
- Fainting

Diagnostic Evaluation

- Blood culture [complete blood count (CBC)]
- Chest X-ray
- CT scan of the chest
- Echocardiogram
- ECG

Treatment and Management

- Defibrillator
- A pacemaker
- CABG
- Heart transplantation

Pharmacological Management

- Angiotensin-converting enzyme (ACE), such as enalapril
- Angiotensin receptor blockers, such as losartan
- Beta blockers
- Digoxin increases the strength of your heart muscle contractions
- Diuretics

Surgical Management

1. **Septal myectomy:** In this the thickened, overgrown heart muscle wall is removed. It improves blood flow and reduces mitral regurgitation.
2. **Pacemaker implantation:** A small battery-operated device that helps the heart beat in a regular rhythm. There are two parts: a generator and wires (leads).
   a. The generator is a small battery-powered unit.
   b. It produces the electrical impulses that stimulate your heart to beat.
   c. The generator may be implanted under your skin through a small incision.
   d. The generator is connected to your heart through tiny wires that are implanted at the same time.
   e. The impulses flow through these leads to your heart and are timed to flow at regular intervals just as impulses from your heart's natural pacemaker would.
3. **Implantable cardioverter defibrillator:** This is a pager-sized device implanted in chest, such as a pacemaker. It provides electrical shocks to restore a normal heart rhythm.
4. **Septal alcohol ablation:** In this, a small portion of the thickened heart muscle is destroyed by injecting alcohol through a catheter into the artery supplying blood to it.
5. **Heart transplant:** The first operation is harvesting the heart from the donor. The donor is usually an unfortunate person who has suffered irreversible brain injury, called "brain death".

   The second operation is removing the recipient's damaged heart. Removing the damaged heart may be very easy or very difficult, depending on whether the recipient has had previous heart surgery (as is often the case). If there has been previous surgery, cutting through the scar tissue may prolong and complicate removal of the heart.
6. The third operation is probably the easiest; the implantation of the donor heart

Nursing Care Plan

1. **Acute pain related to an imbalance of oxygen supply to myocardial demands.**
   Interventions
   - Assessing pain location, duration, and radiation
   - Reviewing the history of previous activities that provoke chest pain
   - Creating a 12-lead ECG
   - Administering oxygen therapy, if necessary
   - Giving analgesics as ordered
   - Maintaining a rest period
   - Checking vital signs.
2. **Decreased CO related to poor myocardial contraction.**
   Interventions
   - Maintaining bed rest
   - Elevating head at 30°
   - Assessing and monitoring vital signs
   - Monitoring and recording ECG
3. **Anxiety related to the needs of the body is threatened.**
   Interventions
   - Assessing signs and verbal expressions of anxiety
   - Taking action to reduce anxiety by creating a calm environment
   - Encouraging patients to express feelings
   - Accompanying patient during periods of high anxiety
   - Providing an explanation of procedures and treatment
   - Referring to the spiritual adviser if necessary

4. **Acute pain related to an impaired ability of blood vessels to supply oxygen to the tissues.**
   Interventions
   - Giving proper bed rest to reduce myocardial oxygen demand
   - Assessing resting pulse rate
   - Maintaining regular ECG tracings
   - Assessing for pericardial friction rub
   - Assessing for the pain or discomfort
   - Administering analgesics as needed
   - Providing postsurgical care, if patient received surgical treatment
   - Providing and encouraging high-protein, and high-carbohydrate diet
   - Providing oral care every 4 hours
   - Providing small and attractive meals
   - Encouraging the client to take good care of the teeth and gums
   - Avoiding visitors who have an upper respiratory tract infection
   - Assessing for signs and symptoms of organ damage
   - Instructing patient and family about activity restrictions, medications, and signs and symptoms of infection

CONGESTIVE HEART FAILURE

It is a physiological condition in which heart's pumping capacity is weaker than normal that results in poor oxygen and nutrients supply to meet the body's metabolic needs. That may be characterized by hypertrophy and thickening of chambers.

Etiology and Types

1. Acute failure
2. Chronic failure
3. Left-sided heart failure
4. Right-sided heart failure
5. Forward failure
6. Backward failure
7. High-output failure
8. Low-output failure

1. **Acute heart failure:** It occurs in response to a sudden decrease in CO, resulting in rapid decrease in tissue perfusion. It can occur due to:
   - Acute viral myocarditis
   - Larger MI
   - Massive pulmonary embolism
   - Valve rupture
   - Cardiac tamponade
2. **Chronic heart failure (CHF):** It occurs when body adjusts to decrease in CO through compensatory mechanisms, resulting in systemic congestion. It develops slowly as in:
   - Pulmonary embolism
   - Emotional stress
   - Progression of acute into chronic failure
   - Systemic arterial hypertension
   - Chronic lung disease
3. **Left heart failure versus right heart failure:** Right heart failure compromises pulmonary flow to the lungs, while left heart failure compromises aortic flow to the body and brain.

Pathophysiology

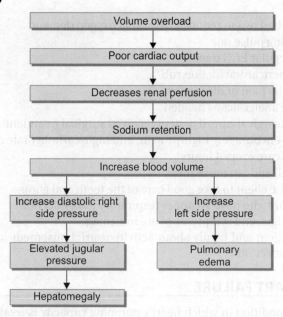

Volume overload
↓
Poor cardiac output
↓
Decreases renal perfusion
↓
Sodium retention
↓
Increase blood volume
↓
Increase diastolic right side pressure → Elevated jugular pressure → Hepatomegaly

Increase left side pressure → Pulmonary edema

Mechanism of Pathophysiology

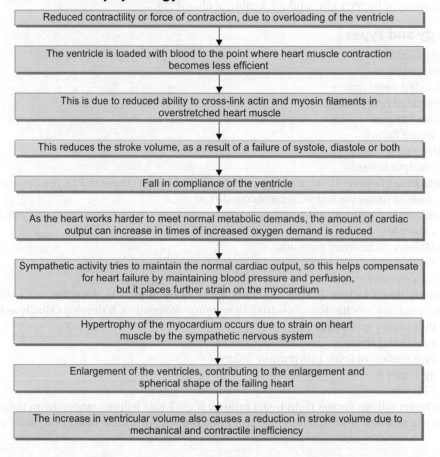

Reduced contractility or force of contraction, due to overloading of the ventricle
↓
The ventricle is loaded with blood to the point where heart muscle contraction becomes less efficient
↓
This is due to reduced ability to cross-link actin and myosin filaments in overstretched heart muscle
↓
This reduces the stroke volume, as a result of a failure of systole, diastole or both
↓
Fall in compliance of the ventricle
↓
As the heart works harder to meet normal metabolic demands, the amount of cardiac output can increase in times of increased oxygen demand is reduced
↓
Sympathetic activity tries to maintain the normal cardiac output, so this helps compensate for heart failure by maintaining blood pressure and perfusion, but it places further strain on the myocardium
↓
Hypertrophy of the myocardium occurs due to strain on heart muscle by the sympathetic nervous system
↓
Enlargement of the ventricles, contributing to the enlargement and spherical shape of the failing heart
↓
The increase in ventricular volume also causes a reduction in stroke volume due to mechanical and contractile inefficiency

Clinical Manifestations

- Congested lungs
- Fluid and water retention weight gain
- Nocturia
- Loss of appetite
- Dizziness, fatigue, and weakness
- Rapid or irregular heartbeats

Left Heart Failure

- Anxiety
- Confusion
- Persistent cough
- Tachycardia
- Tachypnea
- Noisy breathing
- Rales, wheezing
- Dry hacking cough
- Third heart sound
- Pink, frothy sputum
- Dyspnea on exertion
- Paroxysmal nocturnal dyspnea

Right-sided Heart Failure

- Right ventricle fails as an effective pump.
- Right ventricle cannot eject blood returning through vena cava.
- Blood backs up into systemic circulation.
- Increased pressure in systemic capillaries forces fluid out of capillaries into interstitial spaces.
- Tissue edema

Compensatory Mechanism During Chronic Heart Failure

Arterial blood pressure falls

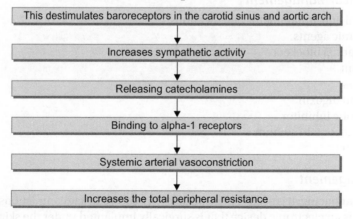

This destimulates baroreceptors in the carotid sinus and aortic arch

↓

Increases sympathetic activity

↓

Releasing catecholamines

↓

Binding to alpha-1 receptors

↓

Systemic arterial vasoconstriction

↓

Increases the total peripheral resistance

Contd...

Contd...

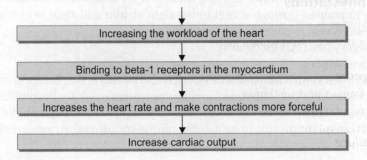

Diagnostic Evaluation

- Blood tests
- B-type natriuretic peptide blood test
- Chest X-ray
- Echocardiogram
- The ejection fraction
- ECG
- Cardiac catheterization
- Stress test

Management

General Measures

- Quitting smoking
- Exercising regularly
- Healthy weight
- Discontinuing alcohol
- Restricting dietary sodium
- Monitoring weight
- Restricting fluids
- Treating high BP
- Low fat diet
- Biventricular pacemaker

Pharmacological Management

- Nonsteroidal anti-inflammatory medications
- Antiarrhythmic agents
- Calcium channel blockers
- Decongestant
- Beta blockers
- Diuretics and digoxin
- An aldosterone inhibitor
- Antacids that contain sodium
- ACE inhibitor

Surgical Management

1. **Biventricular pacing:** It is used to treat the delay in heart ventricle contractions. Biventricular pacemaker is an electronic device that is surgically implanted under the skin by epicardial

approach. The device has two or three leads that are attached to the heart muscles. The leads are implanted through a vein in the right atrium and right ventricle and into the coronary sinus vein to pace the left ventricle.

2. **CABG surgery** (*see* CAD for details).
3. **Heart valve surgery.**
4. **Implantable left ventricular assist device:** It is also known as the "bridge to transplantation" for clients who have not responded to other treatments and are hospitalized with severe systolic heart failure. This device helps heart to pump blood throughout the body.
5. **Stem cell transplantation:** A bone marrow transplant, also called a stem cell transplant, is a treatment for some types of cancer.
   Types:
   a. **Autologous transplant:** This is also called an AUTO transplant or high-dose chemotherapy with autologous stem cell rescue.
   b. **Allogeneic transplantation:** This is also called an ALLO transplant. In an ALLO transplant, you get another person's stem cells.
6. **Heart transplantation**

Complications

- Cardiac asthma
- Nonproductive cough
- Edema
- Hemoptysis
- Hepatomegaly
- Peripheral edema
- Ascites

Nursing Care Plan

1. **Impaired gas exchange related to fluid in the alveoli.**
   Interventions
   - Auscultation of breath sounds
   - Encouraging cough exercise
   - Maintaining Fowler's position
   - Administering oxygen
   - Monitoring ABG
   - Intubation and mechanical ventilation
2. **Decreased CO related to heart failure and dysrhythmias.**
   Interventions
   - Assessing vital signs
   - Auscultating lung and heart sounds
   - Administering oxygen
   - Monitoring urine output
   - Assessing changes in mental status
   - Encouraging small meals
3. **Acute pain related to an imbalance of oxygen supply to myocardial demands.**
   Interventions
   - Assessing pain location, duration, and radiation
   - Reviewing the history of previous activities that provoke chest pain

- Creating a 12-lead ECG
- Administering oxygen therapy if necessary
- Giving analgesics as ordered
- Maintaining a rest period
- Checking vital signs

4. **Decreased CO related to poor myocardial contraction.**
   Interventions
   Maintaining bed rest
   - Elevating head at 30°
   - Assessing and monitoring vital signs
   - Monitoring and recording ECG

5. **Anxiety related to the needs of the body is threatened.**
   Interventions
   - Assessing signs and verbal expressions of anxiety
   - Taking action to reduce anxiety by creating a calm environment
   - Encouraging patients to express feelings
   - Accompanying patient during periods of high anxiety
   - Providing an explanation of procedures and treatment
   - Referring to the spiritual adviser if necessary

6. **Fluid volume excess related to reduced CO, Na and water retention**
   Interventions
   - Monitor IO chart
   - Fowler's position
   - Frequent oral care
   - Daily weighing
   - Assessing jugular vein distension, peripheral edema, and hepatic engorgement
   - Fluid restriction
   - About 2–4 g salt diet

7. **Decreased peripheral tissue perfusion related to reduced CO**
   Intervention
   - Monitoring peripheral pulses
   - Color and temperature of skin
   - Assessing for thrombophlebitis
   - Active or passive range of motion exercise
   - Keeping extremities warm

8. **High risk for digitalis toxicity related to impaired excretion**
   Intervention
   - Assessing for hypokalemia, heart block
   - Serum digitalis levels and potassium

ISCHEMIC HEART DISEASE

Ischemic heart disease is caused by an imbalance between the myocardial blood flow and the metabolic demand of the myocardium. It is characterized by atherosclerosis in the epicardial coronary arteries, which results in progressively narrowing of the coronary artery lumen and minimizes myocardial blood flow. The plaque becomes thick, calcified and solid causing obstruction in coronary blood flow, which results in permanent heart damage or death called acute MI **(Fig. 5.6)**.

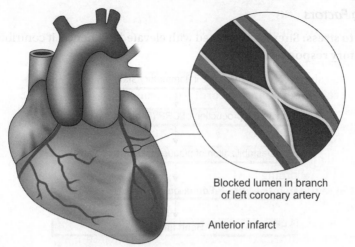

Blocked lumen in branch
of left coronary artery

Anterior infarct

Fig. 5.6: Plaque formation in coronary artery.

Etiology and Pathophysiology

- A reduction in the oxygen-carrying capacity of the blood
- Occlusive intracoronary thrombus
- Vasospasm
- Emboli.

Risk Factors

Nonmodifiable Major Risk Factors

1. **Heredity:** Children whose parents had heart disease, hypertension and diabetes are at higher risk of CAD.
2. **Advance age:** People older than 40 are at greater risk.
3. **Gender:** Men are at higher risk for heart attacks at younger ages. But the risk for women increases significantly at menopause.

Modifiable Major Risk Factors

1. **Cigarette and smoking:** Both active and passive smoking have been strongly implicated as a risk factor in the development of CAD.
2. **Hypertension:** High BP increases the workload of cardiac muscles by increasing stroke volume, enlarging and weakening the left ventricle muscles, hence increase the chances of CAD.
3. **Elevated serum cholesterol level:** The risk of CAD increases as blood cholesterol level increases.
4. **Physical inactivity:** Those who exercise reduce their risk of CAD.
5. **Obesity:** Obesity elevates serum cholesterol and triglyceride levels, high BP, and diabetes so contribute to CAD.
6. **Diabetes:** Patients with diabetes have a two- to eight-fold higher prevalence, incidence and mortality.

Contributing Factors

- **Response to stress:** Stress is associated with elevated BP; hence, it contributes to CAD.
- **Inflammatory responses:**

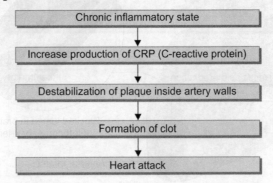

- **Menopause:** The incidence of CHD increases among women after menopause.

Pathophysiology

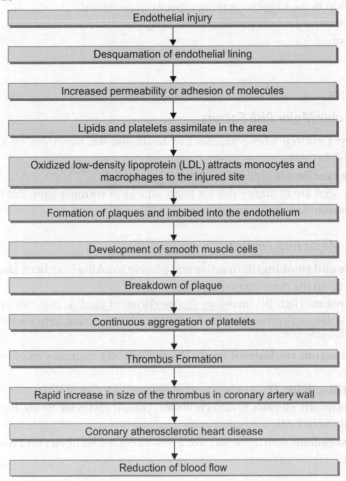

Contd...

Contd...

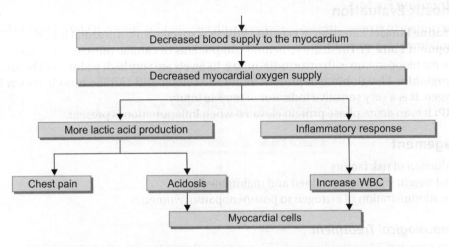

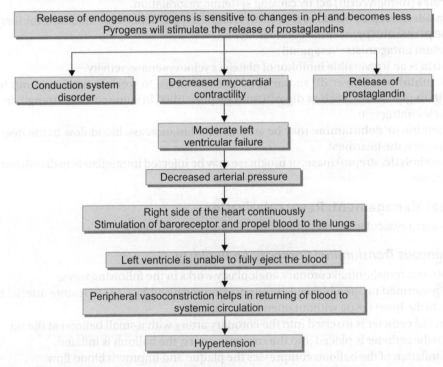

Clinical Manifestation

- Chest pain (unbearable)
- Pain is like punctured pin that can spread to shoulder and continue to left arm also spread to jaw and neck
- Pain does not disappear with the help of rest or nitroglycerin
- Stomach, back, and abdominal pain
- Shortness of breath
- Unexplained anxiety
- Weakness and fatigue
- Palpitations

Diagnostic Evaluation

- **Creatine kinase:** Elevation in **creatine kinase** is specific for myocardial injury.
- **Troponin I and T:** These are structural components of cardiac muscle. They are released into the bloodstream with myocardial injury. Its levels are very high within 3–12 hours of MI.
- **Myoglobin:** Myoglobin is a protein found in skeletal and cardiac muscle which binds oxygen. It is a very sensitive indicator of muscle injury.
- **CRP:** It is an acute phase protein elevated when inflammation is present.

Management

- Reduction of risk factors
- Ideal weight should be attained and maintained
- The administration of estrogen to postmenopausal women

Pharmacological Treatment

- **Nitrates** (nitroglycerin) act by causing systemic vasodilation.
- **Beta-adrenoceptor blockers** reduce myocardial oxygen demand by inhibiting the increases in heart rate and myocardial contractility.
- **Calcium antagonists:** Verapamil
- **Aspirin** is an irreversible inhibitor of platelet cyclooxygenase activity.
- **ACE inhibitors:** Lower BP so the heart does not have to work as hard to pump blood. **Digitalis glycosides**, such as digoxin, may be prescribed in some cases to strengthen heart muscle contraction.
- **Dopamine or dobutamine** may be administered to increase blood flow to the heart and strengthen the heartbeat.
- **Thrombolytic**, streptokinase, or urokinase may be injected immediately to dissolve arterial blockage.

Surgical Management: Revascularization

The primary revascularization options are PCI and CABG surgery.

Percutaneous Transluminal Coronary Angioplasty

Percutaneous transluminal coronary angioplasty works in the following ways:
- It is performed to open blocked coronary arteries caused by CAD to restore arterial blood flow to the heart tissue without open-heart surgery.
- A special catheter is inserted into the coronary artery with a small balloon at the tip.
- Once the catheter is placed into the coronary artery, the balloon is inflated.
- The inflation of the balloon compresses the plaque and improves blood flow.
- Fluoroscope is used to find the location of blockages in the coronary arteries.
- A small sample of cardiac tissue is also taken for further examination for any abnormality.
- Intravascular ultrasound waves are used to visualize and measure the size of the clot.
- Atherectomy is also done during same time to break the hard plaque.
- Atherectomy is used when the plaque is calcified and hardened. It is done with the help of a laser, which opens the artery by "vaporizing" the plaque (*see* **Figs. 5.4A and B**).

ENDOCARDITIS

Endocarditis is an infection of the endocardium layer of the heart, which is characterized by valve dysfunction.

Etiology

- *Streptococcus viridans*
- Dental procedures

Risk Factors

- History of endocarditis
- Congenital heart defect
- Damaged heart valves
- An artificial heart valve
- Hypertrophic cardiomyopathy
- Injected illegal drugs
- HIV
- CABG surgery
- A coronary artery stent
- A pacemaker implantation
- Mitral valve prolapse
- Hemodialysis

Pathophysiology

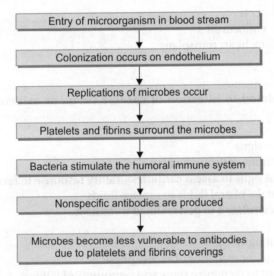

Entry of microorganism in blood stream

↓

Colonization occurs on endothelium

↓

Replications of microbes occur

↓

Platelets and fibrins surround the microbes

↓

Bacteria stimulate the humoral immune system

↓

Nonspecific antibodies are produced

↓

Microbes become less vulnerable to antibodies
due to platelets and fibrins coverings

Clinical Manifestations

- Chills and fever
- Fatigue
- Weight loss
- Night sweats
- Painful joints
- Bleeding under the fingernails
- Red, painless skin spots on the palms and soles (Janeway lesions)
- Persistent cough and shortness of breath
- Tiny purple and red spots under the skin
- Nail abnormalities (splinter hemorrhages)
- Paleness
- Red, painful nodes (Osler's nodes) in the pads of the fingers and toes

Diagnostic Evaluation

A physical examination may reveal:

- Enlarged spleen
- Splinter hemorrhages
- A history of congenital heart disease
- CT scan of the chest
- Echocardiogram
- Chest X-ray
- CBC
- Erythrocyte sedimentation rate
- Echocardiogram

Management

The American Heart Association recommends preventive antibiotics for people at risk for infectious endocarditis before:

- Certain dental procedures
- Surgeries on respiratory tract infection
- Artificial heart valves
- Congenital heart defects
- History of infective endocarditis
- Valve problems after a heart transplant

Nursing Care plan

1. **Hyperthermia related to infection of cardiac tissue as evidenced by temperature elevation.**
   Interventions
   - Monitoring vital signs
   - Administering antipyretic medication
   - Monitoring vital signs to assess cardiorespiratory response to fever
   - Encouraging intake of oral fluids to replace fluids
2. **Activity intolerance related to generalized weakness.**
   Interventions
   - Monitoring vital signs
   - Monitoring client for evidence of excess physical
   - Instructing client to recognize signs and symptoms of fatigue
   - Encouraging alternate rest and activity periods
3. **Decreased CO related to poor myocardial contraction.**
   Interventions
   - Maintaining bed rest
   - Elevating head at 30°
   - Assessing and monitoring vital signs
   - Monitoring and recording ECG
4. **Anxiety related to the needs of the body is threatened.**
   Interventions
   - Assessing signs and verbal expressions of anxiety
   - Taking action to reduce anxiety by creating a calm environment
   - Encouraging patients to express feelings
   - Accompanying patient during periods of high anxiety

- Providing an explanation of procedures and treatment
- Referring to the spiritual adviser if necessary

5. **Deficient knowledge related to lack of experience.**
   - Regarding management protocol and follow-up of therapy
   - Discussing common signs and symptoms of the disease
   - Discussing lifestyle changes that may be required to prevent future complications.

MYOCARDITIS

Myocarditis is the inflammatory process involving the myocardium and characterized by dilation of chamber, infiltration of blood, and degeneration of the muscle fibers.

Etiology

- Viral (HIV, rubella virus)
- Protozoan (*Toxoplasma*)
- Bacterial (*Brucella*)
- Fungal (*Aspergillus*)
- Parasitic
- Drugs
- Allergic reactions
- Rejection after a heart transplant
- Autoimmunity
- Toxins
- Heavy metals
- Electric shock

Pathophysiology

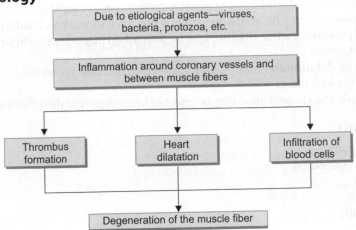

Due to etiological agents—viruses, bacteria, protozoa, etc.

Inflammation around coronary vessels and between muscle fibers

Thrombus formation

Heart dilatation

Infiltration of blood cells

Degeneration of the muscle fiber

Signs and Symptoms

- Chest pain
- Palpitations
- Fever
- Fatigue
- Dyspnea
- Arthralgia

- Edema in leg
- Dysrhythmias
- Syncope
- Oliguria

Diagnostic Evaluations

- **Physical examination** may reveal following:
  - **Auscultation of heart sounds**
  - Fever
  - Fluid in lungs
  - Palpitation
  - Swelling in the legs
- **Chest X-ray**
- **Blood test**
- Elevated cardiac enzymes
- Antibodies are finding against the heart muscle and the body itself
- ECG
- **Cardiac magnetic resonance imaging (MRI)**

Treatment

- Supportive therapy, including bed rest
- Digoxin and diuretics provide clinical improvement
- **Nitrates** (Nitroglycerin) act by causing systemic vasodilation
- **Beta-adrenoceptor blockers** reduce myocardial oxygen demand by inhibiting the increase in heart rate and myocardial contractility
- **Calcium antagonists:** Verapamil
- **Aspirin** is an irreversible inhibitor of platelet cyclooxygenase activity
- **ACE inhibitors:** Lower BP so the heart does not have to work as hard to pump blood. **Digitalis glycosides**, such as digoxin, may be prescribed in some cases to strengthen heart muscle contraction
- **Dopamine or dobutamine** may be administered to increase blood flow to the heart and strengthen the heartbeat.
- **Thrombolytic** and streptokinase may be injected immediately to dissolve arterial blockage.

Complications

- Cardiomyopathy
- Pulmonary congestion
- Pericarditis
- Heart failure
- Sudden death.

PERICARDITIS

Pericarditis is an inflammation of the pericardium.

Classification

The classification of pericarditis is as follows:
A. **Acute pericarditis**
B. **Chronic pericarditis**

- **Bacterial pericarditis:** Caused by bacterial infection
- **Cardiac tamponade:** Fluid builds up between the two layers of the pericardium. Also called pericardial effusion.
- **Abscess:** A pus either within the heart or in the pericardium
- **Constrictive pericarditis:** Pericardium is scarred by the inflammation
- **Viral pericarditis:** Caused by viral infections
- **Chronic effusive pericarditis**: Buildup of fluid within the two layers of the pericardium
- **Traumatic:** Heart surgery or trauma to the chest, esophagus, or heart
- **Pericarditis following heart surgery:** Pericarditis may be a complication of heart surgery
- **Post-heart attack pericarditis**
- **Acute pericarditis:** It is the inflammation of the pericardium characterized by chest pain, pericardial friction rub, and serial of ECG changes (ST elevations).
- **Serous pericarditis:** It is characterized by rheumatic fever, systemic lupus erythematosus, and primary viral infection.
- **Purulent pericarditis:** This is due to bacteria, fungus, or parasitic action.
- **Fibrinous pericarditis**: In this, exudates will be completely resolved or will be organized causing adhesive pericarditis.
- **Caseous pericarditis:** This form is due to tuberculosis by direct extension from lymph nodes.
- **Hemorrhagic pericarditis**: This is composed of an exudate of blood mixed with fibrinous effusion.

Etiology

- Viral, bacterial infection
- Idiopathic
- Immunologic conditions, including systemic lupus erythematosus
- MI
- Trauma to the heart
- Uremia
- Malignancy
- Radiation induced
- Aortic dissection

Pathophysiology

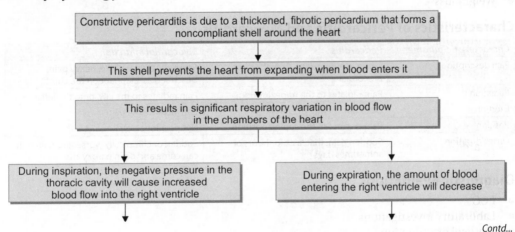

Contd...

Contd...

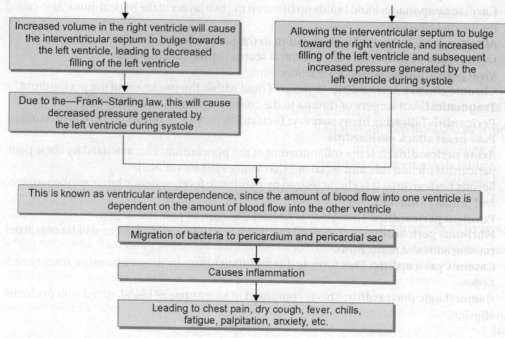

Increased volume in the right ventricle will cause the interventricular septum to bulge towards the left ventricle, leading to decreased filling of the left ventricle

Allowing the interventricular septum to bulge toward the right ventricle, and increased filling of the left ventricle and subsequent increased pressure generated by the left ventricle during systole

Due to the—Frank–Starling law, this will cause decreased pressure generated by the left ventricle during systole

This is known as ventricular interdependence, since the amount of blood flow into one ventricle is dependent on the amount of blood flow into the other ventricle

Migration of bacteria to pericardium and pericardial sac

Causes inflammation

Leading to chest pain, dry cough, fever, chills, fatigue, palpitation, anxiety, etc.

Signs and Symptoms

- Chest pain
- Dry cough
- Fever
- Chills
- Kussmaul's sign
- Fatigue
- Malaise
- Anxiety
- Joint pain
- Anorexia
- Increased heart rate
- Weight loss

Characteristics of Pericarditis and Myocarditis

Characteristic/parameter	Pericarditis	Myocardial infarction
Pain description	Sharp, pleuritic, retrosternal, or left precordial	Crushing, pressure-like, heavy pain. Described as "elephant on the chest"
Radiation	Pain radiates to the trapezius ridge	Pain radiates to the jaw, or to the left arm
Exertion	Does not change the pain	Can increase the pain
Position	Pain is worse in the supine position	Not positional
Onset/duration	Sudden pain, that lasts for hours or sometimes days	Sudden or chronically worsening pain that can come and go in paroxysms

Diagnostic Evaluations

- ECG
- Laboratory investigations
- Physical examination

Acute Complications

- Pericardial effusion
- Cardiac tamponade
- Pulsus paradoxus (decrease of at least 10 mm Hg of the systolic BP upon inspiration)
- Hypotension
- Jugular vein distention

Management

Pharmacological Management

- NSAIDs, such as naproxen
- **Antibiotics to treat tuberculosis**
- Steroids
- **Colchicine**

Surgical Management

Pericardiocentesis: It is a procedure in which pericardial sac is punctured and some of the pericardial fluid is removed to relieve cardiac tamponade.

Chronic pericarditis is a condition in which there is chronic inflammatory thickening of the pericardium that changes the pericardium into thick fibrous band of tissues. Thus, the tissue encircles, encases and compresses the heart, and prevents it from expanding to normal size causing restriction of ventricular filling.

Nursing Care

Assessment

- Assessing signs of pain
- Assessing association of pain with respiratory movements, cough, and swallowing
- Assessing for pericardial friction rub
- Frequently assessing temperature

Nursing Diagnosis

Acute pain related to inflammation of layers of heart
Interventions
- Checking intensity of pain
- Assisting the patient to sit upright or to lean forward to relieve pain
- Restricting the activities of patient
- Providing prescribed analgesics (morphine)

Hyperthermia related to inflammatory process
Interventions
- Monitoring temperature 2–4 hourly
- Observing for basic principles of asepsis, such as handwashing
- Providing cold compression
- Administering antibiotics and antipyretics

Decreased CO related to structural abnormality of valves
Interventions
- Monitoring BP and pulse
- Evaluating jugular vein distension
- Checking laboratory findings

- Maintaining intake–output chart
- Obtaining daily weight
- Administering prescribed drugs, such as digitalis

Risk for complications related to disease process.
Interventions

- Assessing vital signs of patient
- Assessing peripheral edema
- Checking the laboratory findings
- Administering digitalis and digoxin if signs of heart failure appear
- Preparing for emergency pericardiocentesis

RHEUMATIC HEART DISEASE

Rheumatic heart disease is caused by an autoimmune reaction to group A β-hemolytic streptococci that is characterized by valvular damage, fibrosis, and scarring of valve leaflets.

Etiology and Pathophysiology

Autoimmune reaction to group A β-hemolytic streptococci (GAS)

Pathophysiology

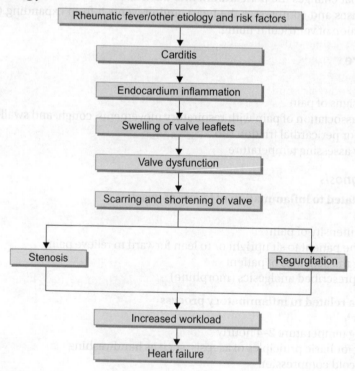

Rheumatic fever/other etiology and risk factors

↓

Carditis

↓

Endocardium inflammation

↓

Swelling of valve leaflets

↓

Valve dysfunction

↓

Scarring and shortening of valve

↓

Stenosis — Regurgitation

↓

Increased workload

↓

Heart failure

Signs and Symptoms

- Polyarthritis
- Raised CRP
- Carditis
- Fever

- Arthralgia
- Subcutaneous nodules
- Erythema marginatum—reddish rash on the trunk or arms
- Chorea—rapid movements without purpose of the face and arms
- ECG showing features of heart block, such as a prolonged PR interval.

Diagnostic Evaluation

- Evidence of recent group A streptococcal infection
- **Physical examination**
  - Checking the joints for signs of inflammation
  - Examining the skin for nodules under the skin or a rash
  - Listening to the heart for abnormal rhythms, murmurs or muffled sounds that may indicate inflammation of the heart.
  - Conducting a series of simple movement tests to detect indirect evidence of inflammation of the central nervous system.
- **CBC**
- **ECG**
- **Echocardiography**

Management

Pharmacological Management

- Antibiotics, penicillin, ampicillin, and amoxicillin
- Salicylates and steroids
- Digoxin and diuretics
- Sodium and fluid restriction

Surgical Management

- Mitral valvulotomy
- Percutaneous balloon valvuloplasty
- Mitral valve replacement may be indicated

Nursing Care Plan

Nursing Assessment

- About heart function
- Nutritional status of patients
- Tolerance to the activities and attitudes of patients toward limiting the activities undertaken
- Disturbances in sleep patterns
- Level of discomfort felt by rheumatic fever patients
- Ability of the patient in terms of troubleshooting
- Knowledge of patients and families will be suffered by rheumatic heart disease.
- History of rheumatic heart disease
- Monitoring of cardiac complications in the event
- Auscultation of heart sounds
- Assessment of the patient's vital signs
- Assessment of pain
- Assessment of the presence of markers of inflammation in the joints
- Assessment of the presence of lesions on the skin

Nursing Diagnosis

Decreased CO related to valvular stenosis

Nursing interventions

- Monitoring vital signs, such as BP, apical pulse and peripheral pulse
- Monitoring cardiac rhythm and frequency
- Semi-Fowler bed rest in a position that is 45°
- Encouraging the patient to stress management techniques (quiet environment, meditation)
- Medical collaboration in terms of oxygen delivery and therapy

Activity intolerance related to decreased CO, oxygen supply and demand imbalance.

Nursing interventions

- Energy saving during the acute patients
- Maintaining bed rest until the results of laboratory and clinical status of patients improved
- Monitoring the gradual increase in the level of activity undertaken
- Teaching the patient to participate in activities of daily necessities
- Creating a schedule of activities and also the breaks

VALVULAR HEART DISEASE

Heart valve disease is characterized by narrowing and stiff valve cusps and leaflets and contracture of valves. Valvular heart disease results in valvular stenosis or regurgitation.

Types

There are several types of valve disease:

Valvular stenosis: This occurs when a valve opening is smaller than normal due to stiff or fused leaflets. The narrowed opening may make the heart work very hard to pump blood through it. This can lead to CHF.

Pathophysiology

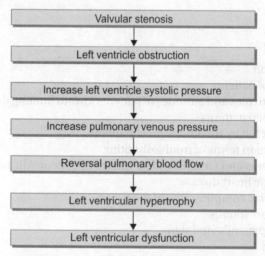

Valvular stenosis

↓

Left ventricle obstruction

↓

Increase left ventricle systolic pressure

↓

Increase pulmonary venous pressure

↓

Reversal pulmonary blood flow

↓

Left ventricular hypertrophy

↓

Left ventricular dysfunction

Valvular regurgitation: It is also called "leaky valve," and this occurs when a valve does not close tightly and some blood will flow backward in the upper chamber.

Pathophysiology

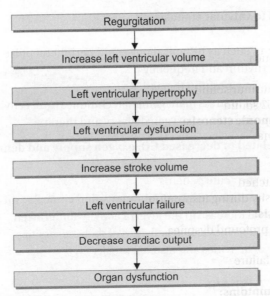

- **Congenital valve disease:** It is characterized by wrong size of valve, leaflets, or has leaflets that are not attached to the annulus correctly.
- **Acquired valve disease:** This includes problems that develop with valves that were once normal. These may involve changes in the structure changes in valve.
- **Mitral valve prolapse:** It is characterized by back flop of valve leaflets into the left atrium during the heart's contraction.

Etiology

- Aging
- Rheumatic heart disease
- Bacterial endocarditis
- Hypertension
- Atherosclerosis

Signs and Symptoms

- **Mitral valve stenosis:**
  - Dyspnea on exertion
  - Palpitation
  - Diastolic murmur sound
  - Arterial fibrillation
  - Hemoptysis
  - Fatigue
- **Mitral valve regurgitation:**
  - Pulmonary edema
  - Shock
  - Systolic murmur
- **Mitral valve prolapse:**
  - Palpitation
  - Dyspnea
  - Chest pain

- ■ Activity intolerance
- ■ Syncope
- **Chronic:**
  - ■ Fatigue
  - ■ Exertional dyspnea
  - ■ Orthopnea
  - ■ High-pitched murmur sound
  - ■ Absent S1 and S2 sound
- **Tricuspid and pulmonic stenosis:**
  - ■ Peripheral edema
  - ■ Ascites
  - ■ Hepatomegaly
  - ■ Diastolic low-pitched
  - ■ Increased intensity during inspiration
- **Aortic valve stenosis:**
  - ■ Abrupt onset of profound dyspnea
  - ■ Chest pain
  - ■ Left ventricular failure
  - ■ Shock
- **Other signs and symptoms:**
  - ■ Hypotension
  - ■ Dizziness
  - ■ Dysrhythmia

Diagnostic Evaluation

- **An ECG (for details** *refer* **CAD)**
- **Stress testing:** Treadmill tests **(for details** *refer* **CAD)**
- **Chest X-ray**
- **Echocardiogram (for details** *refer* **CAD)**
- **Cardiac catheterization (for details** *refer* **CAD)**

Management

Medical Management

- Vasodilators
- ACE inhibitors
- Antibiotic therapy
- Diuretics
- Anticoagulant therapy
- Beta blockers

Surgical Management

- Closed mitral valvotomy
- Open mitral valvotomy
- Mitral valve replacement
- Balloon valvuloplasty

Complications

- Heart failure
- Dysrhythmia

Nursing Care Plan

Assessment
- Auscultate heart sounds
- Place patient in lateral recumbent position with bell hear the low-pitched murmur
- Note radiation of heart sound to axilla and left intrascapular region
- Higher pitch at apex

Nursing Diagnosis
- Decrease CO related to altered preload, afterload
- Activity intolerance related to reduced oxygen supply
- Ineffective coping related to acute and chronic illness

Nursing Intervention
- **Maintaining adequate CO**
  - Change in existing murmur should be assessed frequently
  - Right- and left-sided heart failure should be assessed
  - The dysrhythmia should be monitored and treated as ordered
  - The patient should be prepared for surgical interventions
- **Decreased CO related to poor myocardial contraction**
  Interventions
  - Maintaining bed rest
  - Head elevation of 30°
  - Assessing and monitoring vital signs
  - Monitoring and recording ECG
- **Anxiety related to the needs of the body is threatened**
  Interventions
  - Assessing signs and verbal expressions of anxiety
  - Taking action to reduce anxiety by creating a calm environment
  - Encouraging patients to express feelings
  - Accompanying patient during periods of high anxiety
  - Providing an explanation of procedures and treatment
  - Referring to the spiritual adviser if necessary
- **Improving activity intolerance**
  Interventions
  - Maintaining the bed rest
  - Allowing patient to rest between interventions
  - Assisting in hygiene needs
- **Strength coping abilities**
  Interventions
  - Teaching the client about etiology and therapies
  - Including family member in discussion
  - Stressing the importance of adapting lifestyle to cope up with illness
  - Discussing with patient the surgical intervention as the treatment modality
  - Referring the patient to appropriate counseling services

ARTERIOSCLEROTIC VASCULAR DISEASE

Atherosclerosis is a condition where the arteries become narrowed and hardened due to an excessive buildup of plaque around the artery wall, which results in narrowing of the coronary artery lumen and minimizes myocardial blood flow. The plaque becomes thick, calcified and solid causing obstruction in coronary blood flow **(Fig. 5.8)**.

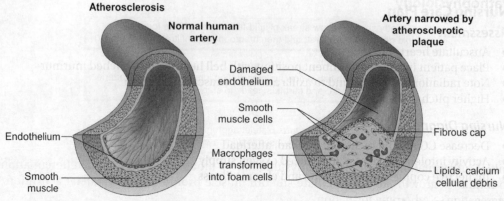

Fig. 5.8: Narrowing of coronary lumen.

Etiology and Risk Factors

- **Nonmodifiable major risk factors include:**
  - **Heredity:** Children whose parents had heart disease, hypertension, and diabetes are at higher risk of CAD.
  - **Advance age:** People older than 40 are at greater risk.
  - **Gender:** Men are at higher risk for heart attacks at younger ages. But the risk for women increases significantly at menopause.
- **Modifiable major risk factors include:**
  - **Cigarette and smoking:** Both active and passive smoking have been strongly implicated as a risk factor in the development of CAD.
  - **Hypertension:** High BP increases the workload of cardiac muscles by increasing stroke volume, enlarging and weakening the left ventricle muscles, hence increase the chances of CAD.
  - **Elevated serum cholesterol level:** The risk of CAD increases as blood cholesterol level increases.
  - **Physical inactivity:** Those who exercise reduce their risk of CAD.
  - **Obesity:** Obesity elevates serum cholesterol and triglyceride levels, high BP and diabetes so contribute to CAD.
  - **Diabetes:** Patients with diabetes have a two- to eight-fold higher prevalence, incidence and mortality.

Contributing Factors

- **Response to stress:** Stress is associated with elevated BP; hence, it contributes to CAD.
- **Inflammatory responses:**

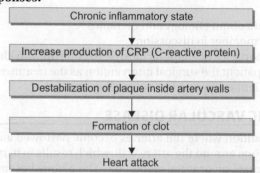

- **Menopause:** The incidence of CHD increases among women after menopause.

Pathophysiology

> Fatty streak (yellow streak of lipid-filled macrophage foam cells. Lipid gets deposited first, and then macrophages infiltrate and ingest it)

↓

> Fibrous plaque (whitish yellow lump occluding lumen of coronary arteries, aorta, and carotids) leads to stable angina

↓

> Thrombus (plaque rupture, platelet aggregation, and thrombus) leads to unstable angina or MI

Initial inflammation → endothelial dysfunction → monocyte recruitment/differentiation to intima → growth factors stimulate smooth muscle proliferation → platelet activation/aggregation → atheroma formation

Pathophysiology

> Arteries contain what is called an endothelium, a thin layer of cells that keeps the artery smooth and allows blood to flow easily. Atherosclerosis starts when the endothelium becomes damaged, allowing LDL cholesterol to accumulate in the artery wall

↓

> The body sends macrophage white blood cells to clean up the cholesterol, but sometimes, the cells get stuck there to the affected site area

↓

> When they stick to an artery they secrete a molecule called netrin-1, this stops normal migration of the macrophages out of the arteries

↓

> Over time this results in plaque being built up, consisting of bad cholesterol (LDL cholesterol) and macrophage white blood cells

↓

> The plaque clogs up the artery, disrupting the flow of blood around the body. This potentially causes blood clots that can result in life-threatening conditions, such as heart attack, stroke and other cardiovascular diseases

↓

> The condition can affect the entire artery tree, but mainly affects the larger high pressure arteries

Signs and Symptoms

- Weakness
- Difficulty breathing
- Headache
- Facial numbness
- Paralysis
- Vomiting
- Extreme anxiety
- Chest pain
- Coughing
- Feeling faint
- Loss of appetite
- Edema

- Poor concentration
- Hair loss
- Male impotence
- Numbness in the legs
- Weakness in the legs.

Diagnostic Evaluation

- Blood tests
- Physical examination
- Ultrasound
- CT scan

Complications

- **Complicated atherosclerotic plaques:** A complicated plaque is characterized by erosion, ulceration, or fissuring of the surface of the plaque.
- **Mural thrombosis:** It results from abnormal laminar and or turbulent blood flow around the plaque that protrudes into the lumen.
- Acute coronary syndromes
- **Aneurysm formation:** Abnormal dilatation of blood vessels
- **Calcification** of plaque

Treatment and Management

Once a cardiac catheterization has been performed, the four most common therapeutic options are:

1. Lifestyle modification
2. Pharmacological therapy
3. Percutaneous coronary intervention
4. Coronary artery bypass grafting (CABG)

Lifestyle Modification

- Quit smoking
- Regular exercise
- Weight control

Pharmacological Therapy

The components of pharmacological therapy include:

- **Antiplatelet agents:** Aspirin
- **Antianginal agents:** Beta blockers, calcium channel blockers, and nitrates are the mainstays of antianginal therapy.

Surgical Management: Revascularization

The primary revascularization options are PCI and CABG surgery **(for details *refer* CAD).**

Nursing Care Plan

Nursing diagnosis

- **Acute pain related to an imbalance of oxygen supply to myocardial demands**
  Interventions
  - Assessing pain location, duration, and radiation
  - Reviewing the history of previous activities that provoke chest pain

- Creating a 12-lead ECG
- Administering oxygen therapy if necessary
- Giving analgesics as ordered
- Maintaining a rest period
- Checking vital signs
- **Decreased CO related to poor myocardial contraction**
  Interventions
  - Maintaining bed rest
  - Head elevation of 30°.
  - Assessing and monitoring vital signs
  - Monitoring and recording ECG
- **Anxiety related to the needs of the body is threatened**
  Interventions
  - Assessing signs and verbal expressions of anxiety
  - Taking action to reduce anxiety by creating a calm environment
  - Encouraging patients to express feelings
  - Accompanying patient during periods of high anxiety
  - Providing an explanation of procedures and treatment
  - Referring to the spiritual adviser if necessary

ARRHYTHMIAS

The term "arrhythmia" refers to any change from the normal sequence of electrical impulses, i.e., rate and rhythm of heart. That can be fatal and life threatening and need immediate medical intervention **(Fig. 5.9)**.

Signs and Symptoms

Signs and symptoms depend on the type of heart block you have. First-degree heart block rarely causes symptoms.

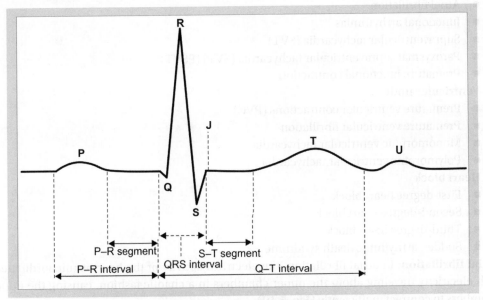

Fig. 5.9: Normal electrocardiogram (ECG) rhythm.

- **Symptoms of second- and third-degree heart block include:**
  - Fainting
  - Dizziness or light-headedness
  - Fatigue (tiredness)
  - Shortness of breath
  - Chest pain
  - Slow heartbeat
  - Irregular heartbeat
  - Arrhythmias
  - Blackouts (Stokes–Adams syndrome)
- **Symptoms of severe case include:**
  - Breathlessness
  - Breathlessness with exertion
  - Breathlessness caused by fever
  - Dizziness
  - Weakness
  - Fainting
  - Fatigue

Classification

- **Sinus node**
  - Sinus bradycardia
  - Sinus tachycardia
  - Sinus arrhythmias
- **Atrial node**
  - Premature atrial contractions
  - Atrial flutter
  - Atrial fibrillation
  - Junctional arrhythmias
  - Supraventricular tachycardia (SVT)
  - Paroxysmal supraventricular tachycardia (SVT) (PSVT)
  - Premature junctional contraction
- **Ventricular node**
  - Premature ventricular contractions (PVC)
  - Premature ventricular fibrillation
  - Monomorphic ventricular tachycardia
  - Polymorphic ventricular tachycardia
- **Heart block**
  - First-degree heart block
  - Second-degree heart block
  - Third-degree heart block
  - Sudden arrhythmic death syndrome

Atrial fibrillation: In atrial fibrillation, the electrical activity of the heart is uncoordinated, with electricity traveling about the upper chambers in a chaotic fashion, causing the upper chambers to contract inefficiently **(Fig. 5.10)**.

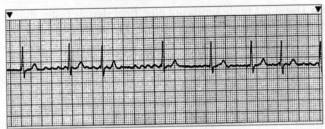

Fig. 5.10: Atrial fibrillation.

Atrial flutter: Atrial flutter causes a rapid but coordinated electrical stimulation of the upper chamber of the heart, often leading to a rapid pulse **(Fig. 5.11)**.

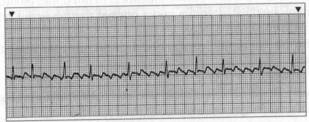

Fig. 5.11: Atrial flutter.

PSVT: This is a fast heart rhythm from the top part of the heart. In this condition, repeated periods of very fast heartbeats begin and end suddenly **(Fig. 5.12)**.

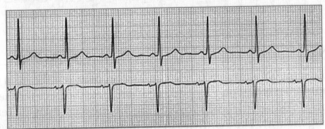

Fig. 5.12: Paroxysmal supraventricular tachycardia (PSVT).

Premature supraventricular contraction or premature atrial contraction (PAC): Premature beats or extra beats frequently cause irregular heart rhythms **(Fig. 5.13)**.

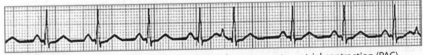

Fig. 5.13: Premature supraventricular contraction or premature atrial contraction (PAC).

Sick sinus syndrome: The sinus node (heart's pacemaker) does not fire its signals properly, so that the heart rate slows down.

Sinus arrhythmia: Cyclic changes in the heart rate during breathing. It is common in children and often found in normal, healthy adults **(Fig. 5.14)**.

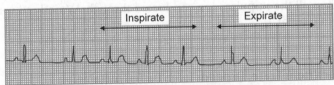

Fig. 5.14: Sinus arrhythmia.

Sinus tachycardia: The sinus node sends out electrical signals faster than usual, speeding up the heart rate. This is a normal response to exercise **(Fig. 5.15)**.

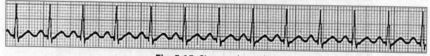

Fig. 5.15: Sinus tachycardia.

Premature ventricular contraction (PVC): An electrical signal from the ventricles causes an early heartbeat that generally goes unnoticed. The heart then seems to pause until the next beat of the ventricle occurs in a regular fashion.

Ventricular fibrillation: It is where electrical signals in the ventricles fire in a very fast and uncontrolled manner. This causes the lower chambers to not pump blood. If the person does not receive immediate medical attention and a normal rhythm is not restored quickly, the patient will suffer brain and heart damage and die.

Ventricular tachycardia: It is a rapid, regular heartbeat arising in the ventricles, and the bottom chamber of the heart.

Paroxysmal atrial tachycardia (PAT): PAT is a very rapid supraventricular rhythm that comes from the atria—usually, it runs at a very rapid rate, about 250–300 bpm **(Fig. 5.16)**.

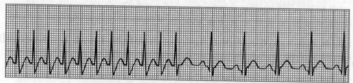

Fig. 5.16: Paroxysmal atrial tachycardia (PAT).

HEART BLOCKS

An AV block involves the impairment of the conduction between the atria and ventricles of the heart. Under normal conditions, SA node in the atria sets the pace for the heart, and these impulses travel down to the ventricles. In an AV block, this message does not reach the ventricles or is impaired along the way. The ventricles of the heart have their own pacing mechanisms, which can maintain a lowered heart rate in the absence of SA stimulation.

Etiology

Etiologies are as follows:
- Ischemia
- Infarction
- Fibrosis
- Drugs
- Strong vagal stimulation may also produce AV block.
  - **AV block:** Conduction block between sinus node and up to and including AV node.
  - **First-degree AV block:** The electrical impulses are slowed as they pass through the conduction system, but they all successfully reach the ventricles. First-degree AV block occurs when all the impulses are conducted through AV node to ventricles at a rate slower than normal.

Characteristics

- **Ventricular or arterial rate:** Depends upon underlying rhythm
- **Ventricular or arterial rhythm:** Depends upon underlying rhythm

- **QRS shape and duration:** Usually normal, but may be abnormal
- **P wave:** In front of the QRS complex; shows sinus rhythm, regular rhythm
- **PR interval:** Greater than 0.20 second
- **P:** QRS ratio: 1:1 **(Fig. 5.17)**

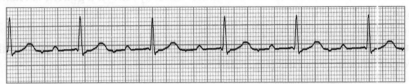

Fig. 5.17: First-degree atrioventricular block.

Interpretation

First-degree AV block
- PR interval: >0.20 second
- Rate: 60 bpm
- Regularity: Regular
- P wave: Normal
- PR interval: >0.20 second (0.36 second)
- QRS duration: Normal 0.08 second

Causes

- Enhanced vagal tone
- Myocarditis
- MI
- Electrolyte disturbances
- Calcium channel blockers, beta blockers, cardiac glycosides
- Hypokalemia or hyperkalemia

Diagnostic Test

- **ECG**
- **Electrolyte and drug screens**

Treatment

- Cautious use of digitalis glycosides
- Atropine is effective if PR interval exceeds 0.26 second or bradycardia develops
- Identifying and correcting electrolyte imbalances and withholding any offending medications
- This condition does not require admission unless there is an associated MI
- It may require outpatient follow-up
- Regular monitoring of the ECG

SECOND-DEGREE ATRIOVENTRICULAR BLOCK

Second-degree AV block is a disease of the electrical conduction system of the heart. It refers to a conduction block between the atria and ventricles. The presence of second-degree AV block is diagnosed when one or more (but not all) of the atrial impulses fail to conduct to the ventricles due to impaired conduction.

Characteristics

- **Ventricular or arterial rate:** Depends upon underlying rhythm
- **Ventricular or arterial rhythm:** PP interval is regular if the patient has an underlying normal sinus rhythm; the RR interval characteristically reflects a pattern of change
- **QRS shape and duration:** Usually normal, but may be abnormal
- **P wave:** In front of the QRS complex
- **PR interval:** PR interval become longer with each succeeding ECG complex until there is a P wave not followed by a QRS **(Fig. 5.18)**.

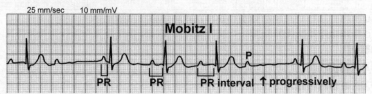

Fig. 5.18: Second-degree atrioventricular (AV) block.

Interpretation: Second-degree AV block type I

- P wave not followed by QRS
- **Rate:** 50 bpm
- **Regularity:** Irregular
- **P wave:** Normal
- **PR interval:** Lengthens
- **QRS duration:** 0.08 second

Etiology

- Inferior wall MI
- Cardiac surgery
- Acute rheumatic fever
- Vagal stimulation
- Digitalis toxicity

Treatment

The types of treatment are as follows:

- This is almost always a benign condition for which no specific treatment is needed.
- Atropine is effective for treating second-degree type I
- Temporary pacemaker implantation for symptomatic bradycardia
- Discontinuation of digitalis glycosides
- In symptomatic cases, IV atropine or isoproterenol may transiently improve conduction.

SECOND-DEGREE ATRIOVENTRICULAR BLOCK

Second-degree AV block occurs when only some of atrial impulses are conducted through the AV node into the ventricles. It is characterized on a surface ECG by intermittently nonconducted P waves not preceded by PR prolongation and not followed by PR shortening.

Characteristics

- **Ventricular or arterial rate:** Depends upon underlying rhythm
- **Ventricular or arterial rhythm:** PP interval is regular

- **QRS shape and duration:** Usually abnormal, but may be normal
- **P wave:** In front of the QRS complex
- **PR interval:** PR interval is constant for those P wave just before QRS complexes **(Fig. 5.19)**.

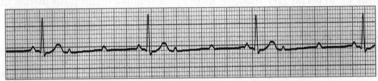

Fig. 5.19: Type II second-degree atrioventricular (AV) block.

Interpretation: Second-degree AV block Type II
- P wave not followed by QRS
- **Rate:** 40 bpm
- **Regularity:** Regular
- **P wave:** Normal
- **PR interval:** 0.14 second
- **PP interval:** Constant
- **QRS duration:** Periodically absent

Etiology

- Conduction is all or nothing (no prolongation of PR interval)
- Typically block occurs in the bundle of His
- Severe CAD
- Anterior wall MI
- Acute myocarditis
- Digitalis toxicity

Treatment

- The definitive treatment for this form of AV Block is an implanted temporary and permanent pacemaker
- Isoproterenol for symptomatic bradycardia
- Discontinuation of digitalis glycosides

SUDDEN ARRHYTHMIC DEATH SYNDROME

Sudden arrhythmic death syndrome is a term (sudden unexpected death syndrome) used to describe sudden death due to cardiac arrest brought on by an arrhythmia.

Etiology

- Viral myocarditis
- Long QT syndrome
- Brugada syndrome
- Ventricular tachycardia
- Hypertrophic cardiomyopathy
- Right ventricular dysplasia

Signs and Symptoms

- Palpitations
- Coagulopathy
- Increased risks stroke

- CHF
- Sudden cardiac death
- Hypotension
- Syncope

Diagnostic Evaluation

- **ECG or EKG:** A picture of the electrical impulses traveling through the heart muscle. An ECG is recorded on graph paper, through the use of electrodes (small, sticky patches) that are attached to your skin on the chest, arms, and legs.
- **Ambulatory monitors**, such as:
  - **Holter monitor:** A small portable recorder that is attached to electrodes on your chest. It continuously records your heart's rhythm for 24 hours.
  - **Transtelephonic monitor:** A small monitor is attached to electrode leads, usually on your finger or wrist. With the help of this device, your heart's rhythm is transmitted over the phone line to your doctor's office.
  - **Transtelephonic monitor with a memory loop:** A small, portable recorder that is worn continuously for an extended period of time to record and save information about your heart's rhythm around the time you experience an arrhythmia. The recording is triggered by pushing a button (event button). The rhythm is recorded, saved and transmitted over the phone line.
- **Stress test** (*refer* **CAD**)
- **Echocardiogram**
- **Cardiac catheterization:** *Refer* **CAD for details**
- **Electrophysiology study:** A special heart catheterization that evaluates your heart's electrical system. Catheters are inserted into your heart to record the electrical activity.
- **Passive head-up tilt test or head upright tilt test:** BP and heart rate on a minute-by-minute basis should be recorded while the table is tilted in a head-up position at different levels.

Management

The goal of management is to:
- Prevent blood clots from forming to reduce stroke risk
- Control your heart rate within a relatively normal range
- Restore a normal heart rhythm, if possible
- Treat heart disease/condition that may be causing arrhythmia
- Reduce other risk factors for heart disease and stroke
  - **Medications:** Antiarrhythmic drugs, amiodarone, bepridil hydrochloride
  - **Beta blockers:** Acebutolol
  - **Anticoagulants:** Anticoagulants (blood thinners) work by making it harder for the blood to clot, or coagulate, warfarin.

Nursing Care Plan

Nursing Assessment

Nursing assessment should be as follows:
- **General complaints:** Palpitations, dizziness, light headedness, chest pain, and syncope
- Physical examination
- Hypotension
- **Mental status:** Confusion, agitation, and anxiety
- Drug history

Nursing Diagnosis

Nursing diagnosis should be as follows:

- **Decreased CO related to electrical and mechanical dysfunction**
  Interventions
  - Assessing the patient continuously for rate, rhythm, and level of consciousness
  - Notifying the physician if any change occurs in normal parameters
  - Administering antidysrhythmic drugs
  - Administering oxygenation therapy
  - Monitoring vital signs frequently
  - Monitoring and recording ECG changes
- **Decreased tissue perfusion related to decreased CO**
  Interventions
  - Monitoring pulse rate
  - Monitoring central venous pressure
  - Providing sterile dressing on wound
  - Giving IV fluid to the patient
  - Giving oxygenation therapy
  - Epinephrine drugs that are first-line drug used for its alpha adrenergic effect to increase perfusion pressure
  - Dopamine is given to stimulate beta adrenergic cell
  - Vagal maneuver induces vagal stimulation of cardiac conduction system
  - Massaging the carotid sinus that causes vagal stimulation
  - Sodium bicarbonate is used for the patients having hyperkalemia
  - Pacemaker should be implanted
- **Chest pain related to electrical and mechanical dysfunction**
  Interventions
  - Assessing for the presence of pain, the scale and intensity of pain
  - Securing the chest tube to restrict movement and avoid irritation
  - Assessing pain reduction measures
- **Ineffective breathing pattern related to disease condition as evidenced by breathlessness**
  Interventions
  - Opening the airway with head tilt, chin lift, and jaw thrust
  - Setting the position to maximize ventilation
  - Using tools airway
  - Performing suction
  - Auscultation of breath sounds
  - Giving bronchodilators
  - Performing chest physiotherapy
  - Teaching to breathe deeply and cough effectively
  - Oxygenation therapy
- **Activity intolerance related to conduction problem as evidenced by tachycardia**
  Interventions
  - Checking the vital signs of the patient
  - Checking for the activity level of the patient
  - Providing small activity
  - Involving in activities of daily living
  - Avoiding staining activity

- **Knowledge deficit about dysrhythmias and its treatment**

  Goal: To provide knowledge about disease and its treatment

  Interventions
  - Explaining the dysrhythmias and its side effects
  - Describing the medications regimen and its rationale
  - Explaining the need for therapeutic serum level of the medication
  - Describing the plan eradicate or limit factors that contribute of the dysrhythmias
  - Stating actions to take in the event of an emergency.

ELECTROCARDIOGRAM—ELECTRICAL CONDUCTION, BASIC ELECTROCARDIOGRAM, 12-LEAD ELECTROCARDIOGRAM, AXIS DETERMINATION

The normal electrical conduction in the heart allows the impulse that is generated by the SA node of the heart to be propagated to the myocardium. The myocardium contracts after stimulation. It is the ordered stimulation of the myocardium that allows efficient contraction of the heart, thereby allowing blood to be pumped throughout the body through aorta.

Conduction Pathway

Signals arising in the SA node stimulate the atria to contract and travel to the AV node. After a delay, the stimulus is conducted through the bundle of His to the Purkinje fibers and the endocardium at the apex of the heart, then finally to the ventricular epicardium.

Depolarization and the Electrocardiogram

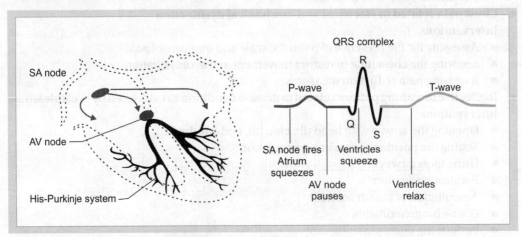

Fig. 5.20: Normal electrocardiogram (ECG).

- **SA node** (P wave): This electrical impulse is propagated throughout the right atrium, stimulating the myocardium of the atria to contract. The conduction of the electrical impulse throughout the atria is seen on the ECG as the P wave **(Fig. 5.20)**.
- **AV node** (PR interval): The AV node functions as a critical delay in the conduction system. The atria and ventricles would contract at the same time, and blood would not flow effectively from the atria to the ventricles. The delay in the AV node forms much of the PR segment on the ECG.

- **QRS complex:** The two bundle branches taper out to produce numerous Purkinje fibers, which stimulate individual groups of myocardial cells to contract. The spread of electrical activity through the ventricular myocardium produces the QRS complex on the ECG.

Ventricular Repolarization

The last event of the cycle is the repolarization of the ventricles. It is the restoration of the resting state. In the ECG, repolarization includes the J wave, ST segment, and T and U waves.

Electrical Signals and Blood Flow

The SA node normally produces 60–100 electrical signals per minute—heart rate or pulse. With each pulse, signals from the SA node follow a natural electrical pathway through heart walls.

- **Depolarization:** Electrical activation of the myocardium
- **Repolarization:** Restoration of the electrical potential of the myocardial cell.

Characteristics of the Normal Basic Electrocardiogram
Characteristics of the normal basic electrocardiogram include:
1. Measurements
2. Rhythm
3. Conduction

Measurements:
- ❖ Heart rate: 60–90 bpm
- ❖ PR interval: 0.12–0.20 second
- ❖ QRS duration: 0.06–0.10 second
- ❖ QT interval (QT$_c$ ≤0.40 second)
- ❖ Bazett's formula: QT$_c$ = (QT)/SqRoot RR (in seconds)

Electrocardiogram Paper

Time is measured from the L to the R—one large box = 0.20 second and one small one = 0.04 second.

The rate of the ECG machine is 25 mm/s. Marks on the upper or lower border of paper fall every 3 seconds or 3 in. **(Fig. 5.21)**.

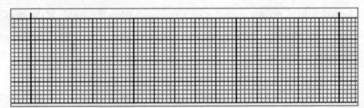

Fig. 5.21: Electrocardiogram (ECG) paper.

Dimensions of grids on ECG paper: Horizontal axis represents time. Large blocks are 0.2 second in duration, while small blocks are 0.04 second in duration. Vertical axis represents voltage. Large blocks are 5 mm, while small blocks represent 1 mm.

Estimation of Heart Rate

Heart rates of 50–300 beats/min: They can be estimated from the number of large squares in an R–R interval. Because there are 300 large blocks in 1 minute, the number of blocks between R–R intervals can be divided into 300 to approximate the rate. For example, one large block between R–R intervals would be determined.

Heart rates of <50 beats/min: They can be estimated with the aid of markings at 3-second intervals along the graph paper. To calculate the rate, the cycles on a 6-second interval (two 3-second markings) are multiplied by 10 (to give the rate per 60 seconds; i.e., per minute).

Definition

A 12-lead ECG will show a short segment of the recording of each of the 12-leads. This is often arranged in a grid of four columns by three rows, the first column being the limb leads (I, II, and III), the second column the augmented limb leads [augmented vector right (aVR), augmented vector left (aVL), and augmented vector foot (aVF)] and the last two columns being the chest leads (V_1-V_6).

Leads

The term "lead" in electrocardiography causes much confusion because it is used to refer to two different things. In accordance with common parlance, the word "lead" may be used to refer to the electrical cable attaching the electrodes to the ECG recorder. As such, it may be acceptable to refer to the "left arm lead" as the electrode (and its cable) that should be attached at or near the left arm. Usually, 10 of these electrodes are standard in a "12-lead" ECG.

Placement of Electrodes

Ten electrodes are used for a 12-lead ECG. The electrodes usually consist of a conducting gel, embedded in the middle of a self-adhesive pad onto which cables clip.

Electrode label (United States)	Electrode placement
RA	On the right arm, avoiding thick muscle
LA	In the same location where RA was placed, but on the left arm
RL	On the right leg, lateral calf muscle
LL	In the same location where RL was placed, but on the left leg
V_1	In the fourth intercostal space (between ribs 4 and 5) just to the right of the sternum (breastbone)
V_2	In the fourth intercostal space (between ribs 4 and 5) just to the left of the sternum
V_3	Between leads V_2 and V_4
V_4	In the fifth intercostal space (between ribs 5 and 6) in the mid-clavicular line
V_5	Horizontally even with V_4, in the left anterior axillary line
V_6	Horizontally even with V_4 and V_5 in the midaxillary line

Additional Electrodes

A posterior ECG can aid in the diagnosis of a posterior MI. This is performed by the addition of leads V_7, V_8, and V_9 extending around the left chest wall toward the back.

Limb Leads

In both the 5- and 12-lead configurations, leads I, II, and III are called limb leads. The electrodes that form these signals are located on the limbs—one on each arm and one on the left leg. The limb leads form the points of is known as Einthoven's triangle.

Unipolar Versus Bipolar Leads

The two types of leads are unipolar and bipolar.

1. Bipolar leads have one positive and one negative pole. In a 12-lead ECG, the limb leads (I, II, and III) are bipolar leads.
2. Unipolar leads also have two poles, as a voltage is measured; however, the negative pole is a composite pole (Wilson's central terminal, or WCT) made up of signals from multiple other electrodes. In a 12-lead ECG, all leads except the limb leads are unipolar (aVR, aVL, aVF, V_1, V_2, V_3, V_4, V_5, and V_6).

Augmented Limb Leads

Leads aVR, aVL, and aVF are augmented limb leads. They are derived from the same three electrodes as leads I, II, and III. However, they view the heart from different angles. This zeroes out the negative electrode and allows the positive electrode to become the "exploring electrode." WCT paved the way for the development of the augmented limb leads aVR, aVL, aVF and the precordial leads V_1, V_2, V_3, V_4, V_5, and V_6.

- **Lead aVR** has the positive electrode (white) on the right arm. The negative electrode is a combination of the left arm (black) electrode and the left leg (red) electrode, which "augments" the signal strength of the positive electrode on the right arm.
- **Lead aVL** has the positive (black) electrode on the left arm. The negative electrode is a combination of the right arm (white) electrode and the left leg (red) electrode, which "augments" the signal strength of the positive electrode on the left arm.
- **Lead aVF** has the positive (red) electrode on the left leg. The negative electrode is a combination of the right arm (white) electrode and the left arm (black) electrode, which "augments" the signal of the positive electrode on the left leg.

Precordial Leads

The electrodes for the precordial leads (V_1, V_2, V_3, V_4, V_5, and V_6) are placed directly on the chest. Because of their close proximity to the heart, they do not require augmentation. Unipolar leads (all have "V" in their names)—aV_R, aV_L, aV_F, and the precordial leads V_1–V_6.

Placement of Electrocardiogram Leads

- Addendum: V_3 is placed halfway between V_2 and V_4
- Right chest (or anterior) leads—V_1, V_2; also aV_R
- Septal leads—V_3 and V_4—located over the interventricular septum
- Left chest (or lateral) leads—V_5, V_6; also I and aV_L
- V_1 and V_2 mirror changes occurring from the posterior side of the heart. None of the usual electrodes are directly adjacent to the posterior surface of the heart
- If additional posterior leads need to be seen (e.g., to diagnose a true posterior infarction) do another 12-lead ECG but move three electrodes to these positions
- V_7 = same horizontal plane as V_4–V_6; posterior axillary line
- V_8 = same horizontal plane as V_4–V_6; mid-scapula
- V_9 = same horizontal plane as V_4–V_6; over spine
- V_3R = halfway between V_1 and V_4R
- V_4R = 5 radioimmunoconjugates (RICS) at mantle cell lymphoma (MCL)
- V_5R = same horizontal plane as V_4R at anterior axillary line
- V_6R = same horizontal plane as V_4R at midaxillary line

Waves and Intervals

Feature	Description	Duration
RR interval	The interval between an R wave and the next R wave; normal resting heart rate is between 60 and 100 bpm	0.6–1.2 s
P wave	During normal atrial depolarization, the main electrical vector is directed from the SA node toward the AV node and spreads from the right atrium to the left atrium. This turns into the P wave on the ECG	80 ms
PR interval	The PR interval is measured from the beginning of the P wave to the beginning of the QRS complex. The PR interval reflects the time the electrical impulse takes to travel from the sinus node through the AV node and entering the ventricles. The PR interval is, therefore, a good estimate of AV node function	120–200 ms
PR segment	The PR segment connects the P wave and the QRS complex. The impulse vector is from the AV node to the bundle of His to the bundle branches and then to the Purkinje fibers. This electrical activity does not produce a contraction directly and is merely traveling down toward the ventricles, and this shows up flat on the ECG. The PR interval is more clinically relevant	50–120 ms
QRS complex	The QRS complex reflects the rapid depolarization of the right and left ventricles. The ventricles have a large muscle mass compared to the atria, so the QRS complex usually has a much larger amplitude than the P wave	80–120 ms
J-point	The point at which the QRS complex finishes and the ST segment begins. It is used to measure the degree of ST elevation or depression present	N/A
ST segment	The ST segment connects the QRS complex and the T wave. The ST segment represents the period when the ventricles are depolarized. It is isoelectric	80–120 ms
T wave	The T wave represents the repolarization (or recovery) of the ventricles. The interval from the beginning of the QRS complex to the apex of the T wave is referred to as the absolute refractory period. The last half of the T wave is referred to as the relative refractory period (or vulnerable period)	160 ms
ST interval	The ST interval is measured from the J-point to the end of the T wave	320 ms
QT interval	The QT interval is measured from the beginning of the QRS complex to the end of the T wave. A prolonged QT interval is a risk factor for ventricular tachyarrhythmias and sudden death. It varies with heart rate and, for clinical relevance, requires a correction for this, giving the QTc	Up to 420 ms in heart rate of 60 bpm
U wave	The U wave is hypothesized to be caused by the repolarization of the interventricular septum. It normally has low amplitude and even more often is completely absent. It always follows the T wave and also follows the same direction in amplitude. If it is too prominent, suspect hypokalemia, hypercalcemia, or hyperthyroidism	
J wave	The J wave that elevated J-point or Osborn wave appears as a late delta wave following the QRS or as a small secondary R wave. It is considered pathognomonic of hypothermia or hypercalcemia	

Normal ECG Waveforms and Intervals

P waves—represent depolarization of the atrial myocardium. (Sinus node depolarization is too small in amplitude to be recorded from the body surface so it is not seen)

The normal P wave is
- Not wider than 0.11 second (under three little boxes on the ECG paper)
- Not taller than 3 mm
- Not notched or peaked; does not have an excessive trough if biphasic
- Positive and rounded in leads I, II, and aV$_F$ in 94% of normal; usually upright in V$_4$–V$_6$.

Electrocardiogram Waveforms

PR Interval

It represents atrial depolarization plus the normal delay at the AV node **(Fig. 5.22)**.
- Normally = 0.12–0.20 second (no longer than one large box)
- Increased in length if AV conduction is prolonged (first-degree AV block)

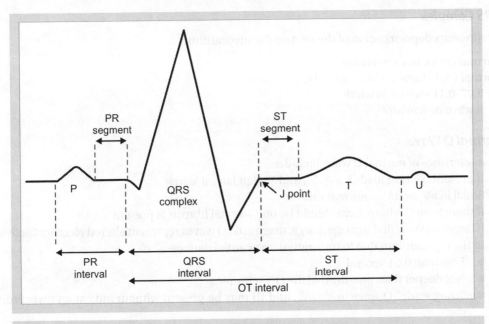

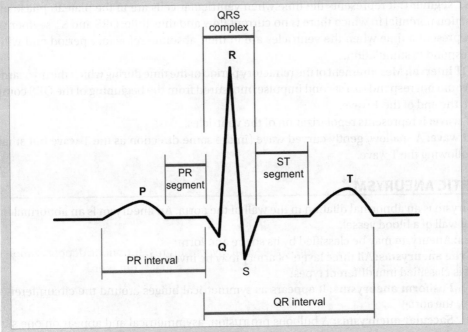

Fig. 5.22: Electrocardiogram (ECG) waveforms.

PR Segment

It begins at the end of the P wave and ends with the onset of the QRS complex and has the following characteristics:

- Should be isoelectric (flat)
- Can be elevated with atrial infarction or pericarditis
- Can be depressed if there is a large repolarization wave (T_p) following the P wave.

QRS Complex

It represents depolarization of the ventricular myocardium.

Normal QRS Characteristics
Normal QRS characteristics include:
- 0.07–0.11 second in width
- R wave progression

Normal Q Wave

Characteristics of normal Q wave include:
- It presents only in leads I, aV_L, V_5, and V_6 (left lateral leads)
- Small in aV_F and V_5—normal variant
- If there is no Q where there should be one—septal fibrosis is present
- If large—myocardial damage. Large, diagnostic Q waves represent altered electrical activity in the myocardium due to transmural myocardial damage.
  - Less than 0.04 second
  - Not deeper than one-third of the QRS complex
  - "Diagnostic" Q wave in V_1, aV_L, and III may be present without indicating myocardial damage.
- **ST segment:** It represents the time when ventricular cells are in the plateau phase of the action potential in which there is no current flow and thus little. QRS and ST segment also represent a time when the ventricles are in their absolute refractory period and will not respond to stimulation.
- **QT interval:** Measurement of the refractory period or the time during which the myocardium would not respond to a second impulse; measured from the beginning of the QRS complex to the end of the T wave.
- **T wave:** It represents repolarization of the ventricles.
- **U wave:** A shallow, gently curved wave (in the same direction as the T wave but smaller) following the T wave.

AORTIC ANEURYSM

Aneurysm is an abnormal dilation in the wall of the aorta. An aneurysm is an abnormal bulge in the wall of a blood vessel.

Types: Aneurysm may be classified by its shape and form:
- **True aneurysms:** All three layers of artery may be involved.
  It is classified into different types:
  1. **Fusiform aneurysms:** It appears as symmetrical bulges around the circumference of the aorta.
  2. **Saccular aneurysms:** A bulbous protrusion, asymmetrical and appear on one side of the aorta.
  3. **Dissecting aneurysms:** A bilateral out pouching in which layers of the vessels wall separate.
- **False aneurysms:** The wall rupture and a blood clot is retained in an out pouching of tissue or there connection between and artery that does not close **(Fig. 5.23)**.

The two types of aortic aneurysm:
1. **Thoracic aortic aneurysms:** They develop in the part of the aorta that runs through the chest.
2. **Abdominal aortic aneurysms:** They develop in the part of the aorta that runs through the abdomen.

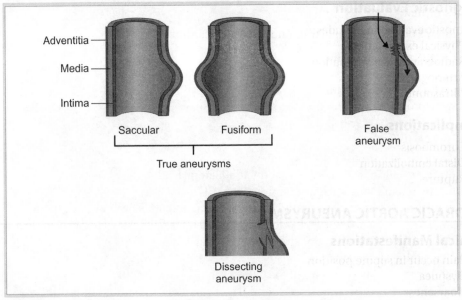

Fig. 5.23: Types of aneurysm.

Etiology

Etiologies are as follows:
- Atherosclerosis
- Hypertension
- Blunt arterial aneurysm
- Pseudoaneurysm
- Hypercholesterolemia
- Tobacco use
- Peripheral vascular disease
- Marfan syndrome
- Bicuspid aortic valve

Pathophysiology

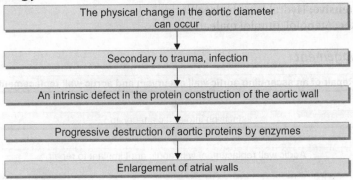

Clinical Manifestations

- Abdominal
  - Flank
  - Back pain

Diagnostic Evaluation

Diagnostic evaluation includes:
- Physical examination
- Radiographical examination
- Arteriography
- Ultrasound

Complications

- Thrombosis
- Distal embolization
- Rupture

THORACIC AORTIC ANEURYSM

Clinical Manifestations

- Pain occur in supine position
- Dyspnea
- Hoarseness
- Stridor
- Weakness
- Aphonia
- Dysphasia

Diagnostic Evaluation

- Physical examination
- Radiographical examination
- Arteriography
- Ultrasound

Treatment

Medical Management

- **Antihypertensive:** Hydralazine hydrochloride
- **Beta blocker:** Atenolol, timolol maleate

Surgical Management

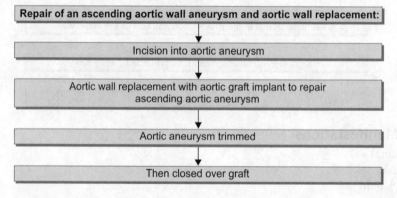

ABDOMINAL AORTIC ANEURYSM

Causes

- The most common cause of abdominal aortic aneurysm is arteriosclerosis
- Congenital weakness
- Trauma or disease

Risk Factors

- Genetic predisposition
- Smoking
- Hypertension

Clinical Manifestations

- Patient can feel their heart beating in abdomen
- Abdominal mass
- Abdominal throbbing

Diagnostic Evaluation

- Physical examination
- Radiographical examination
- Arteriography
- Ultrasound

Medical Management

Medical therapy of aortic aneurysms involves strict BP control. Attention needs to be given to patient's general BP, smoking, and cholesterol risks.

Endovascular Surgery

The endovascular treatment of aortic aneurysms involves the placement of an endovascular stent via a percutaneous technique in portion of the aorta.

DISSECTING AORTA

An aortic dissection is a serious condition in which a tear develops in the inner layer of the aorta, the large blood vessel branching off the heart **classification**.

Etiology

- High BP
- Bicuspid aortic valve
- Marfan syndrome
- Turner syndrome
- Syphilis
- Cocaine use
- Pregnancy
- Trauma
- Surgical complications

Risk Factors

- Aging
- Atherosclerosis
- Blunt trauma to the chest, such as hitting the steering wheel of a car during an accident
- High BP

Pathophysiology

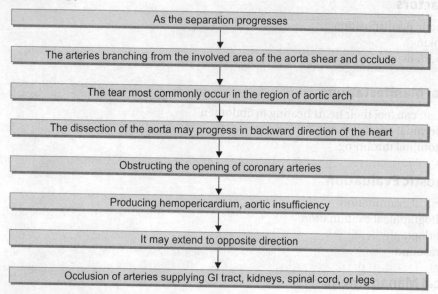

As the separation progresses

↓

The arteries branching from the involved area of the aorta shear and occlude

↓

The tear most commonly occur in the region of aortic arch

↓

The dissection of the aorta may progress in backward direction of the heart

↓

Obstructing the opening of coronary arteries

↓

Producing hemopericardium, aortic insufficiency

↓

It may extend to opposite direction

↓

Occlusion of arteries supplying GI tract, kidneys, spinal cord, or legs

Clinical Manifestations

- Sudden onset of symptoms
- Severe and persistent pain
- Sweating
- Tachycardia
- Appear pale
- Hypertension
- Anxiety and a feeling of doom
- Fainting or dizziness
- Heavy sweating
- Nausea and vomiting
- Orthopnea

Diagnostic Tests

- **Physical examination**
- **D-Dimer:** A blood D-DIMER level less than 500 ng/mL
- **Chest X-ray**
- **CT**
- **MRI**

- **Transesophageal echocardiography**
- **Aortogram:** An aortogram involves placement of a catheter in the aorta and injection of contrast material while taking X-rays of the aorta. The procedure is known as aortography.

Management

Medical Management

- **Antibiotic:** Doxycycline
- **Antihypertensive:** Hydralazine hydrochloride
- **Beta blocker:** Atenolol
- **Vasodilators:** Sodium nitroprusside
- **Calcium channel blockers:** Nifedipine

Surgical Management

1. **Bentall procedure:** Replacement of the damaged section of aorta and replacement of the aortic valve.
2. **David procedure:** Replacement of the damaged section of aorta and reimplantation of the aortic valve.
3. **Tevar:** It is a surgical intervention known as thoracic endovascular aortic repair.
4. **Vascular ring connector (VRC):** Replacement of the damaged section of aorta with a sutureless VRC-reinforced Dacron graft.

RAYNAUD'S PHENOMENON

Raynaud's phenomenon is a vasospastic disorder causing discoloration of the fingers, toes, and occasionally other areas. This condition may also cause nails to become brittle with longitudinal ridges. The result of vasospasms is to decrease blood supply to the respective regions.

Types of Raynaud's Disease

There are two types of Raynaud's disease—primary and secondary

1. **Primary Raynaud's disease:** In these cases, the cause of the condition is unknown.
2. **Secondary Raynaud's disease:** Secondary Raynaud's disease is so called because it occurs secondary to another condition or factor, such as:
   - Medications
   - Hormone imbalance
   - Injury
   - Occupational exposure

Causes

1. **Primary Raynaud's:** Raynaud's disease, or "Primary Raynaud's," is diagnosed if the symptoms are idiopathic or genetics.
2. **Secondary Raynaud's:** It occurs secondary to a wide variety of other conditions, such as **connective tissue disorders, eating disorders, and atherosclerosis; drugs include beta blockers.**

Pathophysiology

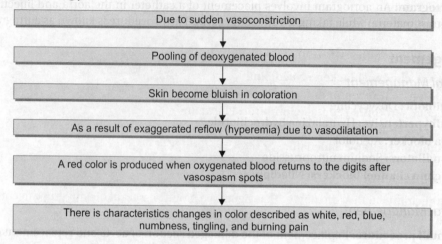

Due to sudden vasoconstriction

↓

Pooling of deoxygenated blood

↓

Skin become bluish in coloration

↓

As a result of exaggerated reflow (hyperemia) due to vasodilatation

↓

A red color is produced when oxygenated blood returns to the digits after vasospasm spots

↓

There is characteristics changes in color described as white, red, blue, numbness, tingling, and burning pain

Signs and Symptoms

- Pain
- Discoloration (paleness)
- Sensations of cold and/or numbness
- Swelling
- Tingling
- Raynaud's also has occurred in breastfeeding mothers, causing nipples to turn white and become extremely painful.

Diagnostic Tests

- Digital artery pressure
- Doppler ultrasound
- Full blood count
- Blood test for urea and electrolytes
- Thyroid function tests

Management

- Environmental triggers should be avoided
- Emotional stress is another recognized trigger
- Consumption of caffeine should be stopped
- Extremities should be kept warm

Emergency Measures

- Keeping warm and maintaining a constant body temperature
- Wearing gloves and warm socks when out in the cold
- No smoking
- Warming the hands and feet
- Medications to thin the blood, for example, aspirin
- Not directly handling cold things
- Keeping the skin supple by using moisturizers
- Managing stress and emotional situations

- Avoiding medications that can aggravate blood vessel spasm, for example, some cold and flu medications
- Alternative therapies, for example, massage and acupuncture

Pharmacological intervention

- **Calcium channel blockers:** Nifedipine
- **Angiotensin II receptor antagonists:** Losartan
- **Selective serotonin reuptake inhibitor:** Fluoxetine
- **Antidepressant medications:** Examples, amitriptyline, nortriptyline, fluoxetine
- **Vasodilator therapy:** Sildenafil

Surgical Intervention

Sympathectomy: In this, the nerves that signal the blood vessels of the fingertips to constrict are surgically cut.

Nursing Care Plan

1. **Risk for hemorrhage related to graft procedure**
   - **Interventions**
     - ♦ Monitoring pulse rate
     - ♦ Monitoring central venous pressure
     - ♦ Providing sterile dressing on wound
     - ♦ Giving vitamin K as physician's order
     - ♦ Preventing infections
2. **Pain related to disease condition as evidenced by verbal communication**
   - **Interventions**
     - ♦ Assessing for the presence of pain, the scale and intensity of pain
     - ♦ Teaching the client about pain management and relaxation with distraction
     - ♦ Securing the chest tube to restrict movement and avoid irritation
     - ♦ Assessing pain reduction measures
     - ♦ Providing NSAIDS as indicated
3. **Risk for impaired gas exchange related to cough and pain from incision**
   - **Interventions**
     - a. *Airway management:*
       - ○ Open the airway with head tilt, chin lift, and jaw thrust
       - ○ Perform chest physiotherapy
       - ○ Perform suction
       - ○ Set the position to maximize ventilation
       - ○ Use tools airway
       - ○ Teach breathing deeply and coughing effectively
       - ○ Auscultation of breath sounds
       - ○ Administer bronchodilators
     - b. *Oxygenation therapy:*
       - ○ Provide humidification system of oxygen equipment
       - ○ Monitor the flow of oxygen and the amount given
       - ○ Monitor signs of oxygen toxicity

MULTIPLE CHOICE QUESTIONS

1. The risk of dying as a result of cardiovascular disease increases with advancing age. Approximately what percent of persons who die of coronary heart disease are older adults—age 65 or older?
   A. >80
   B. 55
   C. 66
   D. 75

2. Modifiable risk factors that increase the risk of acute myocardial infarction (MI) include all of the following, *except*:
   A. Hypertension
   B. Smoking
   C. Food allergies
   D. Lack of physical activity

3. The overwhelming majority of strokes are ischemic. The percentage of strokes attributable to intracerebral hemorrhage is:
   A. 25
   B. 18
   C. 10
   D. <6

4. More than 60% of stroke deaths occur in:
   A. Native Americans
   B. Women
   C. Mexican Americans
   D. Persons age 45–64

5. Risk of ischemic stroke is reduced among women with all of the following characteristics, *except*:
   A. Low BMI
   B. Regular exercise
   C. Healthy diet
   D. Menopause before age 42

6. Transient ischemic attacks (TIA) are associated with all of the following, *except*:
   A. Increased risk of stroke in the first 30 days following the TIA
   B. Increased risk of stroke in the first 90 days following the TIA
   C. Increased risk of death within 1 year of the TIA
   D. Increased risk of congenital heart disease

7. High blood pressure is less common among women who:
   A. Are age 45 and younger
   B. Are obese
   C. Use oral contraceptives
   D. Are African American

8. By definition, prehypertension is untreated systolic or diastolic pressure ranging from:
   A. Systolic pressure of 120–139 mm Hg or diastolic pressure of 80–89 mm Hg
   B. Systolic pressure of 110–129 mm Hg or diastolic pressure of 70–79 mm Hg
   C. Systolic pressure of 130–149 mm Hg or diastolic pressure of 90–99 mm Hg
   D. Systolic pressure of 130-149 mm Hg and diastolic pressure of 90–99 mm Hg

9. The most commonly occurring congenital cardiovascular defect is:
   A. Tetralogy of Fallot
   B. Ventricular septal defect
   C. Coarctation of the aorta
   D. Hypoplastic left heart syndrome

10. Among postmenopausal women with coronary heart disease, the strongest risk factor for heart failure is:
    A. First child after age 30
    B. No children
    C. Diet low in fruits and vegetables
    D. Diabetes

11. Heart disease is the leading cause of death among men and women of all races and ethnic groups; however, mortality varies by ethnicity. The group with the lowest mortality is:
    A. African Americans
    B. Native Americans or Alaska Natives
    C. Hispanics/Latinos
    D. Asian or Pacific Islanders

12. **Reducing cholesterol and blood pressure may reduce all of the following, *except*:**
    A. Heart disease mortality
    B. Incidence of nonfatal myocardial infarction
    C. Risk of developing heart disease
    D. Risk of congenital heart disease

13. **The most commonly occurring arrhythmia is:**
    A. Atrial fibrillation   B. Ventricular tachycardia
    C. Bradycardia   D. Ventricular fibrillation

14. **Symptoms, such as shortness of breath, fatigue, weakness, difficulty breathing when recumbent, weight gain, and swelling in the lower extremities may indicate:**
    A. Atrial fibrillation   B. Heart failure
    C. Cardiac arrest   D. Stroke

15. **To reduce the risk of heart disease total cholesterol levels should be less than:**
    A. 100 mg/dL   B. 60 mg/dL
    C. 200 mg/dL   D. 150 mg/dL

16. **Which condition has a 95% risk of death?**
    A. Myocardial infarction   B. Atrial fibrillation
    C. Heart failure   D. Sudden cardiac arrest

17. **Atrial septal defect is:**
    A. A congenital heart defect in which there is a hole between the heart's two lower chambers
    B. A congenital heart defect in which there is a hole between the heart's two upper chambers
    C. A nonfatal cardiac arrhythmia
    D. Enlargement of the atria

18. **Which of the following groups is not at increased risk of developing endocarditis?**
    A. Patients with artificial heart valve or implanted medical devices in the heart or blood vessels
    B. Patients with congenital heart defects
    C. Persons with poor dental hygiene and gum disease
    D. Persons with elevated cholesterol levels

19. **Which of the following statement about mitral valve prolapse is false?**
    A. It is generally asymptomatic and requires no treatment
    B. It affects less than 3% of the population
    C. It is more common in persons with connective tissue disorders, such as Marfan syndrome
    D. All people with mitral valve prolapse require immediate medical or surgical treatment

20. **The risks associated with stents include all of the following, *except*:**
    A. Blood clot at the stent site
    B. Rupture of an aneurysm
    C. Blocked blood flow to the lower body
    D. Elevated cholesterol or triglyceride levels

Answers

   1. A   2. C   3. C   4. B   5. D   6. D   7. A   8. A   9. B   10. D
   11. B   12. D   13. A   14. B   15. C   16. D   17. B   18. D   19. D   20. D

BIBLIOGRAPHY

1. Brunner S. A textbook of medical surgical nursing, 10th edition. Philadelphia, PA: Lippincott Company; 2007. pp. 1052–60.

2. Edhag O, Swahn A. Prognosis of patients with complete heart block or arrhythmic syncope who were not treated with artificial pacemakers. A long-term follow-up study of 101 patients. Acta Med Scand. 1976;200(6):457–63.

3. Exeer NA. Cardiovascular diseases. In: Conduction disturbances. Aliabad Kabul, Afghanistan: University Hospital, Kabul Medical University; 2010.

4. Hopper P, William L. Understanding of medical surgical nursing, 2nd edition. Davis; 2003. pp. 286–97.

5. Lemone P, Burke K. A textbook of medical surgical nursing, 4th edition. South Asia: Dorling Kindersley; 2007.

Cardiovascular Emergencies

CARDIOVASCULAR ASSESSMENT

An intensive and focused cardiovascular assessment indicates a potential cardiovascular problem.

- **Past health history:** The past health history should include hypertension, elevated blood cholesterol heart murmurs, congenital heart disease, rheumatic fever or unexplained joint pains, and cardiac surgeries.
- **Current lifestyle and psychosocial status:** Current lifestyle and psychosocial issues include:
  - **Nutrition:** Dietary pattern should be determined. Body weight and any recent weight gain or weight loss should be assessed.
  - **Smoking:** Any smoking habits should be informed.
  - **Alcohol:** The quantity of alcohol the patient normally consumes daily should be recorded.
  - **Exercise:** Activity level and exercise regimen should be considered.
  - **Drugs:** Medication history should be queried.
- **Family history:** Any history of hypertension, obesity, diabetes, coronary artery disease, or sudden death should be queried.
- **Assessment of chest pain:** The following characteristics of pain should be informed:
  - Quality of pain: Is it punching, squeezing, throbbing, or chest heaviness?
  - Radiation of pain: If pain radiates toward left side, left arm, left jaw, or left scapula should be queried.
  - Severity: On a scale of 1–10.
  - What worsens the pain, such as cold, emotional stress, or sexual activity.

- **Orthopnea:** Orthopnea is the inability to breathe when in a lying position. Whether the client feels the same during sleep should be asked.
- **Cough:** History of consistent cough, frequency, timing, and severity should be queried.
- **Edema, cyanosis, and pallor:** Assess for any swelling or skin color changes—cyanosis or pallor.
- **Physical examination**
  - **Inspection:** When inspecting the neck vessels, any abnormalities in jugular venous pulse should be looked for. Central venous pressure and cardiac output are estimated.
  - **Auscultation:** The carotid arteries should be auscultated. The presence of a bruit, which is a blowing or swishing sound, indicating turbulent blood flow and blood pressure should be auscultate.
  - **Palpation:** Palpation allows you to assess the neck for tenderness, abnormal temperature, excessive moisture, pulsations, or abnormal masses. The carotid arteries are to be palpated and the contour and amplitude of the pulse should be felt. Also the peripheral arteries, such as brachial, radial, femoral, and popliteal should be palpated.
- **Heart sounds:** The heart sounds and murmurs should be auscultated.
  - S1 is accelerated during exercise, anemia, hyperthyroidism, and mitral stenosis, while it is diminished in first-degree heart block. S1 split is most audible in tricuspid area.
  - Splitting of S2 sound can occur during pulmonic stenosis, left bundle branch block, atrial septal defect, and right ventricular failure.
  - S3 is produced by the rapid filling of the ventricle and is normal in pregnancy and in children.
  - S4 is typically heard in late diastole before S1 due to decreased ventricular compliance.

CARDIOVASCULAR EMERGENCIES

Cardiovascular emergencies are life-threatening conditions that must be diagnosed immediately to avoid any delay in treatment and to minimize morbidity and mortality.

Cardiac emergencies include:

- Cardiopulmonary arrest
- Hypertensive emergency
- Air embolism
- Cardiac tamponade
- Aortic aneurysm
- Aortic dissection
- Cardiac arrhythmia
- Ventricular fibrillation
- Myocardial infarction

CARDIOPULMONARY ARREST

Cardiac arrest is a sudden cessation of circulation of the blood to myocardium muscles due to failure of the heart to contract effectively. It may be associated with myocardial infarction or atherosclerosis.

It is a medical emergency that, in certain situations, is potentially reversible if treated early. Unexpected cardiac arrest can lead to death within minutes.

Classification of Cardiopulmonary Arrest

Cardiac arrest is classified into two types:
1. Shockable
2. Nonshockable.

Shockable:
- In this type, the rhythm is present but abnormal.
- The two "shockable" rhythms are ventricular fibrillation and pulseless ventricular tachycardia.
- Ventricular fibrillation: It is a condition in which there is uncoordinated contraction of the cardiac muscle of the ventricles in the heart, making them quiver rather than contract properly.
- Ventricular fibrillation is a medical emergency that requires prompt advanced life support interventions. If this arrhythmia continues for more than a few seconds, it will likely degenerate further into asystole and result in sudden death.

Nonshockable: These are asystole and pulseless electrical activity.
- **Asystole:** A life-threatening cardiac condition characterized by the absence of electrical and mechanical activity in the heart.
- Pulseless electrical activity.

Treatment

- Emergency team should be activated.
- CPR should be started immediately.
- Heart rhythm should be evaluated and early defibrillation should be performed as indicated.
- Intubation and IV lines should be started.

HYPERTENSIVE EMERGENCY

A hypertensive emergency is an acute, severe elevation in blood pressure more than 120 mm Hg, accompanied by multiple organ dysfunction.

Etiology

- Essential hypertension
- Renal causes
- Renal artery stenosis
- Glomerulonephritis
- Vascular causes
- Pharmacologic causes
- Sympathomimetics
- Endocrine causes
- Cushing's syndrome
- Neurologic causes
- Central nervous system trauma
- Intracranial mass
- Cocaine
- Amphetamines
- Autoimmune cause
- Scleroderma renal crisis

Pathophysiology

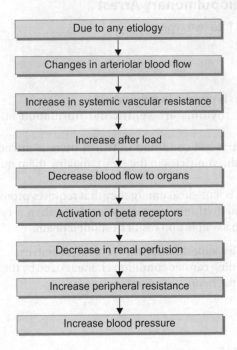

Due to any etiology

↓

Changes in arteriolar blood flow

↓

Increase in systemic vascular resistance

↓

Increase after load

↓

Decrease blood flow to organs

↓

Activation of beta receptors

↓

Decrease in renal perfusion

↓

Increase peripheral resistance

↓

Increase blood pressure

Signs and Symptoms

- Headache
- Blurry vision
- Confusion
- Chest pain
- Shortness of breath
- Back pain

Treatment

- Nitroprusside
- Labetalol

AIR EMBOLISM

An air embolism is a pathological condition characterized by a gas bubble in a vascular system that will result in blockage, which may result in brain, heart, or lung attack.

Etiology

- Injections and surgical procedures
- Lung trauma
- Scuba diving
- Explosion and blast injuries

Signs and Symptoms

- Loss of consciousness
- Cessation of breathing

- Vertigo
- Tremors
- Ataxia
- Loss of control of bodily functions
- Numbness
- Paralysis
- Visual abnormalities
- Hearing abnormalities
- Personality changes
- Cognitive impairment
- Nausea or vomiting
- Extreme fatigue
- Weakness in the extremities
- Areas of abnormal sensation
- Hemoptysis

Diagnostic Evaluation

- Ultrasound
- CT scan
- X-ray

Treatment

- It is important to promptly place the patient in Trendelenburg position.
- The Trendelenburg position keeps a left ventricular air bubble away from the coronary artery and prevents occlusion of coronary arteries.
- Left lateral decubitus positioning helps to trap air in the nondependent segment of the right ventricle.
- Administration of high percentage oxygen is recommended for both venous and arterial air embolism.

CARDIAC TAMPONADE

Cardiac tamponade is accumulation of fluid between the heart muscle between myocardium and pericardium.

Etiology

- Dissecting aortic aneurysm
- End-stage lung cancer
- Heart attack
- Cardiac surgery
- Pericarditis
- Hypothyroidism
- Kidney failure
- Placement of central lines

Signs and Symptoms

- Anxiety and restlessness
- Chest pain

- Radiating to the neck, shoulder, back, or abdomen
- Sharp and stabbing
- Worsened by deep breathing or coughing
- Dyspnea
- Syncope
- Cyanosis
- Palpitation
- Rapid breathing
- Ascites

Diagnostic Evaluation

- Chest CT or MRI of chest
- Chest X-ray
- Coronary angiography
- ECG

Treatment

- **Pericardiocentesis:** It is a procedure that uses a needle to remove fluid from the pericardial sac, the tissue that surrounds the heart.
- **Pericardiectomy:** A procedure to cut and remove part of the pericardium (surgical).

MULTIPLE CHOICE QUESTIONS

1. **Modifiable risk factors that increase the risk of acute myocardial infarction (MI) include all of the following, *except*:**
   A. Hypertension
   B. Smoking
   C. Food allergies
   D. Lack of physical activity

2. **The overwhelming majority of strokes are ischemic. The percentage of strokes attributable to intracerebral hemorrhage is:**
   A. 25
   B. 18
   C. 10
   D. <6

3. **More than 60% of stroke deaths occur in:**
   A. Native Americans
   B. Women
   C. Mexican Americans
   D. Persons aged 45–64

4. **Risk of ischemic stroke is reduced among women with all of the following characteristics, *except*:**
   A. Low BMI
   B. Regular exercise
   C. Healthy diet
   D. Menopause before age 42

5. **Transient ischemic attacks (TIA) are associated with all of the following, *except*:**
   A. Increased risk of stroke in the first 30 days following the TIA
   B. Increased risk of stroke in the first 90 days following the TIA
   C. Increased risk of death within 1 year of the TIA
   D. Increased risk of congenital heart disease

6. **High blood pressure is less common among women who:**
   A. Are age 45 and younger
   B. Are obese
   C. Use oral contraceptives
   D. Are African American

7. **By definition, prehypertension is untreated systolic or diastolic pressure ranging from:**
   A. Systolic pressure of 120–139 mm Hg or diastolic pressure of 80–89 mm Hg
   B. Systolic pressure of 110–129 mm Hg or diastolic pressure of 70–79 mm Hg
   C. Systolic pressure of 130–149 mm Hg or diastolic pressure of 90–99 mm Hg
   D. Systolic pressure of 130–149 mm Hg and diastolic pressure of 90–99 mm Hg

8. **The most commonly occurring congenital cardiovascular defect is:**
   A. Tetralogy of Fallot
   B. Ventricular septal defects
   C. Coarctation of the aorta
   D. Hypoplastic left heart syndrome

9. **Among postmenopausal women with coronary heart disease, the strongest risk factor for heart failure is:**
   A. First child after age 30
   B. No children
   C. Diet low in fruits and vegetables
   D. Diabetes

10. **Heart disease is the leading cause of death among men and women of all races and ethnic groups; however, mortality varies by ethnicity. The group with the lowest mortality is:**
    A. African Americans
    B. Native Americans or Alaska Natives
    C. Hispanics/Latinos
    D. Asian or Pacific Islanders

11. **Reducing cholesterol and blood pressure may reduce all of the following, *except*:**
    A. Heart disease mortality
    B. Incidence of nonfatal myocardial infarction
    C. Risk of developing heart disease
    D. Risk of congenital heart disease

12. **The most commonly occurring arrhythmia is:**
    A. Atrial fibrillation
    B. Ventricular tachycardia
    C. Bradycardia
    D. Ventricular fibrillation

13. **Symptoms, such as shortness of breath, fatigue, weakness, difficulty breathing when recumbent, weight gain, and swelling in the lower extremities may indicate:**
    A. Atrial fibrillation
    B. Heart failure
    C. Cardiac arrest
    D. Stroke

14. **To reduce the risk of heart disease total cholesterol levels should be less than:**
    A. 100 mg/dL
    B. 60 mg/dL
    C. 200 mg/dL
    D. 150 mg/dL

15. **Which condition has a 95% risk of death?**
    A. Myocardial infarction
    B. Atrial fibrillation
    C. Heart failure
    D. Sudden cardiac arrest

16. **Atrial septal defect is:**
    A. A congenital heart defect in which there is a hole between the heart's two lower chambers
    B. A congenital heart defect in which there is a hole between the heart's two upper chambers
    C. A nonfatal cardiac arrhythmia
    D. Enlargement of the atria

17. **Which of the following groups is not at increased risk of developing endocarditis?**
    A. Patients with artificial heart valve or implanted medical devices in the heart or blood vessels
    B. Patients with congenital heart defects
    C. Persons with poor dental hygiene and gum disease
    D. Persons with elevated cholesterol levels

18. **Which of the following statement about mitral valve prolapse is false?**
    A. It is generally asymptomatic and requires no treatment
    B. It affects less than 3% of the population
    C. It is more common in persons with connective tissue disorders, such as Marfan syndrome
    D. All people with mitral valve prolapse require immediate medical or surgical treatment

19. **The risks associated with stents include all of the following, *except*:**
    A. Blood clot at the stent site
    B. Rupture of an aneurysm
    C. Blocked blood flow to the lower body
    D. Elevated cholesterol or triglyceride levels

20. **The risk of dying as a result of cardiovascular disease increases with advancing age. Approximately what percent of persons who die of coronary heart disease are older adults—age 65 or older?**
    A. >80   B. 55
    C. 66   D. 75

Answers

1. C	2. C	3. B	4. D	5. D	6. A	7. A	8. B	9. D	10. B
11. D	12. A	13. B	14. C	15. D	16. B	17. D	18. D	19. D	20. A

Vascular Disorders of Heart

AT THE END OF THIS CHAPTER, THE STUDENTS WILL BE ABLE TO LEARN ABOUT THE NURSING MANAGEMENT OF:

➤ Peripheral vascular disease
➤ Buerger's disease
➤ Takayasu's disease
➤ Syphilitic disease
➤ Aortic aneurysm
➤ Raynaud's disease or Raynaud's syndrome
➤ Varicose veins
➤ Deep vein thrombosis
➤ Hypertension
➤ Hypotension
➤ Chronic venous insufficiency

INTRODUCTION

The primary function of the circulatory system is to transport oxygen, nutrients, and waste products. Hemodynamics of the vessels are governed by a variety of physical properties and laws that explain blood flow through the vascular system. Blood flow is affected by pressure differences, radius of the vessel, length, and viscosity. Flow is directly proportional to the difference in pressure and inversely proportional to resistance. Any disturbance in blood flow in the arterial and venous system disrupts the delivery of oxygen and nutrients and the elimination of waste products. Disturbances of blood flow can be due to compression of the blood vessel, structural changes within the vessel, vasospasm, vasodilatation, or blood clot.

Decrease in perfusion will promote compensatory mechanisms, such as vasodilatation, development of collateral vessels, and anaerobic metabolism. If compensatory mechanisms are unable to meet the oxygen demand by the tissues, ischemia develops, and eventually, tissue death occurs.

ASSESSMENT OF PERIPHERAL VASCULAR SYSTEM

- **General appearance**
  - Does the patient look sick? Are they in any obvious distress?
  - Examine the upper and lower extremities for the following:
    - ◆ Swelling
    - ◆ Erythema
    - ◆ Atrophy/hypertrophy
    - ◆ Deformities
    - ◆ Skin changes

- **Assess for ulcers**
  - Arterial
    - Typically found on finger tips, between the toes and on the heel
    - Are painful, develop acutely, and have discrete borders.
  - Venous
    - Typically found above or over the medial malleolus
    - Are painless, develop slowly, and have poorly defined borders.
- **Varicose veins:** Engorged superficial veins
- **Signs of central or peripheral cyanosis**
  - Central cyanosis—Bluish mucous membranes
  - Peripheral cyanosis—Cool/bluish extremities
- **Capillary refill**
  - Pressure should be applied to the nail bed of the patient's big toe or thumb
  - Upon release, the return of color to the nail bed should be observed:
    - Normal—Return of color within 3–4 seconds
    - Prolonged pallor may indicate arterial insufficiency

Auscultation

Using the diaphragm, auscultation should be done for bruits over the following areas:
- **Carotid arteries:** These auscultate before palpating the carotid arteries.
- **Abdominal aorta:** It auscultates a few centimeters above the umbilicus.
- **Renal arteries:** These auscultate 5 cm above, and 3–5 cm to either side of midline.
- **Femoral arteries:** These auscultate inferior to the midpoint of the inguinal ligament.
- **Popliteal arteries:** These auscultate in the popliteal fossa.

VASCULAR DISEASE

Vascular disease includes any condition that affects the circulatory system. Vascular disease ranges from diseases of arteries, veins, and lymph vessels to blood disorders that affect circulation.

Definition

"Vascular disease is a cardiovascular disorder primarily affecting the blood vessels."

Diagnostic Evaluation

Following are the diagnostic evaluations:
- **The physical examination:** The blood flow in the legs or flow or the blood pressure should be assessed.
- **Tests and examination:**
  - Carotid angiogram
  - **Carotid duplex:** It is a noninvasive procedure that uses ultrasound waves in order to detect plaque.
  - **The Doppler ultrasound:** It is a test used to diagnose both cerebrovascular disease and peripheral vascular disease.
  - **Electroencephalography**
  - **Magnetic resonance imaging (MRI):** This technique is able to obtain 3D images of the body structure.

Nursing Care Plan

Nursing Diagnosis

- Ineffective peripheral tissue perfusion related to impaired arterial circulation
- Pain related to decreased oxygen supply to tissues
- Risk for impaired skin integrity related to compromised tissue perfusion
- Fear and anxiety related to actual or potential lifestyle changes.

Interventions

- **Providing proper positioning:**
  - The legs should be kept in a dependent position to the heart to improve peripheral blood flow.
  - Raising the feet should be avoided.
  - The patient should be kept in a supine position.
- **Promoting vasodilatation:**
  - Warm environment should be provided.
  - Warm drinks or baths should be given.
  - A direct heat source to the extremities should never be applied.
  - Constricting clothes stockings and belts should be avoided.
  - Glucocorticoid should be administered, if indicated.
- **Promoting activity and mobility:** Balanced exercise and rest should be encouraged.
- **Providing care for a client undergoing angiography:**
  - Information regarding procedure should be provided and informed consent should be taken.
  - After the procedure, bed rest should be given.
  - Bleeding, hematoma, or edema at the catheter insertion site should be assessed.
  - Urine output should be monitored.
  - Involved extremity should be kept extended.
  - Vital signs should be monitored.
- **Providing care for a client receiving an autogenous synthetic bypass graft:**
  - The client should be prepared for surgery and the site of the peripheral pulses should be marked safe.
  - The client should be carefully monitored after the procedure for signs of graft rejection.

Common Vascular Disorders
- Peripheral vascular disease
- Syphilitic disease
- Aortic aneurysm
- Raynaud's disease or Raynaud's syndrome
- Varicose veins
- Buerger's disease
- Takayasu's disease
- Deep vein thrombosis

PERIPHERAL VASCULAR DISEASE

It refers to the obstruction of large arteries in extremities that may be associated with atherosclerosis, stenosis, an embolism, or thrombus formation.

Classification

- Mild claudication
- Moderate claudication
- Severe claudication
- Ischemic pain at rest
- Minor tissue loss
- Major tissue loss

Etiology

- Smoking
- Diabetes mellitus
- Elevation of total cholesterol
- Hypertension

Signs and Symptoms

- Pain
- Weakness
- Numbness
- Cyanosis
- Cold extremities
- Diminished hair and nail growth on affected limb and digits.

Diagnostic Evaluation

- **Ankle brachial pressure index:** When the blood pressure readings in the ankles is lower than that in the arms, blockages in the arteries which provide blood from the heart to the ankle are suspected
- **Doppler ultrasound examination:** To rule out the extent of atherosclerosis
- **Angiography**
- **Computerized tomography**

Management

Medical Management

- Smoking cessation
- Management of diabetes
- Management of hypertension
- Management of cholesterol
- Administer antiplatelet drugs
- Regular exercise

Surgical Management

- Percutaneous transluminal angioplasty (*refer* **to coronary artery disease**)
- Coronary artery bypass graft (*refer* **to coronary artery disease**).

THROMBOANGIITIS (BUERGER'S DISEASE)

Thromboangiitis obliterans is a recurring progressive inflammation and thrombosis of small and medium arteries and veins of the extremities.

Etiology

- Autoimmune reaction
- Smoking
- Diabetes mellitus
- Elevation of total cholesterol
- Hypertension

Signs and Symptoms

- Acute and chronic inflammation
- Thrombosis of arteries and veins of the hands and feet
- Ulcerations and gangrene in the extremities
- Claudication
- Pain at rest
- Ischemic ulcers or gangrene

Pathophysiology

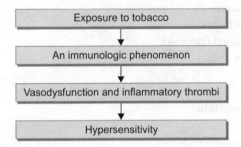

Diagnostic Evaluation

- **Ankle brachial pressure index:** When the blood pressure readings in the ankles is lower than that in the arms, blockages in the arteries which provide blood from the heart to the ankle are suspected
- **Doppler ultrasound examination:** To rule out the extent of atherosclerosis.
- **Angiography**
- **Computerized tomography**

Management

- Smoking cessation
- Management of diabetes
- Management of hypertension
- Management of cholesterol
- Administer antiplatelet drugs
- Regular exercise
- **Surgical management**
  - Percutaneous transluminal angioplasty (*refer* **to coronary artery disease**)
  - Coronary artery bypass graft (*refer* **to coronary artery disease**)

RAYNAUD'S PHENOMENON

Raynaud's phenomenon is a vasospastic disorder causing discoloration of the fingers and toes due to vasospasms.

Types of Raynaud's Disease

a. **Primary Raynaud's disease:** In these cases, the cause of the condition is unknown. It does run in families.

b. **Secondary Raynaud's disease:** Secondary Raynaud's disease is so called because it occurs secondary to another condition or factor, such as:
   - Medications
   - Hormone imbalances
   - Frostbite
   - Occupational exposure

Etiology

- **Connective tissue disorders:**
   - Scleroderma
   - Systemic lupus erythematosus
   - Rheumatoid arthritis
   - Cold agglutinin disease
   - Ehlers–Danlos syndrome
- **Eating disorders:** Anorexia nervosa
- **Obstructive disorders**
   - Atherosclerosis
   - Buerger's disease
   - Thoracic outlet syndrome
- **Drugs**
   - Beta-blockers
   - Cytotoxic drugs—particularly chemotherapeutics and most especially bleomycin.
- **Occupation**
   - Exposure to vinyl chloride, mercury
   - Exposure to the cold
- **Others**
   - Physical trauma, such as that sustained in auto accident or other traumatic events
   - Lyme disease
   - Magnesium deficiency

Signs and Symptoms

- Pain
- Discoloration
- Numbness
- Swelling
- Tingling

Diagnostic Evaluation

- Digital artery pressure
- Doppler ultrasound
- Full blood count
- Blood test for urea and electrolytes
- Thyroid function tests
- Nailfold vasculature

Management

- Environmental triggers should be avoided.
- Emotional stress should be avoided.
- Extremities should be kept warm.
- Consumption of caffeine should be avoided and vasoconstrictors must be prevented.
- **Emergency measures include:**
  - Keeping warm and maintaining a constant body temperature
  - Wearing gloves and warm socks when out in the cold
  - Not smoking
  - Not directly handling cold things
  - Keeping the skin supple by using moisturizers
  - Manage stress and emotional situations
  - Warming the hands and feet with clothing or in warm water.

Pharmacological Management

- Calcium channel blockers
- Angiotensin II receptor antagonists
- Vasodilator therapy
- Selective serotonin reuptake inhibitor
- Antidepressant medications

Surgical Intervention

Sympathectomy: In this, the nerves that signal the blood vessels of the fingertips to constrict are surgically cut.

TAKAYASU'S ARTERITIS

It is a form of large vessel granulomatous vasculitis with massive intimal fibrosis and vascular narrowing.

Etiology

This happens due to obstruction of the main branches of the aorta, including the left common carotid artery, the brachiocephalic artery, and the left subclavian artery.

Pathophysiology

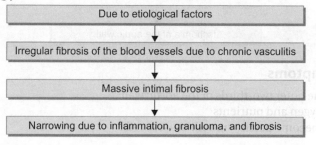

```
Due to etiological factors
          ↓
Irregular fibrosis of the blood vessels due to chronic vasculitis
          ↓
Massive intimal fibrosis
          ↓
Narrowing due to inflammation, granuloma, and fibrosis
```

Signs and Symptoms

- Malaise
- Fever

- Night sweats
- Weight loss
- Arthralgia
- Fatigue
- Anemia

Diagnostic Evaluation

- Elevation of the erythrocyte sedimentation rate (ESR)
- Magnetic resonance angiography
- Computed tomography angiography
- Arterial angiography

Management

Medical Management

Steroids:, such as prednisone

Surgical Management

Surgical management should be as follows:
- Percutaneous transluminal angioplasty (*refer* **coronary artery disease)**
- Coronary artery bypass graft (*refer* **coronary artery disease)**

SYPHILITIC AORTITIS

Syphilitic aortitis is a disease of the aorta associated with the tertiary stage of syphilis infection.

Etiology

It is caused by syphilis infection, which normally occurs in older people.

Pathophysiology

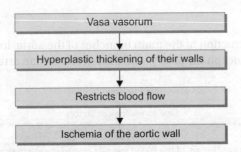

Signs and Symptoms

- Ischemia of the outer two-thirds of the aortic wall
- Starved for oxygen and nutrients
- Elastic fibers become patchy smooth muscle cells
- Necrosis

Treatment

Penicillin treatment is helpful.

AORTIC ANEURYSM

An aneurysm is an abnormal bulge in the wall of a blood vessel.

Types

- **True aneurysms:**
  - **Fusiform aneurysms:** These appear as symmetrical bulges around the circumference of the aorta.
  - **Saccular aneurysms:** These are asymmetrical and appear on one side of the aorta.
  - **Dissecting aneurysms:** A bilateral out pouching in which layers of the vessels wall separate, creating a cavity.
- **False aneurysms:** The wall rupture and a blood clot is retained in an out pouching of tissue or there connection between and artery that does not close.
- **Thoracic aortic aneurysms:** These develop in the part of the aorta that runs through the chest.
- **Abdominal aortic aneurysms:** These develop in the part of the aorta that runs through the abdomen.

Etiology

- Atherosclerosis
- Hypertension

Risk Factors

- Coronary artery disease (CAD)
- Hypertension
- Hypercholesterolemia
- Elevated C-reactive protein
- Tobacco use
- Peripheral vascular disease

Pathophysiology

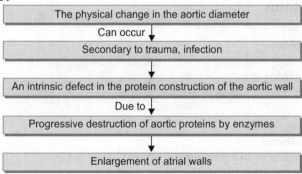

The physical change in the aortic diameter

Can occur ↓

Secondary to trauma, infection

An intrinsic defect in the protein construction of the aortic wall

Due to ↓

Progressive destruction of aortic proteins by enzymes

↓

Enlargement of atrial walls

Management

- **Medical management:** The tetracycline antibiotic doxycycline is currently being investigated for use as a potential drug in the prevention of aortic aneurysm due to its metalloproteinase inhibitor and collagen stabilizing properties.

- **Surgical management:** For abdominal aortic aneurysms suggest elective surgical repair when the diameter of the aneurysm is greater than 5 cm.
- **Open surgery:** Open surgery typically involves dissection of the dilated portion of the aorta and insertion of a synthetic (Dacron or Gore-Tex) patch tube.
- **Endovascular surgery:** The endovascular treatment of aortic aneurysms involves the placement of an endovascular stent via a percutaneous technique (usually through the femoral arteries) into the diseased portion of the aorta.

VARICOSE VEINS

When veins become abnormally thick, full of twists and turns, or enlarged, they are called varicose veins.

Etiology

- Heredity
- Pregnancy
- Obesity
- Menopause
- Aging
- Prolonged standing
- Leg injury
- Abdominal straining
- Crossing legs at the knees

Aggravating Factors of the Varicose Veins

- Pregnancy
- Prolonged standing
- Obesity
- Straining
- Prior surgery
- Age

Signs and Symptoms

- Aching, heavy legs
- Appearance of spider
- Ankle swelling
- A brownish-blue shiny skin
- Redness, dryness, and itchiness of areas of skin
- Cramps
- Prolonged healing
- Restless legs syndrome
- Whitened, irregular scar-like patches can appear at the ankles

Diagnostic Evaluation

- Digital artery pressure
- Doppler ultrasound
- Full blood count
- Blood test for urea and electrolytes

- Thyroid function tests
- Nailfold vasculature

Management

Conservative Management

- Elevating the legs often provides temporary symptomatic relief.
- Advice about regular exercise sounds sensible, but is not supported by any evidence
- The wearing of compression stockings with variable pressure to correct the swelling
- Anti-inflammatory medication

Surgical Management

Stripping: Stripping consists of removal of all or part the saphenous vein main trunk.

Nonsurgical Treatment

Sclerotherapy: A commonly performed nonsurgical treatment for varicose and "spider" leg veins is sclerotherapy in which medicine is injected into the veins to make them shrink.

Complications

- Pain, heaviness
- Inability to walk
- Dermatitis
- Skin ulcers
- Development of carcinoma
- Blood clotting within affected veins
- Acute fat necrosis
- The afflicted person suffers tenderness in that region.

DEEP VEIN THROMBOSIS

Deep vein thrombosis is a blood clot in a deep vein. A clot inside a blood vessel is called a thrombus.

Etiology

- Combination of venous stasis
- Hypercoagulability
- Physical damage or endothelial activation
- Deficiencies in antithrombin

Risk Factors

- Older age
- Immobilization
- Pregnancy
- Antiphospholipid syndrome
- Trauma
- Major surgery
- Cancers
- Oral contraceptives

- Inflammatory diseases
- Nephrotic syndrome
- Obesity
- Infection
- Human immunodeficiency virus (HIV)
- Hormonal replacement therapy
- Central venous catheters
- Chemotherapy

Pathophysiology

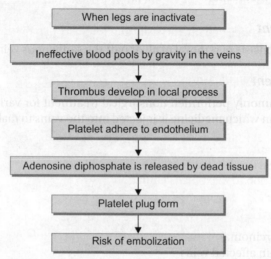

When legs are inactivate

↓

Ineffective blood pools by gravity in the veins

↓

Thrombus develop in local process

↓

Platelet adhere to endothelium

↓

Adenosine diphosphate is released by dead tissue

↓

Platelet plug form

↓

Risk of embolization

Signs and Symptoms

- Swelling in one or both legs
- Pain or tenderness in one or both legs, which may occur only while standing or walking
- Warmth in the skin of the affected leg
- Red or discolored skin in the affected leg
- Visible surface veins
- Leg fatigue

Diagnostic Evaluation

- Physical examination
- CT scan
- D-Dimer test
- Duplex ultrasound

Management

- **Anticoagulation:** Such as heparin
- Graduated compression stockings and walking

Surgical Management

- **Thrombolysis:** This process, which acts to break up clots, can be systemic or catheter-directed.
- **Mechanical thrombectomy:** A mechanical thrombectomy device can remove a thrombosis.

Nursing Care Plan

Nursing Diagnosis

Risk for hemorrhage related to graft procedure

Interventions:
- Monitoring pulse rate
- Monitoring central venous pressure
- Providing sterile dressing on wound
- Giving vitamin K as doctor's order

Pain related to disease condition as evidenced by verbal communication

Interventions:
- Assessing for the presence of pain, the scale and intensity of pain
- Teaching the client about pain management and relaxation with distraction
- Securing the chest tube to restrict movement and avoid irritation
- Assessing pain reduction measures
- Providing analgesics as indicated

Risk for impaired gas exchange related to cough and pain from incision

Interventions:
- **Airway management includes:**
  - Opening the airway with head-tilt, chin-lift, and jaw thrust
  - Setting the position to maximize ventilation
  - Using tools airway
  - Performing chest physiotherapy
  - Teaching the client to breathe deeply and cough effectively
  - Performing suction
  - Auscultation of breath sounds
  - Giving bronchodilators
- **Oxygenation therapy includes:**
  - Providing humidification system of oxygen equipment
  - Monitoring the flow of oxygen and the amount given
  - Monitoring signs of oxygen toxicity

HYPERTENSION

Hypertension is a chronic medical condition in which the blood pressure in the arteries is elevated. High blood pressure is said to be present if it is often at or above 140/90 mm Hg.

Classification of Hypertension

Hypertension may be classified according to type (systolic and diastolic), cause, and degree of severity.

A. **Classification on the basis of type**
   i. **Systolic hypertension:** Systolic hypertension is systolic pressure greater than 140 mm Hg.
   ii. **Diastolic hypertension:** Diastolic hypertension is diastolic pressure greater than 90 mm Hg.

B. **On the basis of etiology:**
   i. **Primary hypertension:** Primary hypertension is also known as **idiopathic hypertension**.
   ii. **Secondary hypertension:** Secondary hypertension results from an identifiable cause.

C. **On the basis of severity**
   i. Borderline hypertension
   ii. Benign hypertension
   iii. Malignant hypertension

TABLE 7.1: Blood pressure classification for adults.*†

Blood pressure classification	SBP‡ (mm Hg§)	DBP¶ (mm Hg)
Normal	<120	and <80
Prehypertension	120–139	or 80–89
Stage 1 Hypertension	140–159	or 90–99
Stage 2 Hypertension	≥160	or ≥100

* *Adapted from* US Department of Health and Human Services; National Institutes of Health; National Heart, Lung, and Blood Institute; National High Blood Pressure Education Program.

† Treatment determined by highest blood pressure category.

‡ SBP: Systolic blood pressure.

§ mm Hg: Millimeters of mercury.

¶ DBP: Diastolic blood pressure.

1. **Borderline hypertension:** Borderline hypertension is defined as intermittent elevation of blood pressure interspersed with normal readings.
2. **Benign hypertension:** Benign hypertension is a term used to describe uncomplicated hypertension, usually of long duration and mild-to-moderate severity.
3. **Malignant hypertension:** Malignant hypertension is a syndrome of markedly elevated BP associated with papilledema **(Table 7.1)**.

Etiology

Primary hypertension has no single or specific cause, rather it may be multifactorial. Secondary hypertension includes the following causes:

- **Renal**
  - Renal parenchymal disease
  - Acute glomerulonephritis
  - Chronic nephritis
  - Polycystic disease
- **Endocrine**
  - Acromegaly
  - Hypothyroidism
  - Hyperthyroidism
  - Hypercalcemia
- **Adrenal**
  - Cortical
  - Cushing's syndrome
- **Exogenous hormones**
  - Estrogen
  - Glucocorticoids
  - Mineralocorticoids
- **Others**
  - Acute stress, including surgery
  - Psychogenic hyperventilation
  - Hypoglycemia
  - Burns

Risk Factors

a. **Nonmodifiable factors**
   1. **Family history**
   2. **Age:** The incidence of hypertension increases with age over 50 years.
   3. **Gender:** Men experience hypertension at higher rates.
   4. **Ethnic Group:** Hypertension is more prevalent in blacks.
b. **Modifiable risk factors**
   1. **Stress:** It has been shown to cause increased peripheral vascular resistance and cardiac output and to stimulate sympathetic nervous system activity.
   2. **Obesity:** Obesity is an important cause of hypertension, the combination may be related to hyperinsulinemia secondary to insulin resistance.
   3. **Nutrients:** A high salt diet may induce excessive release of natriuretic hormone, which may indirectly increase blood pressure.

Pathophysiology

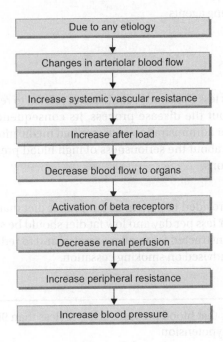

Due to any etiology

↓

Changes in arteriolar blood flow

↓

Increase systemic vascular resistance

↓

Increase after load

↓

Decrease blood flow to organs

↓

Activation of beta receptors

↓

Decrease renal perfusion

↓

Increase peripheral resistance

↓

Increase blood pressure

Signs and Symptoms

- The early stages of hypertension have no clinical manifestations, other than elevations in blood pressure.
- Occipital headache, fatigue, dizziness, flushing, blurred vision, epistaxis, and vertigo.

HYPERTENSIVE CRISIS

Severely elevated blood pressure equal to or greater than a systolic 180 or diastolic of 110—sometimes termed malignant or accelerated hypertension is referred to as a hypertensive crisis.

Treatment of Hypertension

Nonpharmacological Intervention

- Weight reduction
- Sodium restriction

- Modification of dietary fat
- Exercise
- Restriction of alcohol
- Caffeine restriction
- Relaxation techniques
- Smoking cessation.

Pharmacological Management

- Thiazide diuretics
- Loop diuretics
- Aldosterone receptor antagonists
- Nitrates
- β blockers
- Calcium channel blocker
- α_2 agonists: central acting agents
- Vasodilators

Nursing Management

Nursing Diagnosis

- Altered nutrition status less than body requirement related to restriction in dietary pattern
- Knowledge deficit about the disease process, its consequences, and the rationale for intervention and proper administration of prescribed medications.
- Lack of understanding about the seriousness of high blood pressure, cost of therapy, and side effects of medications.

Nursing Intervention

- Education should be provided to patient about proper diet management—sodium intake should be cut to 2.4 g or less per day and low fat diet should be suggested.
- The patient should be instructed for regular exercise, and to reduce the weight.
- The patient should be advised on smoking cessation.

HYPOTENSION

Low blood pressure means that blood pressure is lower (less than 90/60 mm Hg) than normal (<120/80 mm Hg), called hypotension.

Etiology

- Dehydration
- Moderate or severe bleeding
- Severe inflammation of organs inside the body
- Weakened heart muscle
- **Pericarditis:** It is an inflammation of the pericardium
- Pulmonary embolism
- Bradycardia
- Sick sinus syndrome
- Heart block
- Drug toxicity
- Tachycardia

Pathophysiology

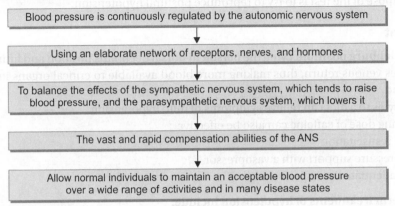

Blood pressure is continuously regulated by the autonomic nervous system

↓

Using an elaborate network of receptors, nerves, and hormones

↓

To balance the effects of the sympathetic nervous system, which tends to raise blood pressure, and the parasympathetic nervous system, which lowers it

↓

The vast and rapid compensation abilities of the ANS

↓

Allow normal individuals to maintain an acceptable blood pressure over a wide range of activities and in many disease states

Signs and Symptoms

- Chest pain
- Shortness of breath
- Irregular heartbeat
- Severe upper back pain
- Cough with phlegm
- Dyspepsia
- Dysuria
- Adverse effect of medications
- Seizures
- Loss of consciousness
- Profound fatigue
- Fever
- Headache
- Stiff neck
- Temporary blurring or loss of vision
- Connective tissue disorder
- Black tarry stools

Diagnostic Evaluation

- Complete blood count
- Blood electrolyte measurements
- Cortisol levels
- Blood and urine culture
- Radiology studies
- Electrocardiogram
- Holter monitor recordings
- Echocardiograms
- **Tilt-table tests:** It used to evaluate patients suspected of having postural hypotension. During a tilt-table test, the patient lies on an examination table with an intravenous infusion administered while the heart rate and blood pressure are monitored. The table then is tilted

upright for 15–45 minutes. Heart rate and blood pressure are monitored every few minutes. The purpose of the test is to try to reproduce postural hypotension.

Treatment

- **Trendelenburg position:** Lying the person in dorsal decubitus position and lifting the legs increases venous return, thus making more blood available to critical organs in the chest and head.
- Electrolytes to a diet can relieve symptoms of mild hypotension
- A morning dose of caffeine can also be effective
- Volume resuscitation
- Blood pressure support with a vasopressor
- Ensure adequate tissue perfusion

Medium-term treatments of hypotension include:
- Blood sugar control
- Early nutrition
- Steroid support

Prevention

- Standing up slowly
- Drinking more water
- Drinking little or no alcohol
- Limiting or avoiding caffeine
- Wearing compression stockings

CHRONIC VENOUS INSUFFICIENCY

Chronic venous insufficiency (CVI) is a condition that occurs when the venous wall or valves in the leg veins are not working effectively, making it difficult for blood to return to the heart from the legs.

Etiology

- Aging
- Extended sitting
- Standing or a combination of aging
- Reduced mobility
- **Phlebitis:** It occurs when a superficial or deep vein becomes swollen and inflamed.

Risk Factors

- Deep vein thrombosis
- Varicose veins
- Obesity
- Pregnancy
- Inactivity
- Smoking
- Extended periods of standing or sitting
- Age over 50

Pathophysiology

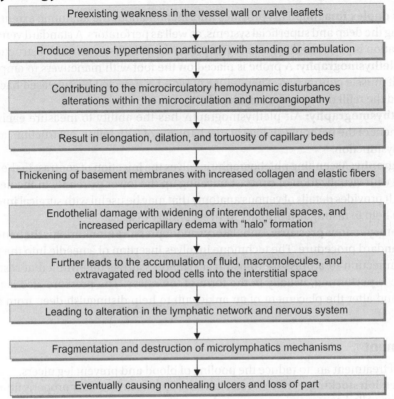

Preexisting weakness in the vessel wall or valve leaflets

↓

Produce venous hypertension particularly with standing or ambulation

↓

Contributing to the microcirculatory hemodynamic disturbances alterations within the microcirculation and microangiopathy

↓

Result in elongation, dilation, and tortuosity of capillary beds

↓

Thickening of basement membranes with increased collagen and elastic fibers

↓

Endothelial damage with widening of interendothelial spaces, and increased pericapillary edema with "halo" formation

↓

Further leads to the accumulation of fluid, macromolecules, and extravagated red blood cells into the interstitial space

↓

Leading to alteration in the lymphatic network and nervous system

↓

Fragmentation and destruction of microlymphatics mechanisms

↓

Eventually causing nonhealing ulcers and loss of part

Clinical Manifestations

- Chronic venous stasis
- Pain
- Tiredness in legs
- Stasis dermatitis
- Superficial vein s may be dilated and tortuous
- Edema in lower legs and ankles
- Altered pigmentation
- Skin ulceration

Diagnostic Evaluations

- **Physical examination:** Inspection and palpation may reveal visual evidence for chronic venous disease.
- **Tourniquet test:** A classic tourniquet test may be performed at bedside to help distinguish deep from superficial reflux. The test is performed with the patient lying down to empty the lower extremity veins.
- **Doppler study:** The use of continuous wave Doppler has often been used to assist in the bedside evaluation. The presence and direction of flow in the veins may be determined after maneuvers, such as the Valsalva maneuver or the sudden release of thigh or calf compression. Minimal signal should be detected toward the feet with these maneuvers. This technique also has been used to assess the great and short saphenous veins, although this is technically more difficult because of the lack of direct visualization.

Noninvasive Testing

- **Venous duplex imaging:** This provides information about the anatomic extent of disease involving the deep and superficial systems, as well as perforators. A standard venous duplex examination is performed to exclude Deep vein thrombosis or venous obstruction.
- **Photoplethysmography:** A probe is placed on the foot with maneuvers to empty the foot with calf muscle contraction. Then return of blood is detected by increased backscatter of light and the refill time may be calculated.
- **Air plethysmography:** Air plethysmography has the ability to measure each potential component of the pathophysiological mechanisms of CVI, reflux, obstruction, and muscle pump dysfunction.
- **Phlebography:** Ascending phlebography involves the injection of contrast in the dorsum of the foot with visualization of contrast traveling up the lower extremity in the deep venous system. It provides details of venous anatomy that may be useful with surgical interventions and can help to distinguish primary from secondary disease.
- **Ambulatory venous pressure:** Ambulatory venous pressure monitoring is the hemodynamic gold-standard procedure. The technique involves insertion of a needle into the pedal vein with connection to a pressure transducer. The pressure is determined at rest and after exercise is performed, usually in the form of toe raises. The pressure also is monitored before and after the placement of an ankle cuff to help distinguish deep from superficial reflux.

Management

The goals of treatment are to reduce the pooling of blood and prevent leg ulcers.
- **Compression stockings:** The most conservative approach is to wear properly fitting support hose (also called compression stockings).
- **Exercise:** Abnormalities in the calf and foot muscle pump functions play a significant role in the pathophysiology of CVI.
- Skin care
- Wound care
- Antibiotics
- Diuretics may be used to reduce swelling
- Pentoxifylline, which improves the flow of blood through the vessels
- Anticoagulation therapy

Nonsurgical Treatment

- **Sclerotherapy** involves the injection of a solution directly into spider veins or small varicose veins that causes them to collapse and disappear.
- **Endovenous thermal ablation** is a newer technique that uses a laser or high-frequency radio waves to create intense local heat in the affected vein. The technology is different with each energy source, but both forms of local heat close up the targeted vessel.

Surgical Treatments

- **Ligation and stripping:** Vein ligation is a procedure in which a vascular surgeon cuts and ties off the problem veins. Stripping is the surgical removal of larger veins through two small incisions.
- **Phlebotomy** is a minimally invasive procedure in which small incisions or needle punctures are made over the veins and a phlebectomy hook is used to remove the problem veins.

- **Subfascial endoscopic perforator surgery:** Subfascial endoscopic perforator surgery provides a means to ligate incompetent perforator veins by gaining access from a remote site on the leg.
- **Valve reconstruction:** Venous valve reconstruction of the deep vein valves has been performed in selected patients with advanced CVI who have recurrent ulceration with severe and disabling symptoms.
- **Angioplasty and stenting:** An angioplasty is the use of a balloon to push open a narrowed or blocked portion of the vein. A stent is a metal-scaffold tube that helps to keep the narrowed areas open.

Prevention of CVI

- Avoiding long periods of standing or sitting
- Exercising regularly
- Losing weight
- Elevating your legs
- Wearing compression stockings
- Taking antibiotics as needed to treat skin infections
- Practicing good skin hygiene
- Losing weight
- Elevating your legs

VARICOSE VEIN

Varicose veins are veins that have become enlarged and tortuous.

Etiology

- Varicose veins are more common in women than in men
- Heredity
- Pregnancy
- Obesity
- Prolonged standing
- High blood pressure
- Leg injury
- Abdominal straining
- Not exercising enough, smoking
- Venous and arteriovenous malformations
- Menopause
- Aging

Pathophysiology

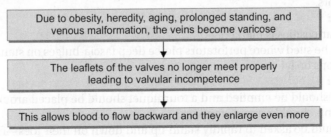

Due to obesity, heredity, aging, prolonged standing, and venous malformation, the veins become varicose

The leaflets of the valves no longer meet properly leading to valvular incompetence

This allows blood to flow backward and they enlarge even more

Contd...

Contd...

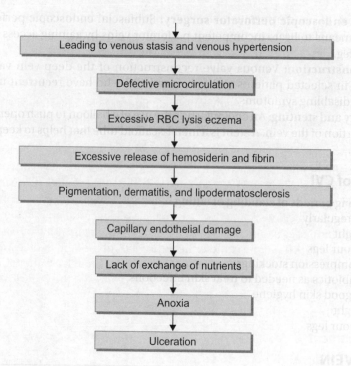

Leading to venous stasis and venous hypertension

↓

Defective microcirculation

↓

Excessive RBC lysis eczema

↓

Excessive release of hemosiderin and fibrin

↓

Pigmentation, dermatitis, and lipodermatosclerosis

↓

Capillary endothelial damage

↓

Lack of exchange of nutrients

↓

Anoxia

↓

Ulceration

Signs and Symptoms

- Aching, heavy legs
- Appearance of spider veins in the affected leg
- Redness, dryness, and itchiness of areas of skin
- Cramps
- Restless legs syndrome
- Ankle swelling
- A brownish-yellow shiny skin discoloration near the affected veins.

Other Tests

- **Trendelenburg's test:**
  - The patient should be lied flat.
  - The leg should be elevated and the veins should be emptied gently.
  - The saphenofemoral junction (SFJ) should be palpated and the patient should be asked to stand while maintaining pressure.
  - Rapid filling after thumb released-SFJ is incompetent.
  - Filling from below upward without releasing thumb—presence of distal incompetent perforators.
- **Fegan's test:**
  - Line of varicosities is marked.
  - It should be sited where perforators pierce deep fascia-bulges on standing and circular depressions on lying.
- **Perthes test:**
  - The vein should be emptied and a tourniquet should be placed around the thigh, and the patients should remain stand up.
  - They should be asked to rapidly stand up and down on their toes—filling of the veins indicated deep venous incompetence. This is a painful and rarely used test.

- **Schwartz test:** In standing position, the lower part of vein should be tapped. Then impulse is felt on saphenofemoral junction.

Treatment

- **Compression stockings**
- **Sclerotherapy:** During sclerotherapy, physician injects a chemical into varicose veins. The chemical irritates and scars veins from the inside out so abnormal veins can then no longer fill with blood.
- **Vein stripping:** To perform vein stripping, physician first makes a small incision in the groin area and usually another incision in calf below the knee. Then physician disconnects and ties off all major varicose vein branches associated with the saphenous vein, the main superficial vein in leg. The physician then removes the saphenous vein from leg. Once physician locates a varicose vein, he passes a suction device through a tiny incision and suctions out the vein.
- **Ablation:** Ablation uses a thin, flexible tube called a catheter inserted into a vein in the leg. Tiny electrodes at the tip of the catheter heat the walls of the vein and destroy it. Similarly, laser treatment uses a tiny fiber that is placed in the vein through a catheter. The fiber sends out laser energy that kills the diseased portion of the vein, and the vein closes off.

Nursing Care Plan

Nursing Assessment

- Inspecting for dilated, tortuous veins
- Performing the manual compression test to determine severity of disorder
- With the fingertips of one hand, feel dilated vein
- With your other hand, compress firmly at least 8 inches higher on the leg
- Feeling for an impulse transmitted towards your lower hand
- Competent saphenous valves should block the impulse. If you feel the impulse, the patient has varicose veins with incompetent valves.
- Perforating veins that are incompetent may be felt as bulging circles at intervals beneath the skin.
- Assessing for any ulceration, CVI or signs of infection.

Nursing Diagnosis

- **Impaired tissue integrity related to chronic changes and postoperative inflammation**
  Interventions:
  - Maintaining elastic compression bandages from toes to groin
  - Monitoring neurovascular status of feet
  - Elevating legs about 30°, providing support for the entire leg
  - Encouraging ambulation
  - Monitoring for signs of bleeding, especially for first 24 hours
  - Elevating the leg, applying pressure, and notifying the physician in case of bleeding
  - Being alert for complaints of pain over bony prominences; if elastic bandage is too tight, loosen it and then reapply it
  - Observing the signs of cellulitis
- **Acute pain related to surgical incisions, inflammation**
  Interventions:
  - Encouraging bed rest on the first day with legs elevated, and the second day, encouraging ambulation for 5–10 minutes every 2 hours.

■ Advising to avoid prolonged standing, sitting, or crossing legs to prevent obstruction.
■ Administering analgesics as prescribed.

Health Education

● **Postoperative instructions:** The patient should be instructed to:
■ Wear pressure bandage or elastic stockings at prescribed—usually for 3-4 weeks after surgery.
■ Elevate legs about 30° and provide adequate support for entire leg
■ Take analgesics for pain as ordered
■ Report such signs as sensory loss, calf pain, or fever to the healthcare providers
■ Avoid dangling of legs
■ Walk as able
■ Note that complaints of patchy numbness can be expected but should disappear in less than 1 year.
■ Follow conservative management instructions to prevent recurrence.
● **Conservative management:** The patient should be instructed to:
■ Avoid activities that cause venous stasis by obstructing venous flow
■ Control excessive weight gain
■ Wear firm elastic support as prescribed, from toe to knee when in upright position
■ Elevate foot of head 6-8 inches for night sleeping
■ Avoid injuring legs

MULTIPLE CHOICE QUESTIONS

1. Maria has PVD. If Maria has cool skin with no edema, what type of PVD does she have?
   A. Chronic arterial PVD   B. Acute arterial PVD
   C. Chronis venous PVD   D. Acute arterial PVD

2. In acute PVD, what would you expect to see?
   A. Full arterial   B. Collapsed arterial
   C. Full venous   D. Collapsed venous

3. Where does PVD often affect the blood flow?
   A. Arms   B. Legs
   C. Heart   D. Kidney

4. In atherosclerosis what is accumulated inside blood vessels?
   A. Lipids   B. Platelets
   C. Reticulocytes   D. Na

5. PVD can be mostly modified by:
   A. Taking medication   B. Losing weight
   C. Quitting smoking   D. Monitoring BP

Answers

1. C   2. C   3. A   4. B   5. C

Blood Disorders

> **AT THE END OF THIS CHAPTER, THE STUDENTS WILL BE ABLE TO LEARN ABOUT NURSING MANAGEMENT OF PATIENT WITH:**
> - Anemia and types
> - Polycythemia
> - Bleeding disorder, clotting factor defects, and platelets defects
> - Thalassemia
> - Leukopenias and agranulocytosis
> - Lymphomas and types
> - Blood transfusion and blood transfusion reaction

REVIEW OF ANATOMY AND PHYSIOLOGY

Blood is a fluid connective tissue. It circulates continually around the body, allowing constant communication between tissues distant from each other. It transports:

- Oxygen from the lungs to the tissues and carbon dioxide from the tissues to the lungs for excretion.
- Nutrients from the alimentary tract to the tissues and cell wastes to the excretory organs principally the kidneys.
- Hormones secreted by endocrine glands to their target glands and tissues.
- Clotting factors that coagulate blood, minimizing bleeding from ruptured blood vessels.

Blood is composed of a clear, straw-colored watery fluid called plasma in which several different types of blood cells are suspended. Plasma normally constitutes 55% of the volume of blood. The remaining 45% is accounted for the cellular fraction of blood.

There are three types of blood cell:

1. Erythrocytes
2. Platelets
3. Leukocytes

Blood cells are synthesized mainly in red bone marrow. Some lymphocytes additionally are produced in lymphoid tissue. In bone marrow, all blood cells originate from pluripotent (i.e., capable of developing into one of a number of cell types) stem cells and go through several developmental stages before entering the blood.

Different types of blood cells follow separate lines of development. The process of blood cell formation is called hemopoiesis.

BLOOD PROFILE

Blood component	Abbreviation used	Reference range	SI reference range
White blood cells	WBC	4500–11,000/mm³	4.5–11.0 × 10⁹/L
Red blood cells	RBC	Male: 4.3–5.9 million/mm³ Female: 3.5–5.5 million/mm³	Male: 4.3-5.9 × 10¹²/L Female: 3.5-5.5 × 10¹²/L
Hemoglobin	HGB	Male: 13.5–17.5 g/dL Female: 12.0–16.0 g/dL	Male: 2.09–2.71 mmol/L Female: 1.86–2.48 mmol/L
Hematocrit	HT	Male: 41–53% Female: 36–46%	Male: 0.41–0.53 Female: 0.36–0.46
Mean corpuscular volume	MCV	80–100 μm³	80–100 fL
Mean corpuscular hemoglobin	MCH	25.4–34.6 pg/cell	0.39–0.54 fmol/cell
Mean corpuscular hemoglobin concentration	MCHC	31–36% Hb/cell	4.81–5.58 mmol Hb/L
Platelets	Platelets	150,000–400,000/mm³	150–400 × 10⁹/L

ANEMIA

Anemia refers to a deficiency in a number of circulating red blood cells (RBCs) available for oxygen transport characterized by overall decrease in the number of erythrocytes, hematocrit and the hemoglobin concentration of the erythrocytes.

Etiology

- Bleeding, such as nose bleed and GI bleed
- Deficiency folic acid, vitamin B$_{12}$, and iron
- Lack of erythropoietin, such as in end-stage renal disease
- Increased destruction of RBCs, such as sickle cell anemia

Classification of Anemia

Morphologic Classification

- Normocytic, normochromic
- Macrocytic, normochromic
- Microcytic, hypochromic

Etiological Classification

- **Decreased erythrocyte production:**
  - Iron deficiency
  - Thalassemia
- **Defective DNA synthesis:**
  - Cobalamin deficiency
  - Folic acid deficiency
- **Decreased number of erythrocyte precursors:**
  - Aplastic anemia
  - Chronic diseases
  - Chemotherapy

IRON DEFICIENCY ANEMIA

Iron deficiency anemia occurs when the intake of dietary iron is inadequate for hemoglobin synthesis.

Etiology and Risk Factors

- Children, adolescents, and pregnant women
- Premenopausal women
- Chronic alcoholics
- Iron malabsorption
- Deficiency folic acid, vitamin B_{12}, and iron
- Lack of erythropoietin, such as in end-stage renal disease
- Increased destruction of RBCs, such as sickle cell anemia.

Clinical Manifestations

Body system	Mild (10–14 g/dL)	Moderate (6–10 g/dL)	Severe (<6 g/dL)
Integumentary	None	None	Pallor, jaundice, pruritis
Eyes	None	None	Icteric conjunctiva and sclera, blurred vision
Mouth	None	None	Glossitis, smooth tongue
Cardiovascular	Palpitation	Increased palpitations, bounding pulse	Tachycardia, systolic murmur, angina, MI
Pulmonary	Exertional dyspnea	Dyspnea	Tachypnea, orthopnea, dyspnea
Neurologic	None	Roaring in ears	Headache, vertigo, irritability, impaired thought process
Gastrointestinal	None	None	Anorexia, hepatomegaly, splenomegaly, difficulty in swallowing, sore mouth
Musculoskeletal	None	None	Bone pain
General	None	Fatigue	Sensitivity to cold, weight loss, lethargy

Diagnostic Evaluation

- **History and physical examination:** Socioeconomic status, injury, etc., should be queried. The vital signs and skin color and signs of anemia should be assessed.
- RBC morphology
- Hematocrit value should be assessed.
- Hemoglobin should be assessed.
- Serum ferritin should be assessed. This protein helps in storing iron in body.
- **Endoscopy:** Bleeding should be checked.
- **Colonoscopy:** Lower intestinal sources of bleeding should be ruled.

Management

To treat iron deficiency anemia, it is recommended of taking iron supplements.

Medical Management

- Oral iron preparations—ferrous sulfate, ferrous gluconate, and ferrous fumarate available.
- Iron dextran
- Emergency medications should be close at hand for allergic reaction.
- IM injection with Z-track technique for administering iron dextran.
- Choose iron-rich foods
- To enhance the body's absorption of iron by drinking citrus juice.

MEGALOBLASTIC ANEMIA

Megaloblastic anemia is a group of disorders caused by impaired DNA synthesis and characterized by the presence of large RBCs evidenced by deficiencies of vitamin B_{12} or folic acid.

Types of Megaloblastic Anemia
1. Cobalamin (vitamin B_{12}) deficiency
2. Folic acid deficiency

Cobalamin (Vitamin B_{12}) Deficiency
It is also known as pernicious anemia. It is caused by the decreased absorption of vitamin B_{12}. Normally, a protein termed "intrinsic factor" is secreted by the parietal cells of the gastric mucosa, which is required for cobalamin absorption. Therefore, secreted and cobalamine will not be released.
- Alcohol increases folic acid requirements
- Chronic hemolytic anemia
- Pregnant women
- Malabsorptive diseases of the small bowel

Vitamin B_{12} Deficiency
- Inadequate dietary intake and meat
- Crohn's disease
- Absence of intrinsic factor

Clinical Manifestations
Signs and symptoms of vitamin deficiency anemia include:
- Fatigue
- Shortness of breath
- Muscle weakness
- Personality changes
- Dizziness
- Pale or yellowish skin
- Irregular heartbeats
- Weight loss
- Numbness or tingling sensation
- Unsteady movements
- Mental confusion or forgetfulness

Diagnostic Evaluation
- **History and physical examination:** The socioeconomic status, injury, etc., should be queried. The vital signs and skin color and signs of anemia should be assessed.
- RBC morphology
- Hematocrit value
- **Methylmalonic acid test:** To measure the presence of a substance called methylmalonic acid. The level of this substance is higher in people with vitamin B_{12} deficiency.
- Hemoglobin should be assessed.
- **Assess for serum ferritin:** This protein helps in storing iron in the body.
- **Endoscopy:** Bleeding should be checked.
- **Colonoscopy:** Lower intestinal sources of bleeding should be ruled out.
- **Antibodies test:** A sample of blood to check for antibodies to intrinsic factor.
- **Schilling test:** In this test, a tiny amount of radioactive vitamin B_{12} is at first ingested. Then blood is checked, if body absorbs the vitamin B_{12} or not. After that, a combination of radioactive vitamin B_{12} and intrinsic factor should be ingested. If the radioactive B_{12} is absorbed only when taken with intrinsic factor, it confirms the lack of intrinsic factor.

Management
- Increasing amount of folic acid in diet
- IM administration of folic acid

- Vitamin B$_{12}$ replacement
- Vegetarian supplements through vitamins or fortified soy milk.

Folic Acid Deficiency Anemia

Folic acid deficiency also causes megaloblastic anemia. Folate deficiency anemia is a decrease in RBCs due to a lack of folate.

Etiology
- Poor nutrition
- Alcohol abuse
- Hemodialysis
- Malabsorption syndrome
- Drugs that impede the absorption
- Pregnancy

Clinical Manifestation
- Headache
- Fatigue
- Abnormal paleness or lack of color in the skin
- Decreased appetite
- Irritability
- Diarrhea
- Pallor
- Sore mouth and tongue

Diagnostic Evaluation
- History and physical examination
- Blood test
- Complete blood count (CBC)
- Serum folate level is low (3–25 mg/mL)

Management
Folic acid deficiency is treated by replacement therapy. The usual dose is 1 mg/day by month and in malabsorption up to 5 mg/day orally.

APLASTIC ANEMIA

Aplastic anemia is characterized by pancytopenia (RBCs, white cells, and platelets) and hypocellular bone marrow. It results in bone marrow aplasia.

Etiology

There are various etiological classifications for aplastic anemia, but they can be divided into two major groups:
1. **Congenital origin:** It is caused by chromosomal alterations.
2. **Acquired aplastic anemia:** It results from exposure to ionizing radiations, chemical agents, viral, and bacterial infections.

Clinical Manifestation

Clinical manifestation includes:
- Fatigue
- Dyspnea
- Arrhythmias
- Pale skin

- Frequent or prolonged infections
- Unexplained or easy bruising
- Epistaxis
- Prolonged bleeding from cuts
- Skin rash
- Dizziness
- Headache

Diagnostic Evaluation

- History and physical examination
- Blood tests; normally, RBC, white blood cell (WBC), and platelet levels
- Bone marrow biopsy

Management

- Blood transfusions
- **RBCs:** Transfusions of RBCs
- Platelets transfusions
- Stem cell transplant
- **Immunosuppressants:** For people who cannot undergo a bone marrow transplant, such as cyclosporine
- **Bone marrow stimulants:** Certain drugs, including colony-stimulating factors, such as sargramostim, and filgrastim.

HEMOLYTIC ANEMIA

Hemolytic anemia is a condition characterized by hemolysis that further causes destruction of RBCs at a rate that exceeds production.

Pathophysiology

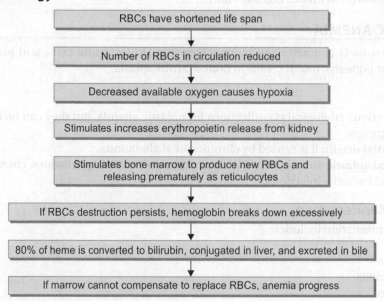

RBCs have shortened life span

↓

Number of RBCs in circulation reduced

↓

Decreased available oxygen causes hypoxia

↓

Stimulates increases erythropoietin release from kidney

↓

Stimulates bone marrow to produce new RBCs and releasing prematurely as reticulocytes

↓

If RBCs destruction persists, hemoglobin breaks down excessively

↓

80% of heme is converted to bilirubin, conjugated in liver, and excreted in bile

↓

If marrow cannot compensate to replace RBCs, anemia progress

Etiology

- Abnormal hemoglobin
- Sickle cell anemia
- Thalassemia
- Hereditary spherocytosis
- Glucose-6-phosphate dehydrogenase deficiency
- Transfusion reaction
- Autoimmune hemolytic anemia
- Trauma
- Mechanical heart valve
- Infection
- Disseminated intravascular coagulation (DIC)

Clinical Features

- Hemoglobin value 7–10 g/dL
- Jaundice
- Enlargement of bones of the face and skull
- Tachycardia
- Cardiac murmurs
- Cardiomyopathy
- Dysrhythmias
- Congestive heart failure

Types of Hemolytic Anemia

Sickle Cell Crisis

There are three types of sickle cell crisis:

1. **Sickle crisis:** It results from the tissue hypoxia and necrosis due to inadequate blood flow to a specific region of tissue or organ.
2. **Aplastic crisis:** It results from infection with human parvovirus. The hemoglobin level falls rapidly and the marrow cannot compensate as evidenced by absence of reticulocytes.
3. **Sequestration crisis:** It results when other organs pool the sickled cells.

Medical Management

There are three primary treatment modalities for sickle cell anemia:

1. **Bone marrow transplantation.**
2. **Hydroxyurea:** It has been shown to be effective in increasing hemoglobin F levels in patients with sickle cell.
3. **Transfusion therapy:** Chronic transfusions with RBCs have been shown to be highly effective in several situations in sickle cell.

GLUCOSE-6-PHOSPHATE DEHYDROGENASE DEFICIENCY

The abnormality in this disorder is in the G-6-PD gene. This enzyme produces an enzyme within the RBC that is essential for membrane stability.

Clinical Manifestation

- Patients are asymptomatic and have normal hemoglobin levels and reticulocyte counts most of the time.
- Pallor

- Jaundice
- Hemoglobinuria

Medical Management

- Stopping the offending medications
- Transfusion is necessary only in the severe hemolytic state.

IMMUNE HEMOLYTIC ANEMIA

Hemolytic anemia can result from exposure of the RBC to antibodies. Alloantibody tends to be large (IgM) and causes immediate destruction of the sensitized RBCs either within the blood vessels or within the liver.

Etiology

- Medication exposure
- Lymphoma
- Collagen vascular disease
- Autoimmune disease
- Infection

Clinical Manifestation

- Patient may be asymptomatic.
- Hemolysis
- Fatigue and dizziness
- Lymphadenopathy
- Jaundice
- Splenomegaly
- Hepatomegaly

Diagnostic Evaluation

- Low hemoglobin level and hematocrit
- RBCs appear abnormal, spherocytes common
- Serum bilirubin level elevated.
- Coombs test, which detects antibodies on the surface of RBCs, shows a positive result.

Management

- Offending medication immediately discontinued
- High doses of corticosteroids
- Blood transfusions
- Splenectomy

HEREDITARY HEMOCHROMATOSIS

Hemochromatosis is a genetic condition in which iron is abnormally absorbed from the gastrointestinal tract. The excessive iron is deposited in various organs, particularly the liver, myocardium, thyroid, and pancreas.

Clinical Manifestation

- Weakness, lethargy
- Arthralgia
- Weight loss

- Loss of libido
- Skin
- Cardiac dysrhythmias
- Cardiomyopathy

Management

Therapeutic phlebotomy (removal of whole blood from a vein)

Nursing Care Plan

Assessment

- Health history and physical examination
- Health history (recent blood loss, trauma, chronic diseases), use of medications, surgery, or other treatment

Nursing Diagnosis

- Activity intolerance related to weakness
- Imbalanced nutrition, less than body requirements, related to anorexia
- Ineffective tissue perfusion related to inadequate blood volume
- Ineffective therapeutic regimen management related to lack of knowledge

Interventions

- **Activity intolerance related to weakness, fatigue, and general malaise includes:**
  - Assessing activity level
  - Planning activity schedule
  - Alternating periods of activity of rest and activity
  - Assisting patient with activities of daily living
  - Monitoring vital signs to evaluate activity tolerance
  - Monitoring hematocrit and hemoglobin as a guide to planning activity
- **Imbalanced nutrition, less than body requirements, related to anorexia includes:**
  - Assessing food tolerance
  - Planning diet schedule
  - Offering the meal in attractive manner
  - Offering meal in calm and relaxed environment
  - Providing small, frequent meals
  - Providing high protein, iron, and calorie diet
  - Teaching about foods high in protein, iron, calories, and other nutrients
  - Teaching and monitoring use of a food diary
- **Ineffective tissue perfusion related to inadequate blood volume includes:**
  - Weighing daily
  - Administering blood transfusions or intravenous (IV) fluids as ordered
  - Administering supplemental oxygen
  - Monitoring vital signs closely
  - Maintaining intake output charting
  - Checking for early sign of dehydration

POLYCYTHEMIA VERA

Polycythemia vera is a chronic myeloproliferative disorder that involves all bone marrow elements, resulting in an increase in RBC mass and hemoglobin.

Etiology and Risk Factors

Some of the chronic risk factors:

- Chronic hypoxia
- Reduction of plasma volume
- Splenomegaly
- Long-term cigarette smoking
- Family history
- High altitudes
- Long-term exposure to carbon monoxide

Pathophysiology

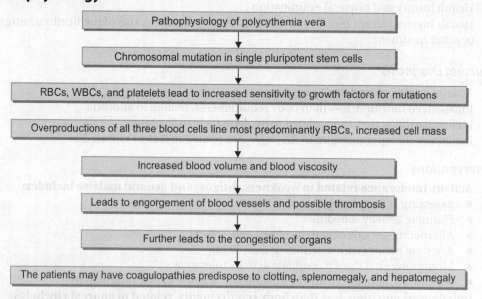

Pathophysiology of polycythemia vera

↓

Chromosomal mutation in single pluripotent stem cells

↓

RBCs, WBCs, and platelets lead to increased sensitivity to growth factors for mutations

↓

Overproductions of all three blood cells line most predominantly RBCs, increased cell mass

↓

Increased blood volume and blood viscosity

↓

Leads to engorgement of blood vessels and possible thrombosis

↓

Further leads to the congestion of organs

↓

The patients may have coagulopathies predispose to clotting, splenomegaly, and hepatomegaly

Types of Polycythemia

- **Primary polycythemia:** Polycythemia vera is known as primary polycythemia. Its cause is unknown.
- **Secondary polycythemia:** Secondary polycythemia is caused by excessive production of erythropoietin disease.
- **Relative polycythemia:** Relative polycythemia describes condition in which red cell volume is high due to increased blood concentration of red cells as a result of dehydration.
- **Stress polycythemia:** This is a condition that may be seen in hardworking, anxious, middle-aged men due to low plasma volume.

Clinical Manifestation

- Pruritus
- Dyspnea
- Excessive bleeding
- Splenomegaly
- Hepatomegaly
- Epigastric discomfort
- Paresthesia
- Headache
- Weakness

- Bleeding tendency
- Hyperuricemia
- Itching
- Hypertension

Diagnostic Evaluation

The following laboratory manifestations are seen in a patient with polycythemia vera:

- Elevated Hb and RBC count with microcytosis
- Low-to-normal erythropoietin (EPO) level
- Elevated WBC count with basophilia
- Elevated platelet
- Elevated leukocyte alkaline phosphatase
- Elevated histamine levels
- Bone marrow examination
- Splenomegaly

Routine blood work includes:

- Clotting profile and metabolic panel
- Chest X-ray
- Electrocardiogram
- Bone marrow examination
- CBC

Management

Medical Management

- **Phlebotomy:** Venesection is a procedure in which a controlled amount of blood is removed from bloodstream.
- **Myelosuppressive drugs:** Myelosuppressive (bone marrow suppressing) drugs are commonly used to reduce blood cell production in the bone marrow.
- **Interferon:** Interferon is a substance produced naturally by the body's immune system.
- **Radioactive phosphorus:** Radioactive phosphorus (32P) is a radioisotope, which may be used for long-lasting control of blood counts in older people.

Nursing Management

- Assessing for cyanosis, reddened face with engorged retinal vein, tinnitus, and weakness
- Assessing for the signs of paresthesia
- Assessing for the hypertension and epistaxis
- Assisting with phlebotomy if acute exacerbation of polycythemia
- Fluid intake and fluid output should be evaluated
- Observing for side effect of myelosuppressive agents

MULTIPLE MYELOMA

Multiple myeloma is the cancer of plasma cells caused by unregulated proliferation of monoclonal plasma cells that finally results in decrease bone marrow function and destruction of bone tissue.

Etiology

- The causes of multiple myeloma are unknown
- Poor immune function
- Exposure to chemicals or radiation

Pathophysiology

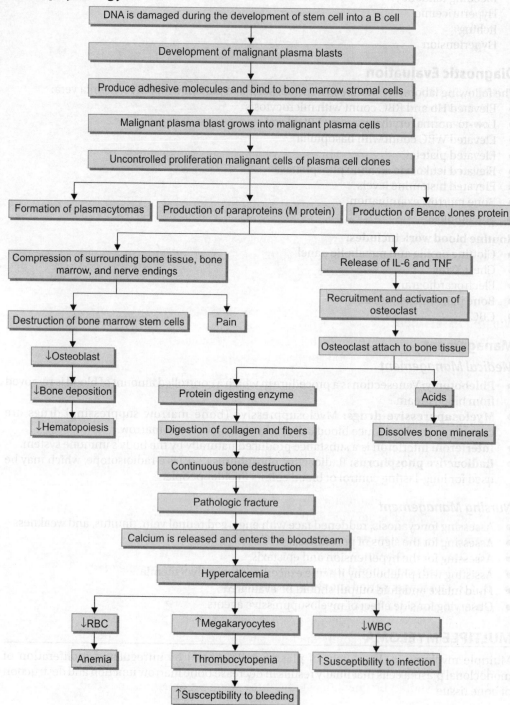

Clinical Manifestation

- Pain in bones
- Fracture

- Renal compromise
- Septicemia
- Weakness
- Fatigue

Diagnostic Evaluation

- Urine analysis for presence of abnormal protein
- Bone marrow biopsy
- Computerized tomography (CT) scan and radiography
- CBC
- MRI to detect the presence of bone abnormalities and fracture
- Estimate myeloma cell mass

Management

Pharmacologic Management

- Prednisone and melphalan given orally for a period of 7.
- Combination chemotherapy, commonly melphalan, cyclophosphamide, carmustine (BCNU), vincristine, and prednisone.

Nursing Care Plan

Nursing Assessment

- Obtaining the health history, focusing on pain, and fatigue
- Evaluating for evidence of bone deformities, bone tenderness, or pain
- Assessing patient's support system and personal coping skills.

Nursing Intervention

To reduce the pain of the client

- The condition of the client should be assessed.
- The severity, duration, and frequency of the pain should be assessed.
- The heat/cold application should be provided.
- The use of nonpharmacologic methods should be taught to help manage pain.
- Nonsteroidal anti-inflammatory drugs should be administered to the client.
- Analgesics should be administered.

To promote the physical mobility of the client

- The client should be encouraged to wear back brace for lumbar lesions.
- Physical and occupational therapy consultation should be recommended.
- Bed rest for longer period should be discouraged.

To reduce the risk of infection

- The vital signs of the client should be monitored.
- The client and his/her family member should be taught about the importance of the handwashing.
- The visitor should be avoided.
- The client should be encouraged about the frequent breathing, position changes, and routine hygiene.

Health Education

- Teaching the client about the risk of infection
- Teaching the client to minimize the risk of fracture

- Using proper body mechanics and assistive devices
- Advising client to report new onset of pain
- Encouraging the patient to maintain high fluid intake

LEUKEMIA

Leukemia is a blood cancer characterized by an abnormal increase of immature WBCs called.

Etiology and Pathophysiology

- Artificial ionizing radiation
- Viruses—HTLV-1 and HIV
- Maternal–fetal transmission
- Hair dyes
- Genetic predisposition
- **Down syndrome**—people with Down syndrome have a significantly higher risk of developing leukemia
- Benzene
- Alkylating chemotherapy agents

Risk Factors of Leukemia

- **Gender:** Men are more likely to develop.
- **Age:** Typically increases with age.
- **Genetics**
- Smoking
- Exposures
- Exposure to high levels of radiation
- Chemical exposure
- Previous cancer treatment

Clinical Manifestation

- Fever and night sweats
- Headache
- Bruising
- Arthralgia
- Splenomegaly
- Swollen lymph nodes
- Feeling very tired or weak
- Anorexia
- Fatigue
- Night sweat
- Hyperthermia

Classification

- Acute lymphatic leukemia
- Acute myelogenous leukemia
- Chronic lymphocytic leukemia
- Chronic myelogenous leukemia.
  - *Acute lymphatic leukemia:* It is a type of leukemia that affects an immature WBC in the bone marrow.

- *Acute myelogenous leukemia:* It is characterized by proliferation of immature myeloid cells.
- *Chronic lymphocytic leukemia:* It is a type of blood cancer that affects mature blood cells.

Pathophysiology

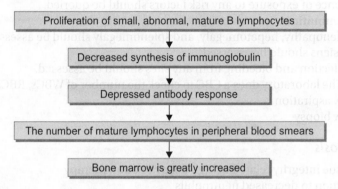

Proliferation of small, abnormal, mature B lymphocytes

↓

Decreased synthesis of immunoglobulin

↓

Depressed antibody response

↓

The number of mature lymphocytes in peripheral blood smears

↓

Bone marrow is greatly increased

Diagnostic Evaluation

- **History:** Assessing the client for the exposure of any risk factors.
- **Physical examination:** Assessing the client for signs and symptoms and assessing client for lymphadenopathy.
- CBC

Management

> **Chemotherapeutic agent, it involves three phases that are as follows:**
> 1. **Induction:** During the induction phase, the client receives an intensive course of chemotherapy designed to induce a complete remission of the disease.
> 2. **Consolidation:** Using modified course of intensive therapy to eradicate any remaining disease.
> 3. **Maintenance:** During the maintenance phase, small doses of different combinations of chemotherapeutic agents are given every 3–4 weeks.

Chemotherapy

Chemotherapy with chlorambucil, cyclophosphamide, and prednisone to decrease lymphadenopathy and splenomegaly.

Supportive Care

- Transfusion therapy to replace platelets and RBCs
- IV immunoglobulins

Nursing Intervention

- Taking measures to prevent infection
- Promoting safety
- Promoting effective coping
- Client and family education
- Providing oral hygiene
- Preventing fatigue

Nursing Care Plan

Nursing Assessment

- **History**
  - Client should be enquired for their family history and past medical history.
  - The presence of exposure to any risk factors should be queried.
- **Physical examination**
  - Lymphadenopathy, hepatomegaly, and splenomegaly should be assessed.
  - The vital signs should be assessed.
  - Sign of infection and bleeding from any sites should be assessed.
- **Blood test:** The laboratory does a CBC to check the number of WBCs, RBCs, and platelets.
- Bone marrow aspiration
- Bone marrow biopsy

Nursing Diagnosis

- Impaired tissue integrity related to high dose radiation therapy
- Risk for infection to decreased neutrophils
- Impaired oral mucous membrane related to low platelet counts
- Risk for injury related to low platelet counts
- Acute pain related to tumor growth
- Activity intolerance related to anemia and adverse effect of chemotherapy.

Interventions

- **Maintain tissue integrity:**
  - Avoiding application of heat and cold to treated areas
  - Encouraging the client to wear loose-fitting clothes
  - Advising the client to protect skin from over and direct exposure to sunlight
  - Encouraging the client to keep the treated area clean and dry
  - Advising the client to clean the area gently
- **Prevent from infection:**
  - Inspecting the client for the signs and symptoms of infection
  - Teaching the client about personal hygiene technique and handwashing
  - Educating the client to report if there is any presence of signs of infection
  - Monitoring granulocyte count and WBC count
  - Maintaining asepsis
  - Instructing the client to take antibiotics
- **Risk for bleeding:**
  - Monitoring lips, tongue, mucous membrane, and gums for moisture, color, texture, and presence of infection
  - Encouraging to use soft, bland, and nonacidic foods
  - Advising to use soft toothbrush
  - Instructing to perform oral hygiene after eating

Complications

- Infections
- Blood problems
- Impaired body function
- Death

DISSEMINATED INTRAVASCULAR COAGULATION

DIC is an acquired thrombotic and hemorrhagic syndrome characterized by abnormal activation of the clotting cascade and accelerated fibrinolysis, so that bleeding and thrombosis occur simultaneously.

Etiology

- Venomous snake bites
- Burns
- Small blood clots
- Inflammation
- Bleeding
- Pancreatitis
- Hemorrhagic skin
- Sepsis and shock
- Incomplete miscarriage

Risk Factor

- Blood transfusion reaction
- Cancer
- Pancreatitis
- Liver disease
- Pregnancy complications
- Severe tissue injury

Pathophysiology

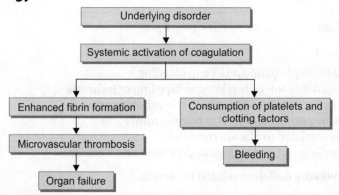

Clinical Manifestation

- Bleeding
- Blood clots
- Bruising
- Hypotension
- Coolness of extremities
- Headache
- Gum bleeding
- Epistaxis

- Tachycardia
- Fever
- Melena
- Arthralgia
- Restlessness
- Altered mental status
- Gangrene

Diagnostic Evaluation

- **History:** Patient should be queried for the presence of any past history of disease.
- **Physical examination:** In physical examination, the patient should be assessed for presence of signs and symptoms.
- **Laboratory tests:** CBC, platelet count, normal value is 150,000–450,000/mm³, there is a decrease in platelet count.
- Prothrombin time increases
- Thrombin time increases
- Fibrinogen decreases

Management

There is no specific treatment for DIC.
- **Supportive treatments may include:**
  - Plasma transfusions to replace blood clotting factors
  - Anticoagulants (heparin) to prevent blood clotting
  - Transfusions of platelets
  - Aspirin to stop blood clots
- **Diet:** Vitamin K-rich food should be provided.

Nursing Care Plan

Nursing Diagnosis

- Risk for deficient fluid volume related to bleeding
- Risk for impaired skin integrity related to bleeding or ischemia
- Risk for injury related to bleeding due to thrombocytopenia
- Ineffective tissue perfusion related to microthrombi
- Anxiety and fear related to disease condition
- Deficient knowledge related to disease condition and treatment.

1. Risk for fluid volume deficient related to bleeding
Interventions
- Monitoring vital signs closely
- Monitoring urine output of the patient
- Avoiding the medications that interfere with platelet count (NSAIDs)
- Avoiding IM injections because it decreases the chance for intramuscular bleeding
- Monitoring the external bleeding
- Avoiding dislodging any clots
- Blood components should be administered.
- Providing packed RBCs is to improve oxygen delivery by increasing the hemoglobin content of the blood.
- Administering platelet transfusion when the platelet count falls below 100,000/mm³.

2. Risk for impaired skin integrity related to bleeding

Interventions

- Assessing the skin of patient
- Repositioning the patient frequently
- Avoiding application of heat and cold to treated areas
- Encouraging the client to wear loose-fitting clothes
- Advising the client to protect skin from over and direct exposure to sunlight
- Encouraging the client to keep the treated area clean and dry
- Advising the client to clean the area gently
- Using pressure-reducing mattress
- Performing skincare every 2 hours
- Providing oral care carefully
- Maintaining personal hygiene

3. Anxiety and fear related to disease condition

Interventions

- Identifying the patient's previous coping mechanisms, if possible
- Encouraging the patient to use that coping mechanisms in this condition
- Explaining all procedures and rationale for those procedures to patient
- Assisting the family in supporting patient
- Explaining about the causes and treatment of the disease to the patient
- Providing psychological support to the patient
- Advising to take medications at right time

HEMOPHILIA (FACTOR VIII DEFICIENCY)

It is a group of hereditary genetic disorders that impair the body's ability to clotting or coagulation.

Etiology

- Hemophilia A is a recessive X-linked genetic disorder involving a lack of functional clotting factor VIII.
- Hemophilia B is a recessive X-linked genetic disorder involving a lack of functional clotting factor IX.
- Hemophilia C is an autosomal genetic disorder involving a lack of functional clotting factor XI.

Clinical Manifestation

- Large bruises
- Hematomas
- Swelling and bruising
- Soft tissue

Complications

- Deep internal bleeding
- Joint damage
- Transfusion transmitted infection
- Intracranial hemorrhage

LYMPHOMAS

The lymphomas are neoplasms of cells of lymphoid cells, which spread to spleen, GI tract, the liver, and the bone marrow.

Lymphomas can be broadly classified into two categories:

1. Hodgkin's lymphoma
2. Non-Hodgkin's lymphoma

HODGKIN'S LYMPHOMA

Hodgkin's lymphoma is a chronic, progressive, and neoplastic disorder of lymphatic tissue characterized by the painless enlargement of lymph nodes with progression to extralymphatic sites, such as the spleen, and liver.

Etiology

- Exact cause of Hodgkin's lymphoma remains unknown
- Infection with Epstein–Barr virus
- Genetic predisposition
- Exposure to occupational toxins

Pathophysiology

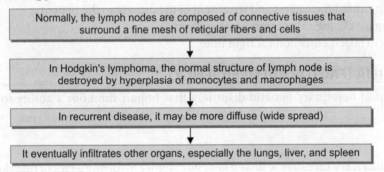

Normally, the lymph nodes are composed of connective tissues that surround a fine mesh of reticular fibers and cells

↓

In Hodgkin's lymphoma, the normal structure of lymph node is destroyed by hyperplasia of monocytes and macrophages

↓

In recurrent disease, it may be more diffuse (wide spread)

↓

It eventually infiltrates other organs, especially the lungs, liver, and spleen

Clinical Manifestation

- Enlargement of nodes
- The enlarged lymph nodes are not painful
- Pruritus
- Cough and pulmonary effusion
- Jaundice
- Abdominal pain
- Retroperitoneal adenopathy
- Bone pain
- Fever
- Weight loss
- Anemia

Diagnostic Evaluation

- **Physical examination:** To assess swollen lymph nodes
- **Complete blood count (CBC)**

- **Imaging tests:** Imaging tests used to diagnose Hodgkin's lymphoma include X-ray, CT scan, and positron emission tomography (PET)
- **Bone marrow biopsy**

Management

The standard for chemotherapy is the ABVD regimen—doxorubicin, bleomycin, vinblastine, and dacarbazine.

NON-HODGKIN LYMPHOMA

Non-Hodgkin lymphomas are a heterogeneous group of malignant neoplasms of primarily B or T cell.

Etiology

Idiopathic

Risk Factors

- Immunosuppressive medicines
- Infection with certain viruses and bacteria

Clinical Manifestation

- Painless, swollen lymph nodes
- Abdominal pain
- Chest pain
- Night sweats
- Weight loss
- Fatigue
- Fever

Diagnostic Evaluation

- **Physical examination:** To assess swollen lymph nodes
- **CBC**
- **Imaging tests:** Imaging tests used to diagnose Hodgkin's lymphoma include X-ray, CT scan, and PET
- **Bone marrow biopsy**

Management

- Chemotherapy
- Radiation therapy
- Stem cell transplant
- **Medications that enhance immune system's ability to fight cancer:** Biological therapy drugs help the body's immune system to fight cancer. For example, one biological therapy called rituximab.
- **Medications that deliver radiation directly to cancer cells:** Radioimmunotherapy drugs are made of monoclonal antibodies that carry radioactive isotopes. This allows the antibody to attach to cancer cells and deliver radiation directly to the cells.

Nursing Care Plan

Nursing Diagnosis

- Activity intolerance related to fatigue
- Impaired tissue integrity related to high-dose radiation therapy
- Risk of infection related to altered immune response

1. Activity intolerance related to fatigue and anemia

Interventions

- Assessing amount of activity that cause fatigue or dyspnea
- Assessed patient with activities as needed
- Providing oxygen therapy as ordered
- Instructing client to space rest with activities

2. Impaired tissue integrity related to high dose radiation therapy

Interventions

- Avoiding rubbing, powder, deodorant, lotion, or ointment
- Encouraging client to keep treated area clean and dry
- Encouraging wearing loose-fitting clothes

3. Risk of infection related to altered immune response

Interventions

- Assessing client for risk factor for infection
- Monitoring client for signs and symptoms of infection
- Teaching the client to avoid exposure to infection
- Teaching client with proper handwashing and good oral and personal hygiene.

THALASSEMIA

Thalassemia is a group of inherited autosomal recessive blood disorders. In thalassemia, the genetic defect, which could be either mutation or deletion, results in reduced rate of synthesis of the globin chains that makes up hemoglobin.

Types of Thalassemia

Alpha-Thalassemia

Alpha-thalassemia is a blood disorder that reduces the production of hemoglobin, the protein in RBCs that carries oxygen to cells throughout the body. Clinically manifested in the form of reduction in hemoglobin

Beta-Thalassemia Minor (Trait)

Beta-thalassemia minor often goes undiagnosed because kids with the condition have no real symptoms other than mild anemia and small RBCs. It is often suspected based on routine blood tests, such as a CBC and can be confirmed with a hemoglobin electrophoresis. No treatment is usually needed.

As with alpha-thalassemia trait, the anemia associated with this condition may be misdiagnosed as an iron deficiency.

Beta-Thalassemia Intermedia

Children with beta-thalassemia intermedia have varying effects from the disease—mild anemia might be their only symptom or they might require regular blood transfusions.

The most common complaint is fatigue or shortness of breath. Some kids also experience heart palpitations, also due to the anemia, and mild jaundice, which is caused by the destruction of abnormal RBCs that result from the disease. The liver and spleen may be enlarged, which can feel uncomfortable for a child. Severe anemia can also affect growth.

Another symptom of beta-thalassemia intermedia can be bone abnormalities. As the bone marrow is working overtime to make more RBCs to counteract the anemia, kids can experience enlargement of their cheekbones, foreheads, and other bones. Gallstones are a frequent complication because of abnormalities in bile production that involve the liver and the gallbladder.

Some kids with beta-thalassemia intermedia may require a blood transfusion only occasionally. They will always have anemia, but may not need transfusions except during illness, medical complications, or later on during pregnancy.

Other children with this form of the disease require regular blood transfusions. In these kids, low or falling hemoglobin levels greatly reduce the blood's ability to carry oxygen to the body, resulting in extreme fatigue, poor growth, and facial abnormalities. Regular transfusions can help alleviate these problems. Sometimes, kids who have this form of the disease have their spleens removed.

Beta-thalassemia intermedia is often diagnosed in the first year of life. Doctors may be prompted to test for it when a child has chronic anemia or a family history of the condition. As long as it is diagnosed while the child is still doing well and has not experienced any serious complications, it can be successfully treated and managed.

Beta-Thalassemia

Beta-thalassemia is due to mutations in the HBB gene on chromosome. It is also inherited in an autosomal-recessive fashion. The severity of the disease depends on the nature of the mutation. Mutations are characterized as either beta-thalassemia major if they prevent any formation of beta-chains.

Diagnostic Evaluation

Microscopic examination of the blood.

Management

- **Medical therapy:** Medical therapy involves iron chelation, such as Deferoxamine.
- **Blood transfusions**
- Iron **chelation therapy:** As the hemoglobin in RBCs is an iron-rich protein, regular blood transfusions can lead to a buildup of iron in the blood. This condition is called iron overload.
- **Folic acid supplements**.

Nursing interventions

- Activity intolerance related to impaired oxygen transport
- High risk for infection related to decreased resistance secondary to hypoxia
- Altered body image related to skeletal changes
- Ineffective management of therapeutic regimen related to lack of knowledge about appropriate nutrition and medication
- Assessing amount of activity that causes fatigue or dyspnea
- Assessed client with activities as needed
- Providing oxygen therapy as ordered
- Instructing client to space rest with activities
- Avoiding rubbing, powder, deodorant, lotion, or ointment

- Encouraging client to keep treated area clean and dry
- Encouraging wearing loose-fitting clothes.

BLOOD TRANSFUSION

A blood transfusion is the transfer of blood or blood products from one person into another person's bloodstream. This is usually done as a lifesaving maneuver to replace blood cells or blood products.

Equipment

- All blood components must be filtered during administration.
- A blood component administration set containing an in-line blood filter is recommended. Either a "Y-type" administration set or a single line set may be used.
- An add-on filter, such as a leukocyte-reduction filter, may be used when the component was not leukocyte reduced by the blood supplier.

Leukocyte-Reduction Filters

With the exception of autologous units, the components stocked by the blood bank are leukocyte reduced by the blood supplier.

Pressure Infusion Devices

- Infusion pumps are available from the patient equipment section of material services.
- Equipment for transfusion must be used in accordance with the manufacturer's instructions.
- Equipment that does not have a current Biomedical Engineering tag should not be used, indicating it has been tested for appropriate function and safety.
- Cuffs for pressure infusion may be used if care is taken not to exceed the designated pressure.

Patient Instructions and Preparation

Blood bank personnel will notify patient unit personnel by telephone when ordered blood is ready for transfusion.

Informed Consent

Informed consent for blood transfusion is a process in which the patient is informed of the medical indications for the transfusion, the possible risks, the possible benefits, the alternatives, and the possible consequences of not receiving the transfusion.

BLOOD TRANSFUSION REACTIONS

- **Hemolytic reactions:** Hemolytic reactions occur when the recipient's serum contains antibodies directed against the corresponding antigen found on donor RBCs. This can be an ABO incompatibility or an incompatibility related to a different blood group antigen. DIC, renal failure, and death are not uncommon following this type of reaction.
- **Allergic reactions**
- **Febrile reactions:** WBC reactions (febrile reactions) are caused by patient's antibodies directed against antigens present on transfused lymphocytes or granulocytes.
- **Transfusion-related acute lung injury**
- **Circulatory overload:** Circulatory overload can occur with administration of blood or any IV fluid, particularly in patients with diminished cardiac function.
- **Massive blood loss**

Nursing responsibilities during blood transfusion reactions include:

- Stopping the transfusion immediately
- Disconnecting the IV line from the needle
- The unit from the IV set should be disconnected
- Attaching a new IV set and prime with saline or flush the line with the normal saline used to initiate the transfusion and reconnect the line.
- Opening the line to a slow drip
- Check to ensure that the patient name and registration number on the blood bag label exactly same as the information regarding the identification of the patient.
- Notifying the blood bank about a transfusion reaction.
- Delaying the transfusion of additional units until the possibility of serological incompatibility has been investigated.
- Initiating the transfusion reaction report form after blood bank personnel have been notified of a transfusion reaction.

MULTIPLE CHOICE QUESTIONS

1. **Production of abnormal and immature white blood cells in body leads to:**
   A. Lungs cancer
   B. Kidney cancer
   C. Skin cancer
   D. Blood cancer

2. **Blood disease that is caused by occurrence of mutations in hemoglobin genes is:**
   A. Leukemia
   B. Bleeding disorders
   C. Thalassemia
   D. Hepatitis

3. **Leukemia is also known as:**
   A. Skin cancer
   B. Blood cancer
   C. Lungs cancer
   D. Kidney cancer

4. **Mutation in hemoglobin genes leads to the production of:**
   A. Defective hemoglobin
   B. Defective antigens
   C. Defective neutrophils
   D. Defective basophils

5. **Cancerous mutation in lymph tissue cells or bone marrow leads to:**
   A. Defective agranulocytes
   B. Defective erythrocytes
   C. Defective leukocytes
   D. Defective thrombocytes

Answers

1. D   2. C   3. B   4. A   5. C

Genitourinary Disorders

AT THE END OF THIS CHAPTER, THE STUDENTS WILL BE LEARN ABOUT THE NURSING MANAGEMENT OF:

➢ Nephritis
➢ Nephrotic syndrome
➢ Renal calculus
➢ Acute renal failure
➢ Chronic renal failure
➢ End-stage renal disease
➢ Dialysis, renal transplant
➢ Benign prostate hypertrophy

REVIEW OF ANATOMY AND PHYSIOLOGY

Anatomy and physiology of kidney: The urinary system is the main excretory system and consists of the following structures:

- Two kidneys, which secrete urine
- Two ureters, which convey the urine from kidney to the urinary bladder.
- The urinary bladder where urine collects and is temporarily stored.
- The urethra through which the urine passes from the urinary bladder to the exterior **(Fig. 9.1)**.

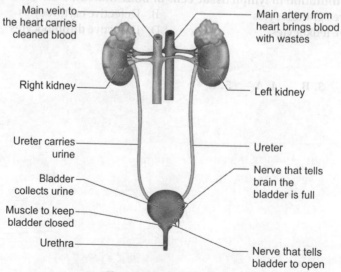

Main vein to the heart carries cleaned blood

Right kidney

Ureter carries urine

Bladder collects urine

Muscle to keep bladder closed

Urethra

Main artery from heart brings blood with wastes

Left kidney

Ureter

Nerve that tells brain the bladder is full

Nerve that tells bladder to open

Fig. 9.1: Structure of kidney.

URINARY SYSTEM

The urinary system plays a vital part in maintaining homeostasis of water and electrolyte concentrations within the body.

- The kidney produces urine that contains metabolic waste products, including nitrogenous compounds urea and uric acid, excess ions, and some drugs.
- Urine is stored in the bladder and excreted by the process of micturation.
- The kidneys lie on the posterior abdominal wall, one on each side of the vertebral column. Behind the peritoneum and below the diaphragm.
- The right kidney is usually slightly lower than the left, probably because of the considerable space occupied by the liver.
- Kidneys are bean-shaped organs, about 11 cm long, 6 cm wide, 3 cm thick and 150 g in weight.
- A sheath of fibrous connective also known as renal fascia encloses the kidney and the renal fat.

Organs associated with the kidneys: As the kidneys lie on either side of the vertebral column, each is associated with a different group of structures.

Right Kidney

- **Superiorly:** The right adrenal gland
- **Anteriorly:** The right lobe of the liver, the duodenum, and the hepatic flexure of the colon.
- **Posteriorly:** The diaphragm and the muscles of the posterior abdominal wall.

Left Kidney

- **Superiorly:** The left adrenal gland.
- **Anteriorly:** The spleen, stomach, pancreas, jejunum, and splenic, flexure of the colon.
- **Posteriorly:** The diaphragm and muscle of the posterior abdominal wall.

Gross structure of the kidney: There are three areas of tissue that can be distinguished when a longitudinal section of kidney is viewed with the naked eye.

- An outer fibrous capsule, surrounding the kidney.
- The cortex, a reddish-brown layer of tissue immediately below the capsule and outside the pyramids.
- The medulla, the inner most layer, consisting of pale conical-shaped striations, the renal pyramids.
- The hilum is the concave medial border of the kidney where the renal blood and lymph vessels, the ureter, and nerves enter.
- The renal pelvis is the funnel structure that collects urine formed by the kidney.

RENAL SYSTEM ASSESSMENT

- **Assess the urinary elimination patterns:** Urethra, assistive devices, catheter, ureterostomy, dialysis, peritoneal catheter or hemodialysis.
- **Assess the characteristics of urine:** Amount, color, dilute or concentrated, timing of passing urine or frequency, odor, pH, frothy, sediment, hematuria, albuminuria (in case of nephrotic syndrome), ketonuria (presence of ketone bodies in urine).
- **Assess the voiding pattern of urine:** Frequency of passing urine, urgency, hesitancy, burning, dysuria, dribbling of urine, nocturia, volume of urine, change in stream, enuresis, and flank pain.

- Assess for urine continence, retention, incontinence, stress incontinence, bladder distention.
- Assess for fluid overload, such as edema.

ACUTE RENAL FAILURE

Definition

Renal failure is a systemic disease and characterized by sudden and almost complete loss of kidney function with decreased glomerular filtration rate (GFR) over a period of hour to days.

Etiology

There are many possible causes of kidney damage:
- Acute tubular necrosis
- Autoimmune kidney disorder
- Blood clot from cholesterol
- Urinary tract blockage
- Kidney stones
- Burns
- Dehydration
- Hemorrhage
- Injury to kidney
- Shock
- Advanced age

Prerenal causes: Prerenal causes interfere with renal perfusion and inadequate supply of blood to a filtered by the glomeruli:
- Decreased output
- Increased vascular resistance
- Fluid volume shifts
- Vascular obstruction
- Renal losses

Intrarenal causes: Renal causes refer to parenchymal changes in kidney due to nephrotoxic substances. It includes:
- Prolonged renal ischemia
- Acute pyelonephritis
- Nephrotoxic agent

Postrenal Causes

Postrenal causes leading to acute renal failure (ARF) arise from obstruction in the urinary tract, anywhere from the tubules to the urethral meatus **(Fig. 9.2)**.

Types of Acute Renal Failure

Following are the types of acute renal failure:
- **Nonoliguric renal failure:** In this client may excrete 2 L/day of urine with hypertension and tachypnea.
- **Oliguric renal failure:** In oliguric renal failure, urine production usually falls below 400 mL/day **(Fig. 9.3)**.

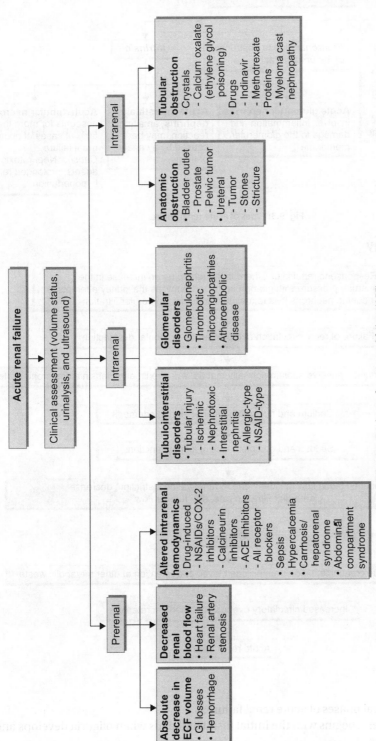

Fig. 9.2: Etiology of acute renal failure (ARF).

(ECF: extracellular fluid; NSAID: nonsteroidal anti-inflammatory drug; GI: gastrointestinal tract)

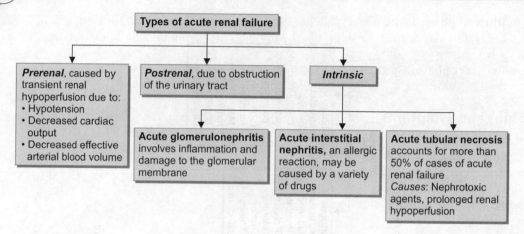

Fig. 9.3: Types of acute renal failure.

Pathophysiology

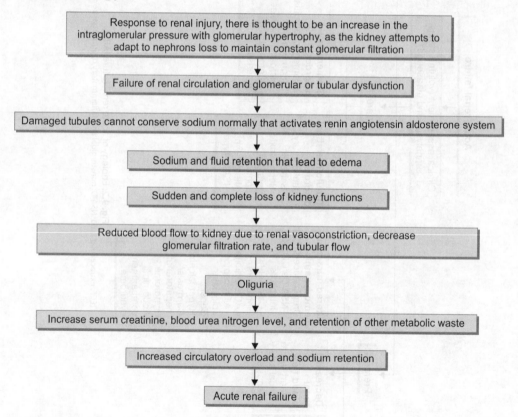

Clinical Phases

There are four clinical phases of acute renal failure:

1. **Initiation phase:** It begins with the initial insult and ends when oliguria develops and can last hours to days.
2. **Oliguria phase:** Usually caused by a reduction in the GFR.

3. **Diuresis phase:** In this phase, patient experiences gradually increasing urine output of 1–3 L/day, but may reach 3–5 L or more, which signals that glomerular filtration has started to recover.

4. **Recovery phase:** The recovery phase signals the improvement of renal function and takes 3–12 months.

Signs and Symptoms

- Dry skin and mucous membrane
- Drowsiness, headache
- Anorexia
- Dyspnea
- Fatigue, slow, sluggish movements
- Flank pain
- Hypertension
- Numbness in hand and feet
- Epistaxis
- Edema in ankle, feet, and legs
- Anuria
- Diarrhea

Diagnostic Evaluation

- Urinalysis
- Urine specific gravity
- Sodium levels
- Serum creatinine
- Urea nitrogen

Urinalysis may reveal the following:

- A fixed specific gravity of 1.010 as the tubules loses the ability to concentrate the filtrate.
- The presence of abnormal protein
- Elevated serum creatinine and BUN
- Elevated serum potassium level
- ABG shows a metabolic acidosis
- CBC demonstrates reduced RBCs.
- Bladder catheterization is performed to rule out urethral obstruction as cause of renal function and obtain urine specimen for culture.
- Computed tomography small kidney size.
- Microscopic examination of the urine sediment may show red blood cells.
- Protein and cellular debris molded in the shape of the tubular lumen.

Management

- **Medical management:** Goal is to prevent complications and restoration of renal function.
- **Collaborative therapy:** Goal is to eliminate cause and manage signs and symptoms and prevent complications:
  - Potassium restriction
  - Calcium supplements
  - Fluid restriction

- **Nutritional therapy:**
  - Adequate protein intake
  - Initiation of dialysis
  - Be active, eat balanced diet, and avoid alcohol and cigarette smoking.
  - It is necessary to provide diet high in carbohydrates, low in protein, salt, and potassium.

Pharmacologic Management

- Fluid replacement must be done very carefully to prevent fluid overload.
- Diuretic therapy may be used, furosemide and mannitol, the most commonly used pharmacologic agents, must be administered cautiously.
- Electrolyte replacement is based primarily on urine and serum electrolyte concentrations.
- Dialysis is usually used for severe acidosis.
- Calcium and phosphorus binders
- Antihypertensive and cardiovascular drugs
- Antiepileptic drugs
- Erythropoietin

Nutritional Therapy

- Foods and fluid that contain potassium or phosphorus (bananas, citrus fruit, juices, and coffee) are restricted.
- Daily weight and record the changes in weight should be monitored.
- Added salts should be avoided.
- It is necessary to provide high calorie, low protein, low sodium, and low potassium snacks between meals.

Nursing Management

- It is important to monitor the vital signs and fluid intake and output.
- It is necessary to assess the general appearance of patient including skin color and edema.
- If patient is receiving dialysis observe or access the site for signs of inflammation.
- It is necessary to assess the mucous membrane for dryness and inflammation.
- It is necessary to assess for any complications, fluid, and electrolyte imbalance.
- Massaging the bony prominences and changing positions frequently.

Nursing Care Plan

Nursing Diagnosis

- Excess fluid volume related to renal failure and fluid retention
- Risk for infection related to alter immune responses
- Imbalanced nutrition pattern less than body requirement related to dietary restrictions
- Impaired skin integrity related to edema
- Anxiety related to disease process and uncertainty of prognosis
- Deficient knowledge regarding disease condition and treatment
- Activity intolerance related to fatigue, retention of waste products.

Excess fluid volume related to renal failure and fluid retention
Interventions

- It is necessary to assess the fluid status of the patient.
- It is necessary to monitor daily weight of patient.
- It is necessary to assess the skin turgor and presence of edema.

- It is necessary to monitor vital signs.
- It is necessary to limit fluid intake to prescribed volume.
- It is necessary to assist patient to cope with the discomforts resulting from fluid retention.
- It is necessary to provide frequent oral care and maintain oral hygiene.
- It is necessary to administer medications and fluids as prescribed by the doctor.

Imbalance nutrition pattern less than body requirement related to dietary restrictions
Interventions

- It is necessary to assess the nutritional status of patient.
- It is necessary to monitor daily weight and record the weight changes.
- It is necessary to provide patient's food preferences within dietary restrictions.
- It is necessary to promote intake of high protein foods, for example, eggs, dairy products, meats.
- It is necessary to encourage high calorie, low protein, low potassium snacks in between meals.
- It is necessary to provide pleasant surrounding at meal times.
- It is necessary to maintain intake–output chart.

Deficient knowledge regarding disease condition and treatment
Interventions

- It is necessary to assess the knowledge of patient.
- It is necessary to assess the understanding of cause of renal failure and its treatment.
- It is necessary to provide explanations of renal function and consequences of renal failure at patient's level of understanding and guided by the patient's readiness to learn.
- It is necessary to assist patient to identify ways to incorporate changes related to illness and its treatment into lifestyle.
- It is necessary to provide oral and written information about disease, fluid and dietary restrictions, medications, follow-up schedule.
- It is necessary to provide psychological support to the patient.

CHRONIC RENAL FAILURE (END-STAGE RENAL DISEASE)

Chronic renal failure is a progressive, irreversible deterioration in renal function in which the body's ability to maintain metabolic and fluid and electrolyte balance fails, resulting in uremia and excessive BUN level.

Etiology

End-stage renal disease (ESRD) is caused by systemic disease, such as:

- Diabetes mellitus
- Hypertension
- Obstruction in urinary tract
- Hereditary lesions
- Polycystic kidney disease
- Vascular disorder
- Toxic agents
- Infections
- Chronic glomerulonephritis
- Pyelonephritis

Pathophysiology

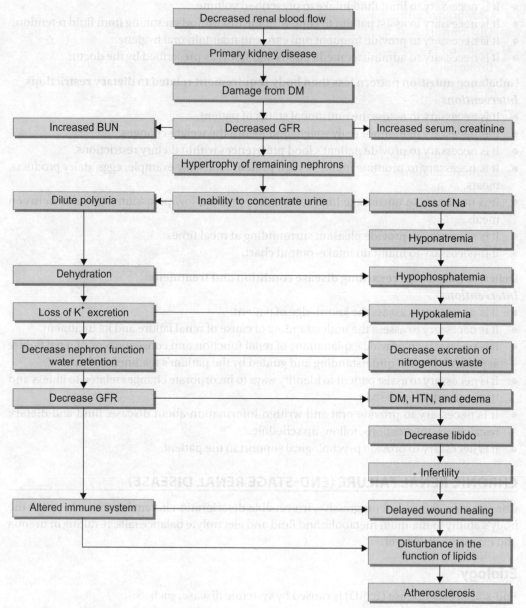

(BUN: blood urea nitrogen; DM: diabetes mellitus; GFR: glomerular filtration rate; HTN: hypertension)

Signs and Symptoms

Neurologic System

- Lethargy
- Apathy
- Decreased ability to concentrate
- Altered mental ability fatigue confusion

Integumentary

- Gray bronze skin color
- Dry pruritus
- Ecchymosis
- Brittle nails
- Thinning hairs

Cardiovascular Disease

- Hypertension
- Pitting edema (feet, hands)
- Periorbital edema
- Pericarditis
- Acceleration of atherosclerotic vascular disease
- Congestive heart failure

Respiratory System

- Dyspnea
- Tachypnea
- Kussmaul-type respiration
- Uremic pneumonitis

Gastrointestinal System

- Ammonia odor to breath
- Metallic taste
- Mouth ulceration and bleeding
- Anorexia
- Nausea and vomiting
- Inflammation of gastrointestinal (GI) tract

Reproductive System

- Amenorrhea
- Testicular atrophy
- Infertility
- Decreased libido

Musculoskeletal System

- Muscle cramp
- Loss of muscle strength
- Osteitis fibrosa
- Osteomalacia

Hematologic

- Anemia
- Thrombocytopenia

Diagnostic Evaluation

- **GFR:** Decreased GFR is obtaining a 24-hour urinalysis for creatinine clearance.
- Sodium and water retention
- **Anemia:** Anemia develops as a result of inadequate erythropoietin production.
- **Calcium and phosphorus imbalance:** The decreased calcium level increased the secretion of parathormone from the parathyroid glands.
- **Acidosis:** Decreased acid secretion primarily caused by the inability of the kidney tubules to excrete ammonia and to reabsorb sodium bicarbonate.

Complication

Following are the list of complications:
- Hyperkalemia
- Pericarditis
- Hypertension
- Anemia

Medical Management

Goal: The goal of management is to maintain the kidney function and homeostasis for as long as possible.

The management is divided into two categories:
1. **Pharmacologic therapy**
2. **Nutrition therapy**
1. **Pharmacologic therapy**
   - **Antacids:** Hyperphosphatemia and hypocalcemia are treated with aluminum-based antacids.
   - **Antihypertensive agents:** Low-sodium diet, diuretic agent, and inotropic agents, such as digitalis, dobutamine.
   - **Antiseizure agents:** Intravenous diazepam or phenytoin is usually administered to control seizure.
   - **Erythropoietin:** It is either administered intravenously or subcutaneously three times a week.
2. **Nutritional therapy**
   - Foods and fluid that contain potassium or phosphorus (bananas, citrus fruit, juices, and coffee) are restricted.
   - Daily weight and record the changes in weight should be monitored.
   - Added salts should be avoided.
   - It is necessary to provide high calorie, low protein, low sodium, and low potassium snacks between meals.

Nursing Management

- It is important to monitor the vital signs and fluid intake and output.
- It is necessary to assess the general appearance of patient including skin color and edema.
- If patient is receiving dialysis observe or access the site for signs of inflammation.
- It is necessary to assess the mucous membrane for dryness and inflammation.
- It is necessary to assess for any complications, fluid, and electrolyte imbalance.
- Massaging the bony prominences, changing positions frequently.

DIALYSIS

Chronic Indications for Dialysis

Following are the list of chronic indications for dialysis:
1. Symptomatic renal failure
2. Low GFR
3. Difficulty in medically controlling fluid overload.

Nursing Diagnosis

- Excess fluid volume related to decreased urine output, dietary excesses, and retention of sodium and water.
- Imbalance nutrition less than body requirement related to anorexia, nausea, vomiting, dietary restrictions, and altered oral membrane.
- Fatigue related to anemia, metabolic state, and dietary restriction.
- Activity intolerance related to fatigue, retention of waste products, and dialysis procedure.
- Grieving related to loss of kidney function as evidenced by expression of feelings of sadness, anger, inadequacy hopelessness.
- Anxiety related to disease process therapeutic interventions and uncertainty of prognosis
- Deficient knowledge regarding condition and treatment.
- Risk of infection related to suppressed immune system, access sites, and malnutrition secondary to dialysis and uremia.

Nursing Care Plan

Nursing Diagnosis

Following are the list of nursing diagnosis:
- Excess fluid volume related to renal failure and fluid retention
- Risk for infection related to alter immune responses
- Imbalanced nutrition pattern less than body requirement related to dietary restrictions
- Impaired skin integrity related to edema
- Anxiety related to disease process and uncertainty of prognosis
- Deficient knowledge regarding disease condition and treatment
- Activity intolerance related to fatigue and retention of waste products.

Excess fluid volume related to renal failure and fluid retention
Interventions
- It is necessary to assess the fluid status of the patient.
- Daily weight of patient should be monitored.
- It is necessary to assess the skin turgor and presence of edema.
- Vital signs should be monitored.
- It is necessary to limit fluid intake to prescribed volume.
- Assist patient to cope with the discomforts resulting from fluid retention.
- It is necessary to provide frequent oral care and maintain oral hygiene.
- It is necessary to administer medications and fluids as prescribed by the doctor.

Imbalance nutrition pattern less than body requirement related to dietary restrictions.

Interventions

- It is necessary to assess the nutritional status of patient.
- It is necessary to monitor daily weight and record the weight changes.
- It is necessary to provide patient's food preferences within dietary restrictions.
- It is necessary to promote intake of high protein foods, for example, eggs, dairy products, and meats.
- It is necessary to encourage high-calorie, low-protein, low-potassium snacks in between meals.
- It is necessary to provide pleasant surrounding at meal times.
- It is necessary to maintain intake–output chart.

Deficient knowledge regarding disease condition and treatment.

Interventions

- It is necessary to assess the knowledge of patient.
- It is necessary to assess the understanding of cause of renal failure and its treatment.
- It is necessary to provide explanations of renal function and consequences of renal failure at patient's level of understanding and guided by the patient's readiness to learn.
- It is necessary to assist patient to identify ways to incorporate changes related to illness and its treatment into lifestyle.
- It is necessary to provide oral and written information about disease, fluid and dietary restrictions, medications, follow-up schedule.

It is a process used to remove fluid and uremic waste products from the body when kidneys cannot do so through diffusion of solute molecules through a semipermeable membrane.

Basic Goals

- To remove the end products of protein metabolism
- To maintain a safe concentration of serum electrolytes
- To correct acidosis and replenish the bicarbonate levels of the blood
- To remove access fluid from the body

Principles of Dialysis

- **Ultrafiltration:** It refers to removal of fluid from blood using either osmotic or hydrostatic pressure to produce the necessary gradient.
- **Diffusion:** It is the process of passage of particles from an area of higher concentration to lower concentration that occurs through a semipermeable membrane.
- **Osmosis:** It the process of passage of particles from an area of lower concentration to higher concentration occurs through a semipermeable membrane.

Types

- **Peritoneal dialysis**
  - Intermittent peritoneal dialysis
  - Intermittent peritoneal dialysis
  - Continuous ambulatory peritoneal dialysis (CAPD)

■ Continuous cycling peritoneal dialysis
■ Automated peritoneal dialysis
● **Hemodialysis**
● **Continuous renal replacement therapies**

Hemodialysis

It is the process of cleansing the blood of accumulated wastes. It is the most commonly used method of dialysis. It is used for patients who are at end-stage renal disease.

Principle

● Diffusion
● Osmosis
● Ultrafiltration

Procedure

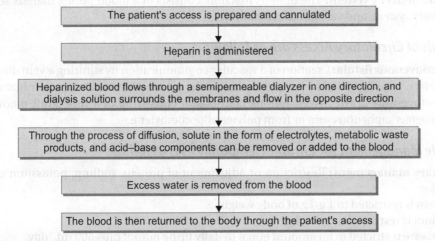

The patient's access is prepared and cannulated

↓

Heparin is administered

↓

Heparinized blood flows through a semipermeable dialyzer in one direction, and dialysis solution surrounds the membranes and flow in the opposite direction

↓

Through the process of diffusion, solute in the form of electrolytes, metabolic waste products, and acid–base components can be removed or added to the blood

↓

Excess water is removed from the blood

↓

The blood is then returned to the body through the patient's access

Requirements for Hemodialysis

● It is necessary to access the patient's circulation.
● Dialysis machine and dialyzer with semipermeable membrane
● Appropriate dialysate bath
● Time—approximately 4 hours, three times weekly.
● Dialysis center

Components to Dialysis

There are three essential components to dialysis:
1. The dialyzer
2. The composition and delivery of the dialysate
3. The blood delivery system.
1. **The dialyzer:** The dialyzer consists of a plastic device with the facility to perfuse blood and dialysate compartments at very high flow rates. These dialyzers are composed of bundles of capillary tubes through which blood circulates while dialysate travels on the outside of the fiber bundle.

There are four categories of dialysis membranes:

i. Cellulose
ii. Substituted cellulose
iii. Cellulosynthetic
iv. Synthetic

2. **Dialysate:** Composition of commercial dialysate is as follows:
- Solute bicarbonate dialysate
- Sodium
- Potassium
- Chloride
- Calcium
- Magnesium
- Acetate
- Bicarbonate
- Glucose

3. **Blood delivery system:** The dialysis machine consists of a blood pump, dialysis solution delivery system, and various safety monitors.

Methods of Circulatory Access are as follows

- **Arteriovenous fistula:** Creation of a vascular communication by suturing a vein directly to an artery. Usually, radial artery and cephalic vein are anastomosed in nondominant arm.
- **Arteriovenous graft:** Arteriovenous connection consisting of a tube graft made from autologous saphenous vein or from polytetrafluoroethylene.

Lifestyle Management for Chronic Hemodialysis is as follows

- **Dietary management:** Restriction or adjustment of protein, sodium, potassium or fluid intake.
- Protein is restricted to 1 g/kg of body weight.
- Sodium is restricted to 2–3 g/kg.
- Fluids are restricted to an amount equal to daily urine output plus 500 mL/day.
- Potassium is restricted to 1.5–2.5 g/day.

Peritoneal Dialysis

It is a type of dialysis that involves repeated cycles of instilling dialysate into the peritoneal cavity, allowing time for substance exchange and then removing the dialysate.

Indications

- Acute renal failure
- To treat overdose of drugs and toxins

Contraindications

- Hypercatabolism
- Abdominal disease
- Respiratory disease
- Abdominal surgery
- Peritonitis
- Abdominal malignancy

Types of Peritoneal Dialysis

CAPD: It is a form of intracorporeal dialysis that uses the peritoneum for the semipermeable membrane.

Procedure

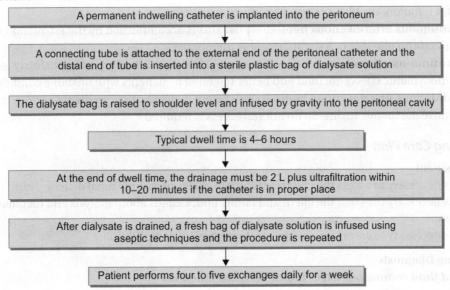

A permanent indwelling catheter is implanted into the peritoneum

A connecting tube is attached to the external end of the peritoneal catheter and the distal end of tube is inserted into a sterile plastic bag of dialysate solution

The dialysate bag is raised to shoulder level and infused by gravity into the peritoneal cavity

Typical dwell time is 4–6 hours

At the end of dwell time, the drainage must be 2 L plus ultrafiltration within 10–20 minutes if the catheter is in proper place

After dialysate is drained, a fresh bag of dialysate solution is infused using aseptic techniques and the procedure is repeated

Patient performs four to five exchanges daily for a week

Complications

- Infectious peritonitis
- Distension
- Nausea
- Catheter malfunction, obstruction, dialysate leak
- Hernia formation

Patient Education

- It is necessary to use strict technique when performing bag exchanges.
- It is necessary to perform bag exchange in clean, closed-off area without pets, etc.
- It is necessary to inspect bag, tubing for defects, and leaks.
- It is necessary to check weight because therapy causes weight gain.
- It is necessary to report sign symptoms of peritonitis.

Continuous Renal Replacement Therapy

These are various therapies that may be indicated for the patients who have acute or chronic renal failure.

Indications

- Those who are too clinically unstable for traditional hemodialysis
- Renal failure
- Acute electrolyte disorders—metabolic crisis
- Septic shock

- Pulmonary edema
- Cerebral edema

Types

1. **Continuous arteriovenous hemofiltration:** Blood flows from an artery to a hemofilter. After filtration, the blood return to body through vein.
2. **Continuous arteriovenous hemodialysis:** This is accomplished by the circulation of the dialysate on one side of a semipermeable membrane.
3. **Continuous venovenous hemofiltration:** Here the filtration occurs slowly so the hemodynamic effects are mild and better tolerated by patients with unstable conditions.
4. **Continuous arteriovenous hemodialysis:** Here concentration gradients are required to remove the uremic toxins. So no arterial access is required.

Nursing Care Plan

Assessment
- It is necessary to assess the client for multiple effects of chronic renal disease.
- It is necessary to assess the client and family understands about dialysis and diet management.
- It is necessary to assess for any sign and symptom of complications.

Nursing Diagnosis

Altered fluid volume related to impaired renal functions
Interventions
- It is necessary to monitor fluid volume status by daily weighting.
- It is necessary to follow the strict diet plan focusing on fluid restrictions.
- It is necessary to monitor blood pressure (BP) regularly.
- It is necessary to maintain input/output chart.

Imbalanced nutrition less than body requirement related to anorexia
Interventions
- It is necessary to assess the clients' status for persistent nausea and vomiting.
- It is necessary to involve the client in planning his/her diet.
- It is necessary to give written diet plan to client.
- It is necessary to help to stimulate client's appetite.
- It is necessary to give dietary counseling to the client.

Risk for impaired skin integrity related to edema
Interventions
- It is necessary to assess the skin condition of the client.
- It is necessary to assess the pressure site frequently.
- It is necessary to apply moisturizers to prevent dryness.
- It is necessary to teach the client about foot care.
- It is necessary to avoid use of soap.

Risk for infections related to presence on indwelling catheter
Interventions
- It is necessary to check the vital signs of patient.
- It is necessary to check the insertion sight of catheter for presence of any redness, etc.

- It is necessary to follow strict aseptic techniques.
- It is necessary to soak the catheter in disinfectant solution if it is needed next time.
- It is necessary to change the dressings on time.

NEPHROTIC SYNDROME

Nephrotic syndrome is a physiological condition characterized by proteinuria, hypoalbuminemia, hyperlipidemia, and edema.

Etiology

The cause of nephrotic syndrome can be divided into three types:
1. Primary
2. Secondary
3. Congenital
1. **Primary cause** of nephrotic syndrome is the disease that affects only the kidneys, such as glomerulosclerosis, membranous nephropathy, diabetic, etc.
2. **Secondary cause** of nephrotic syndrome is diabetes, systemic lupus erythematosus, amyloidosis, blood clot in kidney vein, and heart failure.

Pathophysiology

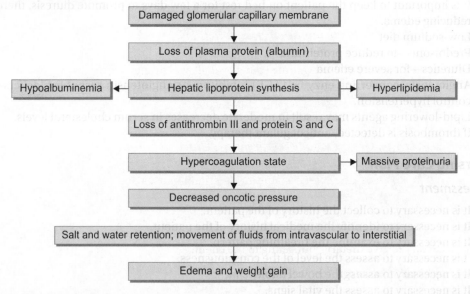

Signs and Symptoms

The major manifestation of nephrotic syndrome is edema. It is usually soft and pitting and is most commonly found around the eyes (periorbital), in dependent areas (sacrum, ankles, and hands) and in the abdomen. Other symptoms include:

- Proteinuria
- Hyperlipidemia
- Hypoalbuminemia
- Pitting edema
- Foamy appearance of the urine
- Hypertension

- Weight gain
- Ascites
- Anorexia
- Malaise

Diagnostic Evaluation

- **Urinalysis:** It shows microscopic hematuria, urinary casts, large amounts of protein and other abnormalities.
- **Needle biopsy of the kidney**
- **Blood analysis:** Creatinine clearance, BUN, creatinine blood test, albumin blood test.

Complications

- Infection
- Thromboembolism
- Pulmonary emboli
- ARF
- Accelerated atherosclerosis

Medical Management

- It is important to keep the patient on bed rest for a few days to promote diuresis, thereby, reducing edema.
- Low-sodium diet
- Prednisone—to reduce proteinuria
- Diuretics—for severe edema
- Angiotensin-converting enzyme (ACE) inhibitors or angiotensin receptor blockers—to control hypertension.
- Lipid-lowering agents may result in moderate decreases in serum cholesterol levels.
- If thrombosis is detected, anticoagulant therapy.

Nursing Care Plan

Assessment

- It is necessary to collect the history of the patient.
- It is necessary to identify the medical history of the patient.
- It is necessary to examine the breathing pattern.
- It is necessary to assess the level of the consciousness.
- It is necessary to assess the bowel habit.
- It is necessary to assess the vital signs.
- It is necessary to assess weight and height.
- It is necessary to assess the frequency, color, and amount of the urine.

Nursing Intervention

Balance the body fluid volume

- It is necessary to monitor intake and output and measure body weight every day.
- It is necessary to monitor blood pressure.
- It is necessary to assess respiratory status including breath sounds.
- It is necessary to give diuretics.
- It is necessary to measure and record the abdominal girth.

Balance the body fluid
- It is necessary to monitor intake and output.
- It is necessary to monitor vital signs.
- It is necessary to monitor laboratory test.
- It is necessary to assess the oral mucous membrane and elasticity of the skin turgor.

Maintenance of adequate nutritional intake
- It is necessary to assess the nutritional status.
- It is necessary to assess patient's nutritional dietary pattern.
- It is necessary to encourage high-calorie, low-protein, low-sodium, and low-potassium snacks between meals.
- Weigh patient daily
- It is necessary to assess for evidence of inadequate protein intake.
- Edema formation, decreased serum albumin levels.

GLOMERULONEPHRITIS

Glomerulonephritis means inflammation of glomeruli. It is an inflammation of tiny filters of kidney that helps to remove excess fluid, and waste from bloodstream and pass them into the urine.

Types: There are two types of glomerulonephritis:
1. Acute glomerulonephritis
2. Chronic glomerulonephritis

Acute Glomerulonephritis

It means active inflammation in glomeruli. Acute glomerulonephritis is most common in children and young adults, but all ages can be affected caused by group A streptococci bacteria.

Pathophysiology

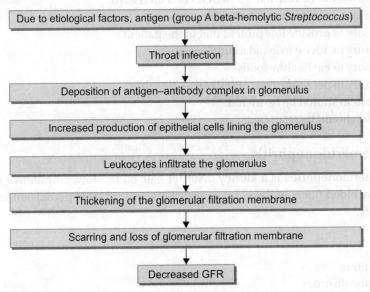

Signs and Symptoms

- Proteinuria
- Anorexia
- Abdominal pain
- Oliguria
- Edema
- Back pain, fatigue
- Weight gain
- Headache, loss of appetite
- Weakness, fatigue
- Hypertension

Diagnostic Evaluation

- **History:** It is necessary to assess and collect history from patient regarding change in pattern of urination frequency, color, or volume.
- **Physical examination:** It is necessary to check vital signs, monitor weight of patient.
- **Urinalysis:** For the presence of hematuria.
- **Needle biopsy:** It reveals obstruction of glomerular capillaries from proliferation of endothelial cells.

Management

Management includes:
- Antihypertensive
- Antibiotics
- Steroids

Nutritional Therapy

Dietary protein should be restricted if BUN level is increased.
- Potassium and sodium should be avoided.
- It is necessary to provide low protein diet to the patient.
- It is necessary to advise to avoid animal products.
- It is necessary to eat healthy foods.
- It is necessary to get proper rest and sleep.
- Dietary protein should be restricted.
- Fluid intake should be restricted.

Chronic Glomerulonephritis

Chronic glomerulonephritis is a kidney disorder caused by slow, cumulative damage and scaring, of tiny blood filters in the kidneys and characterized by hypertension and edema in legs and ankles.

Etiology

- Viral infections
- Autoimmune disorder.

Pathophysiology

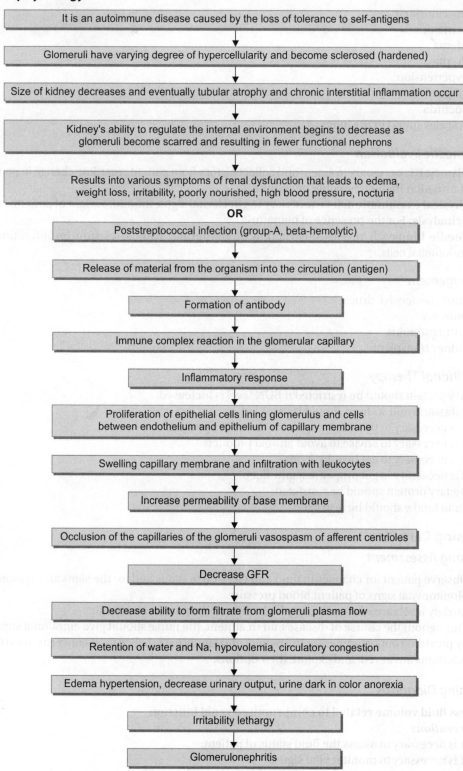

It is an autoimmune disease caused by the loss of tolerance to self-antigens

↓

Glomeruli have varying degree of hypercellularity and become sclerosed (hardened)

↓

Size of kidney decreases and eventually tubular atrophy and chronic interstitial inflammation occur

↓

Kidney's ability to regulate the internal environment begins to decrease as glomeruli become scarred and resulting in fewer functional nephrons

↓

Results into various symptoms of renal dysfunction that leads to edema, weight loss, irritability, poorly nourished, high blood pressure, nocturia

OR

Poststreptococcal infection (group-A, beta-hemolytic)

↓

Release of material from the organism into the circulation (antigen)

↓

Formation of antibody

↓

Immune complex reaction in the glomerular capillary

↓

Inflammatory response

↓

Proliferation of epithelial cells lining glomerulus and cells between endothelium and epithelium of capillary membrane

↓

Swelling capillary membrane and infiltration with leukocytes

↓

Increase permeability of base membrane

↓

Occlusion of the capillaries of the glomeruli vasospasm of afferent centrioles

↓

Decrease GFR

↓

Decrease ability to form filtrate from glomeruli plasma flow

↓

Retention of water and Na, hypovolemia, circulatory congestion

↓

Edema hypertension, decrease urinary output, urine dark in color anorexia

↓

Irritability lethargy

↓

Glomerulonephritis

Signs and Symptoms

- Proteinuria
- Hematuria
- Edema
- Dyspnea
- Hypertension
- Fatigue
- Nocturia
- Crackles sound in the lungs

Diagnostic Evaluation

- **History:** It is necessary to assess and collect history from patient regarding change in pattern of urination frequency, color, or volume.
- **Physical examination:** It is necessary to check vital signs, monitor weight of patient.
- **Urinalysis:** For the presence of hematuria.
- **Needle biopsy:** It reveals obstruction of glomerular capillaries from proliferation of endothelial cells.

Management

- Antihypertensive drugs
- Diuretics
- Corticosteroids
- Kidney transplant.

Nutritional Therapy

Dietary protein should be restricted if BUN level is increased.

- Potassium and sodium should be avoided.
- It is necessary to provide low protein diet to the patient.
- It is necessary to advise to avoid animal products.
- It is necessary to eat healthy foods.
- It is necessary to get proper rest and sleep.
- Dietary protein should be restricted.
- Fluid intake should be restricted.

Nursing Care Plan

Nursing Assessment

- Observe patient for changes in fluid and electrolyte status and for the signs and symptoms
- Monitor vital signs of patient blood pressure.
- Anxiety levels are often extremely high for both the patient and family.
- Throughout the course of disease and treatment, the nurse should give emotional support by providing opportunities for the patient and family to verbalize their concerns, have their questions answered, and explore their options.

Nursing Diagnosis

Excess fluid volume related to compromised renal function
Interventions

- It is necessary to assess the fluid status of patient.
- It is necessary to monitor vital signs.

- It is necessary to limit fluid intake to the patient.
- It is necessary to explain the rationale for restriction of fluid.
- It is necessary to check weight daily and record.
- It is necessary to maintain intake-output chart.

Imbalanced nutrition pattern less than body requirements related to anorexia
Interventions
- It is necessary to assess the nutritional status of the patient.
- It is necessary to monitor weight.
- It is necessary to assess the patient nutritional dietary patterns.
- It is necessary to restrict fluids rich diet to the patient.
- It is necessary to provide adequate diet to patient.
- It is necessary to encourage for proper rest.
- It is necessary to provide pleasant surroundings at the meal time.
- It is necessary to provide patients' food preference within dietary restrictions.
- It is necessary to provide, low salt and protein diet.

Deficient knowledge related to disease condition and treatment
Interventions
- It is necessary to assess the understanding of patient regarding disease condition and treatment.
- It is necessary to provide explanation regarding renal function.
- It is necessary to assist client to identify ways to incorporate changes.
- It is necessary to provide oral and written information.
- It is necessary to clear all the doubts of the client.
- It is necessary to provide psychological support to the client.

NEPHROLITHIASIS

Nephrolithiasis also called the renal calculi obstruct the pathway of urine and characterized by pain. The stones are protein that forms when the urine became supersaturated with a salt capable of forming solid crystals.

Etiology

- Hypercalcemia
- Chronic dehydration
- Chronic infection
- Chronic obstruction with stasis of urine

Risk Factors

- **Metabolic:** Abnormalities that result in increased urine levels of calcium, oxaluric acid, uric acid, or citric acid.
- **Climate:** Warm climate that causes increased fluid loss, low urine volume and increased solute concentration in the urine.
- **Diet:** Large intake of dietary proteins that increases uric acid excretion, excessive amounts of tea or fruit juices that elevate urinary oxalate level, large intake of calcium and oxalate, low fluid intake that increases urinary concentration.
- **Genetic factors:** Family history of stone formation, cystinuria, gout, or renal acidosis
- **Lifestyle:** Sedentary occupation, immobility

Pathophysiology

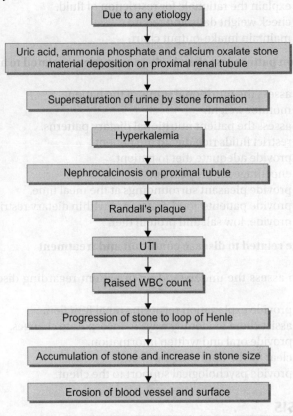

Due to any etiology

↓

Uric acid, ammonia phosphate and calcium oxalate stone material deposition on proximal renal tubule

↓

Supersaturation of urine by stone formation

↓

Hyperkalemia

↓

Nephrocalcinosis on proximal tubule

↓

Randall's plaque

↓

UTI

↓

Raised WBC count

↓

Progression of stone to loop of Henle

↓

Accumulation of stone and increase in stone size

↓

Erosion of blood vessel and surface

Types of Stones

- Calcium oxalate, calcium phosphate, or mixture
- Struvite—magnesium ammonium phosphate
- Uric acid stones
- Cysteine stones

Signs and Symptoms

- Costovertebral angle pain
- Groin pain
- Renal colic
- Anuria
- Restlessness
- Pallor
- Temperature
- Nausea and vomiting
- Flank pain radiating to genitalia
- Hematuria

Diagnostic Evaluation

- History collection
- Physical examination
- Kidney radiography

- Intravenous pyelogram
- Urinalysis
- Ultrasonography
- **Laboratory test:** Serum calcium, phosphorus, sodium, potassium, bicarbonate, uric acid, BUN and creatinine levels are also measured.

Management
Medical Management

- The goals of management are to eradicate the stone.
- It is necessary to relieve the pain.
- Opioid analgesic agents are administered to prevent shock.
- Nonsteroidal anti-inflammatory drugs are effective in treating renal stone pain.

Nutritional Therapy

- It is necessary to encourage fluid intake.
- Client with renal stones should drink 8–10 oz glasses of water daily.
- A urine output exceeding 2 L/day is advisable.

Interventional Procedures

- Ureteroscopy
- Extracorporeal shock wave lithotripsy
- Endourologic stone removal

Ureteroscopy
It involves first visualizing the stone and then destroying it through electrohydraulic lithotripter.

Extracorporeal shock wave lithotripsy
The high energy dry shock waves pass through the skin and fragment the stone.

Endourologic (percutaneous) stone removal
It is used to treat the larger stones. A percutaneous tract is formed and a nephroscope is inserted through it. Then the stone extracted or pulverized.

Chemolysis
Stone dissolution using infusions of chemical solutions (e.g., alkylating agents, acidifying agents).

Nursing Care Plan
Nursing Assessment

- It is necessary to obtain history focusing on family history of calculi.
- It is necessary to assess pain location and radiation.
- It is necessary to monitor for signs and symptoms of urinary tract infection (UTI).
- It is necessary to observe for signs and symptoms of obstruction.

Nursing Diagnosis
Acute pain related to the presence of stone in urinary tract
Interventions

- It is necessary to ask severity, location, and duration of pain.
- It is necessary to encourage fluid intake.

- It is necessary to administer pain medication.
- It is necessary to apply heat to flank pain area to reduce pain and promote comfort.

Impaired urinary elimination related to blockage of urine flow by stones
Interventions
- It is necessary to monitor total urine output and pattern of voiding.
- It is necessary to help patient to walk, ambulation may help move the stone through the urinary tract.
- It is necessary to teach patient to drink eight ounces of liquid with meals.

Risk for infection related to obstruction of urine flow
Interventions
- It is necessary to administer parenteral or oral antibiotics.
- It is necessary to assess urine for color, cloudiness, and odor.
- It is necessary to obtain vital signs, and monitor for fever.

Health Education

- Fluids intake is encouraged.
- It is necessary to teach about analgesics.
- It is necessary to warn that some blood may appear in urine for several weeks.
- Frequent walking is encouraged.

BENIGN PROSTATIC HYPERPLASIA

Benign prostatic hyperplasia also called BPH is a condition in men in which the prostate glands become enlarged and not cancerous. It is also called benign prostate hypertrophy or benign prostatic obstruction.

Etiology

- Low androgen level
- **Some risk factors:** Age 40 years and older
- Family history of BPH
- Medical conditions, such as obesity and lack of physical exercise.
- Erectile dysfunction

Pathophysiology

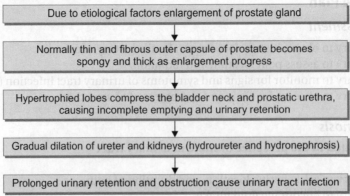

Due to etiological factors enlargement of prostate gland

↓

Normally thin and fibrous outer capsule of prostate becomes spongy and thick as enlargement progress

↓

Hypertrophied lobes compress the bladder neck and prostatic urethra, causing incomplete emptying and urinary retention

↓

Gradual dilation of ureter and kidneys (hydroureter and hydronephrosis)

↓

Prolonged urinary retention and obstruction cause urinary tract infection

Signs and Symptoms

Symptoms of BPH patient result from urinary obstruction. Symptoms fall into two groups:
- Decrease in the force of urine
- Difficulty in initiating voiding
- Dribbling of urine
- Weak and interrupted urine stream
- Smelly urine
- Urinary frequency, urgency
- Dysuria
- Nocturia
- Incontinence

Diagnostic Evaluation

Following are the evaluations made while diagnosis:
- **History:** It is necessary to take personal and family history.
- **Physical examination:** It is necessary to examine patient for discharge from urethra.
- **Urine analysis**.
- **Prostate-specific antigen blood test:** Prostate cells create a protein called prostate-specific antigen (PSA).
- **Uroflowmetry:** It is a test that helps to know urinary flow and urinary flow changes.
- **Cystourethroscopy:** It is a procedure allowing internal visualization of the urethra and bladder.

Management

Management of BPH includes: Men with mildly enlarged prostate need no treatment, unless their symptoms affecting their quality of life.

Pharmacological Management

Medications are used to shrink or stop the growth of prostate and reduce symptoms.
- Drugs used 5-reductase inhibitors
- Alpha-adrenergic receptor blockers
- Phosphodiesterase-5 inhibitors
- Combinations medication

Combination therapy: Combination therapy using both types of drugs has been shown to be more effective in reducing symptoms than using one drug alone; combination includes finasteride and doxazosin.

Surgical Management

- **Transurethral resection of prostate:** In this, rectoscope is inserted through urethra into prostate and cut pieces of enlarged prostate.
- **Transurethral incision of prostate:** Used to widen the urethra by making small cuts in prostate and in the bladder neck.
- **Open prostatectomy:** In this procedure, a cut or incision is made through the skin to reach the prostate. Urologist removes all parts of prostate through the incision.

Lifestyle Changes

- Reducing intake of liquids, particularly before going out or before sleep periods
- Avoiding or reducing intake of caffeine and alcohol

- Exercising pelvic floor muscles
- Preventing or treating constipation
- Eat healthy and adequate diet

Diet Management

- It is essential to eat fruits and vegetables daily.
- It is necessary to limit the consumption of red meat because it is high in fat.
- It is advised to take egg, fish, and beans rich in protein.
- It is advised to eat slowly and not to eat when stomach is full.
- Caffeine should be avoided because it is a diuretic and it increases the urine output.
- Spicy food should be avoided.

Nursing Care Plan

Nursing Assessment

- It is necessary to assess the condition of client.
- It is necessary to monitor vital signs of patient and record.
- It is necessary to maintain intake–output chart.
- It is necessary to monitor daily weight and record.
- If patient is having urinary retention, then insert catheter.
- It is necessary to obtain urine culture if UTI is suspected.
- It is necessary to prepare patient for diagnostic tests and surgery as appropriate.

Nursing Diagnosis

Acute pain related to bladder distension secondary to enlarged prostate
Interventions
- It is necessary to assess the level, location, intensity of pain by using pain relating scale.
- It is necessary to avoid the activities that increase the pain.
- It is necessary to provide comfortable bed, position to the patient.
- It is necessary to initiate bowel to prevent constipation.
- It is necessary to provide opioid analgesics to constipation.
- It is necessary to administer analgesics.

Urinary retention related to urethral obstruction
Interventions
- It is necessary to assess the patient usual pattern of urinary function.
- It is necessary to assess for sign of urinary retention.
- It is necessary to initiate measures to treat retention.
- It is necessary to administer cholinergic agent helps to stimulate bladder contraction.
- It is necessary to monitor the effect of medication.

Anxiety related to concern and lack of knowledge
Interventions
- It is necessary to obtain the history to determine the patients' concerns.
- It is necessary to ask questions regarding disease.
- It is necessary to provide education about diagnosis and treatment.
- It is necessary to answer all the questions asked by the client.
- It is necessary to provide comfortable environment.
- It is necessary to allow the client to ask questions.
- It is necessary to provide psychological support to the client.

Complications

- Urinary retention
- UTI
- Bladder stones
- Kidney damage

MULTIPLE CHOICE QUESTIONS

1. A 74-year-old man is admitted due to inability to void. He has a history of an enlarged prostate and has not voided in 14 hours. When assessing for bladder distention, the BEST method for the nurse to use is to assess for?

   A. Left lower quadrant dullness
   B. Rebound tenderness
   C. Urinary discharge
   D. Rounded swelling above the pubis

2. A client receiving peritoneal dialysis (PD) has outflow that is 100 mL less than the inflow for two consecutive exchanges. Which of the following actions would be best for the nurse to take first?

   A. Continue to monitor third exchange
   B. Change client's position
   C. Check client's blood pressure
   D. Irrigate dialysis catheter

3. A client with a chronic UTI is scheduled for a number of laboratory tests. The nurse would note which test results to best evaluate whether the kidneys are being adversely affected?

   A. Serum potassium 3.8 mEq/L
   B. Urinalysis specific gravity 1.015
   C. Serum creatinine 2.0 mg/dL
   D. Urine culture negative

4. The nurse tells a student nurse that the normal constituents of urine are the following. Select all that apply.

   A. Protein
   B. Urea
   C. Epithelial cells
   D. Water
   E. Ketones

5. A client seen in the emergency department reports painful urination, frequency, and urgency. Which of the following conditions would the nurse suspect?

   A. Renal calculi
   B. Polycystic kidney disease
   C. Glomerulonephritis
   D. Cystitis

Answers

1. D   2. B   3. C   4. B, D, E   5. D

REVIEW OF ANATOMY AND PHYSIOLOGY

Anatomy of thyroid gland: The butterfly shaped of thyroid gland is located just inferior to the larynx (voice box). It is composed of right and left lateral lobes, one on either side of the trachea, that is connected with ISTHMUS anterior to trachea, a small, pyramidal-shaped lobe something extend upward from the isthmus.

Weight: The normal weight of thyroid gland is 30 g.

Blood supply: It is highly vascularized and receives 80–120 mL of blood per minute.

Hormones: Mainly three types of hormones are produced by thyroid gland:

1. **T₃ or triiodothyroxine:** It contains three atoms of iodine
   Normal value: T_3 = 10–26 µg/dL
   T_3 total = 75 ng/dL

2. **T₄ or tertaiodiothyroxine or thyroxine:** It contains four atoms of iodine. It is secreted by follicular cells of thyroid gland.
   Normal value: T_4 = 4–11 µg/dL
   T_4 free = 0.8–1.8 mg/dL

3. **Calcitonin:** It is secreted by parafollicular cells or C-cells
   Function: Lower the level of blood calcium and phosphates by inhibiting bone resorption by osteoclast cell.
   Normal value: 19 mg/L

DISORDERS OF THE ENDOCRINE SYSTEM

HYPOTHYROIDISM

Hypothyroidism is a deficiency of thyroid hormone resulting in low basal metabolic rate (BMR), decreased heat production, and decrease oxygen consumption by the tissues.

Causes

- Iodine deficiency
- Congenital hypothyroidism
- Postpartum thyroiditis
- Genetic factor

Etiology Based on Types of Hypothyroidism

Primary Hypothyroidism

- Gland destruction
  - Surgical removal
  - Irradiation
  - Autoimmune disease (Hashimoto's, atrophic thyroiditis)
  - Idiopathic atrophy
  - Infiltrative process
- Inhibition of thyroid hormone synthesis and release
  - Iodine deficiency
  - Excess iodide in susceptible persons
  - Inherited enzyme defects
- Transient
  - After surgery or therapeutic radioiodine
  - Postpartum
  - Thyroiditis

Secondary Hypothyroidism

- Hypothalamic disease and pituitary disease
  - Genetic forms of pituitary hormone deficiencies
  - Infiltrative disorders
  - Surgery
  - Irradiation
  - Trauma
  - Tumors

Classification

Hypothyroidism is often classified by association with the indicated organ dysfunction.

Type	Origin	
Primary	Thyroid gland	The most common forms include Hashimoto's thyroiditis
Secondary	Pituitary gland	Occurs if the pituitary gland does not create enough thyroid-stimulating hormone (TSH) to induce the thyroid gland to produce enough thyroxine and triiodothyronine
Tertiary	Hypothalamus	Results when the hypothalamus fails to produce sufficient thyrotropin-releasing hormone (TRH)

Pathophysiology

1. Primary hypothyroidism

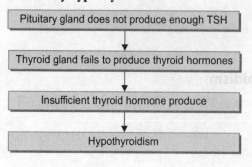

Pituitary gland does not produce enough TSH

↓

Thyroid gland fails to produce thyroid hormones

↓

Insufficient thyroid hormone produce

↓

Hypothyroidism

2. Secondary hypothyroidism

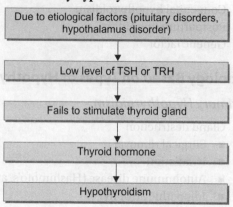

Due to etiological factors (pituitary disorders, hypothalamus disorder)

↓

Low level of TSH or TRH

↓

Fails to stimulate thyroid gland

↓

Thyroid hormone

↓

Hypothyroidism

Signs and Symptoms

- Cold intolerance
- Constipation
- Weight gain
- Elevated serum cholesterol
- Bradycardia
- Fatigue
- Decreased sweating
- Muscle cramps
- Depression
- Poor muscle tone
- Female infertility
- Hyperprolactinemia
- Galactorrhea
- Dry skin
- Thin, brittle fingernails
- Goiter
- Slow speech
- Dry puffy face
- Abnormal menstrual cycles
- Low BMR
- Impaired memory
- Impaired cognitive function.
- Hair loss
- Anemia
- Acute psychosis
- Enlarged tongue

Diagnostic Evaluations

Thyroid function tests: Test reveals high levels of TSH and low level of thyroxine (T_4) and triiodothyronine (T_3).

Complication

- Myxedema
- Infection
- Respiratory failure
- Heart failure
- **Myxedema coma:** It is characterized by hypercalcemia, hypoglycemia and water intoxication, hypoventilation, respiratory acidosis, hypothermia, and hyponatremia.
- **Cretinism** is caused by a decreased production of T_4 and results in mental retardation, stunted growth, short stature and irregularly placed and poorly formed teeth.

Management of Hypothyroidism

Medical Management

- **Thyroid hormones:** Hypothyroidism is treated with the levorotatory forms of thyroxine (levothyroxine) and triiodothyronine.
- **T_4 only:** This treatment involves supplementation of levothyroxine alone, in a synthetic form.

Supportive Management

Arterial blood gases measures especially CO_2 retention and treat with oxygenation.

Nursing Care Plan

Assessment

- Physical assessment findings include a palpable and bilaterally enlarged thyroid; dry.
- It is necessary to assess the signs and symptoms of hypothyroidism.

Nursing Diagnosis

- Constipation, related to decreased peristalsis
- Impaired verbal communication, related to changes in speech pattern
- Low self-esteem related to changes in physical appearance.

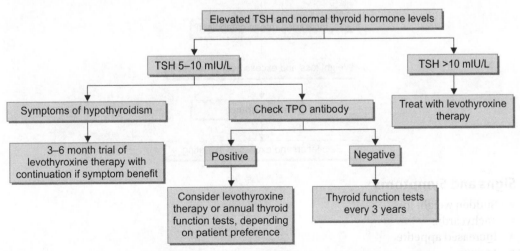

(TSH: thyroid stimulating hormone; TPO: thyroid peroxidase antibody)

Planning and Implementation

- It is necessary to encourage fluids and fiber in the diet.
- It is necessary to take medication as prescribed.
- It is necessary to plan activities around rest periods.
- It is necessary to monitor vital signs, including heart rate and rhythm.
- It is necessary to administer thyroid replacement therapy.
- It is necessary to instruct the client to have low-calorie, low-cholesterol, and low-saturated-fat diet.
- It is necessary to avoid sedatives and narcotic.

HYPERTHYROIDISM

Hyperthyroidism is characteristic by elevated T_3 and T_4 levels that result in increased body mass index (BMI), causing sudden weight loss, a rapid or irregular heartbeat, sweating, and nervousness.

Etiology

- **Graves' disease**: Graves' disease, an autoimmune disorder in which antibodies produced by immune system stimulate thyroid gland.
- Hyperfunctioning thyroid nodules also called Plummer's disease.
- **Thyroiditis**

Pathophysiology

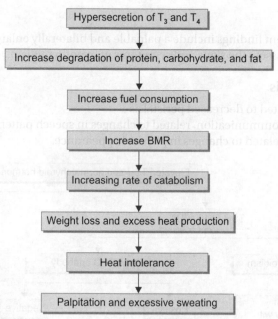

Hypersecretion of T_3 and T_4

↓

Increase degradation of protein, carbohydrate, and fat

↓

Increase fuel consumption

↓

Increase BMR

↓

Increasing rate of catabolism

↓

Weight loss and excess heat production

↓

Heat intolerance

↓

Palpitation and excessive sweating

Signs and Symptoms

- Sudden weight loss
- Tachycardia
- Increased appetite
- Fatigue

- Insomnia
- Nervousness
- Tremor
- Exophthalmos
- Fast tendon reflex
- Sweating
- Changes in menstrual patterns
- Increased sensitivity to heat
- Changes in bowel patterns
- Goiter
- Skin thinning
- Fine, brittle hair
- Reduction in eye movement

Complications

- Atrial fibrillation and congestive heart failure (CHF)
- Osteoporosis
- Graves' ophthalmopathy characterized by bulging, red or swollen eyes, sensitivity to light, and blurring.

Diagnostic Evaluation

- **Radioactive iodine (RAI) uptake test:** High in Graves' disease and toxic nodular goiter, low in thyroiditis.
- **Serum T_4 and T_3:** Increased in hyperthyroidism. Normal T_4 with elevated T_3 indicates thyrotoxicosis.
- **TSH:** Suppressed
- **Thyroglobulin:** Increased
- **TRH stimulation:** Hyperthyroidism is indicated if TSH fails to rise after administration of TRH.
- **Serum glucose:** Elevated (related to adrenal involvement)
- **Plasma cortisol:** Low levels (less adrenal reserve)
- **Alkaline phosphatase and serum calcium:** Increased
- **Serum catecholamines:** Decreased
- **Urine creatinine:** Increased
- Thyroid scan
- **Thyroid T_3 uptake:** Normal to high
- **Protein-bound iodine:** Increased

Management

Medical Management

- **Beta-blockers:** Beta-blockers offer prompt relief of the adrenergic symptoms of hyperthyroidism, such as tremor, palpitations, heat intolerance, and nervousness.
- **Iodides:** Iodides block the peripheral conversion of thyroxine (T_4) to triiodothyronine (T_3) and inhibit hormone release.
- **Antithyroid drugs:** Antithyroid drugs act by suppressing thyroid hormone levels. Methimazole and propylthiouracil
- **Propylthiouracil:** It is preferred for pregnant women.

- **RAI:** RAI is the treatment of choice for most patients with Graves' disease and toxic nodular goiter.
- **Thyroidectomy:** It means the removal of thyroid gland; it may be subtotal thyroidectomy, hemithyroidectomy, or total thyroidectomy.

Nursing Management

Decrease cardiac output related to hypermetabolic state

Interventions

- It is necessary to monitor blood pressure (BP) lying, sitting, and standing.
- It is necessary to monitor central venous pressure.
- It is necessary to assess vital signs.
- It is necessary to monitor electrocardiogram (ECG).
- It is necessary to auscultate heart sounds.
- It is necessary to monitor temperature.
- It is necessary to provide cool environment.
- It is necessary to weigh daily.

Fatigueless related to hypermetabolic state

Intervention

- It is necessary to monitor vital signs.
- It is necessary to document tachypnea, dyspnea, pallor, and cyanosis.
- It is necessary to encourage client to restrict activity and rest in bed as much as possible.
- It is necessary to provide for quiet environment, cool room, decreased sensory stimuli, soothing colors, quiet music.
- It is necessary to encourage client to restrict activity.
- It is necessary to provide comfort measures—touch therapy or massage, cool showers.
- It is necessary to avoid topics that irritate or upset patient and discuss ways to respond to these feelings.

Disturbed thought processes related to altered sleep pattern

Intervention

- It is necessary to assess thinking process.
- It is necessary to determine attention span, orientation level.
- It is necessary to note the changes in behavior.
- It is necessary to assess level of anxiety.
- It is necessary to provide quiet environment.
- It is necessary to provide, calendar, room with outside window, alter level of lighting to simulate day or night.
- It is necessary to administer medication as indicated.
- It is necessary to provide safety measures.

Anxiety related to Central Nervous System (CNS) Stimulation

Intervention

- It is necessary to observe behavior indicative of level of anxiety.
- It is necessary to monitor physical responses, noting palpitations, repetitive movements, hyperventilation, and insomnia.
- It is necessary to stay with patient, maintaining calm manner.
- It is necessary to describe and explain procedures.

- It is necessary to speak in brief statements.
- It is necessary to discuss with patient reasons for emotional liability and psychotic reaction.
- It is necessary to reduce external stimuli.
- It is necessary to administer antianxiety agents or sedatives and monitor effects.

Impaired tissue integrity related to alternation in protective mechanism of eye

Intervention

- It is necessary to encourage use of dark glasses.
- It is necessary to suggest use of eye patch during sleep.
- It is necessary to elevate the head of the bed and restrict salt intake if indicated.
- It is necessary to instruct client in extraocular muscle exercises.

THYROIDITIS

Thyroiditis is inflammation, or swelling of thyroid gland.

Etiology

- **Postpartum thyroiditis**
- **Subacute thyroiditis:** It is characterized by inflammation in the thyroid with pain in the neck, jaw, or ear.
- **Chronic thyroiditis or Hashimoto's disease** is a common thyroid gland disorder.
- **Adrenal insufficiency**
- **Fungal infections**
- **Hyperparathyroidism**

Signs and Symptoms

- Dysphagia
- Fatigue
- Fever
- Hoarseness
- Tenderness to the thyroid gland
- Weakness
- Cold intolerance
- Constipation
- Fatigue

Diagnostic Evaluation

- Low serum TSH level
- High serum free T_4 (thyroid hormone, thyroxine) level
- High erythrocyte sedimentation rate
- High serum TSH level
- Low serum free T_4
- Low RAI uptake
- High serum thyroglobulin level

Management

- Anti-inflammatory medications, such as aspirin or ibuprofen are used to control pain.
- Steroids (prednisone) to control inflammation.
- Antithyroid drugs

HYPOPARATHYROIDISM

Hypoparathyroidism is poor functioning of parathyroid glands which decrease the production of parathyroid hormone. This can lead to low levels of calcium and increased amount of phosphorus.

Etiology and Types

- **Acquired hypoparathyroidism:** This most common cause of hypoparathyroidism develops after accidental damage to or removal of the parathyroid glands during surgery.
- **Hereditary hypoparathyroidism (De-George syndrome):** Congenital absence parathyroid glands at birth.
- **Autoimmune disease:** In this, the immune system creates antibodies against the parathyroid tissues.
- Extensive cancer radiation
- Low levels of magnesium

Signs and Symptoms

Kernig's sign: Patient is kept in supine position, hip and knee are flexed to a right angle, and then knee is slowly extended, if the client experiences resistance or pain during extension of the patient's knees, it indicates meninges irritation and positive Kernig's sign **(Fig. 10.1A)**.

Brudzinski sign: The examiner keeps one hand at the neck and the other on chest in order to prevent the patient from rising. Reflex flexion of the patient's hips and knees after passive flexion of the neck indicates the meninges irritation and positive Brudzinski sign **(Fig. 10.1B)**.

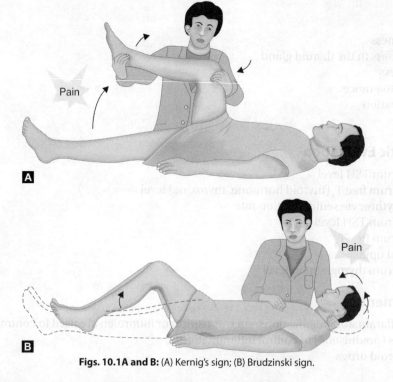

Figs. 10.1A and B: (A) Kernig's sign; (B) Brudzinski sign.

Diagnostic Evaluation

- **History:** Take a history as muscle cramps or tingling sensation.
- **Physical examination:** Looking for signs that suggest hypoparathyroidism, such as facial muscle twitching.
- **Blood tests**
- **ECG:** It can detect arrhythmias.
- **Urine test:** For presence of too much calcium
- **X-rays** and bone density tests

Complication

- **Tetany:** These cramp-like spasms of hands and fingers may be prolonged and painful.
- **Paresthesia:** These are characterized by sensory symptoms of odd, tingling sensations or pins and needles feelings in lips, tongue, fingers, and feet.
- Syncope
- Malformation of the teeth
- Impaired kidney function
- Heart arrhythmias and fainting
- Stunted growth
- Slow mental development in children
- Cataracts

Management

- Oral calcium carbonate tablets
- Vitamin D supplement

Diet

- Diet rich in calcium
  - Low in phosphorus-rich items
  - Intravenous infusion of calcium
- Nutrition and supplements
  - It is necessary to eliminate all potential food allergens.
  - It is necessary to avoid refined foods, such as white breads, pastas, and sugar.
  - It is necessary to use healthy cooking oils, such as olive oil or vegetable oil.
  - It is necessary to reduce or eliminate trans-fatty acids.
  - It is necessary to limit carbonated beverages.
  - It is necessary to avoid coffee and alcohol and tobacco.
  - It is necessary to drink six to eight glasses of filtered water daily.
  - It is necessary to exercise moderately.
  - A multivitamin daily

Nursing Management

- Activity intolerance related to fatigue
- Constipation related to decreased gastrointestinal function
- Ineffective breathing pattern related to depression of ventilation
- Disturbed thought process related to metabolic disorder
- Knowledge deficit related to exposure to information about treatment program for lifelong thyroid replacement therapy.

HYPERPARATHYROIDISM

Hyperparathyroidism is an excess of parathyroid hormone in the bloodstream due to overactivity of parathyroid glands.

Etiology and Types

- **Primary hyperparathyroidism:** It occurs due to noncancerous growth on a gland.
- **Secondary hyperparathyroidism:** Secondary hyperparathyroidism is the result of another condition that lowers calcium levels.

Risk Factors

- Woman who has gone through menopause
- Severe calcium or vitamin D deficiency
- Inherited disorder
- Radiation treatment for cancer that has exposed neck.

Signs and Symptoms

- Osteoporosis
- Renal calculi
- Polyuria
- Abdominal pain
- Weakness
- Depression
- Dementia
- Arthralgia

Diagnostic Evaluation

- **Blood tests:** It indicates elevated calcium level.
- Bone mineral density test (bone densitometry)
- **Urine tests:** How much calcium is excreted in urine?
- **Ultrasound:** Ultrasound uses sound waves to create images of parathyroid glands.
- **Sestamibi scan:** Sestamibi is a especially designed radioactive compound that is absorbed by overactive parathyroid glands and can be detected on computerized tomography (CT) scans.

Complications

- Osteoporosis
- Kidney stones
- Cardiovascular disease (hypertension)
- Neonatal hyperparathyroidism

Management

Medical Management

- **Calcimimetics:** A calcimimetic is a drug that mimics calcium circulating in the blood. Therefore, the drug may trick the parathyroid glands into releasing less parathyroid hormone.
- Hormone replacement therapy
- Bisphosphonates

Prevention

- It is necessary to monitor how much calcium and vitamin D you get in your diet.
- It is necessary to drink plenty of water.
- It is necessary to exercise regularly.
- It is essential to quit smoking.

Nursing Management

- It is necessary to protect the client from injury.
- It is necessary to monitor for possible complications.
- It is necessary to provide client education independence.
- It is necessary to adjust activities and reduce intensity.
- It is necessary to provide positive atmosphere, while acknowledging the difficulty of situation for the client.
- It is necessary to assist client with assistive device, such as walker.
- It is necessary to help minimize frustration.
- It is necessary to protect client from injury.
- It is necessary to remove cause of hypersecretion of parathormones.
- It is necessary to provide at least 3 L of fluid per day.
- It is necessary to take safety precaution to minimize the risk of injury from fall.
- It is necessary to provide comfort measures to alleviate bone pain.
- It is necessary to administer antacids, as appropriate to prevent pelvic ulcers.
- It is necessary to auscultate the lungs regularly.

CUSHING SYNDROME AND ADDISON DISEASE

Cushing Syndrome

Cushing syndrome is also called hypercortisolism, occurs when body is exposed to high levels of the hormone cortisol for a long time. It also refers to over secretion of corticosteroids from adrenal gland, characterized by a fatty hump between shoulders, a rounded face, and pink or purple stretch marks on skin.

Etiology

- A pituitary gland tumor
- An ectopic adrenocorticotropic hormone (ACTH)-secreting tumor
- A primary adrenal gland disease, noncancerous tumor of the adrenal cortex
- Familial Cushing syndrome.

Pathophysiology

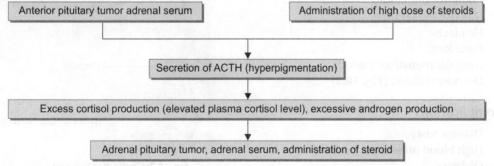

Contd...

Contd...

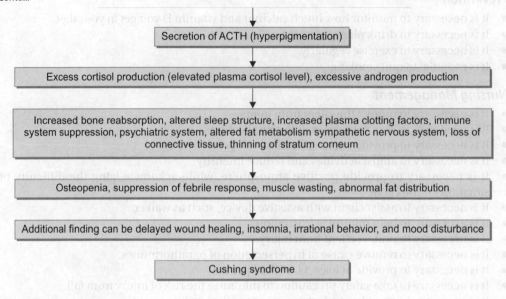

Secretion of ACTH (hyperpigmentation)

↓

Excess cortisol production (elevated plasma cortisol level), excessive androgen production

↓

Increased bone reabsorption, altered sleep structure, increased plasma clotting factors, immune system suppression, psychiatric system, altered fat metabolism sympathetic nervous system, loss of connective tissue, thinning of stratum corneum

↓

Osteopenia, suppression of febrile response, muscle wasting, abnormal fat distribution

↓

Additional finding can be delayed wound healing, insomnia, irrational behavior, and mood disturbance

↓

Cushing syndrome

Signs and Symptoms

- Obesity and skin changes
- Weight gain and fatty tissue deposits at upper back
- Moon face
- Buffalo hump
- Pink or purple stretch marks on the skin of the abdomen, thighs, breasts, and arms
- Depression
- Loss of emotional control
- Slow healing of cuts
- Acne
- Thicker body facial hair
- Decreased fertility
- Erectile dysfunction
- Fatigue
- Muscle weakness
- Cognitive difficulties
- Glucose intolerance
- Headache
- Bone loss
- Irregular menstrual periods
- Decreased libido **(Fig. 10.2)**.

Complications

- Osteoporosis
- High blood pressure
- Diabetes

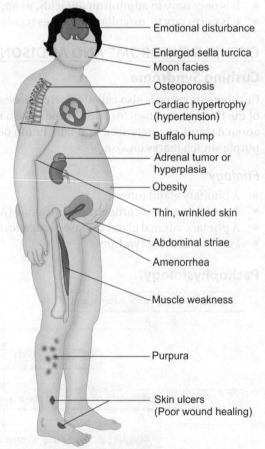

- Emotional disturbance
- Enlarged sella turcica
- Moon facies
- Osteoporosis
- Cardiac hypertrophy (hypertension)
- Buffalo hump
- Adrenal tumor or hyperplasia
- Obesity
- Thin, wrinkled skin
- Abdominal striae
- Amenorrhea
- Muscle weakness
- Purpura
- Skin ulcers (Poor wound healing)

Fig. 10.2: Clinical manifestations.

- Frequent or unusual infections
- Loss of muscle mass and strength

Diagnostic Evaluation

- **24-hour urinary free cortisol level:** Urine is collected over a 24-hour period and tested for the amount of cortisol.
- **Dexamethasone suppression test:** This test helps to distinguish client with excess production of ACTH due to pituitary adenomas from those with ectopic ACTH-producing tumors.
- **Corticotropin-releasing hormone (CRH) stimulation test:** This test helps to distinguish between client with pituitary adenomas and those with ectopic ACTH syndrome or cortisol-secreting adrenal tumors.
- Direct visualization of the endocrine glands
- The dexamethasone-CRH test

Management

The assessment of Cushing syndrome includes:
- Cortisol and aldosterone levels
- The skin is assessed for trauma, infection, edema.
- Changes in physical appearance, such as weight gain or obesity, heavy trunk, thin extremities, buffalo hump.
- It is necessary to assess the client for mood changes.

Medical Management

- **Reducing corticosteroid use**
- **Surgical management:** If the cause of Cushing syndrome is a tumor, doctor may recommend complete surgical removal because the remaining adrenal gland may have atrophied and stopped producing adrenocortical hormones.
- **Radiation therapy**
- **Medications**
  - Metyrapone to control steroid hypersecretion in patient who does not respond to mitotane therapy.
  - Aminoglutethimide blocks cholesterol conversion of pregnenolone, effectively blocking cortisol production.
- **Increase activities slowly**
- **Eat sensibly**
- **Monitor your mental health**
- **Gently soothe aches and pains**

Nursing Care Plan

Nursing Diagnosis

- Risk for injury related to weakness
- Risk for infection related to altered metabolism
- Impaired skin integrity related to edema
- Self-care deficit related to weakness
- Disturbed body image related to altered physical appearance

Nursing Interventions

Risk for injury related to weakness

Intervention

- It is necessary to provide protective environment.
- It is necessary to provide assistance to avoid falling.
- It is necessary to encourage food high in protein, vitamin D and calcium.
- It is necessary to refer the dietician.

Risk for infection related to altered protein metabolism

Intervention

- The client should avoid unnecessary exposure to other with infection.
- The nurse frequently assesses the client for signs of infection.
- It is necessary to use aseptic techniques.
- It is necessary to properly handwash.
- It is necessary to encourage personal hygiene.

Impaired skin integrity related to edema

Intervention

- Use of adhesive tape is avoided.
- The nurse frequently assesses the skin and bony prominence.

Addison's Disease (Adrenal Insufficiency)

Addison's disease is a disorder that occurs when the body produces insufficient amounts of cortisol hormones produced by adrenal glands.

Etiology

- **Primary adrenal insufficiency:** It occurs when the cortex is damaged and does not produce its hormones in adequate quantities.
- Tuberculosis
- Infection to adrenal gland
- Cancer of adrenal glands
- **Secondary adrenal insufficiency**
- Adrenal insufficiency can also occur if pituitary gland is diseased.

Pathophysiology

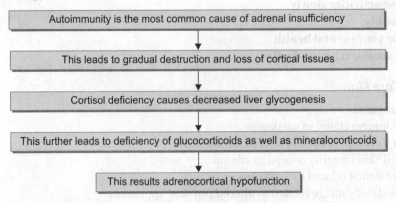

Signs and Symptoms

- Muscle weakness and fatigue
- Weight loss and decreased appetite
- Hyperpigmentation
- Hypotension
- Salt craving
- Hypoglycemia
- Nausea
- Arthralgia
- Irritability
- Depression
- Body hair loss

Diagnostic Evaluation

- **Blood test:** Measuring blood levels of sodium, potassium, cortisol, and ACTH.
- **ACTH stimulation test:** This test involves measuring the level of cortisol in blood before and after an injection of synthetic ACTH.
- CT scan of abdomen to check the size of adrenal glands
- **Insulin-induced hypoglycemia test:** The test involves checking blood sugar and cortisol levels at various intervals after an injection of insulin.

Management

Medical management

- Oral corticosteroids, fludrocortisone to replace aldosterone
- Corticosteroid injections
- Androgen replacement therapy

Management of Addisonian Crisis

Addisonian crisis is a life-threatening condition that results in hypotension, hypoglycemia, and hyperkalemia. Management includes:

- Hydrocortisone
- Saline solution
- Dextrose

Nursing Care Plan

Assessment

- It is necessary to assess the daily weights.
- It is necessary to monitor intake and output.
- It is necessary to assess the pulse.
- It is necessary to assess bone prominences for pressure ulcers.
- It is necessary to monitor for exposure to cold and infections.
- It is necessary to assess serum sodium and potassium imbalance.
- It is necessary to assess skin for changes in color and turgor.

Nursing Diagnosis

Risk for injury
Addisonian crisis related to adrenal insufficiency.

Interventions
- It is necessary to monitor for sudden profound weakness, severe abdominal, back and leg pain.
- It is necessary to administer 1,000 mL of normal saline with water-soluble glucocorticoid added is rapidly infused.
- It is necessary to infuse glucose in case of hypoglycemia.
- It is necessary to monitor vital signs.
- It is necessary to monitor hourly urine output.
- It is necessary to steroid replacement can be administered orally.
- It is necessary to keep bed in lowest position to prevent falling.
- It is necessary to keep side rails.

Deficient fluid volume related to inability to conserve fluid secondary to glucocorticoid deficiency

Interventions
- It is necessary to monitor intake and output hourly.
- It is necessary to monitor vital signs
- It is necessary to monitor hourly urine output.
- It is necessary to monitor weigh daily.
- It is necessary to administer intravenous fluids.
- It is necessary to monitor hemoglobin, blood urea nitrogen and serum creatinine daily.
- It is necessary to administer cortisol as ordered.

Ineffective coping related to inability to respond to stressors.

Interventions
- It is necessary to decrease environmental stressors.
- It is necessary to explain all procedures and interventions to the client to reduce the fair and anxiety.
- It is necessary to provide care in calm environment.

DIABETES MELLITUS, KETOACIDOSIS, AND DIABETIC HYPEROSMOLAR SYNDROME

Diabetes mellitus (DM) is a group of metabolic diseases in which serum sugar level became elevated more than 100 mg/dL in fasting and characterized by polyuria, polydipsia, and polyphagia.

Types of Diabetes Mellitus

- **Type-1 diabetes mellitus:** It is also called insulin-dependent diabetes mellitus; it occurs due to body's failure to produce insulin. It occurs in juveniles. Due to autoimmunity, the immune system mistakenly forms antibodies and inflammatory cells that damage to patients' own body tissues. It may also occur due to certain viral infections (mumps and Coxsackie viruses).
- **Type-2 diabetes mellitus:** It is also called non-insulin-dependent diabetes mellitus or "adult-onset diabetes". In this, client can still produce insulin but do so relatively inadequately for their body's needs.
- **Gestational diabetes:** Gestational diabetes, occurs when pregnant women.

Pathophysiology of Diabetes Mellitus

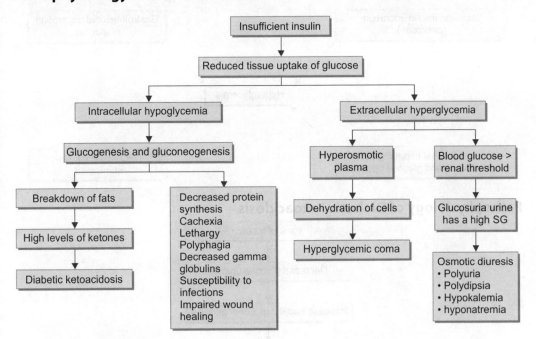

Type 1 Diabetes Mellitus

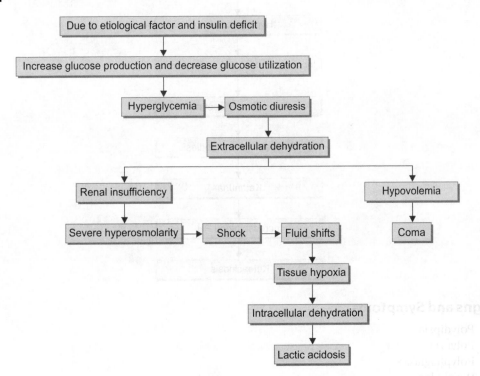

Type 2 Diabetes Mellitus

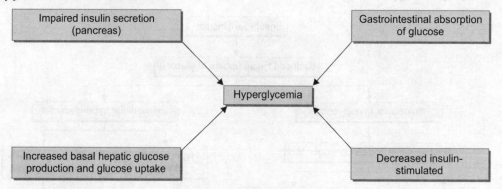

Impaired insulin secretion (pancreas)		Gastrointestinal absorption of glucose

Hyperglycemia

Increased basal hepatic glucose production and glucose uptake		Decreased insulin-stimulated

Pathophysiology of Diabetic Ketoacidosis

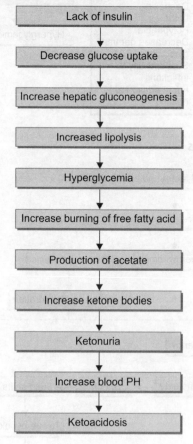

Lack of insulin

↓

Decrease glucose uptake

↓

Increase hepatic gluconeogenesis

↓

Increased lipolysis

↓

Hyperglycemia

↓

Increase burning of free fatty acid

↓

Production of acetate

↓

Increase ketone bodies

↓

Ketonuria

↓

Increase blood PH

↓

Ketoacidosis

Signs and Symptoms

- Polydipsia
- Polyuria
- Polyphagia
- Weight loss
- Fatigue

- Blurred vision
- Slow-healing sores
- Dark skin

Diagnostic Evaluation

- **Glycated hemoglobin test:** This blood test indicates average blood sugar level for the past 2–3 months.
- **Random blood sugar test:** A blood sample will be taken at a random time.
- **Fasting blood sugar test:** A blood sample will be taken after an overnight fast. A fasting blood sugar level less than 100 mg/dL.
- **Oral glucose tolerance test:** It is rarely used test for hyperglycemia, client is asked to fast overnight, and the fasting blood sugar level is measured. Then drink a sugary liquid, and blood sugar levels are tested periodically for the next 2 hours.
- **Urine glucose and ketone levels:** The presence of glucose in urine indicates hyperglycemia.

Complications

- Cardiovascular disease
- Neuropathy
- Nephropathy
- Retinopathy
- Diabetic ketoacidosis
- **Diabetic hyperosmolar syndrome:** This condition occurs when production of insulin is normal, but it does not work properly. Blood glucose levels may become very high—greater than 600 mg/dL.

Management

- Nutrition, meal planning, and weight control are the foundation of diabetes management.
- Regular exercise
- Insulin therapy
- Avoid alcohol
- Avoid stress

Medical Management

- Biguanides
- Sulfonylureas
- Meglitinide derivatives
- Alpha-glucosidase inhibitors
- Thiazolidinediones
- Insulins

Insulin Therapy

Types of insulin:
- Insulin lispro (Humalog)
- Insulin aspart (Novolog)
- Insulin glargine (Lantus)
- Insulin detemir (Levemir)
- Insulin isophane

Nursing Care Plan

Nursing Diagnosis

Fluid volume deficit related to osmotic diuresis

Intervention

- It is necessary to monitor vital signs.
- It is necessary to assess breathing patterns.
- It is necessary to assess body temperature.
- It is necessary to assess peripheral pulses and capillary refill.
- It is necessary to monitor intake and output.
- It is necessary to measure body weight every day.
- It is necessary to collaboration fluid therapy as indicated.

Imbalanced nutrition, less than body requirements related to insulin insufficiency.

Intervention

- It is necessary to measure body weight per day as indicated.
- It is necessary to determine the diet program.
- It is necessary to auscultation of bowel sounds.
- It is necessary to observation of the signs of hypoglycemia.

Risk for infection related to inadequate peripheral defense

Intervention

- It is necessary to observe the signs of infection and inflammation.
- It is necessary to give skin care regularly and earnestly.
- It is necessary to massage depressed bone area.
- It is necessary to position the patient in semi-Fowler position.
- It is necessary to collaborate antibiotics as indicated.
- It is necessary to encourage good handwashing.
- It is necessary to maintain aseptic technique.

MULTIPLE CHOICE QUESTIONS

1. **Acromegaly is most frequently diagnosed in:**
   A. Middle-aged adults
   B. Newborns
   C. Children aged 2–5 years
   D. Adults age 65 and older

2. **Graves' disease is:**
   A. The most common cause of hypothyroidism
   B. The most common cause of hyperparathyroidism
   C. The most common cause of hyperthyroidism
   D. The most common cause of adrenal insufficiency

3. **Symptoms of Graves' ophthalmopathy include all of the following, *except*:**
   A. Bulging eyeballs
   B. Dry, irritated eyes and puffy eyelids
   C. Cataracts
   D. Light sensitivity

4. **An ACTH stimulation test is commonly used to diagnose:**
   A. Graves' disease
   B. Adrenal insufficiency and Addison's disease
   C. Cystic fibrosis
   D. Hashimoto's disease

5. **All of the following are symptoms of Cushing's syndrome, *except*:**
   A. Severe fatigue and weakness
   B. Hypertension and elevated blood glucose
   C. A protruding hump between the shoulders
   D. Hair loss

6. **Which of the following conditions is caused by long-term exposure to high levels of cortisol?**
   A. Addison's disease
   B. Crohn's disease
   C. Adrenal insufficiency
   D. Cushing's syndrome

7. **A "sweat test" or newborn screening may be used to detect:**
   A. Cystic fibrosis
   B. Adrenal insufficiency
   C. Graves' disease
   D. Hypothyroidism

8. **Hashimoto's disease is:**
   A. Chronic inflammation of the thyroid gland
   B. Diagnosed most frequently in Asian-Americans and Pacific Islanders
   C. A form of hyperthyroidism
   D. A rare form of hypothyroidism

9. **Persons at increased risk of developing Hashimoto's disease include all of the following, *except*:**
   A. Persons with vitiligo
   B. Asian-Americans
   C. Persons with rheumatoid arthritis
   D. Persons with Addison's disease

10. **All of the following statements about Hashimoto's disease are true, *except*:**
    A. Many patients are entirely asymptomatic
    B. Not all patients become hypothyroid
    C. Most cases of obesity are attributable to Hashimoto's disease
    D. Hypothyroidism may be subclinical

11. **The most common benign tumor of the pituitary gland is a:**
    A. Glioma
    B. Prolactinoma
    C. Carcinoid tumor
    D. Islet cell tumor

12. **Symptoms of polycystic ovarian syndrome (PCOS) may include all of the following, *except*:**
    A. Pelvic pain
    B. Acne, oily skin, and dandruff
    C. Infertility
    D. Weight loss

13. **Women with PCOS are at increased risk for all of the following, *except*:**
    A. Pregnancy
    B. Diabetes
    C. Cardiovascular disease
    D. Metabolic syndrome

14. **All of the following organs may be affected by multiple endocrine neoplasia type 1, *except*:**
    A. Parathyroid glands
    B. Kidneys
    C. Pancreas and duodenum
    D. Pituitary gland

15. **What is the treatment for hyperparathyroidism?**
    A. Synthetic thyroid hormone
    B. Desiccated thyroid hormone
    C. Surgical removal of the glands
    D. Calcium and phosphate

16. **The most common causes of death in people with cystic fibrosis is:**
    A. Dehydration
    B. Opportunistic infection
    C. Lung cancer
    D. Respiratory failure

17. Untreated hyperthyroidism during pregnancy may result in all of the following, *except*:

A. Premature birth and miscarriage
B. Low birth weight
C. Autism
D. Preeclampsia

18. Short stature and undeveloped ovaries suggest which of the following disorders?

A. Polycystic ovarian syndrome
B. Prolactinoma
C. Graves' disease
D. Turner syndrome

19. Endocrine disorders may be triggered by all of the following, *except*:

A. Stress
B. Infection
C. Chemicals in the food chain and environment
D. Cell phone use

20. An analysis of data from the Women's Health Initiative questioned the use of which therapy to prevent heart disease?

A. Synthetic thyroid hormone
B. Oral contraceptives
C. Weight-loss drugs
D. Postmenopausal hormone replacement therapy

Answers

1. A	2. C	3. C	4. B	5. D	6. D	7. A	8. A	9. B	10. C
11. B	12. D	13. A	14. B	15. C	16. D	17. C	18. D	19. D	20. D

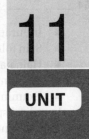

Integumentary Disorders

AT THE END OF THIS CHAPTER, THE STUDENTS WILL BE ABLE TO LEARN ABOUT THE MANAGEMENT OF:

- Pemphigus
- Psoriasis
- Dermatitis, eczema
- Cellulitis
- Acne
- Shingles
- Scabies
- Cold sore
- Impetigo
- Wart
- Alopecia

REVIEW OF ANATOMY AND PHYSIOLOGY

The skin is far more than just the outer covering of human beings; it is an organ just, such as the heart, lung, or liver. Besides providing a layer of protection from pathogens, physical abrasions, and radiation from the sun, the skin serves many other functions. It plays a vital role in homeostasis by maintaining a constant body temperature via the act of sweating or shivering and by making you aware of external stimuli through information perceived within the touch receptors located within the integumentary system. It only takes one visit to a burn unit to see the value of skin and the many complications that arise when this organ is compromised.

The skin, or integument, is considered an organ because it consists of all four types of tissue. The skin also consists of accessory organs, such as glands, hair, and nails, thus making up the integumentary system.

Integumentary System Assessment

- **Inspection and palpation of the skin:** During skin inspection, the general skin changes should be carefully assessed, which may include:
  - Color of skin
  - Temperature, texture, turgor, and tenderness of skin
  - Dryness or moisture skin
  - Scaling over the skin
  - Pigmentation on skin
  - Vascularity over the skin
  - Bruises, petechiae over the skin
  - Edema (pitting or nonpitting)

- Induration of skin
- Skin folds
- Hair, nails, and mucous membranes
- Examining lymph node
- Examining area distal to enlarged lymph nodes
- Jaundice, spider angiomatous skin, and palmar erythema should be assessed.
- The presence of macule and patches (flat, circumscribed, discolored spot, size, and shape) over the skin.
- The presence of nodules over the skin (palpable, solid lesion).

DISORDERS OF INTEGUMENTARY SYSTEM

PEMPHIGUS

Pemphigus vulgaris is an autoimmune disorder that is characterized by painful blisters formation on mucous membranes of mouth, throat, nose, eyes, genitals, and lungs **(Fig. 11.1)**.

Etiology

Autoimmunity: The immune system produces proteins called antibodies. The antibodies break down the bonds between the cells, and fluid, collected between the layers of the skin. This leads to blisters and erosions on the skin.

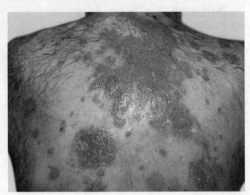

Fig. 11.1: Pemphigus.

Signs and Symptoms and Types

The signs and symptoms of pemphigus depending on its type are as follows:

- **Pemphigus vulgaris:** It usually begins with painful blisters in mouth and membranes of genitals.
- **Pemphigus foliaceus:** Blisters begin on face and scalp and later erupt on chest and back and are not painful.
- **Pemphigus vegetans:** The blisters appear on the groin and under the arms and on the feet.
- **Paraneoplastic pemphigus:** The blisters and sores may appear in the mouth, on the lips, and on the skin.

Diagnostic Evaluation

- **Biopsy:** A small sample of skin may be taken. This is looked at under the microscope and tested to confirm that the blisters are due to pemphigus vulgaris.
- **Blood test for antibodies:** This uses methods called immunofluorescence.

Management

- **Steroids:** The usual treatment is to take steroid tablets, such as prednisolone to reduce inflammation.
- **Immunosuppressant:** It is used to suppress autoimmunity, for example, cyclophosphamide, azathioprine.
- **Topical treatments:** A steroid cream is sometimes used on the skin blisters.
  - Mouthwashes containing antiseptic solution
  - Antifungal medication helps if thrush infects the mouth, throat, or gullet area.

PSORIASIS

Psoriasis is a chronic, autoimmune skin disease characterized by red patches on the skin, silvery-white scales of dead skin cells.

Etiology

- Skin infections
- Injury to the skin
- Stress
- Cold weather
- Smoking

Signs and Symptoms

- Red patches on skin covered with silvery scales
- Small scaling spots
- Dry, cracked skin that may bleed
- Itching, burning, or soreness
- Thickened, pitted, or ridged nails
- Swollen and stiff joints

Types of Psoriasis

Plaque Psoriasis

The most common form, plaque psoriasis causes dry, raised, and red skin lesions (plaques) covered with silvery scales.

Guttate Psoriasis

This primarily affects young adults and children. It is marked by small, water-drop-shaped sores on trunk, arms, legs, and scalp.

Inverse Psoriasis

Mainly affecting the skin in the armpits, in the groin, under the breasts, and around the genitals.

Pustular Psoriasis

It occurs in smaller areas on hands, feet, or fingertips.

Erythrodermic Psoriasis

It covers entire body with a red, peeling rash that can itch or burn intensely.

Psoriatic Arthritis

In addition to inflamed, scaly skin, psoriatic arthritis causes pitted, discolored nails, and the swollen, painful joints.

Nail Psoriasis

Psoriasis can affect fingernails and toenails, causing pitting, abnormal nail growth, and discoloration.

Scalp Psoriasis

Psoriasis on the scalp appears as red, itchy areas with silvery-white scales.

Diagnostic Evaluation

- Physical exam and medical history
- Skin biopsy

Management

Psoriasis treatments aim to:

- **Topical treatments:** Diflorasone Diacetate, fluocinonide
- **Calcineurin inhibitors:** Calcineurin inhibitors minimize the activation of T cells, which, in turn, reduce inflammation and plaque buildup.
- **Vitamin D analogs:** These synthetic forms of vitamin D slow down the growth of skin cell, such as calcipotriene.
- **Anthralin:** This decreases the DNA activity in skin cells and removes scale.
- **Topical retinoids:** These are commonly used to treat acne and sun-damaged skin.
- **Salicylic acid:** It promotes sloughing of dead skin cells and reduces scaling.
- **Coal tar:** It reduces scaling, itching, and inflammation.
- **Moisturizers:** Moisturizing creams would not heal psoriasis, but they can reduce itching and scaling.
- **Phototherapy:** Ultraviolet (UV) light slows skin cell turnover and reduces scaling and inflammation.
- **Narrow band UV therapy:** Narrow band UV therapy may be more effective than broadband UV treatment.
- **Retinoids:** Related to vitamin A, this group of drugs may reduce the production of skin cells.
- **Methotrexate:** Oral methotrexate helps psoriasis by decreasing the production of skin cells and suppressing inflammation.
- **Cyclosporine:** Cyclosporine suppresses the immune system and is similar to methotrexate in effectiveness.
- **Goeckerman therapy:** Combination of UV treatment and coal tar treatment, which is known as Goeckerman treatment.
- **Excimer laser:** This form of light therapy, used for mild-to-moderate psoriasis, treats only the involved skin.

Nursing Management

Nursing interventions include:

- Administering antimicrobial agents if ordered to treat cutaneous infections
- Applying a thin layer of a dry lubricant, such as powder
- Keeping client's skin clean
- Applying topical corticosteroids
- Cleansing infected lesions with antibacterial
- Assisting and preparing client for procedures, such as cryotherapy
- Providing elbow and heel protectors, if indicated
- Increasing activity as allowed and tolerated
- Performing actions to maintain an adequate nutritional status
- Using pressure-reducing or pressure-relieving devices
- Keeping bed linens dry and wrinkle free.

DERMATITIS (ECZEMA)

Dermatitis is inflammation of the skin characterized by red and itchy skin.

Etiology and Types

- **Contact dermatitis:** Contact dermatitis occurs due to allergic reactions and causes pink or red rash over skin.
- **Atopic dermatitis:** Atopic dermatitis is characterized by itch, scale, swell, and blister over the skin.
- **Seborrheic dermatitis:** Seborrheic dermatitis consists of greasy, yellowish, or reddish scaling on the scalp.
- **Stasis dermatitis:** Stasis dermatitis is caused by poor circulation and can happen in people with varicose veins.
- **Nummular dermatitis:** Nummular dermatitis is characterized by coin-shaped red plaques on legs, hands, arms, and torso.

Signs and Symptoms

- A red rash
- Red, itchy, and circular patches over skin
- Greasy, yellowish scales on the scalp and eyebrows, behind the ears, and around the nose.

Diagnostic Evaluation

- Identifying allergens and irritants.
- **Patch testing:** Small amounts of known allergens are applied to the skin. After 2 days, the patches are removed and the skin is assessed to check if there has been any reaction.

Management

There are several ways to treat contact dermatitis, including:
- Avoiding the cause
- Emollients
- Topical corticosteroids
- Oral corticosteroids
- Phototherapy
- Steroid-sparing immunosuppressant therapy.

Nursing Care Plan

Nursing Diagnosis

Impaired skin integrity related to inflammation

Interventions
- Assessing skin, noting color, moisture, texture, and temperature
- Identifying signs of itching
- Encouraging the client to maintain skin care
- Taking bath with lukewarm water
- Allowing the skin to air dry
- Applying topical lubricants to prevent dryness

Disturbed body image related to visible skin lesions

Interventions
- Assessing the client perception of changed appearance
- Assessing the client behavior related to appearance
- Assisting the client in articulating responses to questions

- Allowing client to verbalize feelings
- Assisting client in identifying ways to enhance their appearance

Risk for infection related to severe inflammation

Interventions

- Assessing skin for severity of skin integrity compromise
- Applying topical antibiotics
- Administering oral antibiotics
- Encouraging the client to use appropriate hygiene methods

CELLULITIS

Cellulitis is an infection of the skin and the tissues just below the skin surface (**Fig. 11.2**).

Etiology and Risk Factors

- Athlete's foot
- Skin abrasions
- Swollen legs
- Poor immune system
- Diabetes
- An insect bite
- Skin problems

Signs and Symptoms

- Affected skin feels warm, swollen, red, and inflamed
- Blisters on the skin
- The nearest glands may swell and become tender
- Hyperthermia

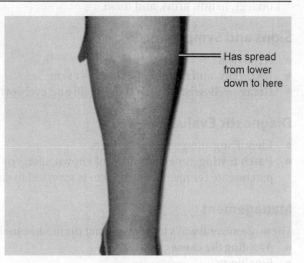

Has spread from lower down to here

Fig. 11.2: Cellulitis.

Management

- Avoiding the cause
- Emollients
- Topical corticosteroids
- Oral corticosteroids
- Maintain personal hygiene

Nursing Care Plan

Impaired skin integrity related to inflammation

Interventions

- Assessing skin, noting color, moisture, texture, and temperature
- Identifying signs of itching
- Encouraging the client to maintain skin care
- Taking bath with lukewarm water
- Allowing the skin to air dry
- Applying topical lubricants to prevent dryness

Disturbed body image related to visible skin lesions

Interventions

- Assessing the client perception of changed appearance
- Assessing the client behavior related to appearance
- Assisting the client in articulating responses to questions
- Allowing client to verbalize feelings
- Assisting client in identifying ways to enhance their appearance

Risk for infection related to severe inflammation

Interventions

- Assessing skin for severity of skin integrity compromise
- Applying topical antibiotics
- Administering oral antibiotics
- Encouraging the client to use appropriate hygiene methods

ACNE VULGARIS

Acne can be blackheads and whiteheads characterized by papules and pustules, nodules and cysts.

Etiology

- Puberty
- Hormonal changes
- Excessive use of oily and fatty food
- Stress
- Poor personal hygiene
- Manipulating acne lesions
- Air pollution
- Fluctuating hormone

Signs and Symptoms

- Whiteheads
- Blackheads
- Small red, tender bumps
- Pimples
- Large, solid, and painful lumps
- Painful, pus-filled lumps

Nursing Care

- Teaching good skin care
- Washing skin with mild soap
- Praising good habits
- Encouraging a balanced diet
- Encouraging application of tretinoin at night
- Encouraging use of nonoil sunscreens of at least sun protection factor (SPF) 15
- Avoiding use of astringents
- Avoiding vigorous scrubbing

Management

- Only acne-affected areas of the skin should be washed twice a day. Too frequent washing may irritate the skin making the symptoms worse.
- A mild soap or cleanser and lukewarm water should be used. Water that is too hot or cold water can make acne worse.
- It is advisable not to squeeze the spots or try to clean out blackheads. This can make things worse or lead to scars.
- It is advisable not to use too much makeup or cosmetics.
- All the makeup should be removed before going to bed.
- A water-based emollient that is fragrance free should be used for any dry skin.
- Shower should be taken after a workout or exercise to stop sweat irritating acne.
- Regular hair washing and keeping hair off the face can also help.

Medical Management

- **Benzoyl peroxide:** This cream helps prevent dead skin blocking follicles and kills bacteria on the skin.
- **Topical retinoids:** These reduce the production of fatty secretions called sebum.
- **Azelaic acid:** This cream or gel may be used to remove dead skin.

SHINGLES (VARICELLA-ZOSTER)

The varicella-zoster virus is responsible for causing chickenpox and shingles characterized by an outbreak of rash or blisters on the skin **(Fig. 11.3)**.

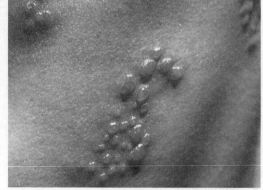

Fig. 11.3: Shingles.

Etiology and Risk Factors

- Age over 50 years
- Immunocompromised clients
- Chronic-ill patient
- Trauma

Signs and Symptoms

- Pain with itching
- Tingling feeling
- High temperature, chills
- Headache

Diagnostic Evaluation

- Physical examination of rashes
- Swab of the fluid

Management

- Antiviral medication, such as acyclovir
- Nonsteroidal anti-inflammatory drugs (NSAIDs), such as ibuprofen.

SCABIES

Scabies is a contagious and itchy skin condition caused by microscopic mites that burrow into the skin **(Fig. 11.4)**.

Etiology

Scabies mites

Signs and Symptoms

- Severe itching
- Small red bumps
- Excessive scratching

Diagnostic Evaluation

A skin scraping may be taken to look for mites, eggs, or mite fecal.

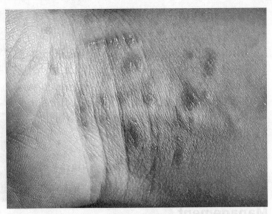

Fig. 11.4: Scabies.

Management

Corticosteroid topical drugs

COLD SORE

Cold sores are common and painful blisters around the lips and mouth caused by the herpes simplex virus (HSV).

Etiology

- HSV
- The virus may be triggered by certain foods, stress, fever, colds, allergies, sunburn, and menstruation.

Signs and Symptoms

- Fluid-filled blisters or red, painful sores on or near the mouth
- Swollen, sensitive gums of deep red color
- Fever
- Swollen lymph nodes
- Tingling and itching

Management

- Avoiding spicy or acidic foods
- Using over-the-counter topical remedies
- Washing hands after touching a cold sore
- It is advisable not to rub eyes after touching cold sore
- It is advisable not to touch genitals after touching cold sore
- Using sunscreen

IMPETIGO

Impetigo is a highly contagious bacterial skin infection characterized by blisters and sores **(Fig. 11.5)**.

Etiology

Staphylococcus aureus

Signs and Symptoms

There are two types of impetigo:

1. **Bullous impetigo** causes large fluid-filled blisters that are painless.
2. **Nonbullous impetigo** is the more contagious form of the condition causing sores that burst leaving a yellow-brown crust.

Other signs are:

- A small patch of blisters
- Formation of a golden or dark-yellow crust

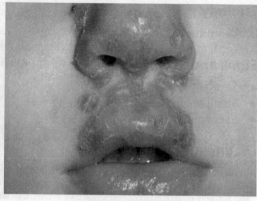

Fig. 11.5: Impetigo.

Management

- Maintaining personal hygiene
- Regular washing with soap and water
- Using topical antibiotic cream
- Avoiding the use of over-the-counter antibacterial ointments
- Using a clean towel each time
- Washing hands properly

WARTS

Warts are skin growths, which are usually fairly small and rough, and are caused by the human papillomavirus **(Fig. 11.6)**.

Types of Warts

- **Plantar warts:** Plantar warts appear on the soles of the feet.
- **Genital warts:** Genital warts can appear in the pubic area.

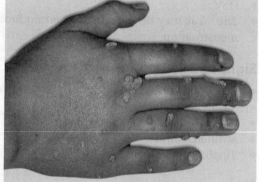

Fig. 11.6: Warts.

Management

- **Cryotherapy:** Liquid nitrogen is used to freeze the wart.
- **Salicylic acid:** The acid "burns" off the top layer of the wart.
- **Minor surgery:** Surgery may be used to cut away the wart.

ALOPECIA

Alopecia simply means hair loss. It may be partial or complete.

Etiology

Etiology of alopecia is based on its type:

1. **Alopecia totalis:** Alopecia totalis is thought to be an autoimmune disorder that causes loss of all head hair.
2. **Alopecia universalis:** Rapid loss of hair all over the body.
3. **Androgenetic alopecia:** It is the most common type of hair loss.

Treatment

- **Corticosteroids:** Anti-inflammatory drugs that are prescribed for autoimmune diseases.
- **Topical corticosteroids, e.g., diflorasone diacetate, fluocinonide**
- **Minoxidil:** This topical drug is already used as a treatment for pattern baldness.

MULTIPLE CHOICE QUESTIONS

1. Which of the following is a longitudinal incision through eschar and down to subcutaneous tissue?
   A. Escharotomy
   B. Dehiscence
   C. Transection
   D. Escharotic's procedure

2. Which of the following types of wounds match the criteria: plantar aspect of foot, heads, heel?
   A. Arterial
   B. Plantar
   C. Venous
   D. Diabetic

3. Which of the following terms match: water and electrolytes (clear)?
   A. Exudate
   B. Transudate
   C. Serosanguineous
   D. Induration

4. Which of the following edema assessment levels correspond with: depression resolving in 10–15 seconds?
   A. +1
   B. +2
   C. +3
   D. +4

5. Which of the following terms match the statement: to increase the fibrous element; to make hard as in the presence of cellulitis?
   A. Induration
   B. Necrosis
   C. Eschar
   D. Maceration

6. Following the rule of nines, what percent would a third-degree burn to the entire arm and back cover?
   A. 28
   B. 27
   C. 20
   D. 18

7. Which of the following matches the definition: a full thickness skin loss involving damage or necrosis of subcutaneous tissue that may extend down to but not through underlying fascia, infection, and/or necrosis may be present?
   A. Stage I wound
   B. Stage II wound
   C. Stage III wound
   D. Stage IV wound

8. Which of the following types of wound is indicated by the definition: relatively painless, decreased with elevation?
   A. Arterial
   B. Plantar
   C. Venous
   D. Diabetic

9. Which of the following matches the definition: the loss of circulatory fluids into interstitial spaces?
   A. Hypovolemia
   B. Necrosis
   C. Eschar
   D. Maceration

10. An emollient has a/an _____ effect.
    A. Pruritic
    B. Antipruritic
    C. Rupture
    D. Impetigo

11. **Which of the following is the outermost layer of the epidermis?**
    A. Stratum spinosum
    B. Stratum corneum
    C. Stratum granulosum
    D. Stratum basale

12. **Which of the following is the deepest layer of the epidermis?**
    A. Stratum spinosum
    B. Stratum corneum
    C. Stratum granulosum
    D. Stratum basale

13. **Which of the following is beneath the stratum corneum?**
    A. Stratum spinosum
    B. Stratum corneum
    C. Stratum granulosum
    D. Stratum basale

14. **Vitamin D is created from _____ by skin cells.**
    A. Dehydrocholesterol
    B. Cholesterol
    C. Hydrocholesterol
    D. Hydrodermis

15. **Which of the following is another name for blackheads associated with acne?**
    A. Pustules
    B. Sebaceous
    C. Eccrine
    D. Comedones

16. **Which of the following identifies skin from a cadaver used in a burn graft?**
    A. Homograft
    B. Autograft
    C. Allograft
    D. Xenograft

17. **Which of the following is a disease characterized by hyperactive sebaceous glands and often associated with dandruff?**
    A. Keloid
    B. Seborrhea
    C. Eczema
    D. Urticaria

18. **Which of the following is a disease characterized by the presence of hives?**
    A. Keloid
    B. Seborrhea
    C. Eczema
    D. Urticaria

19. **Which of the following is a disease characterized by a skin rash that is blistering and itchy?**
    A. Keloid
    B. Seborrhea
    C. Eczema
    D. Urticaria

20. **Sebaceous glands secrete _____.**
    A. Sebum
    B. Impetigo
    C. Serous
    D. Sirius

Answers

1. A	2. D	3. B	4. B	5. A	6. B	7. C	8. B	9. A	10. A
11. B	12. D	13. C	14. A	15. D	16. A	17. B	18. D	19. C	20. A

Musculoskeletal Disorders

AT THE END OF THIS CHAPTER, THE STUDENT WILL BE LEARN ABOUT THE MANAGEMENT OF:

➢ Osteoarthritis
➢ Osteomyelitis
➢ Rheumatic arthritis
➢ Osteomalacia
➢ Paget's disease
➢ Herniated vertebral disk
➢ Spinal cord injury
➢ Hemiplegia, tetraplegia, quadriplegia
➢ Pott's spine
➢ Amputation
➢ Prosthesis
➢ Transplant and replacement surgeries
➢ Rehabilitation
➢ Special therapies and alternative therapies

REVIEW OF ANATOMY AND PHYSIOLOGY

The musculoskeletal system provides support to the body and gives humans, the ability to move. The body's bones (the skeletal system), muscles (muscular system), cartilage, tendons, ligaments, joints, and other connective tissue that supports and binds tissues and organs together comprise the musculoskeletal system.

Most importantly, the system provides form, support, stability, and movement to the body. For example, the bones of the skeletal system protect the body's internal organs and support the weight of the body. The skeletal portion of the system serves as the main storage depot for calcium and phosphorus. It also contains critical components of the hematopoietic system (blood cell production). The muscles of the muscular system keep bones in place; they also play a role in movement of the bones by contracting and pulling on the bones, allowing for movements as diverse as standing, walking, running, and grasping items. To allow motion, different bones are connected by joints. Within these joints, bones are connected to other bones and muscle fibers via connective tissue, such as tendons and ligaments. Cartilage prevents the bone ends from rubbing directly on each other. Muscles contract to move the bone attached at the joint **(Fig. 12.1)**.

MUSCULOSKELETAL EXAMINATION

Musculoskeletal examination is rapid and systematic examination in order to detect deviations from the normal.

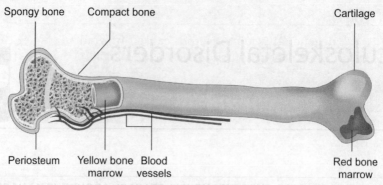

Fig. 12.1: Structure of bone.

Basic Principles

Following are the basic principles:
1. Humans are bilaterally symmetrical, so both the sides should be aligned in symmetry with respect to each other.
2. Observation and comparison, as each area is examined in sequence.

Sequence of Examination

Following are the list of sequence of examination:

Patient Standing

Asking the client to raise the arm, and stand straight with feet slightly apart and now examiner can observe the following:
- Muscle mass of thigh for symmetry
- Alignment of knee
- Swelling in knee
- Alignment of ankle
- Swelling of ankle
- Toe alignment and toe swelling
- Spinal curves in sagittal plane for spine deformity
- Observing calf muscle bulk and symmetry
- Observing spine moment (rotation, flexion, and extension)
- Observing for normal walking pattern ask to walk away and turn around, and walk back
- Inspecting the dorsum of the hands and test finger extension
- Observing for knuckles flexion should be almost 90°
- Assessing arm forward flexion, pronation, then wrist flexion, extension
- Assessing elbow supination and extension and then elbow flexion and extension
- Observing shoulder active range of motion should be smooth, symmetrical, and simultaneous.
- Comparing passive shoulder range of motion with active range of motion

Patient Lying

- Assessing hip flexion, internal rotation, and external rotation knee flexion in supine position
- Assessing ankle dorsiflexion and plantar flexion

OSTEOARTHRITIS

Osteoarthritis is a degenerative joint disorder caused by gradual loss of cartilage and characterized by formation of bony spurs and cysts at the margins of the joints **(Fig. 12.2)**.

Risk Factors

Risk factors are categorized into modifiable and nonmodifiable causes.

Modifiable Factors

- Excess body mass
- Joint injury
- Knee pain
- Heavy lifting
- Muscle weakness

Nonmodifiable Factors

- Gender (women higher risk)
- Increases with age
- Genetic predisposition

Pathophysiology

Pathophysiology of osteoarthritis is explained in five stages:

1. **Buildup:** The surface cartilage starts to show signs of weakness due to lifetime and excessive use. In this stage, no symptoms appear in body.
2. **Cartilage swelling:** Weight-bearing activity causes the weekend cartilage to start swelling. In this stage, mild pain appears during activity but disappears during rest period.
3. **Joint narrowing:** Swollen, weakened cartilage starts to wear causing the joint space to decrease. In this stage, pain and stiffness are main symptoms.
4. **Breakdown:** Continued wearing away the cartilage leads to irregular joint surface. In this stage, swelling and joint clicking are main signs.

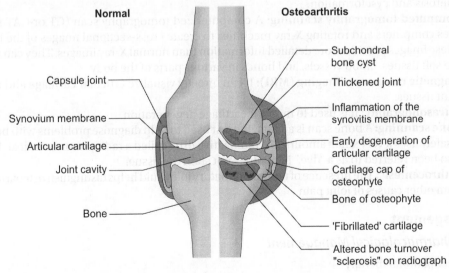

Fig. 12.2: Osteoarthritis.

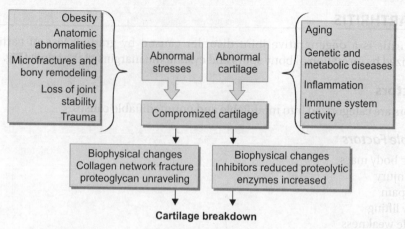

Fig. 12.3: Pathophysiology.

5. **Compensation:** As the joint becomes more painful, this leads to new bone growth on the joint margins. During this phase, deep ache and night pain are present **(Fig. 12.3)**.

Signs and Symptoms

Following are the list of signs and symptoms:
- **Pain:** Pain is the most common symptom of osteoarthritis.
- **Stiffness:** Stiffness of the affected joint.
- **Swelling**
- **Deformity:** Deformity can occur with osteoarthritis due to bone growth and cartilage loss. Degeneration of knee cartilage can result in the outward curvature of knees.
- **Crepitus:** A crackling sound or granting feeling in joint.

Diagnostic Evaluation

Following are the list of diagnostic evaluation:
- **Plain radiography:** Radiographs can depict joint-space loss, as well as subchondral bony sclerosis and cyst formation.
- **Computed tomography scanning:** A computerized tomography scan (CT or CAT scan) uses computers and rotating X-ray machines to create cross-sectional images of the body. These images provide more detailed information than normal X-ray images. They can show the soft tissues, blood vessels, and bones in various parts of the body
- **Magnetic resonance imaging (MRI):** It can directly visualize articular cartilage and other joint tissues.
- **Ultrasonography:** It is used to monitor cartilage degeneration.
- **Bone scanning:** A bone scan is an imaging test used to help diagnose problems with bones. It safely uses a very small amount of a radioactive drug called a radiopharmaceutical. It has also been referred to as a "dye," but it does not stain the tissue.
- **Arthrocentesis:** The presence of noninflammatory joint fluid helps distinguish osteoarthritis from other causes of joint pain.

Management

Nonpharmacological Management

- Occupational therapy
- Unloading in certain joints (e.g., knee, hip) **(Fig. 12.4)**.

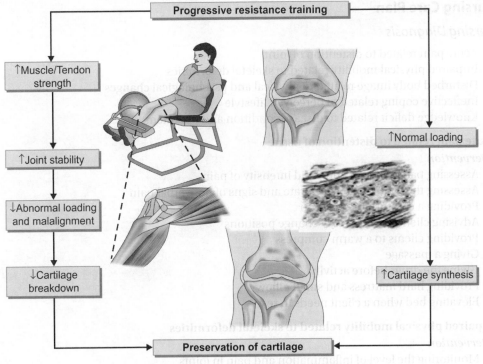

Fig. 12.4: Nonpharmacological intervention.

- Applying heat and cold to the joint
- Protecting joints from injury
- Eating healthy foods
- Getting enough rest
- **Healthy body weight:** Maintaining a healthy body weight will reduce stress on the arthritic joints.
- **Exercise:** Exercise can assist with weight loss, the maintains the muscle strength and mobility of arthritic joints.
- **Physiotherapy:** Physiotherapists can advise on appropriate exercises to improve mobility, increase muscle strength, and decrease pain with the aim of improving function.
- **Synovial fluid supplements** (viscosupplements): Supplement may be injected into the joint. Can also be given orally example, glucosamine.
- **Massage therapy:** Massage therapy may provide short-term pain relief.
- **Braces:** Splints and braces may help support weakened joints.

Pharmacological Management

- Analgesics
- Nonsteroidal anti-inflammatory drugs (NSAIDs)
- Topical pain relievers
- Corticosteroid injections
- Hyaluronic acid injections

Hyaluronic acid: Hyaluronic acid occurs naturally in joint fluid, acting as a shock absorber and lubricant.

Nursing Care Plan

Nursing Diagnosis

- Acute pain related to distention of joint
- Impaired physical mobility related to skeletal deformities
- Disturbed body image related to physical and psychological changes
- Ineffective coping related to perceived lifestyle
- Knowledge deficit related to disease condition and treatment.

Acute pain related to distention of tissue

Intervention

- Assessing pain of the location and intensity of pain
- Assessing the factors that accelerate and signs of nonverbal pain
- Providing a comfortable position
- Advising clients to frequently change positions
- Providing clients to a warm compress
- Giving a massage
- Giving the drugs before activity
- Providing hard mattress and small pillow
- Elevating bed when a client needs to rest

Impaired physical mobility related to skeletal deformities

Intervention

- Monitoring the level of inflammation and pain in joints
- Providing safe techniques
- Engaging in activities
- Assisting in daily living activities

OSTEOMYELITIS

Osteomyelitis is an infection of a bone caused by *Staphylococcus aureus* **(Fig. 12.5)**.

Modes of Transmission

- **Via the bloodstream:** Through hematogenous spread
- **Through an injury:** Bacteria can spread to bone through deep cut on the skin.

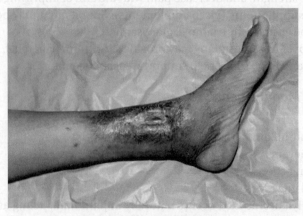

Fig. 12.5: Inflammation of bone.

Pathophysiology

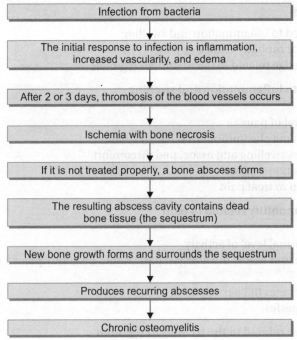

```
┌─────────────────────────────────────────────────┐
│              Infection from bacteria             │
└─────────────────────────────────────────────────┘
                         ↓
┌─────────────────────────────────────────────────┐
│ The initial response to infection is inflammation,│
│        increased vascularity, and edema          │
└─────────────────────────────────────────────────┘
                         ↓
┌─────────────────────────────────────────────────┐
│ After 2 or 3 days, thrombosis of the blood vessels occurs │
└─────────────────────────────────────────────────┘
                         ↓
┌─────────────────────────────────────────────────┐
│            Ischemia with bone necrosis           │
└─────────────────────────────────────────────────┘
                         ↓
┌─────────────────────────────────────────────────┐
│  If it is not treated properly, a bone abscess forms │
└─────────────────────────────────────────────────┘
                         ↓
┌─────────────────────────────────────────────────┐
│        The resulting abscess cavity contains dead │
│            bone tissue (the sequestrum)          │
└─────────────────────────────────────────────────┘
                         ↓
┌─────────────────────────────────────────────────┐
│  New bone growth forms and surrounds the sequestrum │
└─────────────────────────────────────────────────┘
                         ↓
┌─────────────────────────────────────────────────┐
│            Produces recurring abscesses          │
└─────────────────────────────────────────────────┘
                         ↓
┌─────────────────────────────────────────────────┐
│              Chronic osteomyelitis               │
└─────────────────────────────────────────────────┘
```

Etiology and Risk Factors

- Fractured bone
- Have bone prosthesis
- Surgery to a bone
- Have a poor immune system
- History of osteomyelitis
- Poor skin sensation

Signs and Symptoms

- Pain and tenderness over joint
- A lump may develop over a bone
- Redness
- Hyperthermia

Diagnostic Evaluation

- X-ray
- Computed tomography (CT) scan

Medical Treatment

Antibiotics

- An antibiotic is usually started as soon as possible. The initial antibiotic chosen is one that is likely to kill the bacteria which commonly causes osteomyelitis.
- To control pain, you may be given painkillers

Nursing Care Plan

Nursing Diagnosis

- Acute pain related to inflammation and swelling
- Impaired physical mobility related to pain
- Deficient knowledge related to the treatment regimen

Acute pain related to inflammation and swelling

Intervention

- Assessing the level of pain
- The affected part may be immobilized with a splint
- Elevation reduces swelling and associated discomfort
- Comfortable position is given
- Analgesic is given to treat pain

Impaired physical mobility related to pain

Intervention

- Assessing the normal level of activity
- The joints above and below the affected part should be gently placed through their range of motion.
- The nurse encourages full participation in daily activities.
- Administer analgesics

Deficient knowledge related to the treatment regimen

Intervention

- Assessing the level of knowledge by verbalization with the patient
- Answer each question of the patient
- Clarify all doubts of the patient

RHEUMATOID ARTHRITIS

Rheumatoid arthritis is a chronic inflammatory autoimmune disorder affects the small joints in hands and feet.

Etiology and Risk Factors

- Idiopathic
- Genetically inherited.

Risk Factors

- **Age:** Risk increases with age.
- **Gender:** Women are more affected than men.
- **Genetic risk:** There is a strong familial link in some cases.

Pathophysiology

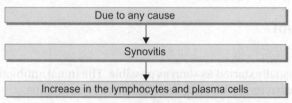

Due to any cause

↓

Synovitis

↓

Increase in the lymphocytes and plasma cells

Contd...

Contd...

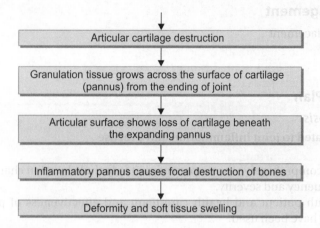

Clinical Manifestations

- Fatigue
- Anorexia
- Weight loss
- Stiffness
- Lack of appetite
- Low-grade fever
- Muscle and joint aches
- Limitation of motion

Complications

- Osteoporosis
- Carpal tunnel syndrome
- Heart problems
- Lung diseases

Diagnostic Evaluation

- **History collection**
- **Physical examination:** Check joints for swelling, redness, and warmth
- **Complete blood count:** Elevated erythrocyte sedimentation rate (ESR)
- X-rays help to track the progression of rheumatoid arthritis in your joints over time.
- **Synovial fluid analysis:** A synovial fluid analysis is performed when pain, inflammation, or swelling occurs in a joint, or when there is an accumulation of fluid with an unknown cause. Taking a sample of the fluid can help diagnose the exact problem causing the inflammation. If the cause of the joint swelling is known, a synovial fluid analysis or joint aspiration may not be necessary.

Treatment

- **NSAIDs:** Brufen
- **Steroids:** Corticosteroid
- **Disease-modifying antirheumatic drugs (DMARDs):** Common DMARDs include methotrexate, leflunomide, hydroxychloroquine, and sulfasalazine.
- **Calcium and vitamin D supplements:** To prevent thinning of the bones due to osteoporosis

Surgical Management

- Total joint replacement
- Tendon repair
- Joint fusion

Nursing Care Plan

Nursing Diagnosis

Chronic pain related to joint inflammation and overuse

Interventions

- Performing a comprehensive assessment of pain to include location characteristics, onset, duration, frequency and severity.
- Evaluating with patient and health-care team and effectiveness of past pain control measures that have been used.
- Reducing or eliminating the factors that increase the pain experience (e.g., fear fatigue lack of knowledge).
- Teaching use of nonpharmacological techniques (relaxation, distraction, massage).
- Providing optimal pain relief with prescribed analgesics.

Impaired physical mobility related to joint pain and stiffness

Interventions

- Determining the limitations of joint movement and functions to establish baseline plan of care.
- Collaborating with physical therapy to establish exercise program to improve the joint function.
- Explaining the plan and purpose of exercises to the patient and family.
- Initiating pain control measures before beginning of joint exercises (hot packs, warm shower).
- Assisting patient to do active, passive joint movements (selection of proper footwear use of assistive devices).

Self-care deficit related to disease progression, weakness

Interventions

- Monitoring patient's ability for independent self-care
- Monitoring patients need for hygiene, dressing, grooming and eating
- Establishing a routine for self-care activities and assisting patient in accepting dependency need to ensure all needs are meet.
- Teaching family to encourage independence and to intervene only when patient is unable.

OSTEOPOROSIS

Osteoporosis is a bone disease, also called porous bone, characterized by honeycomb-like appearance of bone structure under microscope **(Fig. 12.6)**.

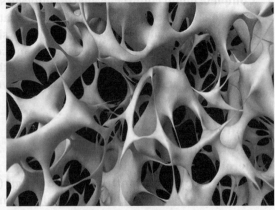

Fig. 12.6: Osteoporosis bone.

Etiology and Risk Factors

- Age
- **Sex:** Females are more prone to get osteoporosis
- Family history
- Body size
- Low-calcium diet
- Eating disorders
- Hormonal imbalance
- Thyroid problem
- Excess use of steroids

Clinical Manifestations

- Back pain
- Loss of height
- Stooped posture
- Bone fracture

Pathophysiology

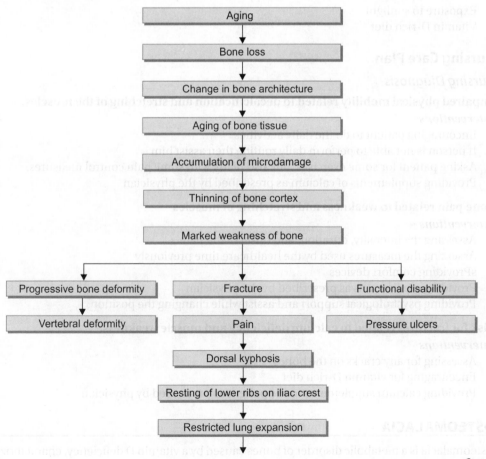

Aging

↓

Bone loss

↓

Change in bone architecture

↓

Aging of bone tissue

↓

Accumulation of microdamage

↓

Thinning of bone cortex

↓

Marked weakness of bone

↓

Progressive bone deformity	Fracture	Functional disability

Vertebral deformity | Pain | Pressure ulcers

↓

Dorsal kyphosis

↓

Resting of lower ribs on iliac crest

↓

Restricted lung expansion

↓

Contd...

Contd...

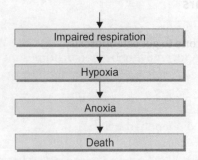

Diagnostic Evaluation

- **Physical examination:** Check for skeletal deformity, such as spinal kyphosis and bowed legs.
- **Blood and urine tests**
- **X-ray:** Slight cracks in bones that are visible on X-rays.
- **Bone biopsy:** Although a bone biopsy is very accurate in detecting osteomalacia.

Management

- Vitamin D, phosphorus, and calcium supplements are prescribed.
- Exposure to sunlight
- Vitamin D-rich diet

Nursing Care Plan

Nursing Diagnosis

Impaired physical mobility related to decalcification and stretching of the muscles.

Interventions

- Encouraging patient to do the daily activities
- If person is not able to perform daily routine then assist him
- Asking patient for some exercises, but also ready with some pain control measures.
- Providing supplements of calcium as prescribed by the physician.

Bone pain related to weakness and stretching of muscles

Interventions

- Assessing the intensity, duration, and onset of the pain
- Assessing the measures used by the healthcare time previously
- sProviding comfort devices
- Providing medications as prescribed by the physician
- Providing psychological support and assist while changing the position.

Risk for fractures related to calcium deficiency and muscle weakness.

Interventions

- Assessing for any cracks on the bones
- Encouraging for vitamin D-rich diet
- Providing calcium supplements to the patient as prescribed by physician.

OSTEOMALACIA

Osteomalacia is a metabolic disorder of bones caused by a vitamin D deficiency, characterized by delayed mineralization of bone.

Etiology

Following are the list of etiology:

- **Vitamin D deficiency:** Vitamin D deficiency is a common cause of osteomalacia.
- **Certain surgeries:** Surgery to remove or bypass small intestine also can lead to osteomalacia.
- **Celiac disease:** It damages intestinal mucosa and does not absorb nutrients, such as vitamin D.
- Kidney or liver disorders
- **Drugs:** Like phenytoin and phenobarbital

Signs and Symptoms

- Bone pain
- Tenderness
- Difficulty in changing position
- Muscle weakness
- Bending of bones
- Pathologic fracture

Pathophysiology

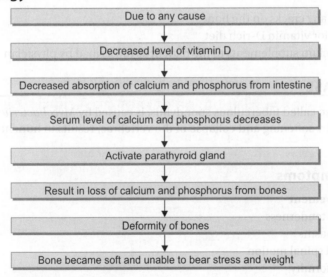

Due to any cause

↓

Decreased level of vitamin D

↓

Decreased absorption of calcium and phosphorus from intestine

↓

Serum level of calcium and phosphorus decreases

↓

Activate parathyroid gland

↓

Result in loss of calcium and phosphorus from bones

↓

Deformity of bones

↓

Bone became soft and unable to bear stress and weight

Diagnostic Evaluation

- **Physical examination:** Assessing skeletal deformity
- **Blood and urine tests:** Assessing vitamin D deficiency and phosphorus loss
- **X-ray:** Slight cracks in bones that are visible on X-rays
- **Bone biopsy:** Taking a sample of bone to rule out abnormalities.

Management

- Vitamin D, phosphorus and calcium supplements
- Exposure to sunlight
- Vitamin D-rich diet

Nursing Care Plan

Nursing Diagnosis

Impaired physical mobility related to decalcification

Interventions

- Encouraging patient to do the daily activities
- If person is not able to perform daily routine, then assist him.
- Asking patient for some exercises, but also ready with some pain control measures.
- Providing supplements of calcium as prescribed by the physician.

Bone pain related to weakness and stretching of muscles

Interventions

- Assessing the intensity, duration and onset of the pain.
- Assessing the measures used by the healthcare time previously.
- Providing comfort devices
- Providing medications as prescribed by the physician
- Providing psychological support and assisting while changing the position.

Risk for fractures related to calcium deficiency and muscle weakness

Interventions

- Assessing for any cracks on the bones
- Encouraging for vitamin D-rich diet
- Providing calcium supplements to the patient as prescribed by physician.

POTT'S DISEASE

Pott's disease, also called tuberculous spondylitis, is caused by *Mycobacterium tuberculosis*. It is characterized by softening and collapse of the vertebrae, results in hunchback curvature of the vertebrae.

Signs and Symptoms

- **Spinal involvement**
  - Localized tenderness
  - Muscle spasms
  - Restricted spinal motion
  - Spinal deformity
  - Neurological deficits
  - Paresis
  - Impaired sensation
  - Nerve root pain
  - Cauda equina syndrome
  - Fever
  - Back pain
  - Paraplegia
  - Night sweats
  - Weight loss
  - Malaise

		SYSTEMIC SIGNS AND SYMPTOMS OF POTT'S DISEASE				
Musculoskeletal	Neurological	Cardiovascular	Integumentary	Urogenital	Constitutional symptoms
Vertebral fractures	Paresthesia	Spinal artery infarction	Pressure ulcers (secondary)	Bowel dysfunction	Fever
Vertebral collapse	Paralysis	Avascularity of intervertebral disks	Sinus (secondary to abscess rupture)	Bladder dysfunction	Night sweats
Spinal ligament destruction	Paresis	Thrombosis	Cutaneous fungal infections		Malaise
Intervertebral disk destruction	Abnormal muscle tone				Weight loss
Paravertebral abscess	Abnormal reflexes				
Osteopenia/ osteoporosis	Cauda equina syndrome				
Bone sequestrations	Myelomalacia				
Dislocated vertebrae	Gliosis				
Kyphotic deformity	Syringomyelia				
Muscle atrophy					
Torticollis					

Diagnostic Evaluation

- **The Mantoux test (tuberculin skin test)** (*refer* **tuberculosis for more detail)** Injection of a purified protein derivative is injected intradermally to check the presence of bacilli.
- **ESR:** ESR may be markedly elevated.
- **Microbiology studies:** Showing acid-fast bacilli
- **Radiography:** Reveal
  - Lytic destruction of anterior portion of vertebral body
  - Increased anterior wedging
  - Collapse of vertebral body
  - Reactive sclerosis on a progressive lytic process
  - Vertebral end plates may be osteoporotic
  - Intervertebral disks may be shrunk or destroyed
  - Vertebral bodies show variable degrees of destruction
  - Fusiform paravertebral shadows suggest abscess formation
  - Bone lesions may occur at more than one level.
- **CT scanning**
- **MRI**
- **Biopsy**
- **Polymerase chain reaction:** Polymerase chain reaction (PCR) techniques amplify species-specific deoxyribonucleic acid (DNA) sequences that are able to rapidly detect and diagnose several strains of *Mycobacterium* without the need for prolonged culture.

Management

Physical Therapy Management

- Spinal stabilization exercises
- Maitland surgery
- Exercise and strengthening

Postspinal Fusion Surgery

- Transcutaneous electrical neuromuscular stimulation
- Aquatic therapy
- Aerobic exercise

Pharmacological Management

- Isoniazid
- Rifampin
- Pyrazinamide
- Ethambutol
- Streptomycin

Nursing Care Plan

Nursing Diagnosis

- Acute pain related to inflammation and swelling
- Impaired physical mobility related to pain
- Deficient knowledge related to the treatment regimen

Acute pain related to inflammation and swelling

Interventions

- Assessing the level of pain
- The affected part may be immobilized with a splint to decrease pain and muscle spasm.
- Elevation reduces swelling and associated discomfort
- Comfortable position is given
- Analgesic given to treat pain

Impaired physical mobility related to pain

Interventions

- Assessing the normal level of activity.
- The joints above and below the affected part should be gently placed through their range of motion.
- The nurse encourages full participation in activities of daily living (ADLs) within the physical limitations to promote general well-being.
- Analgesics are given.

Deficient knowledge related to the treatment regimen

Interventions

- Assessing the level of knowledge by verbalization with the patient
- Answer each question of the patient
- Clarify all doubts of the patient

AMPUTATION AND PROSTHESIS

The surgical removal of a partial or entire limb. It can result from injury, disease or loss of circulation.

Types of Amputation

- **Acquired amputation:** The surgical removal of a limb associated with complications of disease or trauma.

- **Vascular amputation:** The surgical removal of a limb associated with tissue ischemia.
- **Traumatic amputation:** The surgical removal of a limb associated with traumatic injury.
- **Bilateral amputation:** Removal of both limbs on one side.

Levels of Amputation

- **Transhumeral amputation:** An amputation performed at the above the elbow.
- **Transfemoral amputation:** An amputation performed at the level above the knee.
- **Transtibial amputation:** An amputation performed at the level below the knee.
- **Partial foot amputation:** An amputation performed at the level of the foot.
- **Wrist disarticulation:** An amputation performed at the level of the wrist.
- **Syme's amputation:** An amputation performed at the level of the ankle joint that retains the fatty heel pad portion intended to preserve weight-bearing function.

Amputation Recovery

Prosthetic Devices for Amputation

- The goal is to form a round numb so it can be fitted well into a prostatic.
- About 2–3 weeks following removal, replacement limb planning occurs.
- The prostatic fits to the residual limb.

Potential Complications Associated with Amputation

- Infection
- Acute pain and chronic pain
- Abdominal aortic aneurysm
- Emotional issues, such as depression and impaired body image.

Pain Complications

- Phantom pain is a painful sensation in the area where the limb once was; it is believed to be related to neural memory, the nerves have memory of those feelings.
- Adherent scar tissue grows in the area where the removal took place; it often causes pain.
- **Causalgia:** A persistent pain with a burning sensation that results from injury to a peripheral nerve.

Phantom Pain

Phantom pain is the neurological interpretation of noxious stimuli that is commonly associated with amputation. The pain is felt in the region in which the body part was removed. It occurs from nerve damage in the residual limb and is associated with muscle and neural memory. This form of pain is common in veterans who experienced a traumatic injury that resulted in amputation.

Prosthesis

Prosthesis is an artificial extension that replaces a missing body part. It is part of the field of biomechatronics, the science of fusing mechanical devices with human muscle, skeleton, and nervous systems to assist or enhance motor control lost by trauma, disease or defect.

An artificial limb is a type of prosthesis that replaces a missing extremity, such as arms or legs. The type of artificial limb used is determined largely by the extent of an amputation or loss and location of the missing extremity. Artificial limbs may be needed for a variety of reasons, including disease, accidents, and congenital defects.

Types of Prosthesis

There are four main types of artificial limbs. These include the transtibial, transfemoral, transradial, and transhumeral prostheses.

1. **Transradial prosthesis:** A transradial prosthesis is an artificial limb that replaces an arm missing below the elbow. Cable operated limbs work by attaching a harness and cable around the opposite shoulder of the damaged arm. The other form of prosthetics available is myoelectric arms. These work by sensing, via electrodes, when the muscles in the upper arm move, causing an artificial hand to open or close.

2. **Transhumeral prosthesis:** A transhumeral prosthesis is an artificial limb that replaces an arm missing above the elbow. Transhumeral amputees experience some of the same problems as transfemoral amputees, due to the similar complexities associated with the movement of the elbow. This makes mimicking the correct motion with an artificial limb very difficult.

3. **Transtibial prosthesis:** A transtibial prosthesis is an artificial limb that replaces a leg missing below the knee. Transtibial amputees are usually able to regain normal movement more readily than someone with a AK, due in large part to retaining the knee, which allows for easier movement.

4. **Transfemoral prosthesis:** A transfemoral prosthesis is an artificial limb that replaces a leg missing above the knee. Transfemoral amputees can have a very difficult time regaining normal movement. In general, a transfemoral amputee must use approximately 80% more energy to walk than a person with two whole legs. This is due to the complexities in movement associated with the knee. In newer and more improved designs, after employing hydraulics, carbon fiber, mechanical linkages, motors, computer microprocessors, and innovative combinations of these technologies to give more control to the user **(Figs. 12.7A and B)**.

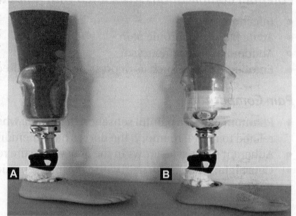

Figs. 12.7A and B: Prosthesis.

Nursing Care Plan

Nursing Interventions

- **Pain:** Assessing and treating pain.
- Determining the risk of suicide and providing an environment that is safe.
- **Altered functioning:** Assisting the patient in performing activities of daily living, which may be altered due to depression.
- **Social functioning:** Assisting the patient in identifying new ways to function socially.
- Ineffective coping patterns for enhanced coping patterns: assessing the patient's coping style and providing education.
- **Knowledge deficit for enhanced learning:** Educating the patient on the healing process, including anticipatory grieving to be expected from the situation, and providing information about limb replacement prostatic and adaptive devices.
- Assessing the patient's pain, including location, onset, characteristics (such as dull, stabbing, or throbbing), and level, preferably using a measurable scale, such as 0–10.
- If assessing the patient after the acute postamputation period, determining what factors worsen pain or relieves pain.

- Administering pain medications as ordered.
- To determine efficacy of the therapeutic regimen, reassessing pain levels 30–60 minutes after administering pain medication by mouth and 15 minutes following intravenous administration.
- Phantom pain can be an extremely isolating and frustrating experience. Acknowledging the individual's pain in order to validate the experience of phantom pain.
- Assessing the patient for suicidal ideation by using an assessment tool, such as sad persons.
- Inquiring about family history, cohabiting mental health conditions, such as depression, and if the patient has ever made any previous suicide attempts.
- Determining if there is a suicide plan in place.
- If a suicide plan is in place, it is essential to enquire to learn about the lethality of the plan and availability to carry it through (such access to a gun or high ledge of a building).
- If the patient is deemed to be suicidal, immediately institute suicide watch, do not leave the patient unattended, ensure that a competent staff member remains no more than an arm's reach away from the patient at all times, remove any potentially harmful objects out of the room, and facilitate referral to the appropriate team members.
- Asking open-ended questions to determine the patient's coping style.
- Learning if the patient was experiencing any other extremely stressful experiences prior to the current crisis.
- Determining what coping patterns the patient is currently using to manage the present crisis.
- Determining if any maladaptive or potentially dangerous coping patterns are being used, which could place the patient at risk for injury.
- Asking about previous coping patterns ones used successfully to manage past crises or stressful situations.

Nursing Diagnosis

Impaired physical mobility related to pain and discomfort and loss of body part

Interventions
- Encouraging him to perform prescribes exercises.
- Providing stump care on a routine basis—inspect area, cleanse and dry thoroughly, and rewrap stump with elastic bandage or air splint, or apply a stump shrinker (heavy stockinette sock), for "delayed" prosthesis.
- Measuring circumference periodically.
- Rewraping stump immediately with an elastic bandage, elevating if "immediate or early" cast is accidentally dislodged. Preparing for reapplication of cast.
- Assisting with specified range of motion (ROM) exercises for both the affected and the unaffected limbs beginning early in the postoperative stage.
- Instructing patient to lie in prone position as tolerated at least twice a day with pillow under abdomen and lower extremity stump.
- Maintaining knee extension
- Providing trochanter rolls as indicated
- Encouraging active and isometric exercises for upper torso and unaffected limbs.
- Demonstrating and assisting with transfer techniques and use of mobility aids, such as trapeze, crutches, or walker.
- Assisting with ambulation
- Instructing patient in stump-conditioning exercises.

Risk for infection related to inadequate primary defenses (broken skin, traumatized tissue), invasive procedures, environmental exposure

Interventions

- During emergency treatment, it is necessary to monitor vital signs (especially in hypovolemic shock), clean the wound, and give tetanus prophylaxis and antibiotics as ordered.
- After a complete amputation, it is necessary to wrap the amputated part in wet dressing soaked in normal saline solution. It is necessary to label the part, seal it in a plastic bag, and float the bag in ice water.
- It is necessary to inspect dressings and wound; note characteristics of drainage.
- It is necessary to maintain aseptic technique when changing dressings and caring for wound.
- It is necessary to flush the wound with sterile saline solution and apply a sterile pressure dressing.
- It is necessary to maintain patency and routinely empty drainage device.
- It is necessary to cover dressing with plastic when using the bedpan or if incontinent.
- It is necessary to expose stump to air; wash with mild soap and water after dressings are discontinued.
- Monitoring vital signs
- Administering antibiotics as indicated.
- Obtaining wound and drainage cultures and sensitivities as appropriate.

Risk for ineffective tissue perfusion related to reduced arterial or venous blood flow, tissue edema, hematoma formation, or hypovolemia

Interventions

- Inspecting dressings and drainage device, noting amount and characteristics of drainage.
- Performing periodic neurovascular assessments (sensation, movement, pulse, skin color, and temperature).
- **Monitoring vital signs:** Palpate peripheral pulses, noting strength and equality.
- Applying direct pressure to bleeding site if hemorrhage occurs. Contacting physician immediately.
- If the patient experiences throbbing after the stump is wrapped, the bandage may be too tight. Removing the bandage and reapply.
- Checking the bandage regularly
- Investigating reports of persistent or unusual pain in operative site.
- Administering IV fluids and blood products as indicated.
- Encouraging and assisting with early ambulation.
- Evaluating nonoperated lower limb for inflammation and positive Homans' sign.
- **Monitoring laboratory studies:** Hb and Hct, etc.

Situational low self-esteem related to loss of body part or change in functional abilities

Interventions

- Encouraging participation in ADLs. Providing opportunities to view and care for stump and using the moment to point out positive signs of healing.
- Helping the amputee cope with his altered body image.
- Encouraging expression of fears, negative feelings, and grief over loss of body part.
- Reinforcing preoperative information including type and location of amputation, type of prosthetic fitting if appropriate (immediate, delayed), expected
- Ascertaining individual strengths and identify previous positive coping behaviors.
- Assessing and considering patient's preparation for and view of amputation.
- Encouraging and providing for visit by another amputee, especially one who is successfully rehabilitating.

- Note withdrawn behavior, negative self-talk, use of denial, or over concern with actual and perceived changes.
- Providing open environment for patient to discuss concerns about sexuality.
- **Discussing availability of various resources:** Psychiatric and sexual counseling and occupational therapist.

OSTEITIS DEFORMANS (PAGET'S DISEASE)

Paget's disease of bone disrupts the body's normal bone recycling process, in which old bone tissue is gradually replaced with the new bone tissue. Over time, the affected bones may become fragile and weak. Paget's disease of bone most commonly occurs in the pelvis, skull, spine, and legs. The involved bone can be soft, leading to weakness and bending of the pelvis, low back (spine), hips, thighs, head, and arms.

Etiology and Pathophysiology

- Both genetic and environmental factors are thought to play a role.
- About 15% of people with Paget's disease have a family history.
- Autosomal-dominant inheritance has also been described in some families.
- Mutations have been identified in four genes that cause Paget's disease.
- Mechanical stress may play a role.
- Paramyxovirus infection (including measles and respiratory syncytial virus) has been suggested as a possible trigger, but this has been disputed.

Pathophysiology

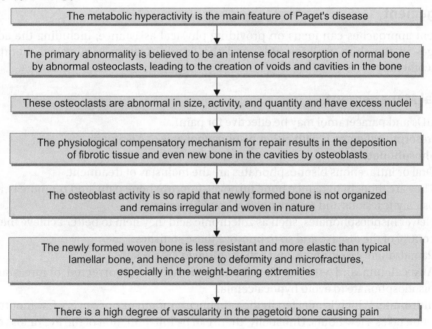

The metabolic hyperactivity is the main feature of Paget's disease

↓

The primary abnormality is believed to be an intense focal resorption of normal bone by abnormal osteoclasts, leading to the creation of voids and cavities in the bone

↓

These osteoclasts are abnormal in size, activity, and quantity and have excess nuclei

↓

The physiological compensatory mechanism for repair results in the deposition of fibrotic tissue and even new bone in the cavities by osteoblasts

↓

The osteoblast activity is so rapid that newly formed bone is not organized and remains irregular and woven in nature

↓

The newly formed woven bone is less resistant and more elastic than typical lamellar bone, and hence prone to deformity and microfractures, especially in the weight-bearing extremities

↓

There is a high degree of vascularity in the pagetoid bone causing pain

Paget's Disease

- An initial, short-lived burst of multinucleate osteoclastic activity causing bone resorption

- A mixed phase of both osteoclastic and osteoblastic activity, with increased levels of bone turnover leading to deposition of structurally abnormal bone.
- A final chronic sclerotic phase, during which bone formation outweighs bone resorption.

Signs and Symptoms

Most people who have Paget's disease of bone experience no symptoms. When symptoms do occur, the most common complaint is bone pain that may include:

- **Pelvis:** Paget's disease of bone in the pelvis can cause hip pain.
- **Skull:** An overgrowth of bone in the skull can cause hearing loss or headaches.
- **Spine:** If spine is affected, nerve roots can become compressed. This can cause pain, tingling, and numbness in an arm or leg.
- **Leg:** As the bones weaken, they may bend. Enlarged and misshapen bones in legs can put extra stress on nearby joints, which may cause wear-and-tear arthritis in knee or hip.

Diagnostic Evaluations

Following are the list of diagnostic evaluations:

- Bone-specific alkaline phosphatase levels are raised.
- Urinary excretion of deoxypyridinoline and N-telopeptide is elevated.
- Serum calcium, phosphorus, and parathyroid hormone levels are usually normal, but immobilization may lead to hypercalcemia.
- X-rays may show a number of signs of both osteolysis and excessive bone formation occur.
- Radionuclide bone scans can show the extent of the disease.
- Bone biopsy may be needed if malignant change is suspected.

Management

Treatment approaches can focus on providing physical assistance, including the addition of wedges in the shoe, walking aids, and the administration of physical therapy and pharmacotherapy.

Medical Management

- NSAIDs and paracetamol may be effective for pain.
- Antiresorptive therapy is with either bisphosphonates or calcitonin.
- **Bisphosphonates:**
  - Oral or intravenous bisphosphonates are the mainstay of treatment.
  - They are thought to reduce bone turnover, improve bone pain, and promote healing of osteolytic lesions and restore normal bone histology.
  - Newer bisphosphonates, such as zoledronic acid may help to better achieve metabolic control of the disease and so to improve these statistics.
  - Pamidronate, risedronate, and zoledronic acid are preferred.
  - Any calcium and vitamin D deficiency needs to be corrected before starting a bisphosphonate to avoid hypocalcemia.
- **Pamidronate:** Which is injected in the vein once a month or once every few months? The injection takes a few hours. Unusually, there can be inflammation of the eye or loss of bone around the teeth (osteonecrosis).
- **Zoledronate:** This is injected in the vein once a year.
- Calcitonin, a hormone that is injected under the skin several times a week.

Complications

Complications from Paget's disease depend on the site affected and the activity of the disease.
- Bone pain
- Bone deformity, kyphosis, frontal bossing of the skull, an enlarged maxilla, an increase in head size
- Pathological fractures
- Osteoarthritis
- Deafness and tinnitus may be due to the compression of cranial nerve VIII
- Spinal stenosis
- Nerve compression syndromes

Nursing Care Plan

Acute pain related to nerve compression and muscle spasm

Interventions
- Assessing complaints of pain, location, duration of attacks, precipitating factors which aggravate.
- Maintaining bed rest, semi-Fowler's position to the spinal bones, hips and knees in a state of flexion, supine position.
- Using log-roll (board) during a change of position
- Auxiliary mounting brace
- Limiting activity during the acute phase according to the needs
- Teaching relaxation techniques
- **Collaboration:** Analgesics, traction, physiotherapy

Impaired physical mobility related to pain, muscle spasms, and damage neuromuscular restrictive therapy

Interventions
- Giving patients to perform passive range of motion exercises and active
- Assisting patients in ambulation activity progressively
- Providing good skin care, massage point pressure after changing the position.
- Checking the state of the skin under the brace with a specific time period
- Noting the emotional responses and behaviors in immobilizing
- Demonstrating the use of auxiliary equipment, such as a cane
- **Collaboration:** Analgesic

PROLAPSED LUMBAR DISK (HERNIATED RUPTURED DISK)

A prolapsed lumbar disk is a spinal condition that can cause lower back pain, as well as numbness, tingling, a "pins and needles" feeling and muscle weakness in the lower body. This condition is also referred to as a herniated or ruptured disk and usually is caused by normal age-related deterioration **(Fig. 12.8)**.

Etiology and Pathophysiology

A prolapsed cervical disk is another name for a herniated, or ruptured, disk in the neck or upper back. It occurs among the seven top-most vertebrae of the spine, known as the cervical

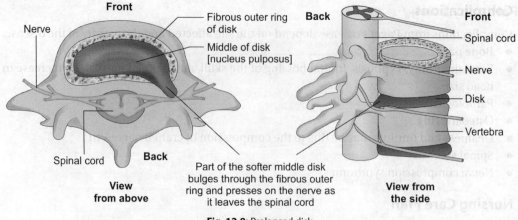

Fig. 12.8: Prolapsed disk.

vertebrae (C1–C7). Although disk herniation is more common in the lower back, the C4–C7 levels of the cervical spine are also vulnerable to disk prolapse as the body ages.

Pathophysiology

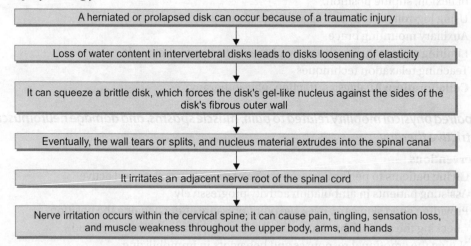

Signs and Symptoms

A prolapsed cervical disk can produce symptoms in the following areas of the body:

- Shoulders
- Upper back
- Deltoid muscles
- Biceps
- Triceps
- Forearms
- Wrists
- Hands
- Fingers
- Head (migraine symptoms)

Pathophysiology

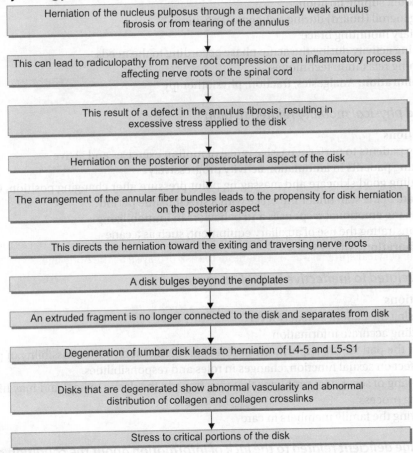

Herniation of the nucleus pulposus through a mechanically weak annulus fibrosis or from tearing of the annulus

↓

This can lead to radiculopathy from nerve root compression or an inflammatory process affecting nerve roots or the spinal cord

↓

This result of a defect in the annulus fibrosis, resulting in excessive stress applied to the disk

↓

Herniation on the posterior or posterolateral aspect of the disk

↓

The arrangement of the annular fiber bundles leads to the propensity for disk herniation on the posterior aspect

↓

This directs the herniation toward the exiting and traversing nerve roots

↓

A disk bulges beyond the endplates

↓

An extruded fragment is no longer connected to the disk and separates from disk

↓

Degeneration of lumbar disk leads to herniation of L4-5 and L5-S1

↓

Disks that are degenerated show abnormal vascularity and abnormal distribution of collagen and collagen crosslinks

↓

Stress to critical portions of the disk

Diagnostic Evaluation

- X-ray
- Computed tomography scan
- MRI
- **Myelogram:** An X-ray of the spinal canal following injection of a contrast material into the surrounding cerebrospinal fluid spaces. By revealing displacement of the contrast material, it can show the presence of structures that can cause pressure on the spinal cord or nerves, such as herniated disks, tumors, or bone spurs.
- Electromyogram and nerve conduction studies

Pharmacological Management

- Anti-inflammatory painkillers
- A stronger painkiller, such as Morphine
- A muscle relaxant, such as diazepam.

Nursing Care Plan

Acute pain related to nerve compression and muscle spasm

Interventions

- Assessing complaints of pain, location, duration of attacks, precipitating factors that aggravate.

- Maintaining bed rest, semi-Fowler's position to the spinal bones, hips, and knees in a state of flexion, supine position.
- Using logroll (board) during a change of position
- Auxiliary mounting brace
- Limiting activity during the acute phase according to the needs
- Teaching relaxation techniques
- **Collaboration:** Analgesics, traction, physiotherapy

Impaired physical mobility related to pain

Interventions
- Giving patients to perform passive range of motion exercises and active
- Assisting patients in ambulation activity progressively
- Providing good skincare and massaging point pressure after changing position. Checking the state of the skin under the brace with a specific time period
- Noting the emotional responses and behaviors in immobilizing
- Demonstrating the use of auxiliary equipment, such as a cane
- **Collaboration:** Analgesic.

Anxiety related to ineffective individual coping

Interventions
- Assessing the patient's anxiety level
- Providing accurate information
- Giving the patient the opportunity to reveal problems, such as the possibility of paralysis, the effect on sexual function, changes in roles and responsibilities.
- Reviewing of secondary problems that may impede the desire to heal and may hinder the healing process.
- Involving the family members in care

Knowledge deficient related to the lack of information about the condition and prognosis

Interventions
- Explaining the process of disease and prognosis, and restrictions on activities.
- Giving information about own body mechanics to stand, lift, and use the shoes backer.
- Discussing about treatment and side effects.
- Suggesting using the board or mat, a small pillow under neck a little flat, bedside with knees flexed.
- Avoiding the use of heaters for a long time.
- Giving information about the signs that need attention, such as puncture pain, loss of sensation, and ability to walk.

Types of Surgeries in Muscular Skeleton System

Various types of total and partial knee replacement surgery:
1. **Total knee replacement (Fig. 12.9):** Total knee replacement (TKR), also referred to as total knee arthroplasty, is a surgical procedure where worn, diseased, or damaged surfaces of a knee joint are removed and replaced with artificial surfaces. It is a common surgical procedure most often performed to relieve the pain and disability from degenerative arthritis, meniscus tears, osteoarthritis, cartilage defects, and ligament tears.

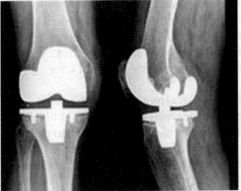

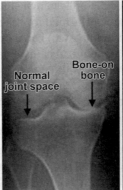

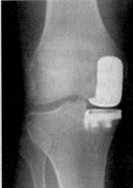

Fig. 12.9: Total knee replacement.

Fig. 12.10: Partial knee replacement.

The most common cause for knee pain, which needs knee replacement surgery, is osteoarthritis. In TKR, the surgeon removes damaged cartilage and bone from the surface of your knee joint and replaces them with a prosthesis or implant of metal and plastic. TKR can help put an end to arthritic pain in knee and enable to resume a functional and active lifestyle.

2. **Partial knee replacement (Fig. 12.10):** Most people are aware of the TKR surgery. This involves replacing the unhealthy surface of the entire knee joint with metal and plastic implants. It is a very successful operation with good long-term results. However, a large percentage of patients have arthritis limited to one part of the joint alone.

Replacing the whole joint in these patients is overkill and unnecessary. Many middle-aged men and women develop osteoarthritis of the knee. Osteoarthritis of the knee affects the inner half or medial compartment to start with and then proceeds to affect the outer half or lateral compartment. In this operation, only that part of the knee, which is unhealthy, is replaced. The normal surfaces are left alone. This operation has several advantages over TKR surgery, such as small incision, longer life of implant, and postoperative hospitalization is reduced and return to normal is much faster than TKR surgery.

3. **Simultaneous bilateral knee replacement—Both knee replacement surgery:** A simultaneous procedure means that both knees are replaced at the same surgery, in 1 day. The benefit of simultaneous knee replacement is that both problems are taken care of at one time. The overall stay and rehabilitation can be done in a shorter time, and there is only one hospitalization. Patients also require one anesthesia.

4. **Revision knee replacement:** TKRs that need to be revised after 15–20 years (post-primary surgery) are also done. The most advanced prosthesis and computer-assisted surgery is also used for the revision knee replacements.

5. **Knee arthroscopic surgery:** Knee arthroscopic surgery is a procedure performed through small incisions in the skin to repair injuries to tissues, such as ligaments, cartilage, or bone within the knee joint area. The surgery is conducted with the aid of an arthroscope, which a very small instrument is guided by a lighted scope attached to a television monitor.

Knee arthroscopy has in many cases replaced the classic arthrotomy that was performed in the past. Today, knee arthroscopy is commonly performed for treating meniscus injury, for the reconstruction of the anterior cruciate ligament, and for cartilage microfracturing. Many knee joint problems are amenable to arthroscopic surgery, such as:

- Trimming a torn meniscus of the knee
- Repairing a torn meniscus of the knee
- Treatment of cartilage damage in the knee

Arthroscopic surgery is a "less invasive" procedure and being a surgical procedure involves risks, but when performed for the right problem, it is often very successful.

6. **Anterior cruciate ligament (ACL) reconstruction:** The ACL keeps the shin bone (tibia) in place. A tear of this ligament can cause knee and hip to give way during physical activity. ACL reconstruction surgery is done to replace the ligament in the center of knee and hip with a new ligament.

7. **Arthroscopic meniscectomy:** Meniscectomy is the surgical removal of all or part of a torn meniscus (rupturing of one or more of the fibrocartilage strips in the knee and hip called menisci). A meniscus tear is a common knee and hip joint injury and can lead to pain and swelling of the knee and hip joint. Menisci can also be torn during innocuous activities, such as walking or squatting. Depending on the location of the tear, a repair may be possible. The outer third of the meniscus, an adequate blood supply exists and a repair will likely heal. Usually, younger patients are more resilient and respond well to this treatment, while older, more sedentary patients do not have a favorable outcome after a repair.

8. **Total hip replacement surgery:** Total hip replacement (THR) is a treatment to all kinds of hip arthritis, improving the quality of life of patients who undergo the operation. The trouble-causing hip is surgically removed and replaced with an artificial one. In THR, the entire femoral head is removed. A new ball and socket are placed as an implant or prosthesis. The new hip ball is attached to a stem that gets machined inside the hip bone. Hip replacement implant can wear out over a period of time due to various reasons.

There are two major types of artificial hip replacements—cemented prosthesis and the uncemented prosthesis. Both types of prosthesis are widely used.

Each prosthesis is made up of two parts

1. The acetabular component or socket portion, which replaces the acetabulum.
2. The femoral component or stem portion, which replaces the femoral head.

The femoral component is made of a metal stem with a metal ball on the end. Some prostheses have a ceramic ball attached to the metal stem. The acetabular component is a metal shell with a plastic inner socket liner that acts, such as a bearing. The type of plastic used is highly cross-linked ultrahigh molecule weight polyethylene that is wear resistant.

A cemented prosthesis is held in place by polymethyl methacrylate (PMMA) cement that attaches the metal to the bone. An uncemented prosthesis has a fine mesh of holes on the surface area that touches the bone. The mesh allows the bone to grow into the mesh and "become part of" the bone.

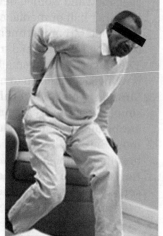

Fig. 12.11: Pain at hip joint after prolong sitting.

Indications of Hip Replacement Surgery

- Progressively worsening severe arthritis in the hip joint.
- Common hip problems resulting into osteoarthritis.
- Bony fractures of the hip joint, rheumatoid arthritis, and death (aseptic necrosis) of the hip bone.
- After pain becomes so severe that it affects normal function.
- Dependency on anti-inflammatory and pain medications.
- Benign and malignant bone tumors.
- Paget's disease occurs mainly in the elderly. Bones become enlarged and weakened, with the potential of a fracture or deformity of the hip bones.

Advantages of Hip Replacement Surgery

- Hip replacement improves quality of life.
- Age is no barrier to hip replacement benefits.
- Hip replacement is cost effective.
- High rate of patient satisfaction associated with hip replacement.
- The artificial hip often improves the movements in a hip joint that has become increasingly stiff from the effects of long-term arthritis and this permits the patient to resume at first gentle activity and then their favorite leisure hobbies.
- Improves mobility
- Independence of arthritis sufferers

Types of Shoulder Surgery

1. **Arthroscopic acromioplasty:** This is an arthroscopic procedure to widen the space between the upper arm and the shoulder blade so that the rotator cuff tendons do not get stuck between them. Arthroscopy with shoulder instability—In case of dislocation of the shoulder, it is normal to have an arthroscopy. It is often possible to repair damage to the shoulder, but sometimes a separate operation is needed.
2. **Rotator cuff repair:** Arthroscopic repair of the shoulder tendons. The goal of these procedures is to minimize the pain and restore strength and functionality.
3. **Total shoulder replacement:** Shoulder arthroplasty—With loss of cartilage, the patient will suffer severe shoulder arthritis. This will eventually make surgical treatment is necessary.

MULTIPLE CHOICE QUESTIONS

1. A client has undergone a lumbar laminectomy and has just returned to the nursing unit. It is essential for the nurse to perform which of the following activities during this period?
   A. Vital sign checks every half-hour
   B. Assessment of bladder function
   C. Early ambulation
   D. Neurovascular checks

2. The nurse is teaching a client with metastatic bone disease about measures to prevent hypercalcemia. It would be important for the nurse to emphasize?
   A. Early recognition of tetany
   B. The importance of walking
   C. The need to restrict fluid intake to less than 1 L/day
   D. The need to have at least five servings of dairy products daily

3. The nurse, assisting in applying a cast to a client with a broken arm, knows that:
   A. The casted extremity should be placed on a cloth-covered surface
   B. The cast should be covered until it dries
   C. The cast material should be dipped several times into the warm water
   D. The wet cast should be handled with the palms of hands

4. Because a client has bursitis, plans for nursing interventions should include:
   A. Aggressive antibiotic therapy
   B. Range-of-motion activities
   C. Rest
   D. A high-protein diet

5. During the first 24 hours after an above-the-knee amputation for vascular disease, nursing priority for stump care would be:
   A. Cleansing with soap and water
   B. Inspecting for redness and pressure points
   C. Initiating fitting for prosthesis
   D. Elevating to reduce edema

6. The client is diagnosed with osteoarthritis. Which sign/symptom should the nurse expect the client to exhibit?

   A. Swan-neck fingers   B. Waddling gait

   C. Severe bone deformity   D. Joint stiffness

7. A complication of Buck's extension traction would be noted by a nurse if:

   A. Toes of affected leg became dusky in color

   B. Skin over the fracture site was flushed

   C. Redness and purulent drainage appeared at the pin site

   D. Dorsiflexion developed in the affected foot

8. A client has been hospitalized after an automobile accident. A full leg cast was applied in the emergency room. The MOST important reason for the nurse to elevate the casted leg is to:

   A. Promote the client's comfort   B. Decrease irritation to the skin

   C. Reduce the drying time   D. Improve venous return

9. A client fractured his femur yesterday. Monitoring for which potential complication must be included by the nurse in the client's plan of care?

   A. Crush injury   B. Disturbed body image

   C. Fat emboli syndrome   D. Chronic pain

10. The nurse assesses which of the following clinical manifestations in a client with osteomyelitis? Select all that apply:

   A. Restlessness   B. Night sweats

   C. Fever   D. Petechial

   E. Cool extremities   F. Nausea

11. The nurse prepares a client for a bone scan. What priority assessment should the nurse perform for this client?

   A. Presence of intravenous (IV) access

   B. Current vital signs

   C. Presence of metallic implants, such as a pacemaker or aneurysm clips

   D. History of claustrophobia

12. The client is being evaluated for osteoporosis. Which diagnostic test is the most accurate when diagnosing osteoporosis?

   A. Serum alkaline phosphatase   B. X-ray of the femur

   C. Serum bone Gla-protein test   D. Dual-energy X-ray absorptiometry (DEXA)

13. A client has bilateral knee pain from osteoarthritis. In addition to taking the prescribed NSAID, the nurse should instruct the client to:

   A. Avoid foods high in citrus acid

   B. Rest the knees as much as possible to decrease inflammation

   C. Keep legs elevated when sitting

   D. Start a regular exercise program

14. A client is admitted following a motor vehicle accident where his left thigh was crushed beneath the vehicle. The nurse must assess for which of the following complications?

   A. Hypokalemia   B. Acute renal failure

   C. Fat emboli syndrome   D. Hypotension

Answers

1. D   2. B   3. D   4. C   5. D   6. D   7. A   8. D   9. C   10. A, B, C, F

11. A   12. D   13. D   14. B

Immunological Disorders

AT THE END OF THIS CHAPTER, THE STUDENTS WILL BE ABLE TO LEARN ABOUT:
- ➤ Assessment of immunological disorders
- ➤ Primary immunodeficiency syndromes
- ➤ Secondary immunodeficiencies
- ➤ Human immunodeficiency virus (HIV)
- ➤ Cycle of human immunodeficiency virus
- ➤ Stages of human immunodeficiency virus

INTRODUCTION

The immune system is the body's natural defense system that helps fight infections. The immune system is made up of antibodies, white blood cells (WBC), and other chemicals and proteins that attack and destroy substances, such as bacteria and viruses that they recognize as foreign and different from the body's normal healthy tissues. The immune system also includes:

- The tonsils and thymus, which make antibodies.
- **The lymph nodes and vessels (the lymphatic system):** This network of lymph nodes and vessels throughout the body carries lymph fluid, nutrients, and waste material between the body tissues and the bloodstream. The lymphatic system is an important part of the immune system. The lymph nodes filter lymph fluid as it flows through them, trapping bacteria, viruses, and other foreign substances, which are then destroyed by special white blood cells called lymphocytes.
- **Bone marrow:** This is soft tissue found mainly inside the long bones of the arms and legs, the vertebrae, and the pelvic bones of the body. It is made up of red marrow, which produces red and white blood cells and platelets, and yellow marrow, which contains fat and connective tissue and produces some white blood cells.
- **The spleen:** It filters the blood by removing old or damaged blood cells and platelets and helps the immune system by destroying bacteria and other foreign substances.
- **White blood cells:** These blood cells are made in the bone marrow and protect the body against infection. If an infection develops, white blood cells attack and destroy the bacteria, virus, or other organisms causing it.

ASSESSMENT OF IMMUNOLOGICAL DISORDERS

- **Confirming diagnosis:** Signs and symptoms may occur at any time after infection, but acquired immunodeficiency syndrome (AIDS) is not officially diagnosed until the patient's CD4+ T-cell count falls below 200 cells/µL or associated clinical conditions or disease.

- **Complete blood count (CBC):** Anemia and idiopathic thrombocytopenia (anemia occurs in up to 85% of patients with AIDS and may be profound). Leukopenia may be present; differential shift to the left suggests infectious process *Pneumocystis jirovecii* (*carinii*) pneumonia (PCP).
- **Purified protein derivative (PPD):** It determines exposure or active tuberculosis (TB) disease. Of AIDS patients, 100% of those exposed to active *Mycobacterium tuberculosis* will develop the disease.
- **Serologic:** Serum antibody test—human immunodeficiency virus (HIV) screen by enzyme-linked immunosorbent assay (ELISA). A positive test result may be indicative of exposure to HIV, but is not diagnostic because false positives may occur.
- **Western blot test:** It confirms diagnosis of HIV in blood and urine.
- **Viral load test:**
  - Polymerase chain reaction (PCR): The most widely used test currently can detect viral RNA levels as low as 50 copies/mL of plasma with an upper limit of 75,000 copies/mL.
  - Branched DNA (bDNA) 3.0 assay: It has a wider range of 50–500,000 copies/mL. Therapy can be initiated, or changes made in treatment approaches, based on rise of viral load or maintenance of a low viral load. This is currently the leading indicator of effectiveness of therapy.
  - T-lymphocyte cells: Total count reduced.
  - CD4+ lymphocyte count (immune system indicator that mediates several immune system processes and signals B cells to produce antibodies to foreign germs): Numbers less than 200 indicate severe immune deficiency response and diagnosis of AIDS.
  - T-cell clones (CTL) (cytopathic suppressor cells): Reversed ratio (2:1 or higher) of suppressor cells to helper cells (T8⁺ to T4⁺) indicates immune suppression.
  - PCR test: It detects HIV-DNA; most helpful in testing newborns of HIV-infected mothers. Infants carry maternal HIV antibodies and therefore test positive by ELISA and Western blot, even though infant is not necessarily infected.
- **Sexually transmitted disease (STD) screening tests:** Hepatitis B envelope and core antibodies, syphilis, and other common STDs may be positive.
- **Cultures:** Histologic, cytologic studies of urine, blood, stool, spinal fluid, lesions, sputum, and secretions may be done to identify the opportunistic infection (OI).
- **Neurological studies:** For example, electroencephalogram (EEG), magnetic resonance imaging (MRI), computed tomography (CT) scans of the brain, and electromyography (EMG)/nerve conduction studies. It indicated changes in mentation, fever of undetermined origin, and changes in sensory or motor function to determine effects of HIV infection or OIs.
- **Chest X-ray:** It may initially be normal or may reveal progressive interstitial infiltrates secondary to advancing PCP (most common opportunistic disease) or other pulmonary complication disease processes, such as TB.
- **Pulmonary function tests:** Useful in early detection of interstitial pneumonias.
- **Gallium scan:** Diffuse pulmonary uptake occurs in PCP and other forms of pneumonia.
- **Biopsies:** It may be done for differential diagnosis of Kaposi's sarcoma (KS) or other neoplastic lesions.

- **Bronchoscopy or tracheobronchial washings:** It may be done with biopsy when PCP or lung malignancies are suspected.
- **Barium swallow, endoscopy, colonoscopy:** It may be done to identify OI [e.g., Candida, cytomegalovirus (CMV)] or to stage KS in the gastrointestinal (GI) system.

Immunodeficiency disorders involve malfunction of the immune system, resulting in infections that develop and recur more frequently, are more severe, and last longer than usual.

Immunodeficiency disorders impair the immune system's ability to defend the body against foreign or abnormal cells that invade or attack it (such as bacteria, viruses, fungi, and cancer cells). As a result, unusual bacterial, viral, or fungal infections or lymphomas or other cancers may develop. Another problem is that up to 25% of people who have an immunodeficiency disorder also have an autoimmune disorder (such as immune thrombocytopenia). In an autoimmune disorder, the immune system attacks the body's own tissue. Sometimes, the autoimmune disorder develops before the immunodeficiency causes any symptoms.

Types of Immunodeficiency Disorders

1. Primary immunodeficiency disorders are congenital immune disorders. Primary disorders include:
   - X-linked agammaglobulinemia
   - Severe combined immunodeficiency
   - Common variable immunodeficiency
   - Alymphocytosis
2. Secondary disorders occur when body is attacked by an outside source, such as a toxic chemical or an infection. Severe burns and radiation also can cause secondary disorders. Secondary disorders include:
   - AIDS
   - Cancers of the immune system, such as leukemia
   - Immune complex diseases, such as viral hepatitis
   - Multiple myeloma.

These are classified as primary and secondary or acquired.

Primary Immunodeficiency Syndromes

- Mostly these are inherited single-gene disorders that present in infancy in early childhood with the exception of common variable immunodeficiency, which usually occurs in adults.
- Mutations or deletions of genes governing stem-cell differentiation.
- They are sometimes classified according to which component is faulty (T-cells, B-cells, phagocytic cells, or complement) or according to individual clinical syndromes.
- About 80% of patients are less than 20 years old when diagnosed, because the majority of cases are inherited or congenital. About 70% occur in males due to X-linked inheritance in many syndromes.
- B-cell defects account for 50% of primary immunodeficiency.
- T-cell defects account for 30%, phagocytic deficiencies 18%, and complement deficiencies 2%.

- **Antibody deficiency syndromes:** This is a group of conditions characterized by an inability to produce antibodies in sufficient quantity or of sufficient quality.
- **Common variable immunodeficiency:** This is a heterogeneous syndrome characterized by various degrees of hypogammaglobulinemia, commonly associated with autoimmunity.
- **Thymoma and hypogammaglobulinemia:** This is characterized by low numbers of B-cells and a distinctive T-cell type.
- **X-linked (Bruton's agammaglobulinemia):** The agammaglobulinemia is an X-linked immunodeficiency in which there is a failure to produce mature B lymphocyte cells. The defect in this disorder is a fault in the enzyme in Bruton's tyrosine kinase, a key regulator in B-cell development.
- Cell-mediated immunity can be subject to a number of genetic defects affecting the function of the T-cells.
- **Thymic aplasia (DiGeorge syndrome):** There are genetic defects of the thymus and often the parathyroid glands and heart, associated with T-cell dysfunction and significant immune deficiency.
- **Severe combined immunodeficiency disease:** This is in fact a group of rare congenital diseases in which there is severe and usually fatal immune deficiency.
- **Inherited syndromes associated with immunodeficiency:** A wide range of inherited immunodeficiency conditions has been identified, many involving a single gene.

Secondary Immunodeficiencies

There are many possible causes and so it is difficult to obtain exact epidemiological data. It is known that the current epidemics of AIDS and tuberculosis have caused global increases in the condition.

Secondary immunodeficiency is common in people who are hospitalized for:

- Lymphoreticular malignancy
- Drugs—particularly cytotoxic drugs and immunosuppressant
- Viruses, for example, HIV
- Malnutrition
- Metabolic disorders, for example, renal disease requiring peritoneal dialysis
- Trauma or major surgery
- Protein loss—for example, due to nephrotic syndrome.

Presentation of Secondary Immunodeficiencies

The most common presenting feature is frequent infections. Recurrent respiratory infections are common.

- The development of severe, persistent recurrent bacterial infection is a better indicator. A common scenario is repeated episodes of sore throat or upper respiratory tract infection which lead to sinusitis, chronic otitis, and bronchitis. Another feature is the ease with which complications develop. For example, bronchitis progresses to pneumonia, bronchiectasis, and respiratory failure.
- Opportunistic infections are common, such as *P. jirovecii* or CMV, especially in patients with T-cell deficiencies. Infection of the skin and mucous membranes occurs frequently, including resistant thrush, oral ulcers, and periodontitis. Conjunctivitis, pyoderma, severe warts, alopecia, eczema, and telangiectasia are also prominent features.

- Common gastrointestinal symptoms include diarrhea, malabsorption and failure to thrive or losing weight. The diarrhea is usually noninfectious, although a range of organisms, including rotavirus, *Giardia lamblia*, *Cryptosporidium*, and CMV, may be involved.
- Less commonly, hematological abnormalities, such as autoimmune hemolytic anemia, leukopenia, or thrombocytopenia can occur.
- Neurological problems, such as seizures and encephalitis, and autoimmune conditions, such as vasculitis and arthritis, are also sometimes seen. There is also a higher incidence of gastric carcinoma and liver disease.
- Paradoxically, autoimmune diseases can be associated with primary immunodeficiencies.

Diagnostic Evaluation

- **Family history:** There may be a familial tendency to early death, similar disease, autoimmunity, allergy, early malignancy, or intermarriage.
- **Check for risk factors:** Diabetes, medications, illicit drug use, and sexual history.
- A history of adverse reactions to immunizations or complications of viral infections may be significant.
- Inquiry should be made about the frequency of previous antibiotic prescriptions and any history of relevant surgery, for example, splenectomy, tonsillectomy, adenoidectomy.
- A history of radiation therapy to the thymus or nasopharynx may also be a pointer to the diagnosis.

Examination

- Patients with immunodeficiency often look ill, with pale skin, general malaise, cachexia, and a distended abdomen. Various skin manifestations may be apparent, such as rashes, vesicles, pyoderma, eczema, and [Telangiectasia is a condition in which widened venules (tiny blood vessels) cause threadlike red lines or patterns on the skin].
- The eyes may be inflamed and infected.
- Signs of chronic ENT disease, such as scarred eardrums, encrusted nostrils, and postnasal drip may be evident.
- There may be a chronic cough with crepitations in both lungs.
- Hepatomegaly and splenomegaly may be detected in the abdomen.
- In infants, crusting around the anus may be a sign of chronic diarrhea. Delayed developmental milestones or ataxia may be evident.

Investigation

Specialist tests are often required to elucidate the exact diagnosis, but screening tests can be done in primary care. These should include:

- Full blood count (FBC), IgG, IgM, and IgA levels and tests to confirm the presence and type of any infection. A systematic review called for screening in patients with recurrent infections, irrespective of age.
- An elevated erythrocyte sedimentation rate (ESR) may indicate chronic infection and chest X-ray (CXR) and sinus X-ray may confirm the source.
- Appropriate microbiological swabs should be taken, as dictated by the clinical picture.
- More advanced investigations include assays of lymphocyte response, antibody response to immunization of diphtheria, tetanus and pneumococcal polysaccharides, and phagocytosis assay.

Management

- General measures include making sure that patients have a healthy lifestyle and are protected as far as possible from infection. This includes having regular dental checks and their own accommodation. There may be an element of social isolation and psychological issues may need to be addressed.
- If there is any evidence of antibody response, the standard regime of killed vaccines should be given. Live vaccines are contraindicated in T-cell deficiency.
- Bacterial and fungal infection should be recognized and treated early. Swabs should be taken before treatment so that empirical treatment failures can be rectified rapidly. Continuous prophylactic antibiotics may be appropriate in some circumstances. Chest infections may require physiotherapy and lung exercises.
- Antiviral therapies, such as amantadine and rimantadine may be lifesaving in the management of viral infections.
- Intravenous or subcutaneous immunoglobulin replacement is the first-line treatment for most immunoglobulin deficiency states. Subcutaneous therapy is preferred by many patients because it is more convenient and they can be more independent. The best treatment for T-cell deficiency conditions is bone marrow transplant, if a donor can be found.
- Other treatment options, some of which are still in the experimental phase, include cytokines, thymic transplants, gene therapy, and stem-cell transplantation.

Prevention

Some of the disorders that can cause immunodeficiency can be prevented and treated, thus helping prevent immunodeficiency from developing. The following are examples:

- **Human immunodeficiency virus infection:** Following safe sex guidelines and not sharing needles to inject drugs can reduce the spread of this infection. Also, antiretroviral (ARV) drugs can usually treat HIV infection effectively.
- **Cancer:** Successful treatment usually restores the function of the immune system unless people need to continue taking immunosuppressant.
- **Diabetes:** Good control of blood sugar levels can help white blood cells function better and thus prevent infections.

Strategies for preventing and treating infections depend on the type of immunodeficiency disorder. For example, people who have an immunodeficiency disorder due to a deficiency of antibodies are at risk of bacterial infections. The following can help reduce the risk:

- Being treated periodically with immune globulin (antibodies obtained from the blood of people with a normal immune system) given intravenously or under the skin.
- Practicing good personal hygiene (including conscientious dental care)
- Not eating undercooked food
- Not drinking water that may be contaminated
- Avoiding contact with people who have infections

Treatment

- **Antibiotics** are given as soon as a fever or another sign of an infection develops and before surgical and dental procedures, which may introduce bacteria into the bloodstream. If a disorder (such as severe combined immunodeficiency) increases the risk of developing serious infections or particular infections, people may be given antibiotics to prevent these infections.

- **Antiviral drugs** are given at the first sign of infection if people have an immunodeficiency disorder that increases the risk of viral infections (such as immunodeficiency due to a T-cell abnormality). These drugs include amantadine and acyclovir.
- **Vaccines** are given if the specific immunodeficiency disorder does not affect antibody production. Vaccines are given to stimulate the body to produce antibodies that recognize and attack specific bacteria or viruses. If the person's immune system cannot make antibodies, giving a vaccine does not result in the production of antibodies and can even result in illness. For example, if a disorder does not affect production of antibodies, people with that disorder are given the influenza vaccine given once a year. Doctors may also give this vaccine to the person's immediate family members and to people who have close contact with the person. Generally, live-virus vaccines are not given to people who have a B- or T-cell abnormality because these vaccines may cause an infection in such people. Live-virus vaccines include rotavirus vaccines, measles–mumps–rubella vaccine, chickenpox (varicella) vaccine, varicella-zoster (shingles) vaccine, bacille Calmette-Guérin vaccine, and influenza vaccine given as a nasal spray.
- **Stem cell transplantation** can correct some immunodeficiency disorders, particularly severe combined immunodeficiency. Stem cells are usually obtained from bone marrow but occasionally from blood (including umbilical cord blood). Transplantation of thymus tissue is sometimes helpful. Gene therapy for a few congenital immunodeficiency disorders has been successful.

HUMAN IMMUNODEFICIENCY VIRUS

As the expanded form of "HIV" suggests:
- **H**—Human—this particular virus can only infect human beings.
- **I**—Immunodeficiency—HIV weaken immune system by destroying important cells that fight disease and infection. A "deficient" immune system cannot protect you.
- **V**—Virus—a virus can only reproduce itself by taking over a cell in the body of its host.

Acquired Immunodeficiency Syndrome

As the expanded form of "AIDS" suggests:
- **A**—Acquired—AIDS is not something inherited from parents. You acquire AIDS after birth.
- **I**—Immuno—body's immune system includes all the organs and cells that work to fight off infection or disease.
- **D**—Deficiency—you get AIDS when the immune system is "deficient" or is not working the way it should.
- **S**—Syndrome—a syndrome is a collection of symptoms and signs of disease. AIDS is a syndrome, rather than a single disease, because it is a complex illness with a wide range of complications and symptoms.

As noted above, AIDS is the final stage of HIV infection, and not everyone who has HIV advances to this stage. People at this stage of HIV disease have badly damaged immune systems, which put them at risk for OIs.

Pathophysiology of Human Immunodeficiency Virus (Fig. 13.1)

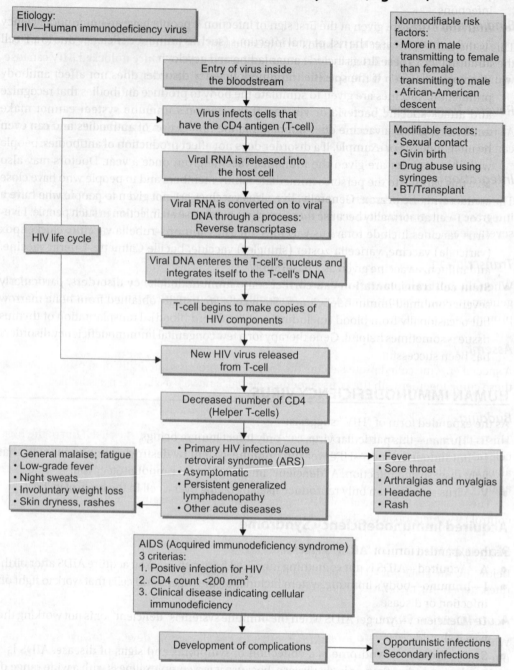

Etiology:
HIV—Human immunodeficiency virus

Nonmodifiable risk factors:
• More in male transmitting to female than female transmitting to male
• African-American descent

Entry of virus inside the bloodstream

Virus infects cells that have the CD4 antigen (T-cell)

Modifiable factors:
• Sexual contact
• Givin birth
• Drug abuse using syringes
• BT/Transplant

Viral RNA is released into the host cell

Viral RNA is converted on to viral DNA through a process: Reverse transcriptase

HIV life cycle

Viral DNA enteres the T-cell's nucleus and integrates itself to the T-cell's DNA

T-cell begins to make copies of HIV components

New HIV virus released from T-cell

Decreased number of CD4 (Helper T-cells)

• General malaise; fatigue
• Low-grade fever
• Night sweats
• Involuntary weight loss
• Skin dryness, rashes

• Primary HIV infection/acute retroviral syndrome (ARS)
• Asymptomatic
• Persistent generalized lymphadenopathy
• Other acute diseases

• Fever
• Sore throat
• Arthralgias and myalgias
• Headache
• Rash

AIDS (Acquired immunodeficiency syndrome)
3 criterias:
1. Positive infection for HIV
2. CD4 count <200 mm^2
3. Clinical disease indicating cellular immunodeficiency

Development of complications

• Opportunistic infections
• Secondary infections

Fig. 13.1: Pathophysiology of human immunodeficiency virus.

Cycle of Human Immunodeficiency Virus

Human immunodeficiency virus can infect multiple cells in body, including brain cells, but its main target is the CD4 lymphocyte, also called a T-cell or CD4 cell. When a CD4 cell is infected with HIV, the virus goes through multiple steps to reproduce itself and create many more virus particles.

The process is broken up into the following steps:

Binding and Fusion

This is the process by which HIV binds to a specific type of CD4 receptor and a coreceptor on the surface of the CD4 cell. This is similar to a key entering a lock. Once unlocked, HIV can fuse with the host cell (CD4 cell) and release its genetic material into the cell.

Reverse Transcription

A special enzyme called reverse transcriptase changes the genetic material of the virus, so it can be integrated into the host DNA.

Integration

The virus' new genetic material enters the nucleus of the CD4 cell and uses an enzyme called integrase to integrate itself into own genetic material, where it may "hide" and stay inactive for several years.

Transcription

When the host cell becomes activated, the virus uses its own enzymes to create more of its genetic material—along with a more specialized genetic material that allows it to make longer proteins.

Assembly

A special enzyme called protease cuts the longer HIV proteins into individual proteins. When these come together with the virus' genetic material, a new virus has been assembled.

Budding

This is the final stage of the virus' life cycle. In this stage, the virus pushes itself out of the host cell, taking with it part of the membrane of the cell. This outer part covers the virus and contains all of the structures necessary to bind to a new CD4 cell and receptors and begin the process again.

These steps of the life cycle of HIV are important to know because the medications used to control HIV infection act to interrupt this replication cycle.

Stages of Human Immunodeficiency Virus

Below are the stages of HIV infection. People may progress through these stages at different rates, depending on a variety of factors.

Acute Infection Stage

Within 2–4 weeks after HIV infection, many, but not all, people develop flu-like symptoms, often described as "the worst flu ever." Symptoms can include fever, swollen glands, sore throat, rash, muscle and joint aches and pains, fatigue, and headache. This is called "acute retroviral syndrome" (ARS) or "primary HIV infection," and it is the body's natural response to the HIV infection.

During this early period of infection, large amounts of virus are being produced in body. The virus uses CD4 cells to replicate and destroys them in the process. Because of this, CD4 count can fall rapidly. Eventually, immune response will begin to bring the level of virus in body back down to a level called a viral set point, which is a relatively stable level of virus in body. At this point, CD4 count begins to increase, but it may not return to preinfection levels. It may be particularly beneficial to health to begin antiretroviral therapy (ART) during this stage.

- It is important to be aware that you are at particularly high risk of transmitting HIV to your sexual or drug using partners during this stage because the levels of HIV in bloodstream are very high. For this reason, it is very important to take steps to reduce risk of transmission.

Clinical Latency Stage

After the acute stage of HIV infection, the disease moves into a stage called the "clinical latency" stage. "Latency" means a period where a virus is living or developing in a person without producing symptoms. During the clinical latency stage, people who are infected with HIV experience no HIV-related symptoms, or only mild ones. (This stage is sometimes called "asymptomatic HIV infection" or "chronic HIV infection.")

During the clinical latency stage, the HIV virus continues to reproduce at very low levels, although it is still active. If patient takes ART, he/she may live with clinical latency for several decades because treatment helps keep the virus in check. For people who are not on ART, the clinical latency stage lasts an average of 10 years, but some people may progress through this stage faster.

It is important to remember that people in this symptom-free stage are still able to transmit HIV to others, even if they are on ART, although ART greatly reduces the risk of transmission.

- If you have HIV and you are not on ART, then eventually your viral load will begin to rise and your CD4 count will begin to decline. As this happens, you may begin to have constitutional symptoms of HIV as the virus levels increase in your body.

Acquired Immunodeficiency Syndrome

This is the stage of HIV infection that occurs when immune system is badly damaged and becomes vulnerable to infections and infection-related cancers called OIs. When the number of CD4 cells falls below 200 cells per cubic millimeter of blood (200 cells/mm^3), you are considered to have progressed to AIDS. (In someone with a healthy immune system, CD4 counts are between 500 and 1,600 cells/mm^3).

- Without treatment, people who progress to AIDS typically survive about 3 years. Once you have a dangerous opportunistic illness, life-expectancy without treatment falls to about 1 year. However, if you are taking ART and maintain a low viral load, then you may enjoy a near normal life span. You will most likely never progress to AIDS.

Factor Affecting the Human Immunodeficiency Virus Progression

- People living with HIV may progress through these stages at different rates, depending on a variety of factors, including their genetic makeup, how healthy they were before they were infected, how soon after infection they are diagnosed and linked to care and treatment, whether they see their healthcare provider regularly and take their HIV medications as directed, and different health-related choices they make, such as decisions to eat a healthful diet, exercise, and not smoke.
- **Factors that may shorten the time between HIV and AIDS:**
    - Older age
    - HIV subtype
    - Coinfection with other viruses
    - Poor nutrition
    - Severe stress
    - Genetic background

- **Factors that may delay the time between HIV and AIDS:**
  - Taking ART
  - Staying in HIV care
  - Closely adhering to doctor's recommendations
  - Eating healthful foods
  - Taking care of yourself
  - Genetic background

Symptoms of Acute Infection

When a person first becomes infected with HIV, they are said to be in the acute stage of infection. The acute stage is a time when the virus is multiplying very rapidly. At this stage, the immune system actively tries to fight off the infection and body will show the following symptoms:

- Tiredness
- Weight loss
- Frequent fever and sweats
- Lymph node enlargement
- Yeast infections
- Persistent skin rashes or flaky skin

Symptoms of AIDS

Acquired immunodeficiency syndrome does not cause many symptoms itself. With AIDS, you will suffer symptoms from OIs. These are infections that take advantage of decreased immune function. Symptoms and signs of common OIs include:

- Dry cough or shortness of breath
- Difficult or painful swallowing
- Diarrhea lasting for more than a week
- White spots or unusual blemishes in and around the mouth
- Pneumonia-like symptoms
- Fever
- Vision loss
- Nausea, abdominal cramps, and vomiting
- Red, brown, pink, or purplish blotches on or under the skin or inside the mouth, nose, or eyelids
- Seizures or lack of coordination
- Neurological disorders, such as depression, memory loss, and confusion
- Severe headaches and neck stiffness
- Coma
- Development of various cancers

Opportunistic infections are signs of a declining immune system. Most life-threatening OIs occur when CD4 count is below 200 cells/mm³. Opportunistic infections are the most common cause of death for people with HIV/AIDS.

The centers for disease control and prevention (CDC) developed a list of more than 20 OIs that are considered AIDS-defining conditions—if one has HIV and one or more of these OIs, you will be diagnosed with AIDS, no matter what CD4 count happens to be:

- Candidiasis of bronchi, trachea, esophagus, or lungs
- Invasive cervical cancer
- Coccidioidomycosis
- Cryptococcosis
- Cryptosporidiosis, chronic intestinal (greater than 1 month's duration)

- CMV disease (particularly CMV retinitis)
- Encephalopathy, HIV related
- **Herpes simplex:** Chronic ulcer (greater than 1 month's duration), or bronchitis, pneumonitis, or esophagitis
- Histoplasmosis
- Isosporiasis, chronic intestinal (greater than 1 month's duration)
- Kaposi's sarcoma
- Lymphoma, multiple forms
- *Mycobacterium avium* complex (MAC)
- Tuberculosis
- *Pneumocystis carinii* pneumonia
- Pneumonia, recurrent
- Progressive multifocal leukoencephalopathy
- *Salmonella* septicemia, recurrent
- Toxoplasmosis of brain
- Wasting syndrome due to HIV

Opportunistic Infections Symptoms on the Basis of CD4 Count

Opportunistic infections can occur all over the body and be relatively **localized** or **systemic** or disseminated. Whether and when you become susceptible to OIs is often related to CD4 count.

Greater than 500 cells/mm³

Opportunistic Infections

In general, people with CD4 counts greater than 500 cells/mm³ are not at risk for OIs. For people with CD4 counts around 500, however, the daily fluctuations in CD4 cell levels can leave them vulnerable to minor infections, such as candidal vaginitis or yeast infections.

500–200 cells/mm³

Opportunistic infections

Candidiasis (thrush)

This is a fungal infection that is normally seen in patients with CD4 counts in this range. It is treatable with antifungal medications. A trained provider can usually diagnose thrush with a visual examination.

Kaposi's sarcoma

Kaposi's sarcoma is caused by Human Herpes Virus-8. Before the introduction of ART, as many as one in five patients with AIDS had KS. It can cause lesions on the body and in the mouth. In addition, this virus can affect internal organs and disseminate to other parts of the body without any external signs.

Symptoms

Oral symptoms include

- White patches on gums, tongue or lining of the mouth
- Pain in the mouth or throat
- Difficulty swallowing
- Loss of appetite

Vaginal symptoms include

- Vaginal irritation
- Itching

- Burning
- Thick, white discharge.

Signs and symptoms of KS can include

- Appearance of a purplish lesion on skin
- Appearance of a purplish lesion in the mouth
- Occasionally gastrointestinal complaints with disseminated KS

200–100 cells/mm³

Opportunistic infections

Pneumocystis jirovecii (carinii) pneumonia

Pneumocystis jirovecii (carinii) pneumonia is a fungal infection and is the OIs that most often cause death in patients with HIV. It is treatable with antibiotic therapy and close monitoring. If necessary, prophylaxis is available for patients who are at risk for PCP. Diagnosing PCP usually involves a hospital stay to ensure proper testing and treatment without complications.

Signs and symptoms of PCP can include:

- Shortness of breath
- Fever
- Dry cough
- Chest pain

Histoplasmosis and coccidioidomycosis

These are fungal infections. They often present as severe, disseminated illnesses in patients with low CD4 counts. Diagnosis consists of blood tests and evaluation for possible exposures related to geographical areas.

Signs and symptoms of histoplasmosis and coccidioidomycosis can include:

- Fever
- Fatigue
- Weight loss
- Cough
- Chest pain
- Shortness of breath
- Headache

Progressive multifocal leukoencephalopathy

Progressive multifocal leukoencephalopathy (PML) is a severe neurological condition and typically occurs in patients with CD4 counts below 200. While there is no definitive treatment for this disease, it has been shown to be responsive to ART. In some cases, the disease resolves without any treatment.

Signs and symptoms of PML can include:

- Dementia
- Seizures
- Difficulty speaking
- Confusion
- Difficulty walking

100–50 cells/mm³

Opportunistic infections

Toxoplasmosis

Toxoplasmosis is caused by the parasite Toxoplasma gondii that can cause encephalitis and neurological disease in patients with low CD4 counts. The parasite is carried by cats, birds, and other animals and is also found in soil contaminated by cat feces and in meat, particularly pork. Toxoplasmosis is treatable with aggressive therapy, and prophylaxis is recommended for patients with low CD4 counts (usually less than 200).

Signs and symptoms of toxoplasmosis can include:

- Headache
- Confusion
- Motor weakness
- Fever
- Seizures.

Cryptosporidiosis

Cryptosporidiosis is a diarrheal disease caused by the protozoa *Cryptosporidium*, and it can become chronic for people with low CD4 counts. Symptoms include abdominal cramps and severe chronic diarrhea. Infection with this parasite can occur through swallowing water that has been contaminated with fecal material (in swimming pools, lakes, or public water supplies); eating uncooked food (such as oysters) that are infected; or by person-to-person transmission, including changing diapers or exposure to feces during sexual contact.

Signs and symptoms of cryptosporidiosis can include:

- Chronic watery diarrhea
- Stomach cramps
- Weight loss
- Nausea
- Vomiting

Cryptococcal infection or cryptococcosis

Cryptococcal infection is caused by a fungus that typically enters the body through the lungs and can spread to the brain, causing cryptococcal meningitis. In some cases, it can also affect the skin, skeletal system, and urinary tract. This can be a very deadly infection if not caught and properly treated with antifungal medication. Although this infection is found primarily in the central nervous system, it can disseminate to other parts of the body, especially when a person has a CD4 count of less than 50.

Signs and symptoms of cryptococcal meningitis include:

- Fever
- Fatigue
- Headache
- Neck stiffness
- Some patients can have memory loss or mood changes.

50–100 cells/mm³

Opportunistic infections

Cytomegalovirus

Cytomegalovirus (CMV) is an extremely common virus that is present in all parts of the world. It is estimated that a majority of the population have had CMV by the time they are 40 years old. Cytomegalovirus can be transmitted by saliva, blood, semen, and other bodily fluids. It can cause mild illnesses when first contracted and many people may never have symptoms. However, it does not leave the body when someone is infected with CMV. In patients with HIV and low CD4 counts, it can cause infections in the eye and gastrointestinal system.

Signs and symptoms of CMV:

- Sore throat
- Swollen glands

- Fatigue
- Fevers

In people with low CD4 counts it can cause:
- Blurred vision (if there is CMV infection is in the eye)
- Painful swallowing
- Diarrhea
- Abdominal pain

Less than 50 cells/mm³

Opportunistic infections
Mycobacterium avium complex

Mycobacterium avium complex is a type of bacteria that can be found in soil, water, and many places in the environment. These bacteria can cause disease in people with HIV and CD4 counts less than 50. The bacteria can infect the lungs or the intestines, or in some cases, can become "disseminated." This means that it can spread to the bloodstream and other parts of the body. If this occurs, it can be a life-threatening infection.

Signs and symptoms of MAC:
- Fevers
- Night sweats
- Abdominal pain
- Fatigue
- Diarrhea

Diagnostic evaluation
- **Confirming diagnosis:** Signs and symptoms may occur at any time after infection, but AIDS is not officially diagnosed until the patient's CD4⁺ T-cell count falls below 200 cells/μL or associated clinical conditions or disease.
- **CBC:** Anemia and idiopathic thrombocytopenia (anemia occurs in up to 85% of patients with AIDS and may be profound). Leukopenia may be present; differential shift to the left suggests infectious process (PCP).
- **PPD:** Determines exposure or active TB disease. Of AIDS patients, 100% of those exposed to active *M. tuberculosis* will develop the disease.
- **Serologic:** Serum antibody test—HIV screen by ELISA. A positive test result may be indicative of exposure to HIV but is not diagnostic because false-positives may occur.
- **Western blot test:** It confirms diagnosis of HIV in blood and urine.
- **Viral load test:**
  - RI-PCR: The most widely used test currently can detect viral RNA levels as low as 50 copies/mL of plasma with an upper limit of 75,000 copies/mL.
  - bDNA 3.0 assay: Has a wider range of 50–500,000 copies/mL. Therapy can be initiated, or changes made in treatment approaches, based on rise of viral load or maintenance of a low viral load. This is currently the leading indicator of effectiveness of therapy.
  - T-lymphocyte cells: Total count reduced.
  - CD4⁺ lymphocyte count (immune system indicator that mediates several immune system processes and signals B cells to produce antibodies to foreign germs): Numbers less than 200 indicate severe immune deficiency response and diagnosis of AIDS.
  - T8⁺ CTL (cytopathic suppressor cells): Reversed ratio (2:1 or higher) of suppressor cells to helper cells (T8⁺–T4⁺) indicates immune suppression.
  - PCR test: It detects HIV-DNA; most helpful in testing newborns of HIV-infected mothers. Infants carry maternal HIV antibodies and therefore test positive by ELISA and Western blot, even though infant is not necessarily infected.

- **STD screening tests:** Hepatitis B envelope and core antibodies, syphilis, and other common STDs may be positive.
- **Cultures:** Histologic, cytologic studies of urine, blood, stool, spinal fluid, lesions, sputum, and secretions may be done to identify the OI.
- **Neurological studies:** For example, EEG, MRI, CT scans of the brain; EMG/nerve conduction studies. It indicated changes in mentation, fever of undetermined origin, and changes in sensory or motor function to determine effects of HIV infection or OIs.
- **Chest X-ray:** It may initially be normal or may reveal progressive interstitial infiltrates secondary to advancing PCP (most common opportunistic disease) or other pulmonary complications, such as TB.
- **Pulmonary function tests:** Useful in early detection of interstitial pneumonias.
- **Gallium scan:** Diffuse pulmonary uptake occurs in PCP and other forms of pneumonia.
- **Biopsies:** It may be done for differential diagnosis of KS or other neoplastic lesions.
- **Bronchoscopy or tracheobronchial washings:** It may be done with biopsy when PCP or lung malignancies are suspected.
- **Barium swallow, endoscopy, colonoscopy:** It may be done to identify OI (e.g., Candida, CMV) or to stage KS in the GI system.

Transmission of Human Immunodeficiency Virus

Certain body fluids from an HIV-infected person can transmit HIV.
These body fluids are:
- Blood
- Semen
- Preseminal fluid
- Rectal fluids
- Vaginal fluids
- Breast milk

These body fluids must come into contact with a mucous membrane or damaged tissue or be directly injected into bloodstream (by a needle or syringe) for transmission to possibly occur. Mucous membranes are the soft, moist areas just inside the openings to body. They can be found inside the rectum, the vagina or the opening of the penis, and the mouth.

How the Human Immunodeficiency Virus Spread?

Having sex with someone who has HIV. In general:
- Anal sex is the highest risk sexual behavior. Receptive anal sex (bottoming) is riskier than insertive anal sex (topping).
- Vaginal sex is the second highest risk sexual behavior.
- Having multiple sex partners or having sexually transmitted infections can increase the risk of HIV infection through sex.
- Sharing needles, syringes, rinse water, or other equipment (works) used to prepare injection drugs with someone who has HIV.

Less commonly, HIV may be spread by

- Being born to an infected mother. HIV can be passed from mother to child during pregnancy, birth, or breastfeeding.
- Being stuck with an HIV-contaminated needle or other sharp objects. This is a risk mainly for healthcare workers.
- Receiving blood transfusions, blood products, or organ transplants that are contaminated with HIV.

- Eating food that has been prechewed by an HIV-infected person. The contamination occurs when infected blood from a caregiver's mouth mixes with food while chewing and is very rare.
- Being bitten by a person with HIV. Each of the very small number of documented cases has involved severe trauma with extensive tissue damage and the presence of blood. There is no risk of transmission if the skin is not broken.
- Oral sex, giving fellatio (mouth to penis oral sex) and having the person ejaculate in mouth is riskier than other types of oral sex.
- Contact between broken skin, wounds, or mucous membranes and HIV-infected blood or blood-contaminated body fluids. These reports have also been extremely rare.
- Deep, open-mouth kissing if the person with HIV has sores or bleeding gums and blood is exchanged. HIV is not spread through saliva. Transmission through kissing alone is extremely rare.

HIV is not spread by

- Air or water
- Insects, including mosquitoes or ticks
- Saliva, tears, or sweat
- Casual contact, such as shaking hands, hugging or sharing dishes, drinking glasses
- Drinking fountains
- Toilet seats
  However, a person with HIV can still potentially transmit HIV to a partner even if they have an undetectable viral load, because:
- HIV may still be found in a person's genital fluids (e.g., semen, vaginal fluids). The viral load test only measures virus in a person's blood.
- A person's viral load may go up between tests. When this happens, they may be more likely to transmit HIV to partners.
- STDs increase viral load in a person's genital fluids.

Signs and Symptoms

The symptoms of HIV vary, depending on the individual and at what stage of the disease is in.

Early Stage

Within 2–4 weeks after HIV infection, many, but not all, people experience flu-like symptoms, often described as the "worst flu ever." This is called ARS or "primary HIV infection," and it is the body's natural response to the HIV infection.
Symptoms can include:

- Fever (this is the most common symptom)
- Swollen glands
- Sore throat
- Rash
- Fatigue
- Muscle and joint aches and pains
- Headache

These symptoms can last anywhere from a few days to several weeks.

Clinical Latency Stage

After the early stage of HIV infection, the disease moves into a stage called the "clinical latency" stage. "Latency" means a period where a virus is living or developing in a person without producing symptoms. During the clinical latency stage, people who are infected with HIV experience no HIV-related symptoms, or only mild ones. (This stage is sometimes called "asymptomatic HIV infection" or "chronic HIV infection").

During the clinical latency stage, the HIV virus reproduces at very low levels, although it is still active. If you take ART, you may live with clinical latency for several decades because treatment helps keep the virus in check.

- It is important to remember that people in this symptom-free period are still able to transmit HIV to others even if they are on ART, although ART greatly reduces the risk of transmission.

Progression from HIV to Aids Symptoms

The onset of symptoms signals the transition from the clinical latency stage to AIDS.

During this late stage of HIV infection, people infected with HIV may have the following symptoms:

- Rapid weight loss
- Recurring fever or profuse night sweats
- Extreme and unexplained tiredness
- Prolonged swelling of the lymph glands in the armpits, groin, or neck
- Diarrhea that lasts for more than a week
- Sores of the mouth, anus, or genitals
- Pneumonia
- Red, brown, pink, or purplish blotches on or under the skin or inside the mouth, nose, or eyelids
- Memory loss, depression, and other neurologic disorders.

Management and Prevention from Human Immunodeficiency Virus

There are several steps can be taken to reduce the risk of getting HIV through sexual contact, and the more of these actions you take, the safer you can be. These actions include:

- **Choosing less risky sexual behaviors:** Oral sex is much less risky than anal or vaginal sex. Anal sex is the highest risk sexual activity for HIV transmission. HIV can be sexually transmitted via blood, semen, preseminal fluid, rectal fluid, and vaginal fluid. Sexual activities that do not involve the potential exchange of these bodily fluids (e.g., touching) carry no risk for getting HIV.
- **Using condoms consistently and correctly:** When used consistently and correctly, condoms are highly effective in preventing HIV.
- **Reducing the number of sexual partners:** The number of sex partners can affect HIV risk. The more partners you have, the more likely you are to have a partner with HIV whose viral load is not suppressed or to have a sex partner with a STD. Both of these factors can increase the risk of HIV transmission.
- **Talking to doctor about preexposure prophylaxis (PrEP):** PrEP is taking HIV medicine daily to prevent HIV infection. PrEP should be considered if you are HIV-negative and in an ongoing sexual relationship with an HIV-positive partner. PrEP also should be considered if you are HIV negative and have had a STD or any anal sex (receptive or insertive) with a male partner without condoms in the past 6 months and are not in an exclusive relationship with a recently tested, HIV-negative partner.
- **Talking to doctor right away (within 3 days) about postexposure prophylaxis (PEP) if you have a possible exposure to HIV**: An example of a possible exposure is if you have anal or vaginal sex without a condom with someone who is or may be HIV positive and you are HIV negative and not taking PrEP. Your chance of exposure to HIV is lower if your HIV-

positive partner is taking ART consistently and correctly, especially if his/her viral load is undetectable. Starting PEP immediately and taking it daily for 4 weeks reduces the chance of getting HIV.
- Get tested and treated for other STDs and encourage your partners to do the same.

Management of Human Immunodeficiency Virus

Preexposure Prophylaxis

The word "prophylaxis" means "to prevent or control the spread of an infection or disease." PrEP is a way for people who do not have HIV to prevent HIV infection by taking a pill every day. The pill contains two medicines that are also used to treat HIV. If you take PrEP and are exposed to HIV through sex or injection drug use, these medicines can work to keep the virus from taking hold in body.

Along with other prevention methods, such as condoms, PrEP can offer good protection against HIV if taken every day.

Postexposure Prophylaxis

Postexposure prophylaxis involves taking anti-HIV medications as soon as possible after being exposed to HIV to reduce the chance of becoming HIV positive. These medications keep HIV from making copies of itself and spreading through body.

There are two types of PEP:

1. **Occupational PEP** (oPEP), taken when someone working in a healthcare setting is potentially exposed to material infected with HIV.
2. **Non-occupational PEP**, taken when someone is potentially exposed to HIV outside the workplace (e.g., from sexual assault, or during episodes of unprotected sex or needle-sharing injection drug use).

   To be effective, PEP must begin within 72 hours of exposure, before the virus has time to make too many copies of itself in body. PEP consists of two to three ARV medications and should be taken for 28 days. PEP is not 100% effective; it does not guarantee that someone exposed to HIV will not become infected with HIV.
3. **ART:** In 1987, a drug called ART became the first approved treatment for HIV disease. Since then, approximately 30 drugs have been approved to treat people living with HIV/AIDS.
   It includes:
   - **"The cocktail"**
   - **ARVs**
   - **Highly active ART**

Each HIV medication is pretty powerful by itself—and the key to treating HIV disease successfully is to pick the right combination of drugs from the different classes of HIV medicines. Antiretrovirals are separated into different classes. The classes include:

1. **Nucleoside or nucleotide reverse transcriptase inhibitors (NRTIs):** Sometimes called "nukes." These drugs work to block a very important step in HIV's reproduction process. Nukes act as faulty building blocks in production of viral DNA production. This blocks HIV's ability to use a special type of enzyme (reverse transcriptase) to correctly build new genetic material (DNA) that the virus needs to make copies of itself. For example, lamivudine, zidovudine, emtricitabine, and abacavir.
2. **Non-NRTIs (NNRTIs):** These are called "nonnukes." They work in a very similar way to "nukes." Nonnukes also block the enzyme, reverse transcriptase, and prevent HIV from making copies of its own DNA. But unlike the nukes (which work on the genetic material),

nonnukes act directly on the enzyme itself to prevent it from functioning correctly. For example, delavirdine, efavirenz, rilpivirine, and etravirine.

3. **Protease inhibitors (PIs):** When HIV replicates inside cells, it creates long strands of its own genetic material. These long strands have to be cut into shorter strands in order for HIV to create more copies of itself. The enzyme that acts to cut up these long strands is called protease. Protease inhibitors (stoppers) block this enzyme and prevent those long strands of genetic material from being cut up into functional pieces. For example, amprenavir, saquinavir, indinavir, and tipranavir.

4. **Entry or fusion inhibitors:** These medications block the virus from entering in cells. HIV needs a way to attach and bond to CD4 cells, and it does that through special structures on cells called receptor sites. Receptor sites are found on both HIV and CD4 cells. Fusion inhibitors can target those sites on either HIV or CD4 cells and prevent HIV from "docking" into healthy cells. For example, enfuvirtide, T-20, and maraviroc.

5. **Integrase inhibitors:** HIV uses cells' genetic material to make its own DNA (a process called reverse transcription). Once that happens, the virus has to integrate its genetic material into the genetic material of body cells. This is accomplished by an enzyme called integrase. Integrase inhibitors block this enzyme and prevent the virus from adding its DNA into the DNA of CD4 cells. Preventing this process prevents the virus from replicating and making new viruses. For example, raltegravir and dolutegravir.

6. **Fixed-dose combinations:** These are not a separate class of HIV medications but combinations of the above classes and a great advancement in HIV medicine. They include ARVs which are combinations of two or more medications from one or more different classes. These ARVs are combined into **one single pill** with specific fixed doses of these medicines. For example, efavirenz, emtricitabine, tenofovir, disoproxil, and fumarate.

Nursing Management

Following are the list of nursing management:

Nursing priorities
- Preventing or minimizing development of new infections
- Maintaining homeostasis
- Promoting comfort
- Supporting psychosocial adjustment
- Providing information about disease process, prognosis, and treatment needs.

Discharge goals
- Infection prevented and resolved
- Complications prevented and minimized
- Pain and discomfort alleviated or controlled
- Patient dealing with current situation realistically
- Diagnosis, prognosis, and therapeutic regimen understood
- Planning in place of meeting needs after discharge

Nursing Diagnosis

1. Imbalanced nutrition
Less than body requirements related to inability or altered ability to ingest, digest metabolize nutrients, nausea, vomiting, hyperactive gag reflex, intestinal disturbances, GI tract infections, fatigue.

Possibly evidenced by
- Weight loss, decreased subcutaneous fat or muscle mass
- Lack of interest in food, aversion to eating, altered taste sensation
- Abdominal cramping, hyperactive bowel sounds, diarrhea
- Sore, inflamed buccal cavity
- **Abnormal laboratory results:** Vitamin, mineral and protein deficiencies, electrolyte imbalances.

Desired outcomes
- Maintaining weight or display weight gain toward desired goal.
- Demonstrating positive nitrogen balance, be free of signs of malnutrition, and display improved energy level.

Interventions
- Assessing patient's ability to chew, taste, and swallow.
- Auscultating bowel sounds
- Weighing as indicated. Evaluating weight in terms of premorbid weight. Comparing serial weights and anthropometric measurements.
- Noting drug side effects
- Planning diet with patient, suggesting foods from home if appropriate. Providing small, frequent meals and snacks of nutritionally dense foods and nonacidic foods and beverages, with choice of foods palatable to patient. Encouraging high-calorie and nutritious foods, some of which may be considered appetite stimulants. Noting time of day when appetite is best, and trying to serve larger meal at that time.
- Limiting food that induces nausea and vomiting is poorly tolerated by patient because of mouth sores or dysphagia. Avoiding serving very hot liquids and foods. Serving foods that are easy to swallow, such as eggs, ice cream, cooked vegetables.
- Scheduling medications between meals (if tolerated) and limiting fluid intake with meals, unless fluid has nutritional value.
- Encouraging as much physical activity as possible.
- Providing frequent mouth care, observing secretion precautions. Avoiding alcohol-containing mouthwashes.
- Providing rest period before meals. Avoiding stressful procedures close to mealtime.
- Removing existing noxious environmental stimuli or conditions that aggravate gag reflex.
- Encouraging patient to sit up for meals.
- Recording ongoing caloric intake.
- Administer, **appetite stimulants**: Dronabinol, megestrol, oxandrolone; **Antibiotic therapy:** Ketoconazole, fluconazole; **Antidiarrheals:** Diphenoxylate, loperamide, octreotide.

2. Fatigue
Fatigue relates to decreased metabolic energy production, increased energy requirements or hypermetabolic state or altered body chemistry: Side effects of medication, chemotherapy
Possibly evidenced by
- Unremitting lack of energy, inability to maintain usual routines, decreased performance, impaired ability to concentrate, lethargy
- Disinteresting surroundings

Desired outcomes
- Reporting improved sense of energy
- Performing activities daily living (ADLs), with assistance as necessary
- Participating in desired activities at level of ability

Intervention
- Assessing sleep patterns and note changes in thought processes and behavior.
- Recommending scheduling activities for periods when patient has the most energy. Planning care to allow for rest periods. Involving patient in schedule planning.
- Establishing realistic activity goals with patient.
- Encouraging patient to do whatever possible: Self-care, sit in chair, short walks. Increasing activity level as indicated.
- **Identifying energy conservation techniques:** Sitting, breaking ADLs into manageable segments. Keeping travel ways clear of furniture. Providing or assisting with ambulation and self-care needs as appropriate.
- **Monitoring physiological response to activity:** Changes in blood pressure (BP), respiratory rate, or heart rate
- Encouraging nutritional intake.
- Referring to physical and occupational therapy
- Providing supplemental O_2 as indicated

3. Acute or chronic pain
Acute or chronic pain related to tissue inflammation, infections, internal or external cutaneous lesions, rectal excoriation, malignancies, necrosis.
Possibly evidenced by
- Reports of pain
- Self-focusing, narrowed focus, guarding behaviors
- Alteration in muscle tone; muscle cramping, ataxia, muscle weakness, paresthesias, paralysis
- Autonomic responses; restlessness

Desired outcomes
- Reporting pain relieved or controlled
- Demonstrating relaxed posture or facial expression
- Be able to sleep or rest appropriately

Interventions
- Assessing pain reports, noting location, intensity (0–10 scale), frequency, and time of onset. Note nonverbal cues, such as restlessness, tachycardia, grimacing.
- Instructing and encouraging patient to report pain as it develops rather than waiting until level is severe.
- Encouraging verbalization of feelings
- **Providing diversional activities:** Providing reading materials, light exercising, visiting, etc.
- **Performing palliative measures:** Repositioning, massage, range of motion (ROM) of affected joints.
- Instructing and encouraging the use of visualization, guided imagery, progressive relaxation, deep-breathing techniques, meditation, and mindfulness.
- Applying warm or moist packs to pentamidine injection and IV sites for 20 minutes after administration.
- Administering analgesics or antipyretics, narcotic analgesics. Using patient-controlled analgesia.

4. Impaired skin integrity
Impaired skin integrity related to decreased level of activity, altered sensation, skeletal prominence, changes in skin turgor.
- **Immunologic deficit:** AIDS-related dermatitis; viral, bacterial, and fungal infections (e.g., herpes, *Pseudomonas*, *Candida*); opportunistic disease processes.

Possibly evidenced by
Skin lesions; ulcerations; decubitus ulcer formation.

Desired outcomes
- Improvement in wound or lesion healing
- Demonstrate behaviors or techniques to prevent skin breakdown and promote healing.

Interventions
- Assessing skin daily. Noting color, turgor, circulation, and sensation.
- Describing and measuring lesions and observing changes. Taking photographs if necessary.
- Maintaining and instructing in good skin hygiene: Washing thoroughly, patting dry carefully, and gently massaging with lotion or appropriate cream.
- Reposition frequently. Using turn sheet as needed.
- Encouraging periodic weight shifts. Protecting bony prominences with pillows, heel, and elbow pads.
- Encouraging ambulation as tolerated.
- Cleansing perianal area by removing stool with water and mineral oil or commercial product.
- Avoiding use of toilet paper if vesicles are present. Applying protective creams: Zinc oxide, A and D ointment.
- Filing nails regularly
- Covering open pressure ulcers with sterile dressings or protective barrier: Tegaderm, DuoDerm, as indicated.
- Providing foam, flotation, alternate pressure mattress or bed.
- Obtaining cultures of open skin lesions.
- Applying and administering medications as indicated.

5. Impaired oral mucous membrane
Impaired oral mucous membrane related to immunologic deficit and presence of lesion-causing pathogens, dehydration, malnutrition, ineffective oral hygiene and side effects of drugs, chemotherapy.

Possibly evidenced by
- Open ulcerated lesions, vesicles
- Oral pain or discomfort
- Stomatitis; leukoplakia, gingivitis, carious teeth

Desired outcomes
- Displaying intact mucous membranes, which are pink, moist, and free of inflammation and ulcerations.
- Demonstrating techniques to maintain integrity of oral mucosa.

Intervention
- Assessing mucous membranes and document all oral lesions. Noting reports of pain, swelling, difficulty with chewing and swallowing.
- Providing oral care daily and after food intake, using soft toothbrush, nonabrasive toothpaste, nonalcohol mouthwash, floss, and lip moisturizer.
- Rinsing oral mucosal lesions with saline and dilute hydrogen peroxide or baking soda solutions.
- Suggesting use of sugarless gum and candy.
- Encouraging oral intake of at least 2,500 mL/day.
- Encouraging patient to refrain from smoking.
- Obtaining culture specimens of lesions.

- Administering medications, as indicated: Nystatin, ketoconazole.
- Referring for dental consultation, if appropriate.
- Planning diet to avoid salty, spicy, abrasive, and acidic foods or beverages. Checking for temperature tolerance of foods. Offer cool or cold smooth foods.

6. Disturbed thought process

Disturbed thought process related to hypoxemia, central nervous system (CNS) infection by HIV, brain malignancies and disseminated systemic OI.

Possibly evidenced by
- Altered attention span and distractibility
- Memory deficit
- Disorientation, cognitive dissonance, delusional thinking
- Sleep disturbances

Desired outcomes

Maintaining usual reality orientation and optimal cognitive functioning.

Intervention
- Assessing mental and neurological status using appropriate tools.
- Considering effects of emotional distress. Assessing for anxiety, grief, and anger.
- Monitoring medication regimen and usage.
- Investigating changes in personality, response to stimuli, orientation, and level of consciousness or development of headache, nuchal rigidity, vomiting, fever, seizure activity.
- Maintaining a pleasant environment with appropriate auditory, visual, and cognitive stimuli.
- Providing reorientation by putting on radio, television, calendars, clocks, room with an outside view if necessary. Using patient's name. Identifying yourself. Maintaining consistent personnel and structured schedules as appropriate.
- Encouraging family to socialize and provide reorientation with current news, family events.
- Encouraging patient to do as much as possible: Dress and groom daily, see friends, and so forth.
- Discussing use of datebooks, lists, and other devices to keep track of activities.
- Encouraging discussion of concerns and fears.
- Providing information about care on an ongoing basis. Answering questions simply and honestly. Repeating explanations as needed.
- Reducing provocative and noxious stimuli. Maintaining bed rest in a quiet, darkened room, if indicated.
- Decreasing noise, especially at night
- Discussing causes or future expectations and treatment if dementia is diagnosed.
- **Maintaining safe environment:** Excess furniture out of the way, call bell within patient's reach, bed in low position and rails up, restriction of smoking, seizure precautions, etc.

7. Anxiety and fear

Anxiety and fear related to threat to self-concept, threat of death, and change in health, separation from support system and fear of transmission of the disease to family and loved ones.

Possibly evidenced by
- Increased tension, apprehension and feelings of helplessness and hopelessness
- Expressed concern regarding changes in life
- Fear of unspecific consequences
- Somatic complaints, insomnia, sympathetic stimulation, and restlessness

Desired outcomes
- Verbalizing awareness of feelings and healthy ways to deal with them
- Displaying appropriate range of feelings and lessened fear and anxiety
- Demonstrating problem-solving skills
- Using resources effectively

Intervention
- Assuring patient of confidentiality within limits of situation.
- Maintaining frequent contact with patient. Talking with and touch patient. Limiting use of isolation clothing and masks.
- Providing accurate, consistent information regarding prognosis. Avoiding arguing about patient's perceptions of the situation.
- Be alert to signs of withdrawal, anger, or inappropriate remarks as these can be signs of in denial or depression. Determining presence of suicidal ideation and assessing potential on a scale of 1–10.
- Providing open environment in which patient feels safe to discuss feelings or to refrain from talking.
- Permitting expressions of anger, fear, despair without confrontation. Giving information that feelings are normal and are to be appropriately expressed.
- Recognizing and supporting the stage patient and family is in the grieving process.
- Explaining procedures, providing opportunity for questions and honest answers. Arranging for someone to stay with patient during anxiety-producing procedures and consultations.
- Identifying and encouraging patient interaction with support systems. Encouraging verbalization and interaction with family.
- Discussing advance directives and end-of-life desires or needs. Reviewing specific wishes and explaining various options clearly.
- **Providing contact with other resources as indicated:** Spiritual advisor or hospice staff
- Referring to psychiatric counseling (psychiatric clinical nurse specialist, psychiatrist, social worker).

8. Social isolation
Social isolation related to altered state of wellness, changes in physical appearance, alterations in mental status, perceptions of unacceptable social or sexual behavior and values.
Possibly evidenced by
- Expressed feeling of aloneness imposed by others and feelings of rejection
- Absence of support from partner, family, acquaintances, and friends

Desired outcomes
- Identifying supportive individual
- Using resources for assistance
- Participating in activities

Intervention
- Ascertaining patient's perception of situation
- Spending time talking with patient during and between care activities. Be supportive, allowing for verbalization. Treating with dignity and regard for patient's feelings.
- Limiting or avoiding use of mask, gown, and gloves when possible and when talking to patient.
- Identifying support systems available to patient, including presence of and relationship with immediate and extended family.
- Explaining isolation precautions and procedures to patient and family.

- Encouraging open visitation, telephone contacts, and social activities within tolerated level.
- **Developing a plan of action with patient:** Look at available resources, support healthy behaviors.
- Helping patient problem-solve solution to short-term or imposed isolation.
- **Be alert to verbal or nonverbal cues:** Withdrawal, statements of despair, sense of aloneness. Asking patient if thoughts of suicide are being entertained.

9. Powerlessness

Powerlessness related to confirmed diagnosis of a potentially terminal disease, incomplete grieving process, social ramifications of AIDS, and alteration in body image.

Possibly evidenced by

- Feelings of loss of control over own life
- Depression over physical deterioration that occurs despite patient compliance with regimen
- Anger, apathy, withdrawal, passivity
- Dependence on others for care/decision making, resulting in resentment, anger, guilt.

Desired outcomes

- Acknowledging feelings and healthy ways to deal with them
- Verbalizing some sense of control over present situation
- Making choices related to care and be involved in self-care

Intervention

- Identifying factors that contribute to patient's feelings of powerlessness: Diagnosis of a terminal illness, lack of support systems, and lack of knowledge about present situation.
- Assessing degree of feelings of helplessness: Verbal or nonverbal expressions indicating lack of control, flat affect, and lack of communication.
- Encourage active role in planning activities, establishing realistic and attainable daily goals.
- Encouraging patient control and responsibility as much as possible. Identifying things that patient can and cannot control.
- Encouraging living will and durable medical power of attorney documents, with specific and precise instructions regarding acceptable and unacceptable procedures to prolong life.
- Discussing desires and assisting with planning for funeral as appropriate.

10. Deficient knowledge

Deficient knowledge related to lack of exposure, information misinterpretation, cognitive limitation, and unfamiliarity with information resources

Possibly evidenced by

- Questions and request for information
- Inaccurate follow-through of instructions, development of preventable complications

Desired outcomes

- Verbalizing understanding of condition and disease process and potential complications
- Identifying relationship of signs and symptoms to the disease process and correlate symptoms with causative factors
- Verbalizing understanding of therapeutic needs
- Correctly performing necessary procedures and explain reasons for actions
- Initiating necessary lifestyle changes and participate in treatment regimen.

Intervention

- Reviewing disease process and future expectations.
- Determining level of independence or dependence and physical condition. Noting extent of care and support available from family and need for other caregivers.

- Reviewing modes of transmission of disease, especially if newly diagnosed.
- Instructing patient and caregivers concerning infection control, using good handwashing techniques for everyone (patient, family, caregivers), using gloves when handling bedpans, dressings or soiled linens, wearing mask if patient has productive cough, placing soiled or wet linens in plastic bag and separating from family laundry, washing with detergent and hot water, cleaning surfaces with bleach and water solution of 1:10 ratio, disinfecting toilet bowl and bedpan with full-strength bleach, preparing patient's food in clean area, washing dishes and utensils in hot soapy water.
- Stressing necessity of daily skincare, including inspecting skin folds, pressure points, and perineum, and of providing adequate cleansing and protective measures—ointments, padding.
- Ascertaining that patient can perform necessary oral and dental care. Reviewing procedures as indicated. Encouraging regular dental care.
- Reviewing dietary needs (high-protein and high-calorie) and ways to improve intake when anorexia, diarrhea, weakness, depression interfere with intake.
- Discussing medication regimen, interactions, and side effects
- Providing information about symptom management that complements medical regimen with intermittent diarrhea; taking diphenoxylate before going to social event.
- Stressing importance of adequate rest
- Encouraging activity and exercise at level that patient can tolerate
- Stressing necessity of continued healthcare and follow-up
- Recommending cessation of smoking
- Identifying signs and symptoms requiring medical evaluation: Persistent fever and night sweats, swollen glands, continued weight loss, diarrhea, skin blotches and lesions, headache, chest pain, and dyspnea.
- **Identifying community resources:** Hospice and residential care centers, visiting nurse, home care services, meals on wheels, peer group support.

11. Risk for injury
Risk for injury related to abnormal blood profile; decreased vitamin K absorption; alteration in hepatic function; and presence of autoimmune antiplatelet antibodies, malignancies, and circulating endotoxins.

Desired outcomes
Displaying homeostasis as evidenced by absence of bleeding.

Intervention
- Avoiding injections, rectal temperatures, and rectal tubes. Administering rectal suppositories with caution.
- Maintaining a safe environment. Keeping all necessary objects and call bell within patient's reach and place bed in low position.
- Maintaining bed rest or chair rest when platelets are below 10,000 or as individually appropriate.
- **Hematest body fluids:** Urine, stool, vomitus, for occult blood
- Observing for or report epistaxis, hemoptysis, hematuria, nonmenstrual vaginal bleeding, or oozing from lesions or body orifices or IV insertion sites.
- **Monitoring for changes in vital signs and skin color:** BP, pulse, respirations, skin pallor, and discoloration.
- Evaluating change in level of consciousness.
- Avoiding use of aspirin products and NSAIDs, especially in the presence of gastric lesions.
- Administering blood products as indicated.

- Reviewing laboratory studies: Partial thromboplastin (PT), activated partial thromboplastin time (aPTT), clotting time, platelets, Hb/Hct.

12. Risk for deficient fluid volume

Risk for deficient fluid volume related to copious diarrhea, profuse sweating, vomiting, and hypermetabolic state.

Desired outcomes

- Maintaining hydration as evidenced by moist mucous membranes, good skin turgor, stable vital signs, and individually adequate urinary output.

Intervention

- Monitoring vital signs, including central venous pressure (CVP) if available. Noting hypotension, including postural changes.
- Noting temperature elevation and duration of febrile episode. Administering tepid sponge baths as indicated. Keeping clothing and linens dry.
- Maintaining comfortable environmental temperature
- Assessing skin turgor, mucous membranes, and thirst
- Measuring urinary output and specific gravity. Measuring and estimating amount of diarrheal loss.
- Weighing as indicated
- Monitoring oral intake and encourage fluids of at least 2500 mL/day
- Making fluids easily accessible to patient; using fluids that are tolerable to patient and that replace needed electrolytes.
- Eliminating foods potentiating diarrhea
- Encouraging use of live culture yogurt or *Lactobacillus acidophilus*
- Administering fluids and electrolytes via feeding tube and IV, as appropriate.
- **Monitoring laboratory studies as indicated:** Serum or urine electrolytes; blood urea nitrogen (BUN), stool specimen collection.
- Maintaining hypothermia blanket, if used.

13. Risk for infection

Risk for infection related to inadequate primary defenses: Broken skin, traumatized tissue, stasis of body fluids, depression of the immune system, chronic disease, environmental exposure and invasive techniques.

Desired outcomes:

- Achieving timely healing of wounds
- Be afebrile and free of purulent drainage or secretions and other signs of infectious conditions
- Identifying participate in behaviors to reduce risk of infection

Intervention

- Assessing patient knowledge and ability to maintain OI prophylactic regimen
- Washing hands before and after all care contacts. Instructing patient and family to wash hands as indicated.
- Providing a clean, well-ventilated environment. Screening visitors and staff for signs of infection and maintaining isolation precautions as indicated.
- Discussing extent and rationale for isolation precautions and maintenance of personal hygiene.
- Monitoring vital signs, including temperature.

- Assessing respiratory rate and depth, noting dry spasmodic cough on deep inspiration, changes in characteristics of sputum, and presence of wheezes or rhonchi. Initiating respiratory isolation when etiology of productive cough is unknown.
- Investigating reports of headache, stiff neck, and altered vision. Noting changes in mentation and behavior. Monitoring for nuchal rigidity and seizure activity.
- Examining skin and oral mucous membranes for white patches or lesions.
- Cleaning patient's nails frequently. Filing, rather than cutting, and avoiding trimming cuticles.
- Monitoring reports of heartburn, dysphagia, and retrosternal pain on swallowing, increased abdominal cramping, and profuse diarrhea.
- Inspect wounds and site of invasive devices, noting signs of local inflammation and infection.
- Wearing gloves and gowns during direct contact with secretions and excretions or any time there is a break in skin of caregiver's hands. Wearing mask and protective eyewear to protect nose, mouth, and eyes from secretions during procedures (suctioning) or when splattering of blood may occur.
- Disposing of needles and sharps in rigid, puncture-resistant containers.
- Labeling blood bags, body fluid containers, soiled dressings and linens, and package appropriately for disposal per isolation protocol.
- Cleaning up spills of body fluids and blood with bleach solution (1:10), add bleach to laundry.

MULTIPLE CHOICE QUESTIONS

1. **To which of the following disease HIV virus leads to:**
   A. Cancer
   B. Brain tumor
   C. AIDS
   D. Hepatitis

2. **What is the full form of HIV?**
   A. Human immunodeficiency virus
   B. Human immunodeficiency vessels
   C. Health interexchange virus
   D. Health immunodeficiency virus

3. **Which cells are destroyed by HIV?**
   A. A-helper cells
   B. K-helper cells
   C. T-helper cells
   D. Y-helper cells

4. **HIV is spread by mosquitoes.**
   A. True
   B. False

Answers

1. C   2. A   3. C   4. B

Communicable Disorders

TUBERCULOSIS

TB is an infectious bacterial disease caused by *Mycobacterium tuberculosis*, which most commonly affects the lungs. It is transmitted from person to person via droplets from the throat and lungs of people with the active respiratory disease.

Etiology

- *M. tuberculosis*
- Immunocompromised person
- Chemical industries

Risk Factor

- Aging
- Alcoholism
- Crowded living conditions

- Diseases that weaken the immune system
- Healthcare workers
- Human immunodeficiency virus (HIV) infection
- Homelessness
- Low socioeconomic status
- Malnutrition, migration from a country with a high number of cases
- Nursing homes
- Unhealthy immune system

Types

1. **Pulmonary TB:** If a TB infection does become active, it most commonly involves the lungs (in about 90% of cases). Symptoms may include chest pain and a prolonged cough producing sputum.
2. **Extrapulmonary TB:** In 15–20% of active cases, the infection spreads outside the lungs, causing other kinds of TB. These are collectively denoted as "extrapulmonary TB." Extrapulmonary TB occurs more commonly in immunosuppressed persons and young children.
3. **Active TB:** Active TB means the bacteria are active in the body. The immune system is unable to stop these bacteria from causing illness. People with active TB in their lungs can pass the bacteria on to anyone they come into close contact with. When a person with active TB coughs, sneezes or spits, people nearby may breathe in the TB bacteria and become infected.
4. **Inactive TB:** Inactive TB infection is also called latent TB. If a person has latent TB, it means their body has been able to successfully fight the bacteria and stop them from causing illness. People who have latent TB do not feel sick, do not have symptoms, and cannot spread TB.

Pathophysiology

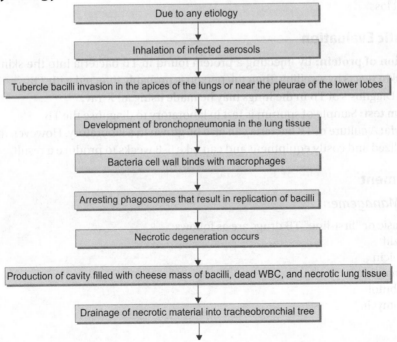

Due to any etiology

↓

Inhalation of infected aerosols

↓

Tubercle bacilli invasion in the apices of the lungs or near the pleurae of the lower lobes

↓

Development of bronchopneumonia in the lung tissue

↓

Bacteria cell wall binds with macrophages

↓

Arresting phagosomes that result in replication of bacilli

↓

Necrotic degeneration occurs

↓

Production of cavity filled with cheese mass of bacilli, dead WBC, and necrotic lung tissue

↓

Drainage of necrotic material into tracheobronchial tree

↓

Contd...

Contd...

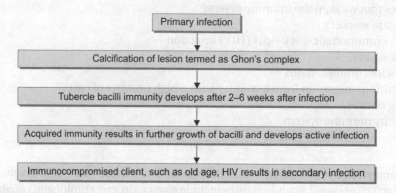

Signs and Symptoms

- A cough lasting for more than 2–3 weeks
- Chest pain
- Chills
- Discolored or bloody sputum
- Fatigue
- Loss of appetite
- Night sweats
- Pain with breathing
- Severe headache
- Shortness of breath
- Slight fever
- Tiredness or weakness
- Weight loss

Diagnostic Evaluation

- **Injection of protein:** By injecting a protein found in TB bacteria into the skin of an arm. If the skin reacts by swelling, then the person is probably infected with TB.
- **X-ray:** Diagnosis of TB in the lungs may be made using an X-ray.
- **Sputum test:** Sample of sputum is test in laboratory to diagnose the TB.
- **Bacteria:** A culture of TB bacteria can also be grown in a laboratory. However, this requires specialized and costly equipment and can take 6–8 weeks to produce a result.

Management

Medical Management

The five basic or "first-line" TB drugs are as follows:
- Isoniazid
- Rifampicin
- Pyrazinamide
- Ethambutol
- Streptomycin

Surgery

If medications are ineffective, there are three surgical treatments for pulmonary TB:

- Pneumothorax, in which air is introduced into the chest to collapse the lung
    - Thoracoplasty, in which one or more ribs are removed
    - Removal of a diseased lung

Nursing Care Plan

Goals

The goal of management is:
- To control the inflammatory process
- To relieve symptoms
- To correct metabolic and nutritional problems and promote healing
- To achieve the previous health status

Nursing Assessment

- Promoting airway clearance
    - Advocating adherence to treatment regimen
    - Promoting activity and adequate nutrition
    - Preventing spreading of TB infection

Nursing Diagnosis

- Ineffective airway clearance related to increased sputum
- Risk for infection related to lower resistance of others who are around people
- Ineffective breathing pattern related to inflammation
- Hyperthermia related to the infection process
- Fluid volume deficit related to fatigue due to lack of fluid intake
- Activity intolerance related to fatigue
- Imbalanced nutrition, less than body requirements related to decreased appetite
- Ineffective management therapeutic regimen related to lack of knowledge about the disease process
- Impaired gas exchange related to alveoli function decline

Intervention

Ineffective airway clearance

- Auscultating lungs for wheezing, decreased breath sounds, coarse sounds
- Using universal precautions if secretions are purulent even before culture reports
- Assessing cough for effectiveness and productivity
- Noting sputum amount, color, odor, consistency
- Sending sputum specimens for culture as prescribed
- Instituting appropriate isolation precautions if cultures are positive
- Using humidity to help loosen sputum
- Administering medications, noting effectiveness, and side effects
- Teaching effective deep breathing and coughing techniques

Risk for infection

- Monitoring sputum for changes indicating infection
- Monitoring vital signs
- Teaching patient and family the purpose and techniques for infection control, such as handwashing, patient covering mouth when coughs, maintaining isolation if necessary

- Teaching patient the purpose, importance, and how to take medications as prescribed consistently over the long-term therapy.

Deficient knowledge
- Determining who will be the learner, patient, or family
- Assessing ability to learn
- Identifying any existing misconceptions about the material to learn
- Assisting the learner to integrate the information into daily life
- Giving clear thorough explanations and demonstrations

Activity intolerance
- Assessing patient's level of mobility
- Observing and documenting response to activity
- Assessing emotional response to change in physical status
- Anticipating patient's needs to accommodate
- Teaching energy conservation techniques
- Referring to community resources as needed.

Ineffective therapeutic regimen management
- Assessing prior efforts to follow regimen
- Assessing patient's perceptions of their health problem
- Assessing other factors that may affect success in a negative way
- Informing patient of the benefits of conforming with the regimen
- Concentrating on the behaviors that will make the most difference to the therapeutic effect
- Including family, support system in teachings, and explanations.

Health Education

- Explaining about the disease condition causes and risk factors
- Using universal precautions if secretions are purulent even before culture reports
- Assessing cough for effectiveness and productivity
- Noting sputum amount, color, odor, consistency
- Sending sputum specimens for culture as prescribed or prn
- Instituting appropriate isolation precautions if cultures are positive
- Using humidity to help loosen sputum
- Administering medications, noting effectiveness and side effects
- Assessing patient's perceptions of their health problem
- Assessing other factors that may affect success in a negative way
- Informing patient of the benefits of conforming with the regimen
- Concentrating on the behaviors that will make the most difference to the therapeutic effect.

Complications

- Miliary TB
- Pleural effusion
- Emphysema
- TB pneumonia

HEPATITIS

Refer page 161 under Gastrointestinal Disorder.

COMPARISON OF MAJOR FORMS OF VIRAL HEPATITIS

Previous name cause	Hepatitis A infectious hepatitis HAV	Hepatitis B serum hepatitis HBV	Hepatitis C non-A, non-B hepatitis	Hepatitis D HDV	Hepatitis E HEV
Mode of transmission	Fecal-oral route, poor sanitation, contact, water and food borne, during sex	Oral and sexual contact, contact T with acute disease, perinatal, and an occupational hazard for healthcare	Blood products, contaminated drug, and blood. Sex with infected partners, STD	Same as HBV, HVB, HBV surface antigen necessary for replication	Fecal-oral route, person-to-person contact
Incubation	15–50 days	28–160 days	15–160 days	21–140 days	15–65 days
Immunity	30 days	70–80 days	50 days	35 day similar	42 days
Signs and symptoms	Flu-like illness preicteric phase headache, malaise, fatigue, anorexia, fever, dark urine, jaundice of sclera, and skin	May develop arthralgias, rash	Similar to HBV, less severe	Similar to HBV	Similar to HAV, very severe in pregnant women
Outcome	Usually mild with recovery. Fatality <1%. No carrier state or increased risk of chronic hepatitis, cirrhosis, cancer	May be severe. Fatality: 1–10%. Increased risk of chronic hepatitis, cirrhosis, and hepatic cancer	Frequent occurrence of chronic carrier state and chronic liver disease. Increase the risk of hepatic cancer	Similar to HBV but greater likelihood of carrier state, chronic, active hepatitis, and cirrhosis	Similar to HAV, except very severe in pregnant women

(STD: sexually transmitted disease; HAV; hepatitis A virus; HDV: hepatitis D virus; HEV: hepatitis E virus; HBV: hepatitis B virus)

CHICKENPOX

Agent
Varicella-zoster virus (VZV), a member of the herpesvirus family.

Symptoms
Varicella (chickenpox): Varicella, the primary infection with VZV, is an acute, generalized disease that occurs most commonly in children and is characterized by a maculopapular rash (few hours), then vesicular rash (3–4 days), often accompanied by fever. Lesions are typically more abundant on trunk; but sometimes present on scalp, mucous membranes of mouth and upper respiratory tract. Lesions commonly occur in successive crops, with several stages of maturity present at the same time. Lesions are discrete, scattered and pruritic. Mild, atypical, and inapparent infections also occur. "Breakthrough" chickenpox which can be seen in previously vaccinated persons is usually a mild illness characterized by few lesions, most of which are papular or papulovesicular.

Zoster (herpes zoster, shingles): Zoster occurs more often in adults or immunocompromised persons and results from reactivation of latent VZV in sensory ganglia. Grouped vesicular lesions appear unilaterally in the distribution of 1–3 sensory dermatomes. Severe pain and paresthesia are common.

Congenital varicella syndrome: Primary varicella infection in the first 20 weeks of gestation is occasionally associated with abnormalities in the newborn that include low birth weight, limb hypoplasia, cicatricial Perinatal Varicella—perinatal varicella occurs within first 10 days of life from a mother infected from 5 days before to 2 days after delivery; it has a 30% fatality rate. The severity of disease results from fetal exposure to the virus without the benefit of passive maternal antibody. Postnatally acquired varicella occurs after 10 days of age and is rarely fatal.

- **Reservoir:** Human
- **Source:** Mucous membranes and vesicles
- **Transmission:** Direct contact with patient with varicella or zoster; droplet or air-borne spread of vesicle fluid (chickenpox and zoster) or secretions of the respiratory tract (chickenpox); indirectly by contaminated fomites. Scabs are not infectious.
- **Communicability:** Communicable 5 days before eruption (especially 1–2 days before eruption) and for up to 5 days after onset of lesions. Communicability may be prolonged in persons with altered immunity.
- **Specific treatment—For cases:** Acyclovir (IV) in susceptible immunocompromised persons, when administered within 24 hours of rash onset, has been effective in reducing morbidity and mortality associated with varicella. The US Food and Drug Administration (FDA) has licensed oral acyclovir for varicella in otherwise healthy children. The American Academy of Pediatrics considers the use of oral acyclovir appropriate in otherwise healthy persons at increased risk of moderate-to-severe varicella, such as those older than 12 years, those with chronic skin or pulmonary disorders, those receiving chronic salicylate therapy or short, intermittent or aerosolized corticosteroids or in secondary case—patients that live in the households of infected children.
- **Immunity:** Infection confers long immunity; second attacks of chickenpox can occur.

Contacts

Note: The following guidelines apply mainly to chickenpox contacts—contact to a shingles case is defined as direct contact with active lesions.

Passive Immunization with VariZIG

Effective in preventing or modifying disease if given within 10 days of first exposure to the case during case's period of communicability. Immunologically normal adults and adolescents should be evaluated on an individual basis. Serologic determination of immune status is advised. Candidates for VariZIG include:

- Immunocompromised, susceptible children
- Susceptible pregnant women. Serologic determination of immune status is advised.
- Newborn infant of a mother who had onset of chickenpox within 5 days before delivery to 48 hours after delivery.
- Hospitalized premature infant (>28-week gestation) whose mother has no history of chickenpox or serologic evidence of immunity.
- Hospitalized premature infants (<28-week gestation or <1,000 g), regardless of maternal history.

Active Immunization with Varicella Vaccine

Susceptible adults and children should be considered for varicella vaccination. The American Academy of Pediatrics recommends varicella vaccine administration to susceptible children up to 5 days after exposure to prevent or modify disease. The Advisory Committee on Immunization Practices has updated its routine varicella recommendations to add a second dose of varicella vaccine for children 4–6 years of age. Especially during varicella outbreaks, persons who have received only one dose of varicella vaccine should receive their second dose, provided the appropriate minimal interval has elapsed since the first dose (3 months for children 12 months through 12 years and 4 weeks for person 13 years and older). Patients should be advised that some contacts may have been exposed at the same time as the index case and that the vaccine will not protect against disease in such circumstances.

SMALLPOX

- **Agent:** Variola virus, a member of the *Poxviridae* family. (This is the agent for both variola major—classic smallpox—and variola minor, a less serious form of the disease).
- **Identification:**
  - **Symptoms:** Most significantly, the rash of smallpox is preceded by a prodrome consisting of 1–4 days of high fever, malaise, headache, muscle pain, prostration; sometimes nausea, vomiting, abdominal pain, and backache. In 90% of cases, smallpox (variola major) presents as an acute infectious disease characterized by a maculopapular rash, which becomes vesicular on day 3 or 4, then slowly evolves into pustular lesions, deeply embedded into the dermis, by day 6. Fourteen days after the initial appearance of the rash, most of the lesions have developed scabs. The rash in smallpox usually appears as a single crop with all lesions progressing from the macular to the pustular stage at about the same time.
  - The mortality rate for smallpox may be as high as 30% in unvaccinated persons and 3% in those with a history of vaccination sometime in the past. (Patients with variola minor have similar signs and symptoms but the disease is less severe and the mortality rate is only about 1%).
  - In a minority of instances, smallpox can present as "flat type" smallpox where lesions remain flush with the skin, never becoming elevated even during the pustular stage. This type of presentation is seen in 5–10% of cases and results in very severe disease. Another severe form of smallpox is "hemorrhagic smallpox," which involves extensive bleeding into the skin and almost always results in death. This form of disease, which can be seen in less than 3% of cases, can easily be mistaken for meningococcal sepsis.
- **Incubation:** Usually 12–14 days (range 7–17 days).
- **Reservoir:** Officially, only in designated laboratory repositories in the United States and Russia. Humans are the only natural host.
- **Source:** Macules, papules, vesicles, pustules, and scabs of the skin and lesions in mouth and pharynx.
- **Transmission:** Inhalation of virus-containing droplet nuclei or aerosols expelled from the oropharynx of an infected person, or less commonly, contact with material from smallpox lesions. Transmission may more easily occur in a hospital setting if isolation of the case is not implemented immediately. The virus is most likely to be disseminated in an aerosol cloud if used in biological warfare.
- **Communicability:** A smallpox case becomes infectious to others when rash lesions first appear in the mouth and pharynx, which usually occurs 24 hours before the rash is noted on the skin. Patients can transmit the virus throughout the course of the rash illness until all scabs have separated.
- **Specific treatment:** None of proven benefit; treatment is supportive
- **Immunity:** Infection is felt to confer lifelong immunity. Immunity from vaccination with the smallpox vaccine (vaccinia virus) gradually wanes over time beginning 5 years after vaccination.

TYPHOID FEVER

- **Agent:** *Salmonella typhi*, a gram-negative bacillus.
- **Identification:**
  - **Symptoms:** Systemic infectious disease with fever, headache, malaise, anorexia, diminished frequency of stool more common than diarrhea, bradycardia, enlargement of spleen and rose spots on trunk. Ulceration of Peyer's patches of ileum in late untreated disease may cause bloody diarrhea.
  - **Differential diagnosis:** Appendicitis, cholecystitis, other diseases with fever or rash, typhoid carrier.
  - **Diagnosis:**
    - ♦ **Culture:** Positive blood, feces, or urine confirms diagnosis. Blood may be positive as early as first week; feces and urine after first week.
    - ♦ **Serum agglutination:** Serologic test for "O" and "H" titers. No single titer or combination is diagnostic and should not be substituted for blood culture.
- **Incubation period:** 2 weeks average; range 1–3 weeks.
- **Reservoir:** Human
- **Source:** Feces and urine of infected person. Possibly infected draining wounds.
- **Transmission:** Fecal–oral route by direct or indirect contact with feces or urine of case or carrier; ingestion of contaminated food or milk; raw shellfish from contaminated water; flies may be vectors.
- **Communicability:** As long as bacilli are shed in excreta, usually after first week of illness into convalescence; 2–5% of acute cases become chronic carriers.
- **Specific treatment:** Ciprofloxacin, ceftriaxone or ofloxacin. Antibiotic sensitivity tests should be obtained on all typhoid isolates. Consult with arterial calcification due to deficiency of CD73 (ACDC) as needed.
- **Immunity:** Generally lifelong

Prevention Education

- Stressing handwashing, personal hygiene and the need to keep fingernails short and clean
- Disposing urine, feces, and fomites in a safe manner
- Preparing, storing, and refrigerating foods properly
- Identify, supervise, and educate typhoid carriers.
- **Typhoid vaccination:** Vaccination is not 100% effective and is not a substitute for careful selection of food/drink especially in areas not on the usual tourist itineraries. Tourists may wish to consider vaccination. There are currently three typhoid vaccines available in the United States—an oral live-attenuated, a parenteral heat-phenol-inactivated vaccine, and a capsular polysaccharide vaccine. All vaccines have approximately 50–80% protection depending on the degree of exposure.

MENINGITIS

Refer page 562 under Neurological Disorders.

LEPROSY

- **Agent:** *Mycobacterium leprae*, an acid-fast, gram-positive bacillus.
- **Identification:**
  - **Symptoms:** Lesions of skin, often enlargement of peripheral nerves, with consequent anesthesia, muscle weakness, and contractures. Major types:

- ♦ **Lepromatous (LL):** Many bacilli present, decreased cell-mediated immunity (CMI), diffuse skin lesions, invasions of upper respiratory tract, lymphoid system, and some viscera. Erythema nodosum leprosum and Lucio reaction may occur.
- ♦ **Borderline (BL, BB, BT):** Bacilli present and CMI unstable; includes features of both major types.
- ♦ **Tuberculoid (TT):** Few bacilli present, increased CMI, usually localized with discretely demarcated lesions, early in nerve involvement; may heal spontaneously in 1–3 years.
- ♦ **Indeterminate:** A benign form, relatively unstable, seldom bacteriologically positive. These cases may evolve toward LL form or the **TT** form or may remain unchanged indefinitely.
- ♦ **Arrested leprosy:** Under control with adequate medication
- ♦ **Complications:** Residual paralysis and anesthesia leading to trophic ulcers; amyloid renal disease; chronic glomerulonephritis. Reversal reactions may destroy tissue abruptly.
- ■ **Differential diagnosis:** Other peripheral neuropathies, chronic dermatological lesions, TB, syphilis, yaws, lymphoma, vitiligo, psoriasis, cutaneous leishmaniasis, etc.
- ■ **Diagnosis:** Characteristic tissue changes, nerve enlargement, history of immigration from endemic area, identification of acid-fast bacilli in tissue.
- **Incubation:** Average 3–6 years; range, 7 months to 20 years
- **Reservoir:** Human. Wild armadillos have been found infected; transmission to humans is uncertain.
- **Source:** Not established. Presumed to be nasal discharges, skin lesions.
- **Transmission:** Not established. Presumed to be via nasal discharges to the skin and respiratory tract of close contacts. Close household contact, genetic factors, and immune response thought to be important.
- **Communicability:** Mildly communicable as long as solid viable bacilli are demonstrable. A single dose of rifampin makes the case noncommunicable.
- **Specific treatment:** Multidrug therapy with dapsone (DDS); rifampin or rifampicin; clofazimine (B663). DDS resistance develops with monotherapy, so multidrug chemotherapy is always used. Rifampin or DDS may be used as prophylaxis for contacts.
- **Immunity:** None.

ANTILEPROSY DRUGS

According to WHO, "Leprosy is a chronic infectious disease caused by *Mycobacterium leprae*, an acid fast, rod-shaped bacillus." The disease mainly affects the skin, the peripheral nerves, mucosa of the upper respiratory tract, and the eyes.

Indications for Multidrug Therapy (MDT)

- **New case of leprosy:** Person with signs of leprosy who have never received treatment before.
- **Other cases:** Persons who need further treatment are recorded as **other cases**.

Classification

Class	Examples
Sulfones	Dapsone, solapsone
Phenazines	Clofazimine
Thiosemicarbazone	Amithiozone
Antitubercular	Rifampicin, ethionamide
Antibiotic	Ofloxacin, clarithromycine

Multidrug Therapy

	Drugs used	Frequency of administration adults	Dosage (adult) 15 years and above	Dosage (children 10–14 years)	Dosage (children below 10 years)	Criteria for RFT
MB leprosy	Rifampicin	Once monthly	600 mg	450 mg	300 mg	Completion of 12 monthly pulses in 18 consecutive months
	Clofazimine	Monthly	300 mg	150 mg	100 mg	
	Dapsone	Daily once	100 mg	50 mg	25 mg	
	Clofazimine	Daily for adults (every other day for children)	50 mg	50 mg (alternate day)	50 mg	
PB leprosy	Rifampicin	Once monthly	600 mg	450 mg	300 mg	Completion of 6 monthly pulses 9 consecutive months
	Dapsone	Daily	100 mg	50 mg	25 mg daily or 50 mg alternate day	

DIPHTHERIA

- **Agent:** *Corynebacterium diphtheriae*, a gram-positive bacillus (Klebs–Löffler).
- **Identification:**
  - **Symptoms:** An acute disease of pharynx, tonsils, larynx or nose, occasionally other mucous membranes or skin, characterized by an adherent grayish membrane. Symptoms include sore throat, large tender cervical lymph nodes, and marked swelling and edema of neck (bull neck). A toxin is responsible for the systemic manifestations. Late effects of the toxin include cranial and peripheral motor and sensory nerve palsies, myocarditis, and nephropathy. Cutaneous diphtheria (wounds, burns) usually appears as a localized ulcer.
  - **Differential diagnosis:** Bacterial and viral pharyngitis, Vincent's angina, infectious mononucleosis, syphilis, and candidiasis.
  - **Diagnosis:** Culture of *C. diphtheriae* from nasopharyngeal, throat, or membrane swabs.
- **Incubation:** 2–5 days, occasionally longer.
- **Reservoir:** Human.
- **Source:** Discharges from nose, throat, skin, eye, and other lesions of infected persons.
- **Transmission:** Contact with patient or carrier; fomites. Raw milk has served as a vehicle.
- **Communicability:** Variable until virulent bacilli disappear; usually 2 weeks or less, seldom more than 4 weeks. Effective antibiotic therapy reduces communicability to less than 4 days. Carriers may shed organisms for 6 months or more.
- **Specific treatment**
  - **Case:** Diphtheria antitoxin (DAT) should be given on the basis of clinical diagnosis; do not wait for bacteriological confirmation. Currently, the only DAT.
  - **Carriers:** Appropriate antibiotic therapy as for all primary contacts to case.
- **Immunity:** None.

DENGUE

- **Agent:** Dengue 1, 2, 3, and 4, four serologically related viruses.
- **Identification:**
  - **Symptoms:** Acute onset with fever, headache, body ache and often a maculopapular rash. Illness generally is self-limited and lasts about 1 week. Minor or severe bleeding manifestations occasionally occur. Dengue hemorrhagic fever, also called dengue shock syndrome, is a distinct clinical entity seen mostly in children with plasma leakage as

its major finding. A platelet count <100,000 and evidence of hemoconcentration are required for the diagnosis. Dengue shock syndrome frequently is fatal unless supportive treatment is given.

- **Differential diagnosis:** Dengue is easily confused in nonepidemic situations with common viral illnesses, for example, enterovirus infection, influenza, measles, and rubella. Dengue can also resemble endemic West Nile virus (WNV) fever and flea-borne murine typhus. Dengue may be confused with chikungunya fever in travelers returning from chikungunya fever-endemic or outbreak areas. Dengue hemorrhagic fever (dengue shock syndrome) may resemble bacterial sepsis, for example, meningococcemia or rickettsial disease.
- **Diagnosis:** Virus may be isolated from acute serum or detected by PCR; demonstration of a four-fold antibody rise by testing paired sera [enzyme-linked immunosorbent assay (EIA) hemagglutination inhibition (HI), complement fixation (CF)] may also confirm the diagnosis.

- **Incubation:** Usually 4–7 days, range 3–14 days.
- **Reservoir:** Humans and mosquitoes, and perhaps monkeys in the jungle of the Malay Peninsula.
- **Source:** The mosquito becomes infectious 8–12 days after the viremic blood meal and remains so for life.
- **Transmission:** Dengue virus is transmitted by the bite of infected *Aedes* mosquitoes, principally *A. aegypti*. *Aedes albopictus*, recently introduced to the United States from Asia, has the potential to become an important vector in this hemisphere.
- **Communicability:** Not directly communicable from person to person. Patients are usually infective for mosquitoes from shortly before to the end of the viremic period, an average of about 3–5 days.
- **Specific treatment:** None. Aspirin may exacerbate bleeding symptoms. Patients with dengue shock syndrome should be hospitalized and treated vigorously with fluid support.
- **Immunity:** Permanent immunity for a specific virus, but infection with other serotypes can occur.

Prevention Education

- Reducing exposure to mosquitoes by using protective clothing, repellents, and avoid outdoor exposure at dawn and dusk.
- Removing water on a regular basis from potential mosquito larval habitats, for example, potted plants, old tires, and pet watering dishes.

PLAGUE

- **Agent:** *Yersinia pestis*, a gram-negative bacillus.
- **Identification**
  - **Symptoms**
    - **Bubonic plague:** It presents as acute lymphadenitis in lymph nodes that drain the site of a fleabite. It occurs more often in inguinal nodes, less commonly in axillary and cervical nodes. It involved nodes become swollen and tender and may suppurate. Fever is usually present.
    - **Septicemic plague:** All forms of plague, including those without lymphadenopathy, may progress to septicemic plague with dissemination by the bloodstream to diverse parts of the body.

♦ **Pneumonic plague:** Often occurs secondarily to hematogenous dissemination of bubonic plague, resulting in pneumonia with mediastinitis or pleural effusion. Inhalation of respiratory droplets or artificially generated aerosols (bioterrorism) can cause primary plague pneumonia, a highly communicable disease that may lead to localized outbreaks. Pneumonia plague is thought to be the most likely presentation in the event of a biological attack.

♦ Untreated bubonic plague has a fatality rate of 50%. Pneumonic and septicemic plagues are invariably fatal if not treated.

■ **Differential diagnosis**

♦ **Bubonic:** Tularemia, granuloma inguinale, staphylococcal or streptococcal lymphadenitis, cat-scratch fever, incarcerated hernia, acute appendicitis, TB adenitis.

♦ **Septicemic:** Enteric fever, meningococcemia.

♦ **Pneumonic and meningitis:** Other bacterial causes of pneumonia and meningitis.

Diagnosis: Confirmed by culture of *Y. pestis* from bubo aspirate, blood, CSF or sputum, or a four-fold or greater change in serum antibody between acute and convalescent specimens. Presumptive diagnosis made by positive EIA, fluorescent antibody test or visualization of bipolar staining dumbbell-shaped organisms on smear of bubo aspirate, blood, spinal fluid, or sputum.

● **Incubation:** About 1–7 days for bubonic plague; primary plague pneumonia in 1–6 days.

● **Reservoir:** Wild rodents, for example, ground squirrels. Lagomorphs (rabbits and hares) and domestic cats can serve as a source of infection to people.

● **Source:** Infected fleas and blood or tissue from an animal infected with *Y. pestis*; respiratory droplets and sputum from patients or animals with pneumonic plague. Intentional release as an agent of bioterrorism.

● **Transmission:**

■ **Bubonic:** Bite from an infected flea, or by handling tissues of an infected animal.

■ **Pneumonic:** Contact with droplets or sputum from an infected patient or animal, Intentional release by terrorist(s).

● **Communicability:** Human to human only in pneumonic form. Fleas may remain infective for months.

● **Specific treatment:** Tetracyclines or sulfonamides

● **Immunity:** Temporary

CASE OF PNEUMONIC PLAGUE

● Droplet precautions and standard precautions

● **Isolation:** Patients should be placed in a private room; persons entering should wear gown gloves and mask. Negative air pressure isolation rooms are not indicated.

● Immediate hospitalization required; arrangements to be made by the ACDC duty officer.

● Eliminating all fleas with an effective insecticide from the patient, clothing, and living quarters.

MALARIA

● **Agent:** Protozoan parasites: *Plasmodium falciparum*, *Plasmodium malariae*, *Plasmodium ovale*, and *Plasmodium vivax*.

● **Identification:**

■ **Symptoms:** Acute or subacute febrile disease, usually with episodes of chills and fever every 2–3 days, separated by afebrile periods. Malaria caused by *P. falciparum* may progress to jaundice, shock, renal failure, coma, and death.

- **Differential diagnosis:** Other febrile illnesses associated with international travel, for example, brucellosis, typhoid fever, and yellow fever.
- **Diagnosis:** Demonstration of parasites in thick or thin blood smears.
- **Incubation:** Variable; 8–12 days for *P. falciparum*, 18 days or up to years for *P. malariae*, and 12–18 days for *P. ovale* and *P. vivax*. Inadequate or inappropriate prophylaxis may extend the incubation period.
  Note: *P. vivax* strains can occur 8–12 months after exposure, due to dormant forms remaining in liver.
- **Reservoir:** Human
- **Source:** Infected female mosquitoes of the genus *Anopheles*.
- **Transmission:** Bite of infective anopheles female mosquito, blood transfusion from infected persons, congenital and parenteral transmission.
- **Communicability**
  - **Mosquito infection:** When gametocytes are present in blood of patient.
  - **Parenteral transmission:** When trophozoites are present in blood.
- **Specific treatment:**
  - *P. ovale, P. vivax:* Chloroquine for acute malaria, primaquine for prevention of relapses (sometimes called "radical cure"). "Terminal prophylaxis" refers to primaquine treatment after leaving regions endemic for these species. Consult centers for disease control and prevention (CDC) yellow book or ACDC physician for details.
  - *P. falciparum, P. malariae:* Chloroquine for nonresistant strains. Patients with resistant *P. falciparum* malaria may require alternative treatment; consult ACDC.
  - Infection by any species transmitted by transfusion, parenteral, or congenital route: chloroquine or consult ACDC physician for suspected resistant strain.
- **Immunity:** Partial immunity for individuals with continuous exposure in endemic areas, for example, Africa, Central America, and Southeast Asia.

Prevention Education

- Appropriate chemoprophylaxis for travelers to areas endemic for malaria.
- Avoiding outdoor exposure during hours of peak mosquito activity, that is, between dusk and dawn.
- Using mosquito repellent (DEET-based up to 35% protective clothing) and mosquito netting at bedtime when traveling to areas with endemic malaria.
- Excluding persons with malaria from blood donor programs for 3 years after becoming asymptomatic and after therapy stopped. Asymptomatic US donors not on antimaterial chemoprophylaxis may donate 6 months after returning from an endemic area.
- IV drug users may acquire malaria by sharing paraphernalia.

PERTUSSIS (WHOOPING COUGH)

- **Agent:** *Bordetella pertussis*, a gram-negative pleomorphic bacillus
- **Identification**
  - **Symptoms:** Acute bacterial disease of the tracheobronchial tree. Insidious onset of mild upper respiratory tract symptoms (catarrhal stage) for 1–2 weeks followed by a cough which becomes paroxysmal within 1–2 weeks, usually lasting 1–2 months (paroxysmal stage). Paroxysms are characterized by repeated violent cough episodes without inhalation followed by characteristic high-pitched inspiratory whoop, frequently ending

with expulsion of clear, tenacious mucus. Fever is usually absent or minimal if present. Cases may not show typical paroxysms or whoop. Post-tussive vomiting is commonly seen and infants can present with apnea.

- **Differential diagnosis:** A whooping cough syndrome may also be caused by *Bordetella parapertussis, Mycoplasma pneumoniae, Chlamydia trachomatis, Chlamydia pneumoniae, Bordetella bronchiseptica* (although rarely), and certain adenoviruses. *B. parapertussis* may cause a portion of the clinical cases of pertussis, especially milder cases, and has been reported as the single agent or as a dual infection with B pertussis in laboratory-confirmed cases.

- **Diagnosis:** Clinical syndrome, isolation of organism from nasopharyngeal swab on Bordet–Gengou media, or Regan–Lowe agar plates. Strikingly elevated white blood cell count with a lymphocytosis occurs in 80% of the cases but may result from other causes. Serological tests may support a probable diagnosis, but only a positive culture, or positive PCR test result in someone with the clinical syndrome, confirms the diagnosis of pertussis.

- **Incubation:** Usually 7–14 days, rarely as short as 5 days or as long as 21 days.
- **Reservoir:** Human
- **Source:** Respiratory tract secretions of infected persons
- **Transmission:** Principally respiratory by droplet spread; indirect spread through articles soiled with discharges is possible.
- **Communicability:** Greater in the catarrhal stage before paroxysms. Tapers off until 21 days after onset of paroxysms, if untreated; only 5 days if treated. There exists a 70–100% secondary attack rate for susceptible household contacts.
- **Specific treatment:** Antibiotic treatment may shorten period of communicability but must be given early to modify clinical manifestations. Initiating treatment 3 or more weeks after cough onset has limited benefit to the patient. *See* section under "Contacts" for medications and recommended dose and duration for each of these agents. Dosage and duration of treatment are the same for treatment and postexposure prophylaxis (PrEP).
- **Immunity:** Immunity due to natural infection has been shown to wane in adolescence and adulthood. Immunity conferred by the pertussis component of the DTP/DTaP vaccine decreases over time with little or no protection 5–10 years following the last dose. Even with full immunizations some exposed infants and children may still develop disease, although much milder.

POLIOVIRUS INFECTION

- **Agent:** Poliovirus, an enterovirus with antigenic types 1, 2, and 3. Type 1 is most often the etiologic agent in paralytic illnesses, type 3 less so and type 2 least commonly. Type 1 most frequently causes epidemics. Most vaccine-associated cases are due to type 3 or 2. The last case of poliovirus infection caused by wild poliovirus in the Americas was reported in 1991 from Peru.

- **Identification**

  - **Symptoms:** Acute viral illness, severity ranging from in-apparent infection to paralytic disease. Over 90% of cases are asymptomatic or only result in nonspecific fever. Symptoms include fever, headache, nausea and vomiting, stiffness in neck and back, with/without paralysis. Paralysis is typically flaccid, asymmetric, and most commonly affecting the lower extremities. Case fatality (paralytic cases) is 2–10% in epidemics and increases with age. Nonparalytic poliovirus infection can present as aseptic meningitis, also common in other enterovirus infections.

- **Differential diagnosis:** Other types of aseptic meningitis, bacterial meningitis, tuberculous or fungal meningitis, brain abscess, leptospirosis, lymphocytic meningitis, encephalitis due to infectious or toxic agents, tick paralysis. Guillain–Barrè syndrome may initially resemble poliovirus infection as can West Nile Virus neurological disease. Other enteroviruses can cause acute flaccid paralysis simulating paralytic poliovirus infection.
- **Diagnosis:** Isolation of poliovirus from stool or pharynx early in the course of the disease is presumptive evidence of poliovirus infection. At least two stool specimens taken 24 hours apart are recommended to increase probability of poliovirus isolation. Recipients of oral live-attenuated polio vaccine (OPV) can excrete virus in feces for several weeks; however,

    OPV is no longer commercially available in the United States. Isolation of virus in CSF, when accomplished, is diagnostic of central nervous system (CNS) disease. CSF shows excess cells; lymphocytes predominate. Neutralizing and complement-fixing antibodies appear during the first 2 weeks of illness.

- **Incubation:** Range 3–6 days for abortive polio (nonspecific febrile illness)—typically 7–21 days for paralytic polio, but occasionally as short as 4 days.
- **Reservoir:** Humans, most frequently in-apparent cases, especially children
- **Source:** Pharyngeal secretions; feces of infected persons
- **Transmission:** Intimate contact with infected persons. Where sanitation is good, oral–oral, and respiratory may be more important than fecal–oral spread; it rarely occurs through milk and water where good sanitary conditions prevail. Transmission from mother to newborn has been reported. Immunodeficient patients may excrete virus for prolonged periods. In temperate climates, poliovirus infections are most common in the summer and fall.
- **Communicability:** Virus demonstrable in pharynx from 36 hours to approximately 1 week after exposure; in feces, from 72 hours to 6 weeks after exposure and occasionally for months. Infectivity is greatest 7–10 days before and after onset of symptoms.
- **Specific treatment:** Supportive
- **Immunity:** Type-specific of long duration

MEASLES

- **Agent:** Measles (rubeola) virus.
- **Identification:**
    - **Symptoms:** Acute, highly communicable febrile illness with cough, high fever, conjunctivitis, coryza, and Koplik's spots on buccal mucosa. Erythematous, maculopapular rash first appears on face (commonly around ears and hairline) about 2–4 days following onset of prodrome. Rash usually spreads to other parts of body and becomes confluent in about 4–7 days. Complications include otitis media, pneumonia, dehydration, convulsions (with/without fever), and acute encephalitis. Subacute sclerosing panencephalitis (SSPE) is extremely rare.
    - **Differential diagnosis:** Distinguish from Kawasaki disease, rubella, scarlet fever, and other childhood exanthems.
    - **Diagnosis:** A presumptive diagnosis is based on clinical and epidemiological grounds. The presence of measles IgM antibody in a person with a febrile rash illness usually confirms the diagnosis of measles and is preferred. (IgM antibodies can also be detected in individuals recently vaccinated against measles for up to 6 weeks after vaccination.) A four-fold or greater increase in specific HI or CF IgG antibody titers between acute and convalescent specimens also confirms the diagnosis.

- **Incubation:** About 10 days, varying from 8 to 13 days from exposure to onset of fever; average 14 days until rash appears; rarely as long as 21 days. Encephalitis can occur 2–6 days after rash.
- **Reservoir:** Human
- **Source:** Respiratory tract secretions and fomites
- **Transmission:** Direct contact with infectious droplets or less commonly, by air-borne spread. Measles is one of the most readily transmitted communicable diseases.
- **Communicability:** From 4 days before beginning of rash to 4 days after its appearance. Patients with SSPE are not contagious.
- **Specific treatment:** Supportive care; no antiviral agent available.
- **Immunity:** Lifelong. Persons can be considered immune to measles only if they have had a documented history of physician-diagnosed measles, have laboratory evidence of immunity, or have documented two doses of a measles-containing vaccine on or after the first birthday. Birth before 1957 is not a reliable indicator of immunity, particularly in healthcare personnel.

INFLUENZA

- **Agent:** Influenza viruses. Only influenza A and B are of public health concern since they are responsible for epidemics.
- **Identification:**
  - **Symptoms:** New acute onset of fever [≥100°F (38°C)], nonproductive cough, sore throat, chills, headache, myalgia, and malaise. Can sometimes also cause gastrointestinal (GI) symptoms. Duration is 2–4 days in uncomplicated cases, with recovery usually in 5–7 days. Infection with nonhuman strains of influenza, such as avian influenza viruses theoretically may cause other illness, such as conjunctivitis, gastroenteritis or hepatitis.
  - **Differential diagnosis:** Other agents that cause febrile respiratory illnesses or community acquired pneumonia including, but not limited to *M. pneumoniae*, adenovirus, respiratory syncytial virus, rhinovirus, parainfluenza viruses, *Legionella* species, and coronavirus.
  - **Diagnosis:** Confirmed by viral isolation, PCR, rapid antigen test, or a direct immuno-fluorescence/indirect immunofluorescence (DFA/IFA) test, and compatible symptoms.
- **Incubation:** 1–4 days; average 2 days
- **Reservoir:** Humans, swine, and migratory birds
- **Source:** Mostly droplet spread by nasal or pharyngeal secretions and sometimes fomites.
- **Transmission:** Large droplet spread from infective persons or sometimes contaminated fomites. Air-borne spread possible, but unlikely.
- **Communicability:** People infected with flu shed virus and may be able to infect others from 1 day before getting sick to 5–7 days after. This can be longer in some people, particularly and people with weakened immune systems.
- **Specific treatment:** Supportive care (e.g., rest, antipyretics, fluids). Antiviral medications may reduce the severity and duration of influenza illness if administered within 48 hours of onset. These same medications may be useful for hospitalized patients or those who are immunocompromised or if vaccine does not cover circulating strain. Streptococcal and staphylococcal pneumonias are the most common secondary complications and should be treated with appropriate antibiotics.
- **Immunity:** Permanent for a specific strain.

TETANUS

- **Agent:** Exotoxin of *Clostridium tetani*, a gram-positive bacillus.

- **Identification:**
  - **Symptoms:** Acute paralytic disease due to tetanus toxin produced by tetanus bacilli growing at site of injury; characterized by painful muscle contractions, principally involving masseter and neck muscles, secondarily muscles of trunk. Muscle contraction sometimes confined to region of injury.
  - **Differential diagnosis:** Hypocalcemic tetany, reaction to antipsychotic and antidepressive medications, CNS disturbances, various types of poisonings.
  - **Diagnosis:** Clinical history, immunization history and anaerobic culture of suspicious wound or debrided tissue. Diagnosis is usually made clinically by excluding other possibilities.
- **Incubation:** Three days to 3 weeks, dependent on character, extent, and location of wound; average 8 days. The further the injury site is from the CNS, the longer the incubation period. In neonatal tetanus, symptoms appear 4–14 days after birth, averaging 7 days.
- **Reservoir:** Organism is normal member of intestinal flora of animals and man; frequently found in soil.
- **Source:** Soil, dust, animal or human feces, plaster, sutures, injection drug use
- **Transmission:** Tetanus spores enter the body usually through wound; occasionally from parenteral injection. Neonatal tetanus occurs through infection of umbilical stump.
- **Communicability:** Not contagious from human to human
- **Specific treatment:**
  - Supportive care including appropriate medications to control tetanus spasms.
  - Tetanus immune globulin in a single total dose of 3,000–6,000 U is recommended for children and adults.
  - Oral (or IV) metronidazole (30 mg/kg/day) given in four divided doses (maximum 4 g/day) for 10–14 days. Parenteral penicillin G, 100,000 U/kg/day, every 4–6 hours can be given as an alternative.
- **Immunity:** The disease does not confer immunity. The primary series of immunizations is needed. Following a properly administered primary series, most people retain antitoxin levels that exceed the minimal protective level for 10 years after the last dose.

YELLOW FEVER

- **Agent:** Yellow fever virus
- **Identification:**
  - **Symptoms:** Acute onset with fever, backache, bradycardia, nausea, vomiting, jaundice, and hemorrhaging. Leukopenia, albuminuria, and anuria can also occur. Duration is short; severity varies.
  - **Differential diagnosis:** Any viral hepatitis, leptospirosis, typhoid fever, dengue, any hemorrhagic fever virus.
  - **Diagnosis:** Serologic tests. EIA or fluorescent antibody (FA) for viral antigen in blood or liver tissue; isolation of virus from blood; CF. Characteristic changes in the liver are also seen.
- **Incubation:** 3–6 days
- **Reservoir:** In urban areas, humans and mosquitoes; in sylvan areas, primates and forest mosquitoes.
- **Source:** Infected mosquitoes
- **Transmission:** Bite of infective mosquitoes
- **Communicability:** Not person-to-person. Human blood can infect feeding mosquitoes during first 3–5 days of illness. Mosquito is infected for life, and can transmit virus 9–12 days after feeding.

- **Specific treatment:** Supportive measures only
- **Immunity:** Permanent

Reporting Procedures

- **Epidemiologic data**
  - Recent travel to endemic areas. The fatality rate in indigenous populations of endemic areas is <5%, but may reach 50% among nonindigenous groups and in epidemics.
  - Exposure to mosquitoes.
  - Reports of febrile illness or unexplained deaths in the area.

Control of Case, Contacts, and Carriers

Immediate investigation required

CASE

Following are the information about case:
- **Isolation:** Blood and body fluid precautions.
- **Precautions:** Patient should be kept in a screened room for at least 5 days after onset.

Contacts

Recommend yellow fever vaccine, if indicated.

Prevention Education

- Vaccine is available for travelers to endemic areas.
- Minimizing contact with mosquitoes in endemic areas by using nets and repellents.

HUMAN IMMUNODEFICIENCY VIRUS

Refer page 401 under Immunological Disorders.

Intraoperative Nursing

ORGANIZATION AND PHYSICAL SET UP OF THE OPERATION THEATER

Introduction

Operation theater (OT) is an area where all surgical operating work is carried out.

OT is highly sterile unit, maintain high standard of performance and perform surgery in safe, aseptic environment.

Classification of OT

OT can be divided into four zones based on specific precaution:
1. Relatively clean area
2. Absolutely clean area
3. Aseptic area
4. Unclean area

1. **Outermost area:** This is a clean zone of OT which is outside the operation theater. It consists of:
   - Operation theater superintendent room
   - Space for surgeons to write OT report
   - X-ray room
   - Changing room
   - Surgeon's room
   - Waiting area for relatives
2. **Intermediate area:** This area is absolutely clean and sterile. It includes:
   - Operating room
   - Anesthesia induction room
   - Scrub room
   - Postoperative recovery room
3. **Inner most area:** This area is absolutely clean and sterile area. No one other than surgeon and assistant should be allowed to enter in this area. This zone includes:
   - Operating room
   - Anesthesia induction room
   - Scrub room
4. **Unclean zone for disposal:** It includes area for keeping used linen and instruments.

Staffing Pattern of Operation Theater (Fig. 15.1)

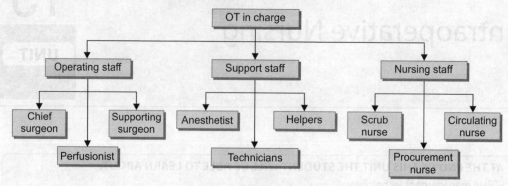

Fig. 15.1: Staffing pattern of operation theater.

Hierarchy of Nursing Personnel in OT (Fig. 15.2)

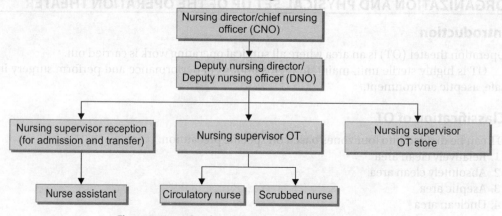

Fig. 15.2: Hierarchy of nursing personnel in operation theater.

Duties and Responsibilities of the Nurse in OT

- **Nursing director and deputy nursing director:** The Nursing Director is responsible for—
    - Maintaining high standards of client care in the OT
    - Professional development of OT staff
    - Forward planning and ordering
    - Liaising with other hospital departments
- **Nursing supervisor:** The Nursing supervisor is responsible for—
    - The day-to-day activity of OT
    - Delegating responsibilities to the scrub and circulatory nurse
    - Liaising with surgeons and anesthetists
    - Evaluating the effectiveness of the performance of the nursing personnel in OT
    - Informing the nursing director of any changes or problems in the OT
    - The continuing education and OT research with staff and student nurses
    - Assessing the OT supplies
    - Weekly stock audit
- **Scrub nurse:**
    - Before an operation
        - Ensures that all the equipment needed during procedure are available
        - Ensures cleanliness of OT

◆ Prepares the surgical trolley
◆ Receives sterile equipment via circulating nurse using sterile technique
◆ Performs initial sponges, instruments and needle count
◆ Preparation for scrubbing, gowning and gloving

■ When surgeon arrives after scrubbing
◆ Provide assistance for gowning and gloving to the surgeon
◆ Assemble the drapes according to use
◆ Assist the surgeon in draping the patient aseptically
◆ Place blade on the knife handle using needle holder, assemble suction tip and suction tube
◆ Secure suction tube
◆ Prepares sutures and needles

■ During an operation
◆ Maintain sterility throughout the procedure
◆ Ensure client's safety
◆ Adhere to the policy regarding sponge, instruments and needles count
◆ Arrange the instrument on the table
◆ Before the incision starts, place two sponges on the operative site prior to incision
◆ Passes the retractor to the assistant surgeon
◆ Anticipate the surgeon's needs
◆ Always keep two sponges on the field throughout the procedure

● **Circulator nurse:**
a. Checks all equipment for proper functioning
b. Make sure that OT is clean
c. Arrange equipments according to the need of the procedure
d. Place a clean sheet OT table
e. Collect necessary stock and equipment
f. Turn on the air conditioner unit and adjust the temperature of the OT room as per the client's need.

Equipment used for Common Surgical Procedures

Surgical instruments are especially designed tools that are used by professional healthcare workers to carry out surgical procedures. Most surgical instruments are made from stainless steel. Some are designed for general use, and others for specific surgical procedures.

Most surgical instruments can be classified into these four basic types:
1. Cutting and dissecting
2. Clamping and occluding
3. Retracting and exposing
4. Grasping and holding

Cutting and dissecting: These instruments are used to cut through skin, tissue and suture material and having sharp edges. Examples, iris scissors **(Fig. 15.3)**.

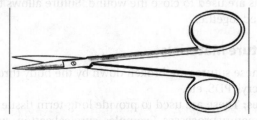

Fig. 15.3: Iris scissors.

Clamping and occluding: These instruments are used for compressing blood vessels, to prevent their contents from leaking.
Example, crile hemostatic forceps **(Fig. 15.4)**.

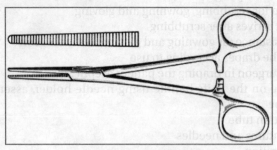

Fig. 15.4: Crile hemostatic forceps.

Retracting and exposing: These surgical instruments are used to retract or to hold the organs and tissue, so that operative area can be assessed. Example, volkman retractor **(Fig. 15.4)**.

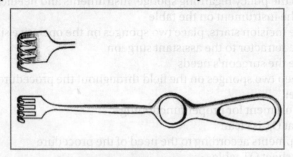

Fig. 15.5: Volkman retractor.

Grasping and holding: These instruments are used to grasp and hold tissue or blood vessels during a surgical procedure. Example, allis tissue forceps **(Fig. 15.6)**.

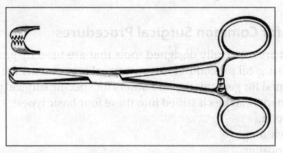

Fig. 15.6: Allis tissue forceps.

Suture and Suture Materials

Surgical suture materials are used to close the wound. Suture allows the healing of tissue by keeping the wound closed together.

Classification of Suture Materials

Absorbable sutures: These sutures are broken down by the body through enzymatic action. Examples, monocryl, vicryl, PDS, etc.

Non-absorbable sutures: These are used to provide long-term tissue support and shredded off by the body's inflammatory processes. Examples, surgical cotton, surgical silk, ethilon, etc.

Scrubbing Procedures

According to CDC guidelines standard safety precaution is defined as control and prevention for reducing the risk of transmission of blood-borne and other pathogens in hospitals. It aims to:

- Reduce the risk of transmission of blood-borne pathogens
- Reduce the risk of pathogens from moist body substances

Gowning

Sterile gowns are worn in the operating room and the delivery room an whenever open wounds are present which necessitate a sterile technique, e.g., to attend to a client with burns. To keep the gowns sterile, they are folded inside out and are touched only on the inside.

Procedure

- Scrub hands thoroughly
- Dry the hands with sterile towel
- Pick up the gown by grasping the folded gown at the neck. Stand well back about one foot from the sterile bundle and the table.
- Unfold it by keeping the gown away from the body. Do not shake the gown.
- Hold the gown at the shoulder seams (inside) and put each hand alternately into the arm holes.
- Extend the arms and hold hands upward at the shoulder height when putting them through the arm hole.
- The circulating nurse the assist her in pulling the sleeves by working from behind and holding the gown from the inside.
- The gown is then fastened at the neck by the circulating nurse and the open edges are then folded or held together.
- The waist ties are then fastened by the circulating nurse from behind.

Cleaning of Article

- Rinse the articles first with cold water to remove the organic material. Hot water coagulates the organic matter and tends to make it stick to the article.
- Then wash the articles in hot water and soap. Soap has an emulsifying action as it reduces surface tension which facilitates the removal of dirt.
- Rinsing with water assists in washing the dirt away
- Use an abrasive such as a stiff bristled brush and a paste or powder to wash the articles. Brush will help to remove the dirt from the grooves and corners.
- Rinse the article with clean water
- Dry them with a towel. There is less chance for the bacteria and dirt to lodge on the cleaned articles when it is dry.
- Disinfect or sterilize if indicated.

Decontamination of Articles

Concurrent disinfection means the immediate disinfection of all contaminated articles and bodily discharges during the course of the disease. It includes:

Procedure

- Cleaning of the isolation unit daily, including the floors using an effective disinfectant.
- Disinfection of all articles including the soiled linen, contaminated articles, etc., before it is sent out of the unit.

- Disposal of all wastes by incineration
- Safe disposal of excreta

Terminal Disinfection

- The terminal disinfection is the disinfection of the client's unit with all the articles used on discharge, transfer or death of a client who had been suffering from an infectious disease.
- Fumigation is often used for this purpose. The commonly used agents are sulfur and formalin. The doors and windows including all crevices are closed prior to fumigation.

Disinfection and Sterilization of Equipment

Autoclave: Autoclaves provide a physical method for disinfection and sterilization. They work with a combination of steam, pressure and time. Autoclaves operate at high temperature and pressure in order to kill microorganisms and spores. They are used to decontaminate certain biological waste and sterilize media, instruments and lab ware. Regulated medical waste that might contain bacteria, viruses and other biological material are recommended to be inactivated by autoclaving before disposal. To be effective, the autoclave must reach and maintain a temperature of 121°C for at least 30 minutes by using saturated steam under at least 15 psi of pressure **(Fig. 15.7)**.

Incineration: A waste treatment technology, which includes the combustion of waste for recovering energy, is called as "incineration". Incineration reduces the mass of the waste from 95 to 96%. Incineration coupled with high temperature waste

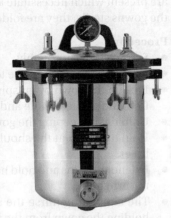

Fig. 15.7: Autoclave.

treatments are recognized as thermal treatments. During the process of incineration, the waste material that is treated is converted into gases, particles and heat. These products are later used for generation of electricity. The gases, flue gases are first treated for eradication of pollutants before going into atmosphere.

Chemical processes: These processes use chemical that act as disinfectants, such as sodium hypochlorite, dissolved chlorine dioxide, peracetic acid, hydrogen peroxide, dry inorganic chemical and ozone are examples of such chemical.

Mechanical processes: These processes are used to change the physical form or characteristics of the waste either to facilitate waste handling or to process the waste in conjunction with other treatment steps. The two primary mechanical processes are:

1. **Compaction:** It is used to reduce the volume of the waste.
2. **Shredding:** It is used to destroy plastic and paper waste to prevent their reuse. Only the disinfected waste can be used in a shredder.

Irradiation processes: It exposes the wastes to ultraviolet or ionizing radiation in an enclosed chamber.

Microwaving: Microwave treatment shall not be used for cytotoxic, hazardous or radioactive wastes, contaminated animal carcasses, body parts and large metal items. The microwave should completely and consistently kill bacteria and other pathogenic organism that is ensured by the approved biological indicator at the maximum design capacity of each microwave unit.

Deep burial: A pit or trench should be dug about 2 m deep. It should be half filled with waste, and then covered with lime within 50 cm of the surface, before filling the rest of the pit with soil.

Therapeutic Environment

Healthcare services are designed in such a way that support and accelerates the art of medicine, technology, patient safety and quality patient care. It also focuses on providing psychosocial support to patient, family, and caregivers in order to maintain therapeutic environment.

'Therapeutic environment can be defined as the total of all the external conditions, environments and influences affecting an individual in the illness situation.'

Therapeutic environment is defined as 'the characteristics of the physical, social, spiritual and emotional environment in which a patient receives care from the care givers and care givers put efforts to maintain a good patient nurse relation that gives good patient outcomes, patient satisfaction, patient safety and good organizational outcomes.

Purpose of the Therapeutic Environment

- To provide for patients' optimal safety and security
- To provide nurses with a healthy surrounding in which nurse are practicing patient care.
- To engage and support everyone concerned with patients' care; patients' family and friends, other health professionals, and assistive personnel
- To achieve clinical excellence in the treatment of patient
- To supports the psychosocial and spiritual needs of the patient

Practical Application of Therapeutic Environment

The application of **therapeutic environment** has been focused on the patient and patient's family. It not only helps to maintain harmonious relation between nurse and patient but also within the healthcare team in terms of satisfaction, effectiveness, and staff retention **(Fig. 15.8)**.

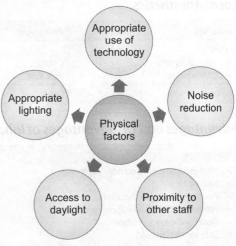

Fig. 15.8: Components of therapeutic environment.

Types of Environmental Hazards in OT

1. **Physical hazards:** Most common physical hazards in the hospitals are heat, noise and vibration. All can be found in excess in some healthcare settings, such as lasers, X-rays, or other forms of radiation.
2. **Biological hazards:** In healthcare facilities healthcare staff may be exposed to a large number of biological hazards. Viruses, such as hepatitis B, bacteria and other biological agents.
3. **Chemical hazards:** Chemicals hazards are most common in healthcare settings, such as disinfectants and antiseptics and chemicals used in laboratories, such as cleaners and anesthetic gases.
4. **Ergonomic hazards**: Lifting and transferring patients, residents, and clients can be very dangerous if the caregiver is not properly trained or if the proper lifting devices are not available. Many caregivers experience sprains and strains related to this kind of activity.
5. **Psychological hazards:** Violence in the workplace can be a hazard to staff in healthcare and community care environments. Aggression from patients, visitors, doctors and clients could take the form of physical, emotional and mental abuse.

General and Local Anesthetics

Class		Example
Inhalation	**Gases**	Nitrous oxide
	Volatile	Halothane , enflurane, isoflurane—propanidid, desflurane, trichloroethylene, ethyl chloride, chloroform
Intravenous		Benzodiazepines, propofol, propanidid, ketamine

General Anesthetics

Subclass	Prototype	*Variants*
Inhaled anesthetics		
➤ Volatile Liquids	Halothane	Enflurane, isoflurane, desflurane, sevoflurane
➤ Gas	Nitric oxide	
Intravenous anesthetics		
➤ Barbiturates (low t ½)	Thiopental	Thiamylal, methohexital
➤ Benzodiazepam	Diazepam	Midazolam
➤ Opioids	Morphine	Fentanyl, sufentanil
➤ Dissociative agent	Ketamine	
➤ Other	Propofol	

Local Anesthetics

Subclass	Prototype	Variants
Esters		
➤ Topical agents	Cocaine	Benzocaine
➤ Intravenous	Procaine	Chloroprocaine
Amides	Lidocaine	Bupivacaine

Advantages and Disadvantages of Inhalation Anesthesia

Advantages	**Disadvantages**
➤ Non-inflammable and non-explosive	➤ Weak analgesic
➤ Non-irritant	➤ Weak muscle relaxants
➤ Produces bronchodilatation	➤ Uterine relaxant
➤ Produces controlled hypotension	➤ Cardiotoxic
➤ Good analgesics in labor	➤ Hepatotoxic
➤ Safe for vital organs	➤ Malignant hyperthermia
	➤ Expensive

Stages of Anesthesia

- **Stage I: Analgesia**
  - Conscious but drowsy
  - Responses to painful stimuli reduced
- **Stage II: Excitment**
  - Lose consciousness
  - No longer responds to non-painful stimuli
  - Responds in a reflex fashion to painful stimuli
- **Stage III: Surgical anesthesia:** Movement ceases and respiration becomes regular
- **Stage IV: Medullary paralysis**
  - Respiration and vasomotor control cease
  - Death occurs

Equipment used in Anesthesia

- The respirator bag valve mask
- Anaesthesia machine
- Oxygen mask
- Laryngoscope
- Tracheostomy tube
- Tuohy needle
- Flexible Endoscope
- Syringe

Nursing Responsibilities during Anesthetic Drug Administration

- Must maintain a good aseptic technique while handling client in intraoperative room and during administering the propofol.
- Before administrating the propofol must check for any discoloration or any precipitates in vial.
- Determine the rate as per the body weight of the client and complete infusion within 6 hours.
- Assess the hemodynamic status before administrating the propofol.
- Tonic-clonic seizures may occur during general anesthesia with propofol.
- Nurse should keep in mind the following during intra operative phase of anesthesia:

  BP: Assess blood pressure.

  GA: Check general anesthetic tray

  HR: Assess heart rate

  MR: Keep muscle relaxants in hands

  PACU: Postanesthetic care unit

  RPAO: Check routine postanesthesia orders

  RR: Assess respiratory rate

  SpO$_2$: Assess oxygen saturations

- **Patient observations in intraoperative room**
  a. Should be documented
  b. Assessment of HR, RR, SpO$_2$, BP and temperature
  c. Presence of drains and patency
  d. Baseline neurological assessment
  e. Observation of client continues ½ hourly for 4 hours if the patient had an endotracheal tube.
  f. Observation of client continues ½ hourly for 2 hours if the patient had a laryngeal mask.

Pain Management Techniques

Noninvasive Non-Drug Pain Management

There is an immense variety of noninvasive non-drug pain management techniques available for treating pain. A few of the most widely accepted in comprehensive pain management programs are the following:

- **Exercise:** Physical exertion with the aim of increasing strength, increasing flexibility, and restoring normal motion. Includes the McKenzie method, water therapy, stretching exercises, aerobic routines and many others. May involve active, passive and resistive elements. Exercise is necessary for proper cardiovascular health, disk nutrition and musculoskeletal health.
- **Manual techniques:** Manipulation of affected areas by applying force to the joints, muscles, and ligaments.

- **Behavioral modification:** Use of behavioral methods to optimize patient responses to back pain and painful stimuli. Cognitive therapy involves teaching the patient to alleviate back pain by means of relaxation techniques, coping techniques and other methods. Biofeedback involves learning to control muscle tension, blood pressure, and heart rate for symptomatic improvement.

- **Superficial heating or cooling of skin:** These pain management methods include cold packs and hot packs, ultrasound, and diathermy and should be used in conjunction with exercise.

- **Complementary and alternative medicine (CAM):** Alternative medicine is an intervention other than conventional medicine for healing practices. It includes AYUSH, naturopathy, chiropractic, herbalism, Chinese medicine, meditation, yoga, biofeedback, hypnosis, homeopathy, and acupuncture, etc.

- **Altered focus:** This is a best technique for demonstrating how powerfully the mind can alter sensations in the body. Focus the attention on any specific non-painful part of the body (hand, foot, etc.) and alter sensation in that part of the body.

- **Dissociation:** As the name implies, this chronic pain technique involves mentally separating the painful body part from the rest of the body, or imagining the body and mind as separate, with the chronic pain distant from one's mind.

- **Sensory splitting:** This technique involves dividing the sensation (pain, burning, pins and needles) into separate parts.

- **Mental anesthesia:** This involves imagining an injection of numbing anesthetic (like Novocain) into the painful area, such as imagining a numbing solution being injected into low back.

- **Mental analgesia:** Building on the mental anesthesia concept, this technique involves imagining an injection of a strong pain killer, such as morphine, into the painful area.

MULTIPLE CHOICE QUESTIONS

1. **Before responding to a first aid scenario, what is the first question you should ask at the scene?**
   A. Age of the injured or ill person   B. Safety of the scene
   C. Nature of the injury   D. Time of the injury

2. **Personal protective equipment consists of the following items:**
   A. Gloves   B. Mask
   C. Eye shield   D. All of the above

3. **A stroke consists of which following signs?**
   A. Confusion   B. Chest pain
   C. Facial droop   D. Nausea

4. **What would be the most likely scenario if a 20-year-old dove headfirst off a dock and once they reached the surface of the water did not appear to be moving?**
   A. Heart attack   B. Low blood sugar
   C. Neck injury   D. Mammalian diving reflex

5. **You are first to the scene and you find an unresponsive person with no pulse that has thrown up. You feel CPR is not something you are comfortable giving them. What would be the next best thing for you to do?**
   A. Wipe off the face or cover with a shirt   B. Compression only CPR
   C. Go and get help   D. Do not initiate resuscitation

6. **What would your next step be after you are performing single-person CPR and the AED (Automatic External Defibrillator) advises a shock?**
   A. Call for help
   B. Resume CPR with chest compressions
   C. Check for a pulse
   D. Resume ventilation

7. **As a daycare provider that is working alone, one of your three-year-old children is not feeling well and laid down for a nap. After checking on the child you notice they are not breathing and are blue in color. What would be the best step to take?**
   A. Do back blows
   B. Do a blind finger sweep
   C. Call 911
   D. Deliver two minutes of CPR

8. **What do you do if an infant is choking and while trying to assist them they become unresponsive?**
   A. Leave the infant to get help
   B. Do a blind finger sweep
   C. Begin CPR
   D. Do abdominal thrusts

9. **AED pads can be used for children at what age?**
   A. 17
   B. 16
   C. 14
   D. Up until puberty

10. **Properly operating an AED include the following steps:**
    A. Power on the AED, attach electrode pads, shock the person, and analyze the rhythm
    B. Power on the AED, attach electrode pads, analyze the rhythm, and shock the person
    C. Analyze the rhythm, attach electrode pads, and shock the person
    D. Power on the AED, shock the person, attach electrode pads, and analyze the rhythm

Answers

1. B   2. D   3. C   4. C   5. B   6. B   7. D   8. C   9. D   10. B

Male Reproductive Disorders

TERMINOLOGY

- **Cryptorchidism** is also called undescended testis.
- **Epispadias** is congenital anomaly in males, the urethra is on the upper surface of the penis.
- **Hypospadias** is a condition in which the opening of the urethra is on the underside of the penis.

ANATOMY AND PHYSIOLOGY

In male reproductive system, male urethra is a tube that connects the lower end of urinary bladder to the exterior, urine stored in the bladder is passed out through it.

The male urethra is divisible into three parts:

1. First part is prostatic part
2. Second part is sphincter urethra externus
3. Third part is spongiose part
   - The male gonads are the right and left testes. They produce the male gametes which are called spermatozoa.
   - From each testis, the spermatozoa pass through a complicated system of genital ducts. The most obvious of these are the epididymis and the ductus deferens. Tests are surrounded by three layers of tissue:
     i. Tunica vaginalis: This double membrane forming the outer covering of the testes and is down growth of the abdominal and pelvic peritoneum.
     ii. Tunica albuginea: This is a fibrous covering beneath the tunica vaginalis that surrounds the testes.
     iii. Tunica vasculosa: This consists of a network of capillaries supported by delicate connective tissue.

Scrotum: The scrotum is a pouch of deeply pigmented skin, fibrous, and connective tissue and smooth muscle. It is divided into two compartments, each of which contains one testis, one epididymis, and the testicular end of the spermatic cord. It lies below the symphysis pubis in front of the upper parts of the thighs and behind the penis.

Functions of Testes

Spermatozoa (sperm) are produced in the seminiferous tubules of the testes, and mature as they pass through the long and epididymis, where they are stored. The hormone controlling sperm production is follicle-stimulating hormone (FSH) from the anterior pituitary.

Spermatic Cords

- The spermatic cords suspend the testes in the scrotum. Each cord contains a testicular artery, veins, lymphatics, deferent duct, and testicular nerves, which come together to form the cord from their various origins in the abdomen.
- The cord that is covered in a sheath of smooth muscle and connective and fibrous tissues extends through the inguinal canal and is attached to the testis on the posterior wall.

Assessment of Male Reproductive System

- **Penis:** It is essential for assessing the discharge, ulceration, pain, size, prepuce, scrotum, size, color nodules, swelling, ulceration, tenderness, pain, erectile function.
- **Testes:** It is essential for assessing the size, shape, swelling, masses, absence, and self-examination practices.
- **Prostate:** It is necessary to ask for the date of last assessment (digital rectal exam, prostate specific antigen).

DISORDERS OF MALE REPRODUCTIVE SYSTEM

CRYPTORCHIDISM

Cryptorchidism is the most common congenital abnormality characterized by undescended testes of one or both to reach the normal position in the scrotum through the inguinal canal.

Etiology

- Impairment of the hypothalamus–pituitary–gonadal axis
- Hereditary and chromosomal abnormalities
- One or both testes (anorchia)
- Short spermatic

Risk Factors

- Low birth weight
- Being born prematurely
- Having a family history of undescended testicles

Types

- **Retractile testis and pseudo-cryptorchidism:** It is because of cremasteric reflex, testis may be temporarily pulled up from the scrotum.
- **True cryptorchidism:** It occurs when the testis is located in the abdominal cavity or inguinal canal "also called intraabdominal testes."
- **Arrested descent:** Descent may stop anywhere along the normal pathway.
- **Ectopic testis:** Testes are found away from the normal line of descent.
- **Absence of testis:** Absence of testis is called anorchia.

Clinical Manifestations

- Undescended testis can be unilateral and bilateral
- Dysgenesis of sperms
- Psychological problems

Diagnostic Evaluation

- **History:** It is necessary to ask the family history of the client related to undescended testis.
- **Physical examination:** Physical examination helps to determine whether the testicles are palpable.
- Ultrasound
- Laparoscopy
- Magnetic resonance imaging (MRI) uses a strong magnetic field and radio waves to create detailed images of the organs and tissues within the body.

Management

- Undescended testicles usually move down into the scrotum naturally by the time when child is 3–6 months old.
- The best time for the therapy is between 1 and 12 years of age to prevent further complications.
- **Administration of hormonal therapy:** It is necessary to administer hormonal therapy with human chorionic gonadotropin (hCG). HCG also results in enlargement of the testis.

Surgical Management

- **Orchiopexy:** It is the surgery to reposition, the testicle from his abdomen into the scrotum. It should be done early by 2 years of age for good result.
- **Herniotomy:** In this, a small cut in the groin region at the natural skin creases the contents of hernia sac that is emptied back into the abdomen and the sac is tied off.
- **In the case of absence of testes,** silastic prosthesis can be inserted at 8–10 years of age to overcome the emotional problems.

Preoperative Management

- It is necessary to explain the whole procedure to the parents of the child.
- It is necessary to clear all the doubts of parents regarding surgery.
- It is necessary to take consent.
- It is necessary to tell to the parents that child surgery will be done under general anesthesia.
- It is necessary to follow the rules for eating or drinking that must be followed in hours before the surgery.
- It is necessary to tell that surgery will take about 45 minutes, but recovery from anesthesia will take several hours.

Postoperative Management

- It is necessary to educate the parents about the diet after the surgery.
- It is necessary to advice to restrict the clear liquids.
- Child should avoid fast foods.
- It is necessary to advise them to maintain hygiene.
- If there is any swelling or redness, pain occurs at the incision site report to the physician.
- It is necessary to advise for the follow-up.

Nursing Care Plan

Nursing Assessment

- It is necessary to assess at the time of birth.
- It is necessary to evaluate by gently compressing both inguinal canal.

Nursing Diagnosis

1. Deficient knowledge (family members) related to the cryptorchidism

Interventions
- It is necessary to assess the knowledge of the family members.
- It is necessary to educate them regarding treatment.
- It is necessary to clear all doubts of family members.

2. Anxiety (family members) related to the possible decreased fertility

Interventions
- It is necessary to assess the level of anxiety in the family members.
- It is necessary to educate the family members regarding the treatment of the disease that early treatment can prevent infertility.
- It is necessary to clear the doubts of the family members related to the disease.
- It is necessary to provide psychological support to family members.
- It is necessary to educate regarding the early treatment.

3. Disturbed body image related to the appearance of genitalia

Interventions
- It is necessary to assess the condition of the client.
- It is necessary to provide emotional support regarding the appearance of genitalia.
- It is necessary to encourage visits by loved ones and understanding friends.
- It is necessary to confirm with the doctor the nature of the treatment anticipated.
- It is necessary to promote the positive acceptance of the condition.
- It is necessary to provide positive reinforcement to the client.
- It is necessary to promote the realistic adaptation to the condition.

Complications
- Testicular cancer
- Fertility problems.

EPISPADIAS

It is a congenital abnormality and rare type of malformation. In this, the urethral opening on the dorsal aspect of the penis due to the abnormal development of the infra umbilical wall and upper wall of the urethra.

Classification

Epispadias in male child can be classified as:
1. **Anterior epispadias:** Anterior epispadias with normal continence
   a. Glandular
   b. Balanitis or penile
2. **Posterior epispadias:** Associated with incomplete bladder neck and incontinence of urine.
   a. Penopubic
   b. Subsymphyseal

In male: Infants with epispadias are having short and broad penis with dorsal curvature.

In female: A cleft extends along the roof or entire urethra involving the bladder neck, urethra is short.

It is classified as:

1. Bifid clitoris with no incontinence of urine
2. Subsymphyseal with incontinence of urine.

Etiology and Risk Factors

- Family history
- Increased maternal age above 32 years
- Low birth weight babies
- Exposure to smoking and drugs during pregnancy

Clinical Manifestation

In Male

- Male usually has a short, wide penis with an abnormal curve.
- The urethra may be open along the whole length of the penis.
- Urinary incontinence
- The urethra usually opens on the top or side of the penis instead of the tip.
- Enlarged pubic bone
- Urinary tract injection (UTI)
- Reflux nephropathy

In Female

- Females have an abnormal clitoris and labia.
- The opening is usually between the clitoris and the labia, but it may be in the belly area.
- Trouble in controlling urination, urinary incontinence.
- Urinary tract infection.
- Enlarged pubic bone.
- Backward flow of urine is present.

Diagnostic Evaluation

- **History:** In history, collect the family history, medical history, birth history of the client.
- **Physical examination:** In physical examination, the child voiding pattern is assessed.
- **Blood test:** Blood test is used to check the level of electrolytes.
- **Intravenous pyelogram:** It helps to detect the abnormalities of upper urinary tract and also the bladder capacity.
- MRI and computed tomography (CT) scan
- Ultrasound

Management

- **Bladder exstrophy:** It includes penile lengthening, elongation of urethral strip, and chordee correction.
- **Cystoplasty:** It can be done to enhance the bladder capacity.

Nursing Management

Preoperative Care

- It is necessary to prepare the child's parents and child for the surgery.
- The parents must be assured that if surgery is done in early child life.
- They should also be prepared for appearance of surgical area postoperatively.
- The procedure is explained to the parents.
- Written consent is taken.

Postoperative Care

- If the surgery is done, the nurse must also help the child to handle the anxiety.
- It is necessary to keep the operated area clean and dry.
- It is necessary to provide more emphasis on the prevention of infection.
- It is necessary to provide emotional support for long-term management schedule.
- It is necessary to maintain health of the child.
- It is necessary to provide adequate, balanced diet and healthy nutrition to child.
- It is necessary to maintain hygiene.

HYPOSPADIAS

Hypospadias is most common congenital anomaly of the penis in which the opening of the urethra is on the underside of the penis, instead of the tip.

Classification

Hypospadias can be classified depending upon the sites of the urethral meatus:
- a. Anterior hypospadias
- b. Middle penile shaft hypospadias
- c. Posterior hypospadias

Etiology and Risk Factors

- Family history
- Increased maternal age above 32 years
- Low birth weight babies
- Exposure to smoking and drugs during pregnancy

Clinical Manifestations

- Presence of the painful downward curvature of the penis
- Deflected stream of urine
- Abnormal spraying during the urination
- Hooded appearance of penis
- Having to sit down to urinate
- Inability to void urine while standing
- Urethral stricture

Diagnostic Evaluation

- **History:** In history, collect the family history, medical history, birth history of the client.
- **Physical examination:** In physical examination, the child voiding pattern is assessed.
- **Blood test:** Blood test is used to check the level of electrolytes.
- **Intravenous pyelogram:** It helps to detect the abnormalities of upper urinary tract and also the bladder capacity.
- MRI and CT scan
- Ultrasound

Management

- **Meatotomy:** It can be done at any age after birth of child. Chordee correction and advancement of prepuce can be done at the age of 2–3 years.

- **Meatoplasty and glanuloplasty:** It is a reconstruction of meatus and glans to achieve meatus at the tip of penis.
- **Urethroplasty:** It is a reconstruction of missing distal urethra.

Nursing Management

Preoperative Care

- It is necessary to prepare the child's parents and child for the surgery.
- The parents must be assured that if surgery is done in early in child life, there will be no influence on his self-image.
- They should also be prepared for appearance of surgical area postoperatively.
- It is necessary to explain the procedure to the parents.
- Written consent is taken from client and parents.

Postoperative Care

- If the surgery is done, the nurse must also help the child to handle the anxiety.
- It is important that the nurse helps both the parents and child to relieve their anxieties so that they are not transmitted from one family to the other family members.
- It is necessary to keep the operated area clean and dry, to prevent from infection and urinary tract infection.
- It is necessary to provide play therapy to child to divert the mind.
- It is necessary to be with the client.

Other Supportive Nursing Care includes

- It is necessary to provide more emphasis on the prevention of infection.
- It is necessary to provide emotional support for long-term management schedule.
- It is necessary to maintain health of the child by giving more emphasis on child growth and development.
- It is necessary to provide adequate, balanced diet and healthy nutrition to child.
- It is necessary to maintain hygiene.
- It is necessary to provide parental guidance and educate them how to cope with the problem.

Nursing Care Plan

Nursing Assessment

- Nurse has to assess the condition of child.
- Nurse has to inspect the genitalia of child that helps to show the location of abnormal urethra and other problems associated with this condition.
- It is necessary to assess that baby or a boy cannot urinate at a normal position.

Nursing Diagnosis

Acute pain related to physical factors (damage to tissue), incision.

Interventions

- It is necessary to assess the level of pain in the client.
- It is necessary to provide diversional therapy to the client, such as play and music therapy.
- It is necessary to provide comfortable environment to the client.
- It is necessary to monitor the vital signs.
- It is necessary to provide emotional support to the client and their parents.

Altered family process related to the diagnosis of disease condition.

Interventions

- It is necessary to assess the anxiety of parents and fear level of the child by asking questions.
- It is necessary to provide emotional support to the child.
- Allowing parents involvement in the treatment.
- Allowing play and self-care as tolerated by the child.
- Encouraging child interaction with other child.
- Answering the questions asked by the parents and allowing expressing their frustration.

Knowledge deficit related to the disease condition and prognosis.

Interventions

- It is necessary to assess the ability of the parents to take care of the child.
- Discussing about the care after discharge from the hospital, regarding rest, diet, hygiene, continuation of medication, need for medical help, and follow up.
- Teaching about features of infections, signs of relapse and precautions to prevent complications.
- It is necessary to provide parental guidance and educate them how to cope with the problem.

INFERTILITY

According to the WHO Infertility is a disease of the reproductive system defined by the failure to achieve a clinical pregnancy after 12 months or more of regular unprotected sexual intercourse.

Types of Infertility

1. **Primary:** Primary infertility means where someone who has never conceived a child in the past has difficulty in conceiving.
2. **Secondary:** When a person has had one or more pregnancies in the past but is having difficulty in conceiving again.

Etiological Factors

In Female

- Ovulation disorders
- Polycystic ovary syndrome
- Thyroid problems
- Premature ovarian failure
- Womb and fallopian tubes
- **Scarring from surgery:** Pelvic surgery
- Cervical mucus defect
- **Endometriosis:** It is a condition where small pieces of the womb lining.
- Pelvic inflammatory disease
- **Medicines and drugs:** Nonsteroidal inflammatory drugs, long-term use cause difficulty in conceiving, such as aspirin, ibuprofen.
- Chemotherapy

In Male

- Due to abnormal semen
- Decreased number of sperm
- Decreased sperm mobility
- Testicular cancer

- Testicular surgery
- Hypogonadism
- Alcohol
- Smoking
- Stress
- Cryptorchidism
- Trauma to testicles
- Sterilization

Clinical Manifestations

The main symptom of infertility is not getting pregnant.

In Female

- In women, changes in the menstrual cycle and ovulation may be a symptom of infertility.
- Abnormal periods, bleeding may be heavy or low
- Acne
- Change in sex drive and desire
- Weight gain
- Milky discharge from nipples but unrelated to breastfeeding
- Pain during sex

In Male

- In male, it includes problems with the sexual functions, i.e., difficulty in ejaculation, reduced desire, and erectile dysfunction.
- Pain and swelling in testicles
- Having a lower normal sperm count

Diagnostic Evaluation

- **History**
  - It is necessary to collect the history related to irregular menstruation.
  - It is necessary to collect the history related to the known problems with uterus, tubes or other problems, such as endometriosis.
  - It is necessary to collect history related to male infertility problems.
  - It is necessary to ask about the history of drugs uses and about the alcohol and smoking use.
  - It is necessary to ask the couple about their relationship.
- **Physical examination:** In physical examination, patients need to be assessed for any abnormalities, such as abnormalities of penis, vas deferens, testicles.
  - It is necessary to assess the client for skin changes.
  - It is necessary to check the weight of patient.
  - It is necessary to ask the client for their menstrual history.
- **Male partner semen analysis:** A complete semen analysis measures the quantity and quality of the fluid released during ejaculation. It evaluates both the liquid portion, called semen or seminal fluid, and the microscopic, moving cells called sperm. It is often used in the evaluation of male infertility. A shorter version of this test checks solely for the presence of sperm in semen a few months after a man has had a vasectomy to determine whether the surgery was successful.
- **Hysterosalpingogram:** This is an X-ray procedure to see if the fallopian tubes.
- **Transvaginal ultrasonography:** A transvaginal ultrasound, or endovaginal ultrasound, is a procedure that doctors use to examine the internal organs in the female pelvic region.

- **Sonohysterography:** This procedure uses transvaginal ultrasound after filling the uterus with saline. This improves detection of intrauterine problems, such as endometrial polyps, fibroids.
- **Hysteroscopy** is used to diagnose or treat problems of the uterus. A hysteroscope is a thin, lighted telescope-like device. It is inserted through your vagina into your uterus.
- **Laparoscopy:** Visualization of internal organs during surgery.

Management

In management, limited numbers of medical treatments are aimed at improving chances of conception for patients with known cause of infertility.

- **Artificial androgen, such as testosterone**
- **Artificial insemination:** Depositing semen into the female genital tract

Pharmacological Therapy

- Clomiphene used when hypothalamus not stimulating pituitary gland to release FSH and luteinizing hormone (LH).
- Menotropin is a combination of FSH or LH is used for women with deficiencies in these hormones.
- Urofollitropin containing FSH with a small amount of LH, used in polycystic ovarian syndrome to stimulate follicle growth.
- Chronic gonadotropin used to stimulate release of egg from ovary.

Lifestyle Modifications

- Healthy lifestyle and daily exercise may restore fertility
- Body weight management
- It is necessary to avoid smoking and alcohol.
- Caffeine and drugs should be avoided.
- It is necessary to take a healthy diet.
- A high intake of vitamin C and E increases sperm count.

Nursing Care Plan

Nursing Assessment

- It is necessary to assist the client in reducing stress in the relationship.
- It is necessary to encourage cooperation, protect privacy, foster understanding, and refer the couple to appropriate resources when necessary.
- Infertility workups are expensive, time consuming, stressful so couples need support in working together to deal with these problems.

Nursing Diagnosis

Anticipatory grieving related to loss of pregnancy

Interventions

- It is necessary to assess the client's condition.
- Client distress may not be expressed verbally, and not by partner.
- Nurse should be present to listen and provide support.
- The client partner should also participate in this process.
- If the client is having severe distress, counseling should be referred.

Anxiety related to the diagnosis of fertility

Interventions

- It is necessary to assess the level of anxiety in client.
- The patient must be allowed to talk and ask questions.

- It is necessary to assist the patient in expressing their feelings.
- It is necessary to provide support.
- It is necessary to educate them about the disease condition and also about the treatment.
- Tell the client partner to be with the patient.

Disturbed body image related to the altered fertility and fears about sexuality and relationship between partner and family

Interventions

- It is necessary to assess the condition of patient.
- The patient may have strong emotional reactions related to the diagnosis of infertility, view the others who may be involved (family, partner, religious beliefs, and fears about prognosis).
- It is necessary to provide reassurance to the client.
- It is necessary to provide psychological support.
- If the fear or stress level is high, then patient should be referred for counseling.

MULTIPLE CHOICE QUESTIONS

1. **The primary sex organ is known as** _____
   A. Regulate blood volume and composition
   B. Synthesize glucose
   C. Regulate blood pressure
   D. Gonads

2. **The incomplete descent of the testes into the scrotum is called cryptorchidism.**
   A. True   B. False

3. **Name the site of sperm maturation.**
   A. Epididymis   B. Ductus deferens
   C. Spermatic cord   D. Urethra

4. **Which of the following produces the male sex hormone?**
   A. Rete testis   B. Seminiferous tubule
   C. Leydig cell   D. Scrotum

5. **Which of the following is an energy source for the sperm?**
   A. Somatostatin   B. Prostaglandin
   C. Proteins   D. Fructose

6. **Mark the INCORRECT statement about prostate gland?**
   A. Located inferior to the urinary bladder
   B. Secretion is thin and milky colored
   C. Secretion is acidic in nature
   D. Function in increasing the mobility of the sperm

7. **The fluid from which of the following accessory gland neutralizes the acidity in a vagina of the female?**
   A. Seminal vesicle   B. Prostate gland
   C. Cowper's gland   D. Urethra

Answers

1. D   2. A   3. A   4. C   5. D   6. C   7. C

Ear, Nose, and Throat Disorders

AT THE END OF THIS CHAPTER, THE STUDENTS WILL BE ABLE TO LEARN ABOUT NURSING MANAGEMENT OF PATIENT WITH:

➤ Otitis media
➤ Tympanic membrane perforation
➤ Otosclerosis
➤ Mastoiditis
➤ Meniere's disease
➤ Labyrinthitis
➤ Epistaxis
➤ Cancer of the larynx
➤ Speech defects and speech therapy
➤ Hearing aids, implanted hearing devices
➤ Role of nurse communicating with hearing impaired and muteness

---

REVIEW OF ANATOMY AND PHYSIOLOGY

The Outer Ear

The outer ear includes the portion of the ear that we see—the pinna or auricle and the ear canal.

Pinna

The pinna or auricle is a concave cartilaginous structure, which collects and directs sound waves traveling in air into the ear canal or external auditory meatus.

Ear Canal

The ear canal or external auditory meatus is approximately 1.25 inches long and .25 inch diameter. The inner two thirds of the ear canal are embedded in the temporal bone. The outer one third of the canal is cartilage. Although the shape of each ear canal varies, in general the canal forms an elongated "s"-shaped curve. The ear canal directs airborne sound waves toward the tympanic membrane (TM) (eardrum). The ear canal resonates sound waves and increases the loudness of the tones in the 3,000–4,000 Hz range.

The ear canal maintains the proper conditions of temperature and humidity necessary to preserve the elasticity of the tympanic membrane. Glands, which produce cerumen and tiny hairs in the ear canal, provide added protection against insects and foreign particles from damaging the tympanic membrane.

Middle Ear

The middle ear is composed of the tympanic membrane and the cavity, which houses the ossicular chain.

Tympanic Membrane

The tympanic membrane or eardrum serves as a divider between the outer ear and the middle ear structures. It is gray-pink in color when healthy and consists of three very thin layers of living tissue.

The eardrum is very sensitive to sound waves and vibrates back and forth as the sound waves strike it. The eardrum transmits the airborne vibrations from the outer to the middle ear and also assists in the protection of the delicate structures of the middle ear cavity and inner ear.

Middle Ear Cavity

The middle ear cavity is located in the mastoid process of the temporal bone. The middle ear cavity extends from the tympanic membrane to the inner ear. It is approximately 2 cm³ in volume and is lined with mucous membrane. The middle ear cavity is actually an extension of the nasopharynx via the Eustachian tube.

Eustachian Tube

The Eustachian tube acts as an air pressure equalizer and ventilates the middle ear. Normally, the tube is closed but opens while chewing or swallowing. When the Eustachian tube opens, the air pressure between the outer and middle ear is equalized. The transmission of sound through the eardrum is optimal when the air pressure is equalized between the outer and middle ear. When the air pressure between the outer and middle ear is unequal, the eardrum is forced outward or inward causing discomfort and the ability of the eardrum to transmit sound is reduced.

ASSESSMENT OF THE EARS, NOSE, THROAT, AND MOUTH

History

During history of client focus on the following:
- Onset of symptoms
- Location (ear, nose, or mouth)
- Radiation of pain in surrounding area
- Any aggravating factors
- Relieving factors
- Quality of pain
- Frequency and duration of symptom
- Effects on daily activities
- Previous treatments

Family History

Keeping a record of history for any seasonal allergies, asthma, or hearing loss.

Ears

- **Inspection:** Evaluating the position of external ear, congenital defects, presence of lesions, discharge, swelling, redness, odor, presence of wax, or foreign bodies.
- **Palpation:** Tenderness over tragus or mastoid process—tenderness on manipulation of the pinna.

Nose

- **Inspection:** Assessing for inflammation, deformity, discharge, bleeding
- **Palpation:** Assessing for sinus and nasal tenderness.

Neck

- **Inspection:** Assessing for symmetry, redness, enlargement of thyroid, active range of motion, and swelling
- **Palpation:** Tenderness, enlargement, mobility, symmetry, and presence of masses.

Mouth and Throat

- **Inspection:** Assessing for symmetry and color of lips, presence of lesions oral mucosa and tongue, redness, swelling, caries on gums and tooth
- **Palpation:** Assessing for tenderness, enlargement, mobility, contour, and consistency of nodes.

OTITIS MEDIA

Otitis media refers to inflammation of the middle ear. Acute otitis media (AOM) occurs when a cold, allergy, or upper respiratory infection, and the presence of bacteria or viruses lead to the accumulation of pus and mucus behind the eardrum, blocking the Eustachian tube and characterized by earache and swelling.

When fluid accumulates in the middle ear, the condition is known as "**otitis media with effusion.**" This occurs in a recovering ear infection.

Types

Following are the types of otitis media:

Acute Otitis Media

It is usually of rapid onset and short duration. AOM is typically associated with fluid accumulation in the middle ear together with signs or symptoms of ear infection and may associates with drainage of purulent material (pus, also termed suppurative otitis media).

Chronic Otitis Media

It is a persistent inflammation of the middle ear, typically for a minimum of a month. Following an acute infection, fluid may remain behind the eardrum for up to 3 months before resolving. Chronic otitis media may develop after a prolonged period with fluid or negative pressure behind the eardrum.

Etiology

Winter is high season for ear infections. They often follow a cold. Some factors that increase a risk for middle ear infections include:
- Crowded living conditions
- Attending daycare
- Exposure to secondhand smoke
- Respiratory illnesses, such as the common cold
- Close contact with siblings who have colds
- Having a cleft palate

- Allergies that cause congestion on a chronic basis
- Premature birth
- Not being breast-fed
- Bottlefeeding while lying down

Signs and Symptoms

Symptoms of an ear infection may include:

Acute otitis media (AOM)

- Pulling at ears
- Excessive crying
- Fluid draining from ears
- Sleep disturbances
- Fever
- Headaches
- Problems with hearing
- Irritability
- Difficulty balancing

Symptoms of fluid buildup may include:

- Popping, ringing, or a feeling of fullness or pressure in the ear
- Trouble hearing
- Balance problems and dizziness

Diagnostic Evaluation

Following are the information about diagnostic evaluation:

- History, a physical examination and an ear examination
- Pneumatic otoscope to look at the eardrum for signs of an ear infection or fluid buildup.
- **Tympanometry:** It measures how the eardrum responds to a change of air pressure inside the ear.
- Hearing tests
- **Tympanocentesis:** This test can remove fluid if it has stayed behind the eardrum (chronic otitis media with effusion).
- Blood tests, which are done if there are signs of immune problems.

Complications

Infratemporal infections can include:

- Tympanic membrane perforation
- Mastoiditis
- Facial nerve palsy
- Acute labyrinthitis
- Petrositis
- Acute necrotic otitis
- Chronic otitis media

Intracranial infections can include:

- Meningitis
- Encephalitis
- Brain abscess
- Otitic hydrocephalus

- Subarachnoid abscess
- Subdural abscess
- Sigmoid sinus thrombosis

Management

Antibiotic is the only treatment for otitis media (**Table 17.1**).

TABLE 17.1: Agents used in the treatment of otitis media.

Agent	Dosage	Comments
Antimicrobials		
Amoxicillin	80–90 mg/kg/day, given orally in two divided doses	First-line drug. Safe, effective, and inexpensive
Amoxicillin (Augmentin)	90 mg of amoxicillin per kg per day given orally in two divided doses	Second-line drug. For patients with recurrent or persistent acute otitis media, those taking prophylactic amoxicillin, those who have used antibiotics within the previous month, and those with concurrent purulent conjunctivitis
Azithromycin	30 mg/kg, given orally	For patients with penicillin allergy. One dose is as effective as longer courses
Azithromycin (3-day course)	20 mg/kg once daily, given orally	For patients with recurrent acute otitis media
Azithromycin (5-day course)	5–10 mg/kg once daily, given orally	For patients with penicillin allergy (type 1 hypersensitivity)
Cefdinir	14 mg/kg/day, given orally in one or two doses	For patients with penicillin allergy, excluding those with urticaria or anaphylaxis to penicillin (i.e., type 1 hypersensitivity)
Cefpodoxime	30 mg/kg once daily, given orally	For patients with penicillin allergy, excluding those with urticaria or anaphylaxis to penicillin (i.e., type 1 hypersensitivity)
Ceftriaxone	50 mg/kg once daily, given intra-muscularly or intravenously. One dose for initial episode of otitis media, three doses for recurrent infections	For patients with penicillin allergy, persistent or recurrent acute otitis media, or vomiting
Cefuroxime	30 mg/kg/day, given orally in two divided doses	For patients with penicillin allergy, excluding those with urticaria or anaphylaxis to penicillin (i.e., type 1 hypersensitivity)
Clarithromycin	15 mg/kg/day, given orally in three divided doses	For patients with penicillin allergy (type 1 hyper-sensitivity). May cause gastrointestinal irritation
Clindamycin	30–40 mg/kg/day, given orally in four divided doses	For patients with penicillin allergy (type 1 hypersensitivity)
Topical agents		
Ciprofloxacin/ hydrocortisone	3 drops twice daily	–
Hydrocortisone/ neomycin	4 drops three to four times daily	–
Ofloxacin	5 drops twice daily (10 drops in patients older than 12 years)	–
Analgesics		
Acetaminophen	15 mg/kg every 6 hours	–
Antipyrine/ benzocaine	2–4 drops three to four times daily	–
Ibuprofen	10 mg/kg every 6 hours	–

Nursing Care Plan

Nursing Diagnosis

1. Acute pain related to inflammation of the middle ear tissue
2. **Disturbed sensory perception:** Auditory conductive disorder related to the sound of the organ.

Acute pain related to inflammation of the middle ear tissue

Intervention

- Assessing the level of intensity of the client and client's coping mechanisms
- Giving analgesics as indicated
- **Distracting the patient by using relaxation techniques:** Distraction, guided imagination, touching, etc.

Disturbed sensory perception

Auditory conductive disorder related to the sound of the organ.

Intervention

- Reducing noise in the client environment.
- Looking at the client when speaking.
- Speaking clearly and firmly on the client without the need to shout.
- Providing good lighting when the client relies on the lips.
- Using the signs of nonverbal (e.g., facial expressions, pointing, or body movement) and other communications.
- Instructing family or the people closest to the client on how techniques of effective communication so that they can interact with clients.
- If the client wants, the client can use hearing aids.

TYMPANIC MEMBRANE PERFORATION

The eardrum serves two important functions in ear. It senses vibrating sound waves and converts the vibration into nerve impulses that convey the sound to brain. It also protects the middle ear from bacteria as well as water and foreign objects. Normally, the middle ear is sterile. But when the eardrum is ruptured, bacteria can get into the middle ear and cause an infection known as otitis media.

A ruptured eardrum is a tear in the thin membrane that separates outer ear from inner ear and when there is any abnormal opening or perforation in tympanic membrane is termed as perforated tympanic membrane.

Etiology

Traumatic causes of TM perforation include:

- A number of things can cause the eardrum to rupture; one of the most common causes is an ear infection. When the middle ear is infected, pressure builds up and pushes against the eardrum. When the pressure gets too great, it can cause the eardrum to perforate.
- Insertion of objects into the ear canal purposely, another common cause of a ruptured eardrum is poking the eardrum with a foreign object, such as a cotton-tipped swab or a bobby pin that's being used to clean wax out of the ear canal. Sometimes, children can puncture their own eardrum by putting objects, such as a stick or a small toy in their ear.
- Concussion caused by an explosion or open-handed slap across the ear.
- Head trauma

- Sudden negative pressure (e.g., strong suction applied to the ear canal)
- **Barotrauma:** This happens when the pressure inside the ear and the pressure outside the ear are not equal. That can happen, for example, when an airplane changes altitude, causing the air pressure in the cabin to drop or rise. The change in pressure is also a common problem for scuba divers.
- Iatrogenic perforation during irrigation or foreign body removal.

Signs and Symptoms

Some people do not notice any symptoms of a ruptured eardrum. Others complain only after several days of general discomfort in their ear and feeling that "something's not quite right with the ear." Some people are surprised to hear air coming out their ear when they blow their nose. Forcefully blowing nose causes air to rise up to fill the space in middle ear. Normally, this will cause the eardrum to balloon outward. But if there is a hole in the eardrum, air will rush out. Sometimes, the sound is loud enough for other people to hear.

Other symptoms of a ruptured eardrum include:
- Sudden sharp ear pain or a sudden decrease in ear pain
- Drainage from the ear that may be bloody, clear, or resemble pus
- Ear noise or buzzing
- Hearing loss that may be partial or complete in the affected ear
- Episodic ear infections
- Facial weakness or dizziness

Diagnostic Evaluation

Audiometry

This hearing test checks how sensitive ears are to sounds at different volumes. The hearing tests may include pure-tone audiometry and speech audiometry tests. The tests help measure the quietest sounds or speech that can hear. They also help measure how well one can understand words when they are spoken at a normal sound level. These tests may check type of hearing loss.

Otoscopy

An otoscope helps to see inside the ear and visualize the eardrum.

Tuning Fork Test

For this test, a vibrating tuning fork is held against the bone behind the ear. The tuning fork may also be held against the forehead, nose, or outside the opening of ear. You will be asked if you can hear certain sounds. Your hearing may be tested holding the tuning fork in more than one place. When this is done, you will be asked to state which area you heard the sound best.

Management

- Ear kept dry
- Oral or topical antibiotics

Often, no specific treatment is needed. The ear should be kept dry, routine antibiotic ear drops are unnecessary. However, prophylaxis with oral broad-spectrum antibiotics or antibiotic ear drops is necessary if contaminants may have entered through the perforation as occurs in dirty injuries. If the ear becomes infected, amoxicillin 500 mg is given for 7 days. Although most perforations close spontaneously, surgery is indicated for a perforation persisting.

Surgical Management

Surgery is required to repair eardrum and prevent future ear infections. This is done when the hole in eardrum is large or does not heal on its own.

Myringoplasty

This type of surgery uses a tissue graft to cover torn eardrum. A tissue graft may be taken from own body, another person, an animal, or is man-made. A procedure called a mastoidectomy may also be done with a myringoplasty. A mastoidectomy is removal of infected bone from behind ear.

Tympanoplasty

This surgery repairs torn eardrum and any damage to inner ear. A tympanoplasty also helps prevent ear infections that stop and come back. The hole in eardrum will be covered with a tissue graft.

OTOSCLEROSIS AND HEARING LOSS

Otosclerosis is a term derived from oto, meaning "of the ear," and sclerosis, meaning "abnormal hardening of body tissue." The condition is caused by abnormal bone remodeling in the middle ear. Bone remodeling is a lifelong process in which bone tissue renews itself by replacing old tissue with a new characterized by abnormal remodeling of ear bone that disrupts the ability of sound to travel from the middle ear to the inner ear.

Types of Hearing Impairment

The external ear and the middle ear conduct sound; the inner ear receives it. If there is some difficulty in the external or middle ear, a conductive hearing impairment occurs. If the trouble lies in the inner ear, a sensorineural or nerve hearing impairment is the result. When there is difficulty in both the middle and the inner ear a mixed or combined impairment exists. Mixed impairments are common in otosclerosis.

Cochlear Otosclerosis

When otosclerosis spreads to the inner ear a sensorineural hearing impairment may result due to interference with the nerve function. This nerve impairment is called cochlear otosclerosis and one it develops it may be permanent. On occasion, the otosclerosis may spread to the balance canals and may cause episodes of unsteadiness.

Stapedial Otosclerosis

Usually, otosclerosis spreads to the stapes or stirrup, the final link in the middle ear transformer chain. The stapes rests in the small groove, the oval window, in intimate contact with the inner ear fluids. Anything that interferes with its motion results in a conductive hearing impairment. This type of impairment is called stapedial otosclerosis and is usually correctable by surgery.

Etiology

The most commonly affected portion of the bone around the inner ear (otic capsule) is the anterior oval window. It can also involve the round window niche, the internal auditory canal, and occasionally ossicles other than the stapes. Otosclerosis is thought to begin with otospongiosis, which is a localized softening of the normally very hard bone of the otic capsule.

There appear to be three stages of otosclerosis—resorptive osteoclastic stages with signs of inflammation, followed by an osteoblastic stage involving immature bone, followed by mature bone formation.

- Genetic
- Viral

Diagnostic Evaluation

1. Tympanometry can show stiffening of the ossicular chain.
2. Acoustic reflexes are very useful in otosclerosis, as they show a characteristic "inversion" pattern.
3. The temporal bone computerized tomography (CT) scan is both nonspecific and insensitive.

Treatment of Otosclerosis

There are four treatment options:

1. Do Nothing is a Reasonable Option

Otosclerosis does not have to be treated, as there are no medications that have been shown to work, and it will progress or not independent of any treatment. It is advisable to have a formal hearing test repeated once a year.

2. Hearing Aids

Hearing aids are effective for conductive hearing loss and certainly are less risky than having ear surgery. Hearing aid technology has undergone tremendous advances since the invention of surgical treatment for otosclerosis. Bone implanted hearing aids can be especially convenient.

3. Medical Treatment

Fluorides

Fluoride therapy is no longer a recommended primary treatment for otosclerosis, because of its effect on other bones including the possibility of increasing the risk of hip fractures. After 2 years of fluoride treatment, the dose of fluoride is reduced from three times a day to once a day. Once the otospongiosis phase of otosclerosis is over and there is a clear cut otosclerosis documented by conductive hearing loss, fluoride may be stopped. The treatment is continued after surgery. Biphosphonates can also be recommended in some cases.

Other Approaches

Avoidance of estrogens or use of estrogen blockers might be helpful in individual with otosclerosis as otosclerosis frequently worsens during pregnancy, suggesting hormonal modulation. Similarly, hormone supplements in menopause might be adverse to hearing in persons with otosclerosis.

4. Surgical Treatment

For conductive hearing loss, stapedectomy can be done, which produced excellent hearing results, which remain good for many years after the surgery. This procedure may allow avoidance of hearing aids. It, however, does not help the sensory component of the hearing loss and at best, may close the "air–bone" gap.

The stapes operation (stapedectomy) is recommended for patients with otosclerosis who are candidates for surgery. This operation is usually performed under local anesthesia and requires but a short period of hospitalization and convalescence. Over 90% of these operations are successful in restoring the hearing permanently.

Stapedectomy or stapedotomy is performed through the ear canal under local or general anesthesia. A small incision may be made behind the ear to remove muscle or fat tissue for use in the operation.

Complications of Surgery

- **Hearing loss**
- **Tinnitus:** Most patients with otosclerosis notice tinnitus (head noise) to some degree. The amount of tinnitus is not necessarily related to the degree or type of hearing impairment. Following successful stapedectomy, tinnitus is often decreased in proportion to the hearing improvement, but occasionally may be worse.
- **Dizziness:** Dizziness is normal for a few hours following a stapedectomy and may result in nausea and vomiting. Some unsteadiness is common during the first few postoperative days, dizziness on sudden head motion may persist for several weeks.
- **Taste disturbance and mouth dryness:** Taste disturbance and mouth dryness are not uncommon for a few weeks following surgery.
- **Eardrum perforation:** A perforation in the eardrum membrane is an unusual complication of the surgery. If healing does not occur, surgical repair (myringoplasty) may be required.
- **Weakness of the face:** A very rare complication of stapedectomy is temporary weakness of the face. This may occur as the result of an abnormality or swelling of the facial nerve.

Nursing Management

Successful communication requires the efforts of all people involved in a conversation. Even when the person with hearing loss utilizes hearing aids and active listening strategies, it is crucial that others involved in the communication process consistently use good communication strategies, including the following:

- Facing the hearing impaired person directly, on the same level and in good light whenever possible. Position yourself so that the light is shining on the speaker's face, not in the eyes of the listener.
- Do not talk to client from other room, not being able to see each other when talking is a common reason people have difficulty understanding what is said.
- Speak clearly, slowly, distinctly, but naturally, without shouting or exaggerating mouth movements. Shouting distorts the sound of speech and may make speech reading more difficult.
- Saying the person's name before beginning a conversation. This gives the listener a chance to focus attention and reduces the chance of missing words at the beginning of the conversation.
- Avoiding talking too rapidly or using sentences that are too complex. Slow down a little, pause between sentences or phrases, and wait to make sure you have been understood before going on.
- Keeping your hands away from your face while talking. If you are eating, chewing, smoking, etc., while talking, your speech will be more difficult to understand. Beards and moustaches can also interfere with the ability of the hearing impaired to speech read.
- If the hearing impaired listener hears better in one ear than the other, try to make a point of remembering which ear is better so that you will know where to position yourself.
- Be aware of possible distortion of sounds for the hearing impaired person. They may hear your voice, but still may have difficulty understanding some words.
- Most hearing impaired people have greater difficulty understanding speech when there is background noise. Trying to minimize extraneous noise when talking.
- Some people with hearing loss are very sensitive to loud sounds. This reduced tolerance for loud sounds is not uncommon. Avoiding situations where there will be loud sounds when possible.

- If the hearing impaired person has difficulty understanding a particular phrase or word, try to find a different way of saying the same thing, rather than repeating the original words over and over.
- Acquainting the listener with the general topic of the conversation. Avoiding sudden changes of topic. If the subject is changed, explain the patient clearly what you are going to discuss with him/her. In a group setting, repeat questions or key facts before continuing with the discussion.
- If you are giving specific information—such as time, place, or phone numbers—to someone who is hearing impaired, have them repeat the specifics back to you. Many numbers and words sound alike.
- Whenever possible, providing pertinent information in writing, such as directions, schedules, work assignments.
- Recognizing that everyone, especially the hard-of-hearing, has a harder time hearing and understanding when ill or tired.
- Paying attention to the listener. A puzzled look may indicate misunderstanding. Tactfully asking the hearing impaired person if they understood you, or asking leading questions so you know your message got across.
- Taking turns speaking and avoid interrupting other speakers.
- Enrolling in aural rehabilitation classes with your hearing impaired spouse or friend.

MENIERE'S DISEASE

Meniere's disease is a disorder of the inner ear that causes spontaneous episodes of vertigo, a sensation of a spinning motion, along with fluctuating hearing loss, ringing in the ear (tinnitus), and sometimes a feeling of fullness or pressure in ear.

Etiology

The cause of Meniere's disease is not well understood. It appears to be the result of the abnormal volume or composition of fluid in the inner ear.

The inner ear is a cluster of connected passages and cavities called a labyrinth. The outside of the inner ear is made of bone (bony labyrinth). Inside is a soft structure of membrane (membranous labyrinth) that's a slightly smaller, similarly shaped version of the bony labyrinth. The membranous labyrinth contains a fluid (endolymph) and is lined with hair-like sensors that respond to movement of the fluid.

Meniere's disease may occur because of the following reasons:
- Improper fluid drainage, perhaps because of a blockage or anatomic abnormality
- Abnormal immune response
- Allergies
- Viral infection
- Genetic predisposition
- Head trauma
- Migraines

Signs and Symptoms

The primary signs and symptoms of Meniere's disease are as follows:
- **Recurring episodes of vertigo:** Vertigo is similar to the sensation experience if you spin around quickly several times and suddenly stop. Patient feels as if the room is still spinning, and he loses his balance. Episodes of vertigo occur without warning and usually last 20 minutes to 2 hours or more, up to 24 hours. Severe vertigo can cause nausea and vomiting.

- **Hearing loss:** Hearing loss in Meniere's disease may fluctuate, particularly early in the course of the disease. Eventually, most people experience some degree of permanent hearing loss.
- **Ringing in the ear (tinnitus):** Tinnitus is the perception of a ringing, buzzing, roaring, whistling, or hissing sound in ear.
- **Feeling of fullness in the ear:** People with Meniere's disease often feel aural fullness or increased pressure in the ear.

Diagnostic Evaluation

A diagnosis of Meniere's disease requires:
- Two spontaneous episodes of vertigo, each lasting 20 minutes or longer
- Hearing loss verified by a hearing test on at least one occasion
- Tinnitus or aural fullness
- Exclusion of other known causes of these sensory problems

Physical Examination and Medical History

Physical examination may include:
- The severity, duration, and frequency of the sensory problems
- History of infectious diseases or allergies
- Medication use
- Past ear problems
- General health
- History of inner ear problems in family

Hearing Assessment

A hearing test (audiometry) assesses how well you detect sounds at different pitches and volumes and how well you distinguish between similar-sounding words. The test not only reveals the quality of hearing but may also help to determine if the source of hearing problems is in the inner ear or the nerve that connects the inner ear to the brain.

Balance Assessment

Between episodes of vertigo, the sense of balance returns to normal for most people with Meniere's disease. But there may be some degree of ongoing balance problems.

There are several tests that assess function of the inner ear. Some or all of these tests can yield abnormal results in a person with Meniere's disease.

Videonystagmography (VNG): This test evaluates balance function by assessing eye movement. Balance-related sensors in the inner ear are linked to muscles that control movement of the eye in all directions. This connection is what enables us to move head around while keeping our eyes focused on a single point.

In a VNG evaluation, warm and cool water or warm and cool air are introduced into the ear canal. Measurements of involuntary eye movements in response to this stimulation are performed using a special pair of video goggles. Abnormalities of this test may indicate an inner ear problem.

Rotary-chair testing: Like a VNG, this measures inner ear function based on eye movement. In this case, stimulus to inner ear is provided by movement of a special rotating chair precisely controlled by a computer.

Vestibular evoked myogenic potentials (VEMP) testing: VEMP testing measures the function of sensors in the vestibule of the inner ear that help to detect acceleration movement.

These sensors also have a slight sensitivity to sound. When these sensors react to sound, tiny measurable variations in neck or eye muscle contractions occur. These contractions serve as an indirect measure of inner ear function.

Posturography: This computerized test reveals which part of the balance system, vision, inner ear function, or sensations from the skin, muscles, tendons, and joints. While wearing a safety harness, you stand in bare feet on a platform and keep your balance under various conditions.

Magnetic resonance imaging (MRI): This technique uses a magnetic field and radio waves to create images of soft tissues in the body. It can be used to produce either a thin cross-sectional "slice" or a 3D image of brain.

CT: This X-ray technique produces cross-sectional images of internal structures in body.

Auditory brainstem response audiometry: This is a computerized test of the hearing nerves and hearing centers of the brain. It can help detect the presence of a tumor disrupting the function of auditory nerves.

Management

No cure exists for Meniere's disease, but a number of strategies may help to manage some symptoms.

Medications for Vertigo

- **Motion sickness medications**, such as meclizine or diazepam, may reduce the spinning sensation of vertigo and help control nausea and vomiting.
- **Antinausea medications,** such as promethazine, may control nausea and vomiting during an episode of vertigo.
- **Diuretic**, these drugs reduces the amount of fluid the body retains and helps to regulate the fluid volume and pressure in inner ear.

Noninvasive Therapies and Procedures

Some people with Meniere's may benefit from other noninvasive therapies and procedures, such as:
- **Rehabilitation:** Problems with balance between episodes of vertigo may be reduced by vestibular rehabilitation therapy. The goal of this therapy, which may include exercises and activities that perform during therapy sessions and at home, is to help your body and brain regain the ability to process balance information correctly.
- **Hearing aid:** A hearing aid in the ear affected by Meniere's disease may improve hearing.
- **Meniett device:** For vertigo that is hard to treat, this therapy involves the application of positive pressure to the middle ear to improve fluid exchange. A device called a Meniett pulse generator applies pulses of pressure to the ear canal through a ventilation tube. The treatment is performed at home, usually three times a day for 5 minutes at a time. Meniett device shows improvement in symptoms of vertigo, tinnitus, and aural pressure.

Middle Ear Injections

Medications injected into the middle ear, and then absorbed into the inner ear, may improve vertigo symptoms. For example, **gentamicin, steroids,** such as dexamethasone, also may help control vertigo attacks in some people.

Surgical Management

If vertigo attacks associated with Meniere's disease are severe and debilitating and other treatments do not help, surgery may be an option. Procedures may include:

- **Endolymphatic sac procedures:** The endolymphatic sac plays a role in regulating inner ear fluid levels. These surgical procedures may alleviate vertigo by decreasing fluid production or increasing fluid absorption.

   In endolymphatic sac decompression, a small portion of bone is removed from over the endolymphatic sac. In some cases, this procedure is coupled with the placement of a shunt, a tube that drains excess fluid from inner ear.
- **Vestibular nerve section:** This procedure involves cutting the nerve that connects balance and movement sensors in inner ear to the brain (vestibular nerve). This procedure usually corrects problems with vertigo while attempting to preserve hearing in the affected ear.
- **Labyrinthectomy:** With this procedure, the surgeon removes the balance portion of the inner ear, thereby removing both balance and hearing function from the affected ear. This procedure is performed only if one already has near-total or total hearing loss.

Nursing Management

Nursing Diagnosis

- Risk for injury related to altered mobility because of gait disturbed and vertigo.
- Impaired adjustment related to disability requiring change in lifestyle because of unpredictability of vertigo.
- Risk for fluid volume imbalance and deficit related to increased fluid output, altered intake, and medications.
- Anxiety related to threat of, or change in, health status and disabling effects of vertigo.
- Ineffective coping related to personal vulnerability and unmet expectations stemming from vertigo.
- Self-care deficits related to labyrinth dysfunction and episodes of vertigo.

Nursing Interventions

- Providing nursing care during acute attack.
- Providing a safe, quiet, dimly lit environment, and enforce bed rest.
- Providing emotional support and reassurance to alleviate anxiety.
- Administering prescribed medications, which may include antihistamines, antiemetic, and possibly, mild diuretics. Instructing the client on self-care instructions to control the number of acute attacks.
- Discussing the nature of the disorder.
- Discussing the need for a low-salt diet.
- Explaining the importance of avoiding stimulants and vasoconstrictions (e.g., caffeine, decongestants, and alcohol).
- Discussing medications that may be prescribed to prevent attacks or self-administration of appropriate medications during an attack, which may include anticholinergics, vasodilation, antihistamines, and possibly, diuretics or nicotinic acid.
- Discussing, preparing, and assisting the client with surgical options.
- A labyrinthectomy is the most radical procedure and involves resection of the vestibular nerve or total removal of the labyrinth performed by the transcanal route, which results in deafness in that eat.
- An endolymphatic decompression consists of draining the endolymphatic sac and inserting a shunt to enhance the fluid drainage.

LABYRINTHITIS

Labyrinthitis is a disorder of the inner ear. The two vestibular nerves in inner ear send information to brain about head movement. When one of these nerves becomes inflamed, it creates a condition known as labyrinthitis.

Etiology

Labyrinthitis can happen to people of all ages. It can be caused by a variety of factors, including:

- Respiratory illnesses (such as bronchitis)
- Viruses of the inner ear
- Stomach viruses
- Herpes viruses
- Bacterial infections (including bacterial middle ear infections)
- Infectious organisms (like the one that causes Lyme disease)

Risk Factors

- Smoking
- Drink large quantities of alcohol
- Have a history of allergies
- Are habitually fatigued
- Extreme stress
- Over-the-counter medications

Signs and Symptoms

- Dizziness
- Nausea
- Loss of hearing
- Vertigo can interfere with driving, working, and other activities
- Loss of balance
- Tinnitus
- Difficulty focusing eyes

Diagnostic Evaluation

Labyrinthitis can be diagnosed during a physical examination.

- Hearing tests
- CT or MRI scan of the head to record images of cranial structures
- EEG (brain wave test)
- Electronystagmography (ENG) (eye movement test)
- Blood tests.

Management

Symptoms can be relieved with medications, including:

- Antihistamines, such as Clarinex or Allegra, Benadryl, and Claritin.
- Medications that can reduce dizziness and nausea, such as Antivert.
- Sedatives, such as diazepam.
- Corticosteroids, to reduce the inflammation.
- Avoiding quick changes in position or sudden movements.
- Sitting still during a vertigo attack.
- Getting up slowly from a lying down or sitting position.
- Avoiding television, computer screens, and bright or flashing lights during a vertigo attack.
- If vertigo occurs while you are in bed, try sitting up in a chair and keeping head still. Low lighting is better than darkness or bright lights.

Nursing Management

See nursing care plan for acute otitis media (AOM).

EPISTAXIS

The purpose of the nose is to warm and humidify the air that we breathe in. The nose is lined with many blood vessels that lie close to the surface where they can be injured and bleed. Epistaxis is defined as bleeding from the nostril, nasal cavity, or nasopharynx. Nosebleeds are due to the bursting of a blood vessel within the nose.

Etiology

- Dry, heated, indoor air, which dries out the nasal membranes and causes them to become cracked or crusted and bleed when rubbed or picked or when blowing the nose
- Dry, hot, low-humidity climates, which can dry out the mucus membranes
- Colds (upper respiratory infections) and sinusitis, especially episodes that cause repeated sneezing, coughing, and nose blowing
- Vigorous nose blowing or nose picking
- The insertion of a foreign object into the nose
- Injury to the nose or face
- Allergic and nonallergic rhinitis (inflammation of the nasal lining)
- Use of drugs that thin the blood (aspirin, nonsteroidal anti-inflammatory medications, warfarin, and others)
- High blood pressure
- Chemical irritants (e.g., cocaine, industrial chemicals)
- Deviated septum
- Tumors or inherited bleeding disorders
- Facial and nasal surgery.

Nosebleeds can be divided into two categories, based on the site of bleeding:

1. **Anterior hemorrhage:** The source of bleeding is visible in about 95% of cases—usually from the nasal septum, particularly Little's area which is where Kiesselbach's plexus forms (an anastomotic network of vessels on the anterior portion of the nasal septum).
2. **Posterior hemorrhage:** This emanates from deeper structures of the nose and occurs more commonly in older individuals. Nosebleeds from this area are usually more profuse and have a greater risk of airway compromise.

Diagnostic Evaluation

History

- Determining if blood is running out of the nose and one nostril (usually anterior) or if blood is running into the throat or from both nostrils (usually posterior)
- Asking about trauma (including nose picking)
- Noting family or past history of clotting disorders or hypertension
- Noting whether there has been previous nasal surgery
- Discussing medication—especially, warfarin, aspirin
- Enquiring about any facial pain or otalgia—these may be presenting signs of a nasopharyngeal tumor
- In young male patients, ask about nasal obstruction, headache, rhinorrhea, and anosmia—signs of juvenile nasopharyngeal angiofibroma.

Investigation

- Coagulation studies and blood typing
- Quite marked anemia can result but a hematological malignancy may also be revealed.

Management

Initial Assessment First Aid

- Resuscitating the patient (if necessary)—remember the ABCD of resuscitation.
- Asking the patient to sit upright, leaning slightly forward, and to squeeze the bottom part of the nose (NOT the bridge of the nose) for 10–20 minutes to try to stop the bleeding. The patient should breathe through the mouth and spit out any blood or saliva into a bowl. An ice pack on the bridge of the nose may help.
- Monitoring the patient's pulse and blood pressure.
- If bleeding has stopped after this time proceeds to inspect the nose, using a nasal speculum, consider cautery.
- If the history is of severe and prolonged bleeding, get expert help—and watch carefully for signs of hypovolemia.

Cautery

- Nasal cautery is a common treatment of epistaxis. A caustic agent, such as silver nitrate or an electrically charged wire, such as platinum is used to stop bleeding in the nasal mucous membrane.
- Chemical cautery of the visible blood vessels on the anterior part of the nasal septum is the most popular treatment method for idiopathic recurrent nosebleeds.
- Carefully examining the nasal cavity, looking for any bleeding points, which can usually be seen on the anterior septum—either an oozing point or a visible clot. Noting whether there is any pus, suggesting local bacterial infection.
- Blowing the nose decreases the effects of local fibrinolysis and removes clots, permitting a clearer examination. Applying a vasoconstrictor before examination may reduce hemorrhage and help locate the bleeding site. A topical local anesthetic reduces pain from examination and nasal packing.
- Applying a silver nitrate cautery stick for 10 seconds, working from the edge and moving radially—never both sides of the septum at the same session.
- Topical application with 0.5% neomycin + 0.1% chlorhexidine cream or with Vaseline petroleum jelly is alternative topical treatments.
- If bleeding continues, packing may be considered.
- A topical application of injectable form of tranexamic acid has been shown to be better than anterior nasal packing in the initial treatment of idiopathic anterior epistaxis.
- It may be necessary to ligate the sphenopalatine artery endoscopically, or occasionally the internal maxillary artery and ethmoid arteries, or perform endovascular embolization of the internal maxillary artery, when packing fails to control a life-threatening hemorrhage. Ligation of the external carotid artery is the last resort.

Complications of Packing

- Anosmia
- Pack falling out and continued bleeding
- Breathing difficulties and aspiration of clots
- Posterior migration of the pack, causing airway obstruction and asphyxia
- Perforation of the nasal septum or pressure necrosis of cartilage.

Follow these Steps to stop a Nosebleed in Emergency when you are Alone

- Relax
- Sitting down and leaning your body and your head slightly forward. This will keep the blood from running down your throat, which can cause nausea, vomiting, and diarrhea.
- Breathing through your mouth.
- Using a tissue or damp washcloth to catch the blood.
- Using your thumb and index finger to pinch together the soft part of your nose. Making sure to pinch the soft part of the nose against the hard bony ridge that forms the bridge of the nose. Squeezing at or above the bony part of the nose will not put pressure where it can help stop bleeding.
- Keeping pinching your nose continuously for at least 5 minutes before checking if the bleeding has stopped. If your nose is still bleeding, continue squeezing the nose for another 10 minutes.
- You can spray an over-the-counter decongestant spray, such as oxymetazoline into the bleeding side of the nose and then applies pressure to the nose.
- WARNING: These topical decongestant sprays should not be used over the long term.
- Once the bleeding stops, do not bend over, strain or lift anything heavy and do not blow, rub, or pick your nose for several days.

Nursing Management

Providing Nursing Interventions to Control Bleeding

- Having the client sit upright, breathing through the mouth, and refraining from talking
- Compressing the soft outer portion of the nares against the septum for 5–10 minutes
- Instructing the client to avoid nose blowing during or after the episode
- If pressure does not control bleeding, preparing to assist the health-care provider in inserting an anterior packing or posterior packing as appropriate
- Keeping scissors and a hemostat on hand to cut the strings and removing the packing in the event of airway obstructions.

Providing Ongoing Assessment to Monitor for Bleeding

- Inspecting for blood trickling into the posterior pharynx
- Observing for hemoptysis, hematemesis, and frequent swallowing or belching
- Instructing the client not to swallow but to spit out any blood into emesis basins
- Monitoring the client's vital signs

Providing Oral and Written Instructions for Treatment and Prevention

- Discussing ways to prevent epistaxis, including avoiding forceful nose blowing, straining, high altitudes, and nasal trauma
- Instructing the client to have adequate humidification to prevent drying of nasal passages
- Instructing the client on the proper way to stop bleeding
- Instructing the client to not put anything up the nasal passages
- Instructing the client to contact a health-care provider if the bleeding does not stop.

LARYNX CANCER

Throat cancer refers to cancerous tumors that develop in throat (pharynx), voice box (larynx), or tonsils.

Types of Larynx Cancer

Throat cancer is a general term that applies to cancer that develops in the throat (pharyngeal cancer) or in the voice box (laryngeal cancer). The throat and the voice box are closely connected, with the voice box located just below the throat.

Though most throat cancers involve the same types of cells, specific terms are used to differentiate the part of the throat where cancer originated.

- **Nasopharyngeal cancer** begins in the nasopharynx.
- **Oropharyngeal cancer** begins in the oropharynx.
- **Hypopharyngeal cancer (laryngopharyngeal cancer)** begins in the hypopharynx.
- **Glottic cancer** begins in the vocal cords.
- **Supraglottic cancer** begins in the upper portion of the larynx and includes cancer that affects the epiglottis.
- **Subglottic cancer** begins in the lower portion of voice box and below vocal cords.
- Cancers that start in gland cells (adenocarcinoma), adenocarcinoma is uncommon compared to squamous cell laryngeal cancer. It starts in the adenomatous cells that are scattered around the surface of the larynx. Adenomatous cells are gland cells that produce *mucus*.
- Connective tissue cancers (sarcoma), sarcomas are cancers that start in the body's connective tissues. These are the supporting tissues of the body, such as bone, muscle, and nerves. Cartilage is the supporting tissue of the larynx. Cancers that develop from cartilage are called chondrosarcomas.

TNM Classification of Cancer of Larynx

TNM stands for tumor, node, and metastasis. The system describes:
- The size of a primary tumor.
- Whether the lymph nodes have cancer cells in them.
- Whether the cancer has spread to a different part of the body.

The exact T staging of laryngeal cancer varies depending on which part of the larynx is involved. The cancer may start on the vocal cords (glottis), above the vocal cords (supraglottis), or below the vocal cords (subglottis).

Early-Stage Laryngeal Cancer (T0–T2)

- **T stage 0, Tis (tumor in situ):** In very early cancer of the larynx, this means there are abnormal cells that may be precancerous. Tis means an early cancer that has not broken through the basement membrane of the tissue it is growing in.
- **T stage 1:** T stage 1 means the tumor is in only one part of the larynx and the vocal cords are able to move normally.
- **T stage 2:** T stage 2 means the tumor which may have started on the vocal cords (glottis), above the vocal cords (supraglottis), or below the vocal cords (subglottis) has grown into another part of the larynx. In cancer of the vocal cords (glottic cancer) stage T2a means that the vocal cords move normally.

Locally Advanced Laryngeal Cancer (T2b–T4)

- **Glottic cancer T stage 2b:** In T stage 2b in cancer that starts in the vocal cords (glottis), the vocal cord movement is limited.
- **T stage 3:** T stage 3 means the tumor is throughout the larynx but has not spread further than the covering of the larynx.
- **T stage 4:** T stage 4 means the tumor has grown into body tissues outside the larynx. It may have spread to the thyroid gland, windpipe (trachea) or food pipe.

N Stages of Laryngeal Cancer

There are four main lymph node stages in cancer of the larynx. N2 is divided into N2a, N2b, and N2c. The important points here are whether there is cancer in any of the nodes and if so, the size of the node and which side of the neck it is on.

- N0 means there are no lymph nodes containing cancer cells.
- N1 means there are cancer cells in one lymph node on the same side of the neck as the cancer, but the node is less than 3 cm across.
- N2a means there is cancer in one lymph node on the same side of the neck and it is between 3 and 6 cm across.
- N2b means there is cancer in more than one lymph node, but none are more than 6 cm across. All the nodes must be on the same side of the neck as the cancer.
- N2c means there is cancer in lymph nodes on the other side of the neck from the tumor, or in nodes on both sides of the neck, but none is more than 6 cm across.
- N3 means that at least one lymph node containing cancer is larger than 6 cm across.

M Stages of Laryngeal Cancer

There are two stages to describe whether cancer of the larynx has spread:

1. M0 means there is no cancer spread.
2. M1 means the cancer has spread to other parts of the body, such as the lungs.

Cancer Grading

The grade of a cancer tells how much the cancer cells look like normal cells under a microscope. There are three grades of laryngeal cancer:

1. **Grade 1 (low grade):** The cancer cells look very much like normal larynx cells (they are well differentiated).
2. **Grade 2 (intermediate grade):** The cancer cells look slightly like normal larynx cells (they are moderately differentiated).
3. **Grade 3 (high grade):** The cancer cells look very abnormal and very little like normal larynx cells (they are poorly differentiated).

Etiology and Risk Factors

- Age, as with most cancers, cancer of the larynx is more common in older people than in younger. There are very few cases in people under 40 years of age.
- Drinking alcohol and smoking, smoking tobacco and drinking a lot of alcohol are the main risk factors for cancer of the larynx in the western world.
- Alcohol and cigarettes contain chemicals that increase the risk of cancer.
- Heavy drinking and smoking are particularly linked to cancer above the vocal cords (the supraglottis) and the area around the vocal cords (the glottis). Compared to nondrinkers, heavy drinkers have about three times the risk of developing cancer of the larynx. Even drinking less than two drinks a day (e.g., two pints of beer or two small glasses of wine) gives a slightly increased risk of laryngeal cancer. But nonsmokers are unlikely to have an increased risk of laryngeal cancer at this level of drinking.
- HPV infection, HPV stands for human papilloma virus (HPV). There are many types of HPV. Some types can affect the lining of the larynx and cause small, wart-like growths.
- Diet, poor eating patterns are common in people who are heavy drinkers. This may be one reason why alcohol increases the risk of cancer. A poor diet may increase risk of cancer of the larynx. This may be due to a lack of vitamins and minerals. A diet high in fresh fruit and vegetables seems to reduce the risk of cancer of the larynx. This may be because these foods

contain high levels of the antioxidant vitamins A, C, and E. Vitamins and other substances in fresh foods may help to stop damage to the lining of the larynx that can lead to cancer.

- Family history and people who have a first-degree relative diagnosed with a head and neck cancer have double the risk of laryngeal cancer of someone without a family history.
- Immunocompromised patient
- Exposure to substances, some chemicals may increase risk of cancer of the larynx like, wood dust, soot or coal dust, or paint fumes, exposure to coal as a fuel source in the home.
- Acid reflux, reflux happens when stomach acid comes back up the esophagus and irritates the lining. In the long-term, this can cause damage to the cells in the esophagus. This irritation and damage can extend to the larynx and may increase cancer risk.

Signs and Symptoms

- A cough
- Changes in voice, such as hoarseness
- Difficulty swallowing
- Ear pain
- A lump or sore that does not heal
- A sore throat
- Weight loss

Diagnostic Evaluation

- **Flexible endoscopy of the larynx:** This test means the back of mouth and throat (including the larynx) examined with a narrow, flexible telescope (a nasendoscope). This is passed up the nose to look at all upper air passages, including the larynx from above. This may be a bit uncomfortable, but can have an *anesthetic* spray to numb throat first. This test is sometimes called a nasoendoscopy.
- **Endoscopy:** An endoscope is a series of connected telescopes that an ENT specialist uses to look at the back of throat. There is a camera and light at one end, and an eyepiece at the other. Through the endoscope, doctor can see the inside of nose and throat very clearly and will take biopsies of any abnormal-looking areas.
- **Transnasal esophagoscopy:** The doctor inserts a flexible tube (endoscope) through nose and down throat. This test is sometimes used instead of having an endoscope under general anesthetic. The tip of the tube has a digital video system and self-contained light. This test is done under a *local anesthetic*. It gives clear pictures of the inside of the throat and larynx.
- **Fine-needle aspiration:** This is sometimes written as FNA. A FNA is done to aspirate the fluid to evaluate any cancerous property.
- **Physical examination**
- **CT scan:** This is a computerized scan using X-rays to evaluate the size of the cancer and any enlarged lymph nodes in the neck.
- **MRI scan:** Magnetic Resonance Imaging is a non-invasive imaging technology that produces three dimensional detailed anatomical images. It is often used for disease detection, diagnosis, and treatment monitoring.
- **PET-CT scan:** Positron emission tomography (PET) uses small amounts of radioactive materials called radiotracers or radiopharmaceuticals, a special camera and a computer to evaluate organ and tissue functions. By identifying changes at the cellular level, PET may detect the early onset of disease before other imaging tests can.

Management

The main treatments for cancer of the voice box are radiotherapy or surgery.

Radiotherapy

Radiotherapy can shrink a large tumor in the larynx and make it easier to remove. Or it can kill off any cancer cells that might have been left behind after surgery. This lowers the risk of the cancer coming back.

Radiotherapy may be used to treat the lymph nodes after surgery; if there is a risk these may contain cancer cells. This may be instead of lymph node dissection.

Surgical Management

- **Partial laryngectomy:** Tumors that are limited to one vocal cord are removed, and a temporary tracheotomy is performed to maintain the airway. After recovery from surgery, the patient will have a voice but it will be hoarse.
- **Hemilaryngectomy:** When there is a possibility the cancer includes one true and one false vocal cord, they are removed along with an arytenoid cartilage and half of the thyroid cartilage. Temporary tracheotomy is performed, and the patient's voice will be hoarse after surgery.
- **Supraglottic laryngectomy:** When the tumor is located in the epiglottis or false vocal cords, radical neck dissection is done and tracheotomy performed. The patient's voice remains intact; however, swallowing is more difficult because the epiglottis has been removed.
- **Total laryngectomy:** Advanced cancers that involve a large portion of the larynx require removal of the entire larynx, the hyoid bone, the cricoid cartilage, two or three tracheal rings, and the strap muscles connected to the larynx. A permanent opening is created in the neck into the trachea, and a laryngectomy tube is inserted to keep the stoma open. The lower portion of the posterior pharynx is removed when the tumor extends beyond the epiglottis, with the remaining portion sutured to the esophagus after a nasogastric tube is inserted. The patient must breathe through a permanent tracheostomy, with normal speech no longer possible.

Biological Therapy

Biological therapy is treatment that changes the activity of substances made naturally in the body. These therapies can control or destroy cancer cells. Example:

Cetuximab: Cetuximab (Erbitux) is a type of biological therapy known as a monoclonal antibody. It is designed to block areas on the surface of cancer cells that can trigger growth. These are called epidermal growth factor receptors. Blocking these receptors can stop the signals that tell the cancer to grow.

Side Effects of Biological Therapies

- Tiredness
- Diarrhea
- Skin changes (rashes or discoloration)
- A sore mouth
- Weakness
- Loss of appetite
- Low blood counts
- Swelling of parts of the body, due to fluid build-up

Nursing Management

- Maintaining patent airway, adequate ventilation
- Assisting patient in developing augmentative and alternative communication (AAC) methods

- Restoring and maintaining skin integrity
- Re-establishing and maintaining adequate nutrition
- Providing emotional support for acceptance of altered body image
- Providing information about disease process and prognosis and treatment

Discharge Goals

- Ventilation and oxygenation adequate for individual needs
- Communicating effectively
- Complications prevented or minimized
- Beginning to cope with change in body image
- Disease process, prognosis, and therapeutic regimen understood

Nursing Diagnosis

Ineffective Airway Clearance and Risk for Aspiration Related to Partial or Total Removal of the Glottis, Altering Ability to Breathe, Cough, and Swallow

Intervention

- Monitoring respiratory rate, depth. Auscultate breath sounds
- Elevating the head of the bed 30–45
- Encouraging swallowing, if patient is able
- Encouraging effective coughing and deep breathing
- Do suctioning and note the amount and color of secretions
- Demonstrating and encouraging the patient to being self-suction
- Maintaining the proper positioning of laryngectomy tube
- Changing patient position to check pooling of blood behind neck.

Impaired Verbal Communication Related to Removal of Vocal Cord and Tracheostomy

Intervention

- Reviewing preoperative instructions and discussion of why speech and breathing are altered, using anatomical drawings or models to assist in explanations.
- Determining whether patient has other communication impairments, for example, hearing, vision, literacy.
- Providing immediate and continual means to summon nurse, for example, call light/bell.
- Let patient know the summons will be answered immediately. Stop by to check on patient periodically without being summoned.
- Post noticing at central answering system or nursing station that patient is unable to speak.
- Providing alternative means of communication appropriate to patient need, for example, pad and pencil, magic slate, alphabet, picture board, sign language.
- Allowing sufficient time for communication.
- Providing nonverbal communication, for example, touching and physical presence. Anticipating needs.
- Encouraging ongoing communication with the world, for example, newspapers, television, radio, calendar, clock.
- Referring to loss of speech as temporary after a partial laryngectomy and depending on availability of voice prosthetics, vocal cord transplant.
- Caution patient not to use voice until physician gives permission.
- Arranging for meeting with other persons who have experienced this procedure, as appropriate.
- Prearranging signals for obtaining immediate help.

Skin and Tissue Integrity, Impaired Related to Surgical Removal of Tissues, and Radiation or Chemotherapeutic Agents

Intervention
- Assessing skin color, temperature and capillary refill in operative and skin graft areas.
- Keeping head of bed elevated 30–45°. Monitoring facial edema (usually peaks by third to fifth postoperative day).
- Protecting skin flaps and suture lines from tension or pressure. Providing pillows, rolls, and instruct patient to support head and neck during activity.
- Monitoring bloody drainage from surgical sites, suture lines, and drains.
- Reporting any milky-appearing drainage.
- Cleansing incisions with sterile saline and peroxide (mixed 1:1) after dressings have been removed.
- Monitoring donor site if graft performed and check dressings as indicated.
- Cleansing thoroughly around stoma and neck tubes, avoiding soap or alcohol. Showing patient how to do self-stoma or tube care with clean water and peroxide, using soft, lint-free cloth, not tissue or cotton.
- Monitoring all sites for signs of wound infection, for example, unusual redness, increasing edema, pain, exudates, and temperature elevation.

Oral Mucous Membrane, Impaired Related to Dehydration, Absence of Oral Intake, Decreased Saliva Production Secondary to Radiation or Surgical Procedure

Intervention
- Suction oral cavity gently and frequently
- Having patient perform self-suctioning when possible or using gauze wick to drain secretions
- Showing patient how to brush inside of mouth, palate, tongue, and teeth frequently
- Applying lubrication to lips and provide oral irrigations as indicated
- Avoiding alcohol-based mouthwashes
- Using normal saline or mixture of saltwater and baking soda for rinsing
- Suggesting use of artificial saliva preparations (e.g., pilocarpine hydrochloride) if mucous membranes are dry.

Pain, Acute Related to Surgical Incisions and Tissue Swelling

Intervention
- Supporting head and neck with pillows. Showing patient how to support neck during activity.
- Providing comfort measures (e.g., back rub, position change) and diversional activities (e.g., television, visiting, and reading).
- Encouraging patient to expectorate saliva or to suction mouth gently if unable to swallow.
- Investigating changes in characteristics of pain. Checking mouth, throat suture lines for fresh trauma.
- Noting nonverbal indicators and autonomic responses to pain.
- Evaluating effects of analgesics
- Medicating before activity and treatments as indicated.
- Scheduling care activities to balance with adequate periods of sleep and rest.
- Recommending use of stress management behaviors, for example, relaxation techniques, guided imagery.
- Providing oral irrigations, anesthetic sprays, and gargles. Instructing patient in self-irrigations.

- Administering analgesics, for example, codeine, acetylsalicylic acid, and propoxyphene as indicated.

Nutrition: Imbalanced, Less than Body Requirements Related to Temporary or Permanent Alteration in Mode of Food Intake

Intervention

- Auscultating bowel sounds.
- Maintaining feeding tube, for example, check for tube placement, flush with warm water as indicated.
- Monitoring intake and weigh as indicated. Showing patient how to monitor and record weight on a scheduled basis.
- Instructing patient in self-feeding techniques, for example, bulb syringe, bag and funnel method, and blending soft foods if patient is to go home with a feeding tube. Making sure patient and family member are able to perform this procedure before discharge and that appropriate food and equipment are available at home.
- Beginning with small feedings and advance as tolerated. Noting signs of gastric fullness, regurgitation, and diarrhea.
- Providing supplemental water by feeding tube or orally if patient can swallow.
- Encouraging patient when relearning swallowing, for example, maintaining a quiet environment, having suction equipment on standby, and demonstrating appropriate breathing techniques.
- Encouraging patient when relearning swallowing, for example, maintaining a quiet environment, having suction equipment on standby, and demonstrating appropriate breathing techniques.
- Resuming oral feedings when feasible. Staying with patient during meals the first few days.
- Developing and encouraging a pleasant environment for meals.
- Helping patient to develop nutritionally balanced home meal plans.
- Consulting with dietitian and nutritional support team as indicated. Incorporating and reinforcing dietitian's teaching.
- Providing nutritionally balanced diet (e.g., semisolid/soft foods) or tube feedings (e.g., blended soft food or commercial preparations) as indicated.
- Monitoring laboratory studies, for example, blood urea nitrogen, glucose, liver function, prealbumin, protein, electrolytes.

Disturbed Body Image and Role Performance Related to Loss of Voice

Intervention

- Discussing meaning of loss or change with patient, identifying perceptions of current situation and future expectations.
- Noting nonverbal body language, negative attitudes, and self-talk.
- Assessing for self-destructive and suicidal behavior.
- Noting emotional reactions, for example, grieving, depression, anger.
- Allowing patient to progress at own rate.
- Maintaining calm, reassuring manner. Acknowledging and accepting expression of feelings of grief, hostility.
- Allowing but do not participate in patient's use of denial, for example, when patient is reluctant to participate in self-care (e.g., suctioning stoma). Providing care in a nonjudgmental manner.
- Setting limits on maladaptive behaviors, assisting patient to identify positive behaviors that will aid recovery.

- Encouraging family member to treat patient normally and not as an invalid.
- Alerting staff that facial expressions and other nonverbal behaviors need to convey acceptance and not revulsion.
- Encouraging identification of anticipated personal and work conflicts that may arise.
- Recognizing behavior indicative of overconcern with future lifestyle and relationship functioning.
- Encouraging patient to deal with situation in small steps.
- Providing positive reinforcement for efforts and progress made.
- Encouraging patient and family to communicate feelings to each other.

Knowledge, Deficient Regarding Prognosis, Treatment, Self-care, and Discharge Needs Related to Lack of Information

Intervention

- Assessing amount of preoperative preparation and retention of information.
- Assessing level of anxiety related to diagnosis and surgery.
- Providing and repeat explanations at patient's level of acceptance.
- Providing written directions for patient to read and have available for future reference.
- Discussing inaccuracies in perception of disease process and therapies with patient and family.
- Educating patient and family about basic information regarding stoma, shower with stoma collar, shampoo by leaning forward, no swimming or water sports.
- Covering stoma with foam or fiber filter (e.g., cotton or silk).
- Covering stoma when coughing or sneezing.
- Reinforcing necessity of not smoking.
- Discussing inability to smell and taste as before surgery.
- Discussing importance of reporting to caregiver and physician immediately such symptoms as stoma narrowing, presence of—lump in throat, dysphagia, or bleeding.
- Recommending wearing medical-alert identification tag or bracelet identifying patient as a neck breather.
- Encouraging family members to become certified in cardiopulmonary resuscitation if they are interested or able to do so.
- Giving careful attention to the provision of needed rehabilitative measures, for example, temporary, permanent prosthesis, dental care, speech therapy, surgical reconstruction. Vocational, sexual or marital counseling, and financial assistance.
- Identifying homecare needs and available resources.

SPEECH DISORDERS

Types of Speech Impairment

Speech impairments may be present in different forms. Adult-impaired speech is a symptom of several different speech disorders. They include:

- **Spasmodic dysphonia:** It is identified by involuntary movements of the vocal cords when speaking. Voice may be hoarse, airy, and tight.
- **Aphasia:** The inability to express and comprehend language. Individuals with aphasia may find it difficult to think of words. They may also mispronounce words.
- **Dysarthria:** Weak vocal muscles. These weak muscles cause slurred and slow speech. The larynx and vocal cords have difficulty coordinating to make a fluent sound.

- **Vocal disturbances:** Any factor that changes the function or shape of vocal cords can cause changes in the sound and ease of speech.

Etiology and Types of Speech Disorders

Speech impairment can occur suddenly or can gradually progress. Each speech impairment type has a different cause.

Spasmodic Dysphonia

This is abnormal brain functioning. Though scientists are not sure, it is believed this condition originates in the **basal ganglia** (part of the brain that controls muscle movement in the body).

Aphasia

Brain damage from a stroke or blood clot is a common cause of aphasia. Other causes include:
- Head trauma
- Brain tumor
- Cognitive degenerative conditions, such as Alzheimer's disease or dementia.

Dysarthria

Degenerative muscle and motor conditions, such as multiple sclerosis, muscular dystrophy, cerebral palsy, and Parkinson's disease may cause this condition. Other causes may include:
- Stroke
- Head trauma
- Brain tumor
- Lyme disease
- Drinking alcohol
- Facial weakness, such as Bell's palsy
- Tight or loose dentures

Vocal Disturbances

- Throat cancer can affect the sound of the voice.
- Polyps, nodules, or other growths on vocal cords can cause vocal concerns.
- Heavy use of the voice can cause a hoarse voice, as in the case of a singer, performer, or coach.
- Ingestion of certain drugs, such as caffeine, antidepressants, and amphetamines can cause a dry, tight voice.

Clinical Manifestation

Changes in speech will depend on the type of speech disorder.

Apraxia of Speech

Individuals with apraxia may demonstrate:
- Difficulty imitating and producing speech sounds, marked by speech errors, such as sound distortions, substitutions, or omissions
- Inconsistent speech errors
- Groping of the tongue and lips to make specific sounds and words
- Slow speech rate
- Impaired rhythm

- Better automatic speech (e.g., greetings) than purposeful speech
- Inability to produce any sound at all in severe cases

Dysarthria

A person with dysarthria may demonstrate the following speech characteristics:
- "Slurred," "choppy," or "mumbled" speech that may be difficult to understand
- Slow rate of speech
- Rapid rate of speech with a "mumbling" quality
- Limited tongue, lip, and jaw movement
- Abnormal pitch and rhythm when speaking
- Changes in voice quality, such as hoarse or breathy voice or speech that sounds "nasal" or "stuffy."

Stuttering

- The person is having difficulty moving from the "w" in "where" to the remaining sounds in the word. On the fourth attempt, he successfully completes the word.
- The person is having difficulty moving from the "s" in "save" to the remaining sounds in the word. He continues to say the "s" sound until he is able to complete the word.
- The person expects to have difficulty smoothly joining the word "you" with the word "around." In response to the anticipated difficulty, he produces several interjections until he is able to say the word "around" smoothly.

Aphasia

- Difficulty producing language
- Experiencing difficulty coming up with the words they want to say
- Substituting the intended word with another word that may be related in meaning to the target (e.g., "chicken" for "fish") or unrelated (e.g., "radio" for "ball")
- Switching sounds within words (e.g., "wish dasher" for "dishwasher")
- Using made-up words (e.g., "frigilin" for "hamburger")
- Having difficulty putting words together to form sentences
- Stringing together made-up words and real words fluently but without making sense
- Difficulty understanding language
- Misunderstanding what others say, especially when they speak fast (e.g., radio or television news) or in long sentences
- Finding it hard to understand speech in background noise or in group situations
- Misinterpreting jokes and taking the literal meaning of figurative speech (e.g., "it's raining cats and dogs")
- Difficulty reading forms, pamphlets, books, and other written material
- Problems spelling and putting words together to write sentences
- Difficulty understanding number concepts (e.g., telling time, counting money, adding/subtracting)

Management

Augmentative and Alternative Communication

It includes all forms of communication (other than oral speech) that are used to express thoughts, needs, wants, and ideas. We all use AAC when we make facial expressions or gestures, use symbols or pictures, or write.

People with severe speech or language problems rely on AAC to supplement existing speech or replace speech that is not functional. Special augmentative aids, such as picture and symbol communication boards and electronic devices, are available to help people express themselves. This may increase social interaction, school performance, and feelings of self-worth.

Types of AAC Systems

When children or adults cannot use speech to communicate effectively in all situations, there are options.

a. **Unaided communication systems:** It is necessary to rely on the user's body to convey messages. Examples include gestures, body language, and sign language.

b. **Aided communication systems:** It is necessary to require the use of tools or equipment in addition to the user's body. Aided communication methods can range from paper and pencil to communication books or boards to devices that produce voice output (speech generating devices) and written output. Electronic communication aids allow the user to use picture symbols, letters, or words and phrases to create messages. Some devices can be programmed to produce different spoken languages.

Hearing Aids and Cochlear Implant

Hearing aids differ in design, size, and the amount of amplification, ease of handling, volume control, and availability of special features. However, they do have similar components that include the following:

- Microphone to pick up sound
- Amplifier circuitry to make the sound louder
- Receiver (miniature loudspeaker) to deliver the amplified sound into the ear
- On/off switch and batteries to power the electronic parts

Types of Hearing Aid

In-the-canal and completely-in-the-canal aids

These aids are contained in a tiny case that fits partly or completely into the ear canal. They are the smallest aids available and offer some cosmetic and listening advantages **(Fig. 17.1)**.

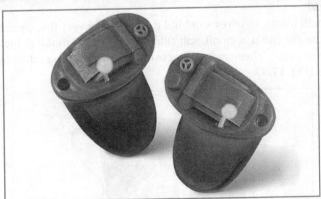

Fig. 17.1: In-the-canal and completely-in-the-canal aids.

In-the-ear aids

All parts of the aid are contained in a shell that fills in the outer part of the ear. These aids are larger than canal aids and, for some people, may be easier to handle than smaller aids **(Fig. 17.2)**.

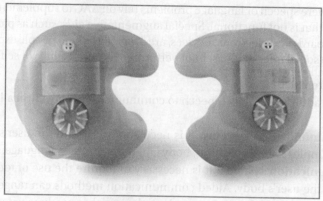

Fig. 17.2: In-the-ear aids.

Behind-the-ear (BTE) aids

All parts of the aid are contained in a small plastic case that rests behind the ear. The case is connected to an earmold by a piece of clear tubing. This style is often chosen for young children for safety and growth reasons **(Fig. 17.3)**.

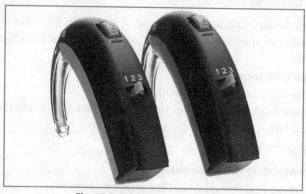

Fig. 17.3: Behind-the-ear (BTE) aids.

Behind-the-ear aid

Open fitting—a small plastic case rests behind the ear, and a very fine clear tube runs into the ear canal. Inside the ear canal, a small, soft silicone dome or a molded, highly vented acrylic tip holds the tube in place. These aids offer cosmetic and listening advantages and are used typically for adults **(Fig. 17.4)**.

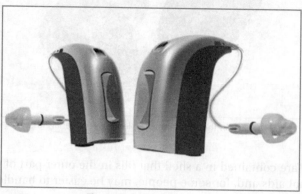

Fig. 17.4: Behind-the-ear aid.

Receiver-in-canal aids

These aids look very similar to the behind-the-ear hearing aid with a unique difference: the speaker of the hearing aid is placed inside the ear canal, and thin electrical wires replace the acoustic tube of the BTE aid. These aids also offer cosmetic and listening advantages and are typically used for adults **(Fig. 17.5)**.

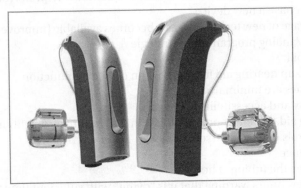

Fig. 17.5: Receiver-in-canal aids.

Extended wear hearing aids

These aids are devices that are nonsurgically placed in the ear canal by an audiologist. They are worn up to several months at a time without removal. The devices are made of soft material designed to fit the curves of the ear. They are worn continuously and then replaced with a new device. They are very useful for active individuals because their design protects against moisture and earwax, and they can be worn while exercising, showering, etc.

Middle ear implants

These hearing systems implanted in the space behind the eardrum that mechanically vibrate the middle ear structures. This device has two parts: an external portion and an implanted portion.

Features Available in Hearing Aids

Many hearing aids have optional features that can be built into assist in different communication situations. Some options are:

- **Directional microphone:** Some hearing aids have a switch to activate a directional microphone that responds to sound coming from a specific direction. When set to the normal, nondirectional setting, the aid picks up sound almost equally from any direction. When the directional microphone is activated, the aid focuses on a sound coming from in front of you and reduces sound coming from behind you. This can be especially helpful in a noisy room or for face-to-face conversation.
- **Telephone (telecoil) switch:** This feature is something that everyone should consider adding to their hearing aid. This switch allows you to move from the normal microphone "on" setting to a "T" (telecoil) setting to hear better on the telephone. You can talk on the phone without your hearing aid "whistling" because the hearing aid's microphone is turned off! This feature can also be used with other hearing assistive technology that is telecoil-compatible. The T setting can be used in settings, such as theaters, auditoriums, and houses of worship that have induction loop or frequency modulation (FM) installations. Some hearing aids have a combination "M/T" (microphone/telephone) switches so that, while listening with an induction loop, you can still hear nearby conversation.
- **Direct audio input:** Some hearing aids have a direct audio input capability that allows you to plug in a remote microphone or an FM assistive listening system. This enables you to

connect directly to a TV or other device, such as your computer, CD player, MP3 player, or radio.

Advantages of Hearing Aids

- Greater control over the prosthetic device
- Can try different hearing aids to see which is qualitatively preferred, so that user can conceivably purchase a new device
- Can take advantage of new technology as it becomes available (improved earmolds, tubing, telecoils, digital/analog programming strategies)
- Greater affordability
- Can have a back-up hearing aid for times when device malfunction
- Cost of accessories are minimal
- Greater flexibility and accessibility for repairs
- Can use hearing aid dispenser or audiologist in just about any neighborhood
- Can adjust controls on some personal device
- Easier maintenance
- Can easily change the tubing at home
- Battery gives a few hours warning that it is "dying" with sufficient time to change batteries at a more convenient time or place.

Disadvantages of Hearing Aids

- Limited hearing assistance in high frequency range
- Earmolds and their acoustic feedback issues may be repetitive, time-consuming, aggravating.
- Loud noises are bothersome for those using linear amplification.
- Hearing aids for those with severe loss need to be fitted carefully, assertively, and well monitored.

Daily Care for the Hearing Aid

Hearing aids require special care to ensure that they function properly. It includes:

- **Perform listening checks:** Listening to the hearing aid every day. Using a listening tube, you can listen to the hearing aids to be sure that they sound clear and not weak or scratchy.
- **Check batteries:** Batteries should last about 1 or 2 weeks. Using a battery tester, checking that the batteries are at full strength so that the hearing aids are working at peak performance. It always keep sparing batteries with you. Storing them in a cool, dry place. Discarding batteries one at a time.
- **Cleaning the hearing aids regularly with a soft, dry cloth:** Checking for dirt and grime. Earmolds can be removed from the hearing aids and cleaned with a mild soap solution. Drying them carefully using a forced air blower (not a hairdryer). Be sure they are dry before reattaching them to the hearing aids.
- **Minimizing moisture in the hearing aids:** This is important for proper function. A hearing aid drying container will help keep moisture from building up inside the hearing aids and will lengthen their life. Be sure to take the batteries out of the hearing aid before placing them in the storage containers.
- **Avoid feedback:** Feedback is the whistling sound that can be heard from the hearing aid. It occurs when amplified sound comes out of the earmold and re-enters the microphone.

Cochlear Implants

A cochlear implant is a small, complex electronic device that can help to provide a sense of sound to a person who is profoundly deaf or severely hard-of-hearing. The implant consists of an external portion that sits behind the ear and a second portion that is surgically placed under the skin. An implant has the following parts:

- A microphone, which picks up sound from the environment
- A speech processor, which selects and arranges sounds picked up by the microphone
- A transmitter and receiver or stimulator, which receives signals from the speech processor and convert them into electric impulses
- An electrode array, which is a group of electrodes that collects the impulses from the stimulator and sends them to different regions of the auditory nerve.

Functioning of Cochlear Implant

A cochlear implant is very different from a hearing aid. Hearing aids amplify sounds so they may be detected by damaged ears. Cochlear implants bypass damaged portions of the ear and directly stimulate the auditory nerve. Signals generated by the implant are sent by way of the auditory nerve to the brain, which recognizes the signals as sound. Hearing through a cochlear implant is different from normal hearing and takes time to learn or relearn. However, it allows many people to recognize warning signals, understand other sounds in the environment, and enjoy a conversation in person or by telephone.

Advantages of Cochlear Implants

- It can enable one to hear conversation and thus learn spoken language with relative ease, particularly for those with severe-profound hearing loss.
- It may enable one to use a regular telephone when otherwise not possible.
- It avoids problems of acoustic feedback and earmold issues.
- Greater ease in high-frequency consonant perception.
- Distance hearing is likely better than with hearing aids.
- It may be a greater potential for incidental learning.
- Greater opportunity for natural-sounding voice.
- Understanding women on the telephone may be easier as compared to understanding them with a cochlear implant for a severe-profound loss.

Disadvantages of Cochlear Implants

- Environmental and practical living issues
- **Static:** Radar detector, playgrounds, trampolines, computers, carpeting
- **Pressure:** Some recommended restrictions, such as scuba diving.
- **Magnetic:** Suggested MRI restriction.
- **Trauma:** Some restrictions from rough sports, such as football.
- Surgical issues, such as staphylococcal infection, vertigo, tinnitus, partial facial nerve paralysis.

Hearing-assistive Technology

Hearing-assistive technology systems (HATS) are devices that can help to function better in day-to-day communication situations. HATS can be used with or without hearing aids or cochlear implants to make hearing easier and thereby reduce stress and fatigue. Hearing aids + HATS = Better listening and better communication.

ROLE OF NURSE WITH HEARING IMPAIRED AND MUTE CLIENTS

- **Facing the client directly:** Be sure to look directly at the client, they must be able to see you to hear you. Avoid talking from behind the client, backs or from another room and never turn away face when speaking. Smiles, frowns, head shakes, and hand signals are great conversational aides.
- **Spotlighting your face:** Face a window or a lamp so the light illuminates your mouth as you speak. If the room is dark, move to another area with more lighting. People with hearing loss rely a great deal on lip-reading.

- **Avoiding noisy backgrounds:** A conversation is difficult to hear over background noises. Do not try to talk above loud noises. Always ask to suggest things you can do, such as speaking to a better ear or moving to a better light, to facilitate communication.
- **Getting attention first:** Be sure that client is aware of you before you start talking. One can get their attention by gently touching them, flicking on a light switch, or moving a window shade.
- **Not shouting:** Shouting only makes things worse. It can distort the face, making lip-reading impossible. Also, shouting which is amplified by a hearing aid can greatly shock and upset the client.
- **Clearly speaking at a moderate pace:** Speak more slowly and pause occasionally to help the client keep up with the word flow. Do not mouth or exaggerate expressions, as this simply makes it harder for the client to understand.
- Giving clues when changing subjects. Hearing-impaired people may become confused if you change the subject without warning. Keeping them on track by saying something like, "Now I want to talk to you about our upcoming family night" so that they can become ready for a new topic.
- Using longer phrases, which tend to be easier to understand and give more "meaning" clues than shorter phrases. For example, "Will you get me a drink of water?" Presents much less difficulty than "Will you get me a drink?"
- Using a different choice of words. After repeating something a second time without the client understanding, try a different choice of words for the third try.
- Facing the hearing-impaired person directly, on the same level and in good light whenever possible. Position yourself so that the light is shining on the speaker's face, not in the eyes of the listener.
- Not talking from another room, not being able to see each other when talking is a common reason people have difficulty understanding what is said.
- Speaking clearly, slowly, distinctly, but naturally, without shouting or exaggerating mouth movements. Shouting distorts the sound of speech and may make speech reading more difficult.
- Saying the person's name before beginning a conversation. This gives the listener a chance to focus attention and reduces the chance of missing words at the beginning of the conversation.
- Avoiding to talk too rapidly or using sentences that are too complex. Slow down a little, pause between sentences or phrases, and wait to make sure you have been understood before going on.
- Keeping your hands away from your face while talking. If you are eating, chewing, smoking, etc., while talking, your speech will be more difficult to understand. Beards and moustaches can also interfere with the ability of the hearing impaired to speech read.
- If the hearing-impaired listener hears better in one ear than the other, trying to make a point of remembering which ear is better so that you will know where to position yourself.
- Be aware of possible distortion of sounds for the hearing-impaired person. They may hear your voice but still may have difficulty understanding some words.
- Most hearing-impaired people have greater difficulty understanding speech when there is background noise. Trying to minimize extraneous noise when talking.
- Some people with hearing loss are very sensitive to loud sounds. This reduced tolerance for loud sounds is not uncommon. Avoid situations where there will be loud sounds when possible.
- If the hearing-impaired person has difficulty understanding a particular phrase or word, it is necessary to try to find a different way of saying the same thing, rather than repeating the original words over and over.

- Acquainting the listener with the general topic of the conversation. Avoiding sudden changes of topic. If the subject is changed, it is necessary to tell the hearing-impaired person what you are talking about now. In a group setting, repeating questions or key facts before continuing with the discussion.
- If you are giving specific information—such as time, place or phone numbers—to someone who is hearing impaired, have them repeat the specifics back to you. Many numbers and words sound alike.
- Whenever possible, providing pertinent information in writing, such as directions, schedules, work assignments, etc.
- Recognizing that everyone, especially the hard-of-hearing, has a harder time hearing and understanding when ill or tired.
- Paying attention to the listener. A puzzled look may indicate misunderstanding. Tactfully asking the hearing-impaired person if they understood you, or ask leading questions so you know your message got across.
- Taking turns speaking and avoid interrupting other speakers.
- Enrolling in aural rehabilitation classes with your hearing-impaired spouse or friend.

MULTIPLE CHOICE QUESTIONS

1. **The nurse correctly tells a client that the priority goal in the treatment for Meniere's disease is to:**
   A. Promote a quiet environment
   B. Eliminate environmental noise
   C. Preserve the remaining hearing
   D. Maintain a sodium-free diet

2. **Which of the following should the nurse include in the assessment of the client's cranial nerves and extraocular eye muscles?**
   A. Six cardinal fields of gaze
   B. Disc characteristics
   C. Macular characteristics
   D. Red reflex

3. **The nurse implements which of the following in the plan of care for a client who is hearing impaired?**
   A. Speaks in a raised voice
   B. Speaks slowly
   C. Has the light behind the nurse
   D. Uses exaggerated facial expressions

4. **Which of the following nursing measures should receive priority in the client's plan of care after eye surgery?**
   A. Instruct on the importance of follow-up
   B. Pain management
   C. Prevent increased intraocular pressure and infection
   D. Instruct on how to perform the Valsalva maneuver

5. **Nurse collects a history from a client suspected of a sensorineural hearing loss. Which of the following findings supports the diagnosis and should be reported?**
   A. A history of exposure to excessive noise over a period of time
   B. The ability to hear high-pitched sounds
   C. The client speaks softly
   D. Frequent ear irrigations for dry, hard cerumen

6. **The nurse should consider which of the following drugs taken by a client with glaucoma? Drugs that:**
   A. Increase intraocular pressure
   B. Decrease vitreous humor
   C. Cause anesthesia
   D. Decrease intraocular pressure

7. **For a client who sustained a chemical burn from battery acid, the nurse should include which of the following in the emergency procedures?**
   A. Irrigate the eye with sterile normal saline
   B. Swab the eye with antibiotic ointment
   C. Cover the affected eye with an eye patch
   D. Assess the visual acuity

8. **During the initial assessment, the nurse observes the presence of bright red drainage on the eye dressing. Which of the following should be the nurse's first action?**
   A. Continue to monitor the vital signs and pain
   B. Note the amount of drainage on the client's record
   C. Mark the drainage on the dressing and monitor the amount and color
   D. Report the findings to the physician

9. **The nurse is admitting a client in the emergency room with a foreign body in the ear identified as an insect. Which of the following interventions is a priority for the nurse to perform?**
   A. Irrigate the affected ear
   B. Instill a cortisone ointment into the affected ear
   C. Instill diluted alcohol in the affected ear
   D. Instill an antibiotic ointment into the affected ear

10. **The nurse implements which of the following interventions to reduce intraocular pressure following eye surgery?**
    A. Keeps the head of the bed elevated
    B. Provides bright lighting in the room
    C. Applies hot compresses
    D. Applies gentle pressure on the affected eye

11. **In planning the preoperative care for a client with a retinal detachment, the nurse should include which of the following in the plan of care?**
    A. Maintain flat bed rest
    B. Have client wear dark glasses for reading and television
    C. Restrict ambulation
    D. Place a patch over the affected eye

12. **When completing a measurement of the client's visual acuity, which of the following would be appropriate?**
    A. Snellen chart   B. Visual field
    C. Penlight   D. Ophthalmoscope

Answers

1. C   2. A   3. B   4. C   5. A   6. A   7. A   8. D   9. C   10. A
11. D   12. A

BIBLIOGRAPHY

1. Acuin J, for the World Health Organization. Chronic suppurative otitis media. burden of illness and management options. Geneva: World Health Organization; 2004.

2. Acuin J. Extracts from "Concise clinical evidence": chronic suppurative otitis media. BMJ. 2002;325:1159.

3. American Academy of Family Physicians, American Academy of Otolaryngology-Head and Neck Surgery, American Academy of Pediatrics Subcommittee on Otitis Media With Effusion. Otitis media with effusion. Pediatrics. 2004;113:1412-29.

4. American Academy of Pediatrics Subcommittee on Management of Acute Otitis Media. Diagnosis and management of acute otitis media. Pediatrics. 2004;113:1451-65.

5. Arrieta A, Singh J. Management of recurrent and persistent acute otitis media: new options with familiar antibiotics. Pediatr Infect Dis J. 2004;23(2 suppl):S115-24.

6. Gehanno P, Lenoir G, Barry B, Bons J, Boucot I, Berche P. Evaluation of nasopharyngeal cultures for bacteriologic assessment of acute otitis media in children. Pediatr Infect Dis J. 1996;15:329-32.

7. Hendley JO. Clinical practice. Otitis media. N Engl J Med. 2002;347:1169-74.

8. Karma PH, Penttila MA, Sipila MM, Kataja MJ. Otoscopic diagnosis of middle ear effusion in acute and non-acute otitis media. I. The value of different otoscopic findings. Int J Pediatr Otorhinolaryngol. 1989;17:37-49.

9. Kemaloglu YK, Sener T, Beder L, Bayazit Y, Goksu N. Predictive value of acoustic reflectometry (angle and reflectivity) and tympanometry. Int J Pediatr Otorhinolaryngol. 1999;48:137-42.

10. Klein JO, Pelton S. Epidemiology, pathogenesis, clinical manifestations, and complications of acute otitis media.

11. Kontiokari T, Koivunen P, Niemela M, Pokka T, Uhari M. Symptoms of acute otitis media. Pediatr Infect Dis J. 1998;17:676-9.

12. Marcy M, Takata G. Management of acute otitis media. Evidence report/technology assessment no. 15. Rockville, MD: Agency for Healthcare Research and Quality, Southern California Evidence-Based Practice Center/RAND; 2001. AHRQ publication no. 01-E 010.

13. McCracken GH Jr. Diagnosis and management of acute otitis media in the urgent care setting. Ann Emerg Med. 2002;39:413-21.

14. Niemela M, Uhari M, Jounio-Ervasti K, Luotonen J, Alho OP, Vierimaa E. Lack of specific symptomatology in children with acute otitis media. Pediatr Infect Dis J. 1994;13:765-8.

15. Onusko E. Tympanometry. Am Fam Physician. 2004;70:1713-20.

16. Rothman R, Owens T, Simel DL. Does this child have acute otitis media? JAMA. 2003;290:1633-40.

17. Rovers MM, Schilder AG, Zielhuis GA, Rosenfeld RM. Otitis media. Lancet. 2004;363:465-73. [Published correction appears in Lancet 2004;363:1080].

18. University of Michigan Health System. Guidelines for clinical care. Otitis media; 2007. [Accessed May 15, 2007]

Eye Disorders

REVIEW OF ANATOMY AND PHYSIOLOGY

Eye is like a camera. The external object is seen via eye like the camera takes the picture of any object. Light enters the eye through a small hole called the pupil and is focused on the retina, which is like a camera film. Eye also has a focusing lens, which focuses on images from different distances on the retina. The colored ring of the eye, the iris, controls the amount of light entering the eye. It closes when light is bright and opens when light is dim. A tough white sheet called sclera covers the outside of the eye. Front of this sheet (sclera) is transparent in order to allow the light to enter the eye, the cornea. Ciliary muscles in ciliary body control the focusing of lens automatically. Choroid forms the vascular layer of the eye supplying nutrition to the eye structures. Image formed on the retina is transmitted to brain by optic nerve. The image is finally perceived by brain. A jelly-like substance called vitreous humor fills the space between lens and retina.

The lens, iris, and cornea are nourished by clear fluid, aqueous humor, formed by the ciliary body and fill the space between lens and cornea. This space is known as anterior chamber. The fluid flows from ciliary body to the pupil and is absorbed through the channels in the angle of anterior chamber. The delicate balance of aqueous production and absorption controls pressure within the eye.

EYE ASSESSMENT

1. **Inspect the eyes, eyelids, pupils, sclera, and conjunctiva**
   - For swelling of the eyelids
   - Color of sclera must be white and shiny.
   - Color of conjunctiva must be pink and not swollen.
2. **Looking for strabismus**: Do the eyes line up with another.
3. **Looking for anisocoria**: Are the pupils equal in size.
4. **Testing cranial nerves III (oculomotor), IV (trochlear), VI (abducens) (*see* neurological assessment for details)**:
   - Have the patient follow penlight by moving it 12–14 inches from the face
   - Assessing **nystagmus**
   - Assessing the pupil's reaction toward light.
5. **Assessing vision with visual acuity test:** A visual acuity test uses an eye chart to measure how well an eye can read a series of letters.

REFRACTIVE ERRORS

A refractive error is a very common eye disorder. It occurs when the eye cannot clearly focus the images from the outside world. The result of refractive errors is blurred vision, which is sometimes so severe that it causes visual impairment **(Fig. 18.1)**.

The four most common refractive errors are as follows:

1. **Myopia:** It is also known as nearsightedness. This occurs when the distance between the cornea and the retina is too long. Light rays entering the eye are focused in front of the retina causing the image that falls on the retina to be blurred.
2. **Hypermyopia:** It is also known as farsightedness and occurs when the distance between the cornea and the retina is too short. Light rays entering the eye have not yet come into focus when they reach the retina. So again the image is blurred.
3. **Astigmatism:** It is a condition in which the cornea is curved unevenly. A cornea that is curved the same in each direction is shaped like a basketball, while a cornea with astigmatism is more curved in one direction than the other like a football. Light passing through this uneven cornea is not properly focused on the retina.
4. **Presbyopia:** It is a normal condition associated with age that causes problems with near vision.

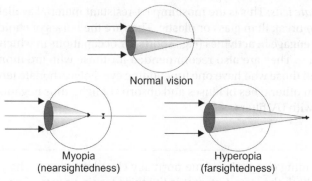

Fig. 18.1: Refractive errors.

Treatment of Refractive Errors

1. **Eyeglasses:** Eyeglass lenses correct refractive errors by focusing light directly on the retina. The type of lens depends on the type and severity of the refractive error. The type of refractive error determines the lens's shape. A concave lens is used to correct myopia. In myopia, light rays fall in front of the retina rather than on it. Because a concave lens is thin in the center and thicker on the edges, it diverges light rays so that the eye's lens focuses them directly on the retina.

   - A convex lens is used to correct hypermyopia. In hypermyopia, light rays fall behind the retina. The lens is thickest in the center and thinnest on the outer edges. The convex lens converges light rays so that the eye's lens focuses them on the retina.
   - To correct astigmatism, which is caused by distortions in the shape of the lens or cornea, a cylinder lens is frequently used. The cylinder lens has two refractive powers on one lens. One power is placed over the entire lens and the other is oriented in one direction. This corrects the scattered pattern in which light enters the eye and creates one focal point on the retina.

2. **Multifocal lenses:** People that have more than one refractive error may require two pairs of eyeglasses or glasses with multifocal lenses. Multifocal lenses contain two or more vision-correcting prescriptions.

   - Bifocals are the most common type of multifocal lenses. The lens is split into two sections; the upper part is for distance vision and the lower part for near vision. They are usually prescribed for people over the age of 40 whose focusing ability has declined due to presbyopia.
   - Trifocals have a third section used for middle distance vision (i.e., objects within arm's reach, such as a computer screen).

3. **Eyeglass frames:** The choice of frames usually depends on personal preference, fashion, comfort, and cost. Frames are made from metals, plastic, nylon, and other synthetics. Each material has its advantages.

4. **Eyeglass lenses:** Traditionally, lenses have been made from glass, but today, they are more commonly made from plastic. Glass lenses are breakable and are about twice as heavy as plastic ones. They are more resistant to scratches. Plastic lenses scratch more easily, even with scratch-resistant coatings, but they are much lighter, less likely to break, and can be treated with ultraviolet (UV) filters and antiglare coatings.

   - *Photochromic lens:* This type of lens changes from colorless to dark, depending on the amount of UV exposure. The lenses are clear, but in sunlight a tint appears, eliminating the need for prescription sunglasses. Photochromic lenses are available in plastic and glass and for nearly every type of refractive error.
   - *Polycarbonate lens:* This is the most impact-resistant material available and is 10 times less likely to break than glass or plastic. They are the lenses of choice for children and adults who engage in activities (e.g., sports) or occupations in which eyeglasses can be easily broken. They are also recommended for those who are monocular (have only one eye) and those who have one functioning eye. Polycarbonate lenses are lighter and thinner than other types of lenses and absorb UV light, thus negating the need to treat eyeglasses with UV filters.

CATARACT

A cataract is a clouding or opacity of the normally clear lens of eye. The patient may have a cataract in one or both the eyes. Cataract is the third leading cause of preventable blindness **(Figs. 18.2A and B).**

Risk Factors and Etiology

- Increasing age
- Diabetes
- Drinking excessive amounts of alcohol
- Excessive exposure to sunlight
- Exposure to ionizing radiation, such as that used in X-rays and cancer radiation therapy
- Family history of cataracts
- High blood pressure
- Obesity
- Previous eye injury or inflammation
- Previous eye surgery
- Prolonged use of corticosteroid medications
- Smoking

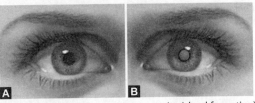

Figs. 18.2A and B: Cataract is an opacity (cloud formation) of the eye lens, develops due to aging. (A) Normal eye; (B) Cataract eye.

Pathophysiology

Following are the various mechanisms involves in the occurrence of cataract:

- Caused by degeneration and opacification of existing lens fibers, formation of aberrant fibers or deposition of other material in their place.
- Loss of transparency occurs because of abnormalities of lens protein and consequent disorganization of the lens fibers.
- Any factor that disturbs the critical intra- and extracellular equilibrium of water and electrolytes, the colloid system within the fibers causing opacification.
- Fibrous metaplasia of lens fibers occurs in complicated cataract.
- Epithelial cell necrosis occurring in angle-closure glaucoma leads to focal opacification of the lens epithelium.
- Abnormal products of metabolism, drugs or metals can be deposited in storage diseases, metabolic diseases, and toxic reactions.

Three biochemical changes during cataract:

1. **Hydration**: Seen particularly in rapidly developing forms. Actual fluid droplets collect under the capsule forming lacunae between fibers, the entire tissue may swell and becomes opaque, and this process is reversible in early stage, as in juvenile insulin-dependent diabetes. Hydration may be due to osmotic changes in the lens or due to changes in the semipermeability of the capsule.
2. **Denaturation of lens proteins**: If the proteins are denatured with an increase in insoluble protein, a dense opacity is produced. This stage is irreversible and opacity does not clear, this change is seen in young lens or the cortex of the adult nucleus where metabolism is active.
3. **Sclerosis**: Inactive fibers of the nucleus suffer from degenerative change of slow sclerosis.

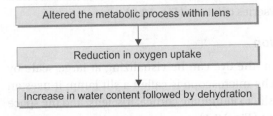

Altered the metabolic process within lens

↓

Reduction in oxygen uptake

↓

Increase in water content followed by dehydration

Contd...

Contd...

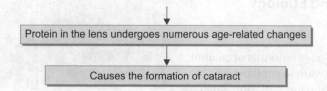

Protein in the lens undergoes numerous age-related changes

↓

Causes the formation of cataract

Types of Cataract

1. **Nuclear cataracts:** A nuclear cataract may at first causes more nearsighted. But with time, the lens gradually turns more densely yellow and further cloudy. As the cataract slowly progresses, the lens may even turn brown. Advanced yellowing or browning of the lens can lead to difficulty distinguishing between shades of color.

2. **Cortical cataracts:** A cortical cataract begins as whitish, wedge-shaped opacities or streaks on the outer edge of the lens cortex.

3. **Posterior subcapsular cataracts:** A posterior subcapsular cataract starts as a small, opaque area that usually forms near the back of the lens, right in the path of light on its way to the retina.

4. **Congenital cataracts (aphakia):** Some people are born with cataracts or develop them during childhood. Such cataracts may be the result of the mother having an infection during pregnancy.

5. **Hypermature shrunken cataract:** When cortex disintegrates and transforms into mass. The lens becomes inspissated and shrunken, the anterior capsule becomes thickened.

6. **Morgagnian hypermature cataract:** Sometimes, cortex becomes liquefies and nucleus sinks into the bottom. The liquefied cortex becomes milky and nucleus is seen as brown mass, visible as semicircular line in pupillary area altering its position with change in position of the head.

Signs and Symptoms

- Clouded, blurred or dim vision
- Increasing difficulty with vision at night
- Sensitivity to light and glare
- Seeing "halos" around lights
- Frequent changes in eyeglass or contact lens prescription
- Fading or yellowing of colors
- Double vision in a single eye

Diagnostic Evaluation

Visual acuity test: A visual acuity test uses an eye chart to measure how well an eye can read a series of letters **(Fig. 18.3)**.

Slit-lamp Examination

With this examination, the eye can be visualizing at large scale by magnifying the eye. The microscope is called a slit lamp; it uses an intense line of light, a slit, to illuminate cornea, iris, lens, and the space between iris and cornea **(Fig. 18.4)**.

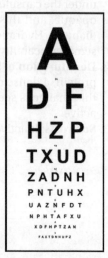

Fig. 18.3: Visual acuity test.

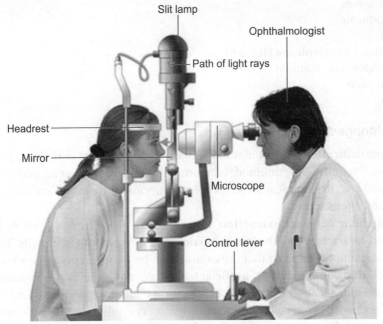

Slit lamp
Ophthalmologist
Path of light rays
Headrest
Mirror
Microscope
Control lever

Fig. 18.4: Slit-lamp examination.

Retinal Examination

To visualize the retina.

Other Tests

- Snellen visual acuity test
- Ophthalmoscopy
- Slit-lamp bimicroscopic examination
- Glare testing
- Keratometry
- Ocular examination
- Perimetry: To determine the scope of visual fields

Management

Objectives of Cataract Surgery

- To remove the opacified lens
- Successful treatment of acute attack and prompt alleviation of manifestations
- Prevention of complications and further attacks
- Rehabilitation and education of the clients and significant others

Pharmacologic Therapy

- Beta carotene
- Vitamins C and E
- Antioxidant supplements
- Selenium
- Multivitamin supplements

- Contact lenses
- Strong bifocals
- Glasses
- Mydriatics: Phenylephrine HCl acid
- Cycloplegics: Tropicamide
- Homatropine
- Atropine

Surgical Management

- **Phacoemulsification:** In this method, surgery can usually be performed in <30 minutes and usually requires only minimal sedation. Numbing eyedrops or an injection around the eye is used and, in general, no stitches are used to close the wound, and often no eye patch is required after surgery.
- **Extracapsular cataract extraction surgery:** This procedure is used mainly for very advanced cataracts where the lens is too dense to dissolve into fragments. This technique requires a larger incision so that the cataract can be removed in one piece without being fragmented inside the eye. An artificial lens is placed in the same capsular bag as with the phacoemulsification technique. This surgical technique requires a various number of sutures to close the larger wound, and visual recovery is often slower. Extracapsular cataract extraction usually requires an injection of numbing medication around the eye and an eye patch after surgery.
- **Intracapsular cataract surgery:** This surgical technique requires an even larger wound than extracapsular surgery, and the surgeon removes the entire lens and the surrounding capsule together. This technique requires the intraocular lens to be placed in a different location, in front of the iris.
- **Aphakia** (absence of the lens) is corrected by the use of eyeglasses and contact lenses.

Nursing Management

Nursing Assessment
Assessing knowledge level regarding procedure
- Assessing the level of fear and anxiety
- Determining visual limitations

Postoperative Assessment
Assessing pain level
- Sudden onset: May be due to ruptured vessel or suture and may lead to hemorrhage
- Severe pain: Accompanied by nausea and vomiting may be caused by intraocular pressure (IOP)
- Assessing visual acuity in unoperated eye
- Assessing patient's ability to ambulate
- Assessing patient's level of independence

Nursing Diagnoses
- Self-care deficit related to visual deficit
- Anxiety related to lack of knowledge about the surgical and postoperative experience
- Risk for injury related to blurred vision
- Risk for infection related to trauma to incision
- Acute pain related to trauma to incision

Nursing Intervention
Relieving pain
- Giving medication to reduce pain as analgesics
- Giving cold compression demand for blunt trauma
- Encouraging the use of sunglasses in strong light
- Vital signs must assess frequently
- Physical rest in bed with backrest elevated to provide comfort

Relieving anxiety
- Assessing the degree and duration of visual impairment
- Orienting the patient to a new environment
- Explaining the preoperative routines
- Pushing to perform daily living habits when able
- Encouraging the participation of family

Prevention of injury
- Providing a comfortable position to the patient
- Helping the patient to set the environment
- Orienting the patient in a room
- Discussing the need for use of goggles when instructed
- Not putting pressure over the affected eye trauma
- Using the proper procedures when providing eye drugs

Promoting self-care
- Clearing all the doubts of patient regarding the disease condition
- Maintaining good interpersonal relation (IPR) with the patient
- Providing a calm and cool environment to the patient
- Music therapy and pet therapy given to patient
- Relaxation therapy also provided to relieve the anxiety of patient

Improving knowledge
- Providing adequate knowledge about a disease condition
- Providing the sunglasses to patient during exposure to sunlight
- Providing medications to patient on proper time
- Advising the patient to talk with doctor
- Following the recommendations that ensure regular eye checkup by the ophthalmologist

Health Education
- Advising the patient to wear sunglasses during exposure
- Advising the patient to take analgesics to reduce pain
- Advising the patient to take proper diet
- Advising the patient to take care of eyes after surgery
- Advising patient to prevent eyes from dirt and dust
- Advising patient to preventing eyes from trauma
- Advising patient to report to doctor for early complications
- Advising patient to increase activities gradually as directed by health care provider
- Caution against activities that cause patient to strain
- Instructing patient and family in proper use of medications
- Advising patient to apply plastic shield over the eye at night to avoid accidental injury during sleep
- Infirming about fitting temporary corrective lenses for the first 6 weeks.

Complications

- Capsular rupture
- Vitreous loss
- Endophthalmitis is a purulent inflammation of the intraocular fluids (vitreous and aqueous)
- Pseudoexfoliation
- Myopia

Aftercare

Before the patient goes home, he or she may receive the following:
- A patch to wear over eye until the follow-up examination.
- Eyedrops to prevent infection, treat inflammation, and help with healing.
- Wear dark sunglasses outside after removing the patch.
- Washing hands well before and after using eyedrops and touching eye. Try not to get soap and water in eye when are bathing or showering for the first few days.

GLAUCOMA

Glaucoma is a disease of the major nerve of vision, called the optic nerve. Glaucoma is characterized by a particular pattern of progressive damage to the optic nerve that generally begins with a subtle loss of side vision **(Figs. 18.5A and B)**.

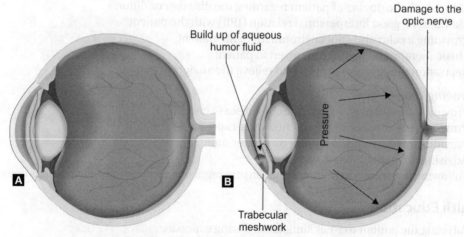

Figs. 18.5A and B: (A) Normal eye; (B) Eye with glaucoma.

Etiology and Risk Factors

- Age
- Elevated eye pressure
- Thin cornea
- Family history of glaucoma
- Nearsightedness
- Past injuries to the eyes
- Steroid use
- A history of severe anemia or shock

Pathophysiology

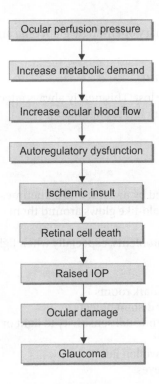

```
Ocular perfusion pressure
          ↓
Increase metabolic demand
          ↓
Increase ocular blood flow
          ↓
Autoregulatory dysfunction
          ↓
Ischemic insult
          ↓
Retinal cell death
          ↓
Raised IOP
          ↓
Ocular damage
          ↓
Glaucoma
```

Types

1. **Open-angle glaucoma (chronic):** Chronic open-angle glaucoma is the most common form of glaucoma. The "open" drainage angle of the eye can become blocked leading to gradual increased eye pressure. If this increased pressure results in optic nerve damage, it is known as chronic open-angle glaucoma. The optic nerve damage and vision loss usually occur so gradually and painlessly.

2. **Angle-closure glaucoma:** Angle-closure glaucoma results when the drainage angle of the eye narrows and becomes completely blocked. In the eye, the iris may close off the drainage angle and cause a dangerously high eye pressure. When the drainage angle of the eye suddenly becomes completely blocked, pressure builds up rapidly, and this is called acute angle-closure glaucoma.

3. **Exfoliation syndrome:** Exfoliation syndrome is a common form of open-angle glaucoma that results when there is a buildup of abnormal, whitish material on the lens and drainage angle of the eye. This material and pigment from the back of the iris can clog the drainage system of the eye, causing increased eye pressure.

4. **Pigmentary glaucoma:** Pigmentary glaucoma is characterized by the iris bowing backwards, and coming into contact with the support structures that hold the lens in place. This position disrupts the cells lining the back surface of the iris containing pigment, and results in a release of pigment particles into the drainage system of the eye. This pigment can clog the drain and can lead to an increase in eye pressure.

5. **Low-tension glaucoma:** This is another form that experts do not fully understand. Even though eye pressure is normal, optic nerve damage still occurs. Perhaps the optic nerve is over-sensitive or there is atherosclerosis in the blood vessel that supplies the optic nerve.

Signs and Symptoms

The signs and symptoms of primary open-angle glaucoma and acute angle-closure glaucoma are quite different.

Primary Open-Angle Glaucoma

- Peripheral vision is gradually lost. This nearly always affects both eyes.
- In advanced stages, the patient has tunnel vision.

Closed-Angle Glaucoma

- Eye pain, usually severe
- Blurred vision
- Eye pain is often accompanied by nausea, and sometimes vomiting
- Lights appear to have extra halo-like glows around them
- Red eyes
- Sudden, unexpected vision problems, especially when lighting is poor

Common Symptoms

- Unusual trouble adjusting to dark rooms
- Difficulty focusing on near or distant objects
- Squinting or blinking due to unusual sensitivity to light or glare
- Change in color of iris
- Red-rimmed, encrusted, or swollen lids
- Recurrent pain in or around eyes
- Double vision
- Dark spot at the center of viewing
- Lines and edges appear distorted or wavy
- Excess tearing or "watery eyes"
- Dry eyes with itching or burning
- Sudden loss of vision in one eye
- Sudden hazy or blurred vision
- Flashes of light or black spots
- Halos or rainbows around light.

Stages of glaucoma is shown in **Figures 18.6A to D**.

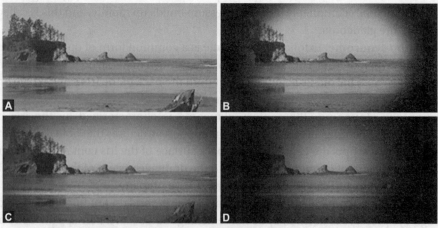

Figs. 18.6A to D: Stages of glaucoma. (A) Normal vision; (B) Advanced glaucoma; (C) Early glaucoma; (D) Extreme glaucoma.

Diagnostic Evaluation

Eye-pressure Test

Tonometer, a device that measures IOP. Some anesthetic and a dye are placed in the cornea, and a blue light is held against the eye to measure pressure. This test can diagnose ocular hypertension; a risk factor for open-angle glaucoma.

Gonioscopy

This examines the area where the fluid drains out of the eye. It helps determine whether the angle between the cornea and the iris is open or blocked (closed).

Perimetry Test

Also known as a visual field test. It determines which area of the patient's vision is missing. The patient is shown a sequence of light spots and asked to identify them. Some of the dots are located where the person's peripheral vision is; the part of vision that is initially affected by glaucoma. If the patient cannot see those peripheral dots, it means that some vision damage has already occurred.

Optic Nerve Damage

The ophthalmologist uses instruments to look at the back of the eye, which can reveal any slight changes which may also point towards glaucoma onset.

Visual Acuity Test

This eye chart test measures how well you see at various distances.

Visual Field Test

This test measures peripheral (side vision).

Dilated Eye Examination

In this examination, drops are placed in eyes to widen, or dilate, the pupils. Eye care professional uses a special magnifying lens to examine retina and optic nerve for signs of damage and other eye problems.

Management

Medical Management

- **Prostaglandin analogs:** These medications have prostaglandin-like compounds as their active ingredient. They increase the outflow of the fluid inside the eye. Examples include Xalatan and Lumigan.
- **Beta-blockers:** These medications reduce the amount of fluid the eye produces. Some patients may experience breathing problems, hair loss, fatigue, depression, memory loss, a drop in blood pressure. Examples of such medications include timolol, betaxolol, and metipranolol.
- **Carbonic anhydrase inhibitors:** These also reduce fluid production in the eye. Side effects may include nausea, eye irritation, dry mouth, frequent urination, tingling in the fingers or toes, and a strange taste in the mouth. Examples include brinzolamide and dorzolamide.
- **Cholinergic agents:** Also known as miotic agents.

Surgery

- **Trabeculoplasty:** A high-energy laser beam is used to unblock clogged drainage canals, making it easier for the fluid inside the eye to drain out. This procedure nearly always reduces inner eye pressure. However, the problem may come back.

- **Filtering surgery (viscocanalostomy):** If eyedrops and laser surgery are not effective in controlling eye pressure, trabeculectomy is required. This procedure is performed in a hospital or an outpatient surgery center. Patient receives a medication to help relax and usually an injection of anesthetic to numb eye. Using small instruments under an operating microscope, an opening is created in the sclera and removes a small piece of eye tissue at the base of cornea through which fluid drains from eye (the trabecular meshwork). The fluid in eye can now freely leave the eye through this opening. As a result, eye pressure will be lowered.

- **Drainage implant (aqueous shunt implant):** This option is sometimes used for children or those with secondary glaucoma. A small silicone tube is inserted into the eye to help it drain out fluids better.

- **Laser cycloablation** (ciliary body destruction, cyclophotocoagulation or cyclocryopexy) is another form of laser treatment generally reserved for patients with severe forms of glaucoma with poor visual potential. This procedure involves applying laser burns or freezing to the part of the eye that makes the aqueous fluid. This therapy destroys the cells that make the fluid, thereby reducing the eye pressure.

- **Aqueous shunt devices:** They are artificial drainage devices used to lower the eye pressure. They are essentially plastic microscopic tubes attached to a plastic reservoir. The reservoir is placed beneath the conjunctival tissue. The actual tube is placed inside the eye to create a new pathway for fluid to exit the eye. This fluid collects within the reservoir beneath the conjunctiva creating a filtering bleb. This procedure may be performed as an alternative to trabeculectomy in patients with certain types of glaucoma.

Nursing Care Plan

Nursing Assessment

- Evaluating the patient for any of the clinical manifestations
- Assessing patient's level of anxiety and knowledge base
- Assessing the patient's knowledge of disease process

Nursing Diagnosis

- Pain related to increased IOP
- Fear related to pain and potential loss of vision
- Self-care deficit related to visual deficit
- Anxiety related to lack of knowledge about the surgical and postoperative experience
- Risk for injury related to blurred vision
- Risk for infection related to trauma to incision
- Acute pain related to trauma to incision

Nursing Intervention

1. **Relieving pain**
   - Notifying health care provider immediately
   - Administering medications as directed
   - Explaining to patient that the goal of treatment is to reduce IOP as quickly as possible

- Explaining procedures to patient
- Reassuring patient that with reduction in IOP, pain and other signs and symptoms should subside.

2. **Relieving fear**
   - Providing reassurance and calm presence to reduce anxiety and fear
   - Preparing patient for surgery, if necessary

3. **Relieving anxiety**
   - Assessing the degree and duration of visual impairment
   - Orienting the patient to a new environment
   - Explaining the preoperative routines
   - Pushing to perform daily living habits when able
   - Encouraging the participation of family

4. **Prevention of injury**
   - Providing a comfortable position to the patient
   - Helping the patient to set the environment
   - Orienting the patient in a room
   - Discussing the need for use of goggles when instructed
   - Not putting pressure over the affected eye trauma
   - Using the proper procedures when providing eye drugs

5. **Promoting self-care**
   - Clearing all the doubts of patient regarding the disease condition
   - Maintaining good IPR with the patient
   - Providing a calm and cool environment to the patient
   - Music therapy and pet therapy given to patient
   - Relaxation therapy also provided to relieve the anxiety of patient

6. **Improving knowledge**
   - Providing adequate knowledge about a disease condition
   - Providing the sunglasses to patient during exposure to sunlight
   - Providing medications to patient on proper time
   - Advising the patient to talk with doctor

Complications

If left untreated, glaucoma will cause progressive vision loss, normally in these stages:
- Blind spots in peripheral vision
- Tunnel vision
- Total blindness

RETINAL DETACHMENT

The retina is a light-sensitive membrane located at the back of the eye. When retina is detached from its pigmented epithelium, it is called retinal detachment. It is characterized by partial or total loss of vision **(Fig. 18.7)**.

Types and Causes

1. **Rhegmatogenous retinal detachment:** It is characterized by tear or hole in retina. This allows fluid from within the eye to slip through the opening and get behind the retina. The fluid separates the retina from the membrane that provides it with nourishment and oxygen. The pressure from the fluid can push the retina away from the retinal pigment epithelium, causing the retina to detach.

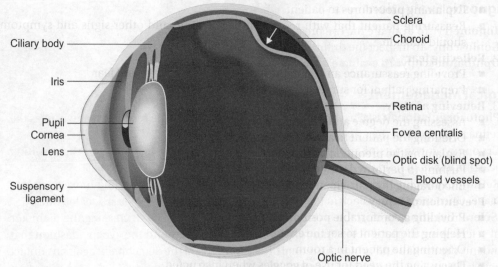

Fig. 18.7: Retinal detachment.

2. **Tractional retinal detachment:** It occurs when scar tissue on the retina's surface contracts and causes the retina to pull away from the back of the eye. This is a less common type of detachment that typically affects people with diabetes.

3. **Exudative detachment:** This type of detachment is caused by retinal diseases such as inflammatory disorder or Coats disease, which causes abnormal development in the blood vessels behind the retina.

Risk Factors

Risk factors for retinal detachment include:

- Posterior vitreous detachment—a common condition in aging individuals, in which the fluid in the retina breaks down, putting strain on the retinal fibers.
- Extreme nearsightedness because:
  - Family history of retinal detachment
  - Trauma to the eye
  - Being over 40 years old
  - Prior history of retinal detachment
  - Complications from cataract surgery
  - Diabetes

Signs and Symptoms

There is no pain associated with retinal detachment, but there are usually symptoms before the retina becomes detached. Primary symptoms include:

- Blurred vision
- Partial vision loss
- Flashes of light when looking to the side
- Areas of darkness in field of vision
- Suddenly seeing many floaters (small bits of debris that appear as black flecks or strings floating before the eye).

Diagnostic Evaluation

- **Tonometry:** To evaluate the eye pressure
- **Gonioscopy:** To inspect the drainage angle of eye
- **Ophthalmoscopy:** To evaluate the optic nerve

Surgical Management

- **Photocoagulation:** It is a laser burn around the tear site and the resulted scar will fixes the retina to the back of the eye.
- **Cryopexy:** It consists of application of freezing probe to the tear site and the resulting scarring will help hold the retina in place.
- **Retinopexy:** In this, doctor will put a gas bubble in eye to help the retina move back into place. Once the retina is back in place, with the help of laser, the holes are sealed out.
- **Scleral buckling:** In this, the sclera is pulled near the retina by decreasing the diameter of sclera. A small piece of silicone may be sutured on or around the eye in a fashion that indents the eyeball and brings the retinal break that caused the detachment again in contact with it. This allows the subretinal fluid to reabsorb and the retina to reattach. Sometimes, an air or gas bubble is injected at the time of surgery to aid reattachment of the retina.
- **Vitrectomy:** By making tiny incisions into the eyeball, instruments are able to remove all the vitreous and subretinal fluid and reattach the retina. The retinal tear or tears that caused the detachment are then treated with laser to cause a permanent adhesive scar in this area and prevent a future detachment. A gas bubble, or less frequently an oil bubble, is instilled in the eye at the end of surgery to maintain the retina in contact with the eye wall as the laser scar matures.

Nursing Management

Nursing Diagnosis

- Anxiety related to possible vision loss
- Disturbed sensory perception related to visual impairment
- Ineffective health maintenance related to knowledge deficit
- Risk for injury related to impaired vision
- Self-care deficit related to impaired vision

Nursing Interventions

- Preparing the patient for surgery
- Instructing the patient to remain quiet in prescribed (dependent) position, to keep the detached area of the retina in dependent position
- Patching both eyes
- Washing the patient's face with antibacterial solution
- Instructing the patient not to touch the eyes to avoid contamination
- Administering preoperative medications as ordered
- Taking measures to prevent postoperative complications
- Caution the patient to avoid bumping head
- Encouraging the patient not to cough or sneeze or to perform other strain-inducing activities that will increase IOP
- Encouraging ambulation and independence as tolerated

- Administering medication for pain, nausea, and vomiting as directed
- Providing quiet diversion activities, such as listening to a radio- or audiobooks
- Teaching proper technique in giving eye medications
- Advising patient to avoid rapid eye movements for several weeks as well as straining or bending the head below the waist
- Advising patient that driving is restricted until cleared by ophthalmologist
- Teaching the patient to recognize and immediately report symptoms that indicate recurring detachment, such as floating spots, flashing lights, and progressive shadows
- Advising patient to follow-up

OTHER EYE DISORDERS

Stye (External and Internal Hordeolum)

An external stye or hordeolum is an infection of a lash follicle and its associated gland of Zeis or Moll. Internal styes are infections of the meibomian sebaceous glands lining the inside of the eyelids (**Fig. 18.8**).

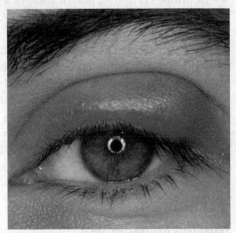

Fig. 18.8: Stye.

Causes

- *Staphylococcus aureus* bacterial infection
- Blocking of an oil gland
- Triggered by poor nutrition, sleep deprivation, lack of hygiene or rubbing of the eyes.

Signs and Symptoms

- A lump on the top or bottom eyelid
- Localized swelling of the eyelid
- Localized pain
- Redness
- Tenderness to touch
- Crusting of the eyelid margins
- Sensation of a foreign body in the eye

Treatment

- Application of warm compresses
- Cleansing must be done gently
- Topical antibiotic ointments or antibiotic or steroid combination

Prevention

- Proper handwashing
- Proper eye hygiene
- Application of a warm washcloth
- Never share cosmetics
- Removing makeup every night before going to sleep
- People are often advised to avoid touching their eyes or sharing towels and washcloths.

CHALAZION (MEIBOMIAN CYST)

A chalazion also known as a meibomian gland lipogranuloma is a cyst in the eyelid that is caused by inflammation of a blocked duct of meibomian gland, usually on the upper eyelid **(Fig. 18.9)**.

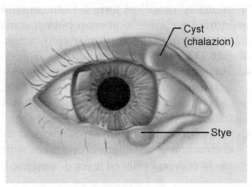

Cyst (chalazion)

Stye

Fig. 18.9: Chalazion.

Signs and Symptoms

- Swelling on the eyelid
- Eyelid tenderness
- Sensitivity to light
- Increased tearing
- Heaviness of the eyelid

Treatment

- Chalazia will often disappear without further treatment within a few months and virtually all will resorb within 2 years.
- Topical antibiotic eye drops or ointment (e.g., chloramphenicol or fusidic acid) are sometimes used.
- A home remedy is to have a hot, wet flannel, and rub gently, until the heat has reached the cyst.

BLEPHARITIS

Blepharitis is an ocular condition characterized by chronic inflammation of the eyelid **(Fig. 18.10)**.

Signs and Symptoms

- Redness of the eyelids
- Flaking of skin on the lids
- Crusting at the lid margins, this is generally worse on waking
- Cysts at the lid margin (hordeolum)
- Red eye
- Debris in the tear film, seen under magnification (improved contrast with use of fluorescein drops)
- Gritty (sandy) sensation of the eye
- Reduced vision

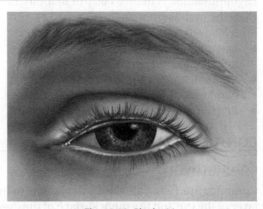

Fig. 18.10: Blepharitis.

Treatment

- The single most important treatment principle is a daily routine of lid margin hygiene.
- After lid margin cleaning, spread small amount of prescription antibiotic ophthalmic ointment with fingertip along lid fissure while eyes closed. Using prior to bedtime as opposed to in the morning to avoid blurry vision.
- Avoiding the use of eye make-up until symptoms subside

TRICHIASIS

Trichiasis is a medical term for abnormally positioned eyelashes that grow back toward the eye, touching the cornea or conjunctiva **(Fig. 18.11).**

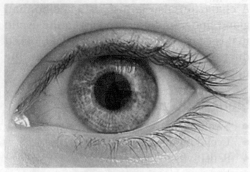

Fig. 18.11: Trichiasis.

- This can be caused by infection, inflammation, autoimmune conditions, congenital defects, eyelid agenesis, and trauma such as burns or eyelid injury.
- Standard treatment involves removal or destruction of the affected eyelashes with electrology, specialized laser, or surgery.

ENTROPION

Entropion is a medical condition in which the eyelid (usually the lower lid) folds inward.

ECTROPION

- Ectropion is a medical condition in which the lower eyelid turns outwards.
- Ectropion can occur due to any weakening of tissue of the lower eyelid. The condition can be repaired surgically.

LAGOPHTHALMOS

Lagophthalmos is defined as the inability to close the eyelids completely **(Fig. 18.12).**

- It leads to corneal drying and ulceration.
- Lagophthalmos can arise from a malfunction of the facial nerve.
- Lagophthalmos can also occur in comatose patients.
- Blepharoplasty can be done as a treatment.

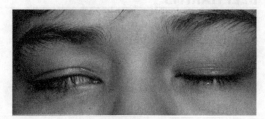

Fig. 18.12: Lagophthalmos.

CONJUNCTIVAL DISORDERS

Conjunctivitis

Conjunctivitis (also called pink eye) refers to inflammation of the conjunctiva (the outermost layer of the eye and the inner surface of the eyelids).

Types of Conjunctivitis

- Allergic conjunctivitis
- Bacterial conjunctivitis
- Viral conjunctivitis
- Chemical conjunctivitis
- Neonatal conjunctivitis

Signs and Symptoms

- Red eye (hyperemia)
- Irritation (chemosis)

- Watering (epiphora)
- Pain
- Crusting of the eyelid margins
- Burning in the eye
- Droopiness of the eyelid
- Scratchy sensation on the eyeball
- Mucous discharge in the eye
- Light sensitivity
- Discomfort during blinking
- Sensation of a foreign body in the eye

Management

- Conjunctivitis resolves in 65% of cases without treatment, within 2–5 days. The prescribing of antibiotics to most cases is not necessary.
- Symptomatic relief may be achieved with cold compresses and artificial tears.

Prevention

- People with conjunctivitis should not touch their eyes, regardless of whether or not their hands are clean, as they run the risk of spreading the condition to another eye.
- With either type of conjunctivitis, handwashing is the best means of preventing the spread of disease.
- People are often advised to avoid touching their eyes or sharing towels and washcloths.
- During home care, eyes should be cleansed gently to remove exudates and the cleansing tissues disposed of using standard precautions.
- Avoiding shaking hands with other people.
- Using separate medication bottles or tubes for each eye.

PTERYGIUM

- Pterygium (Surfer's eye) most often refers to a benign growth of the conjunctiva.
- A pterygium commonly grows from the nasal side of the sclera.
- It is associated with, and thought to be caused by UV-light exposure (e.g., sunlight), low humidity, and dust.

Symptoms

- Persistent redness
- Inflammation
- Foreign body sensation, which can cause bleeding, dry and itchy eyes
- Tearing
- In advanced cases, the pterygium can affect vision as it invades the cornea.

Treatment

- Some of the irritating symptoms can be addressed with artificial tears.
- However, no reliable medical treatment exists to reduce or even prevent pterygium progression.
- Definitive treatment is achieved only by surgical removal, that is, irradiation, conjunctival autografting or amniotic membrane transplantation, along with glue and suture application.
- Long-term follow-up is required as pterygium may recur even after complete surgical correction.

Prevention

- As it is associated with excessive sun or wind exposure, wearing protective sunglasses with side shields and wide-brimmed hats may help prevent their formation.
- Surfers and other water-sport athletes should wear eye protection that blocks 100% of the UV rays from the water, as is often used by snow-sport athletes.

SUBCONJUNCTIVAL HEMORRHAGE

- A subconjunctival hemorrhage is bleeding underneath the conjunctiva.
- Although its appearance may be alarming, a subconjunctival hemorrhage is generally a painless and harmless condition.
- It may be associated with high blood pressure, trauma to the eye, or a base of skull fracture.

Causes

- Blood dyscrasia
- Blood thinners: These can also make the vessels in the eye more susceptible to the pressure.
- Diving accidents
- Severe hypertension
- Laser-assisted in situ keratomileusis (LASIK).
- Minor eye trauma
- Spontaneously with increased venous pressure
- Strenuous exercising
- Straining
- Vomiting
- Prolonged stress
- Severe thoracic trauma, leading to increased pressure in the extremities, including around the eyes
- Subconjunctival hemorrhages in infants may be associated with scurvy (a vitamin C deficiency), abuse or traumatic asphyxia syndrome.

Treatment and Management

- Self-limiting condition that requires no treatment in the absence of infection or significant trauma.
- The elective use of aspirin and nonsteroidal anti-inflammatory drugs (NSAIDs) is typically discouraged.

CORNEAL DISORDERS

Keratitis

- Keratitis is a condition in which the eye's cornea, the front part of the eye, becomes inflamed.
- The condition is often marked by moderate to intense pain and usually involves impaired eyesight.

Types

1. Superficial keratitis involves the superficial layers of the cornea. After healing, this form of keratitis does not generally leave a scar.
2. Deep keratitis involves deeper layers of the cornea, and the natural course leaves a scar upon healing that impairs vision if on or near the visual axis. This can be reduced or avoided with the use of topical corticosteroid eyedrops.

Causes

- Viral: Infection of herpes simplex virus secondary to an upper respiratory infection, involving cold sores.
- Amoebic keratitis, amoebic infection of the cornea is the most serious corneal infection, usually affecting contact lens wearers. It is usually caused by *Acanthamoeba*.
- Bacterial keratitis, bacterial infection of the cornea can follow from an injury or from wearing contact lenses. The bacteria involved are *S. aureus* and for contact lens wearers, *Pseudomonas aeruginosa*. *P. aeruginosa* contains enzymes that can digest the cornea.
- Fungal keratitis, filamentous fungi are most frequently the causative organism for fungal keratitis.
- Onchocercal keratitis, which follows *Onchocerca volvulus* infection by infected blackfly bite. These blackflies usually dwell near fast-flowing African streams, so the disease is also called "river blindness."

Treatment

- Treatment depends on the cause of the keratitis. Infectious keratitis generally requires antibacterial, antifungal, or antiviral therapy to treat the infection.
- In addition, contact lens wearers are typically advised to discontinue contact lens wear and discard contaminated contact lenses and contact lens cases.
- With proper medical attention, infections can usually be successfully treated without long-term visual loss.

CORNEAL DYSTROPHIES

- Corneal dystrophies comprise a group of hereditary and acquired disorders of unknown cause, characterized by deposits in the layers of the cornea and alteration of the corneal structure.
- Corneal dystrophies are associated with all five layers of the cornea. Although the disease usually originates in the inner layers (Descemet's membrane, the stroma, and Bowman's membrane), the degeneration, erosion, and deposits affect all layers.

Management

The goal of treatment is to restore visual clarity for both safety and improved quality of life.

Medical Management

Dystrophies cannot be cured; however, with certain medications, blurred vision resulting from corneal swelling can be controlled.

Surgical Management

Corneal transplantation: Corneal transplantation (keratoplasty) is the use of donor corneas to improve the clarity of vision.

NURSING PROCESS—INFLAMMATION AND INFECTION OF THE EYE

Assessment

Assessment of symptoms for any eye problem includes asking the client for subjective data using the WHAT'S UP acronym:

- **W**here is it? What part of the eye is affected? Eyelid, conjunctiva, cornea?
- **H**ow does it feel? Pressure? Itchy? Painful? No pain? Irritated? Spasm?
- **A**ggravating and alleviating factors. Worse when rubbing eyes, blinking? Photosensitivity?
- **T**iming: Was there exposure to a pathogen? Previous infection or irritation? Length of time symptoms has persisted?
- **S**everity: Is there visual impairment? Does pain affect activities of daily living (ADL)?
- **U**seful data for associated symptoms. Immunosuppression drugs? Do other members of the family or peer group have symptoms? Are decongestant eyedrops used? Is there exudate? Are the eyelids sticks together on awakening? Does client wear contact lenses, soft contact lenses overnight, disposable contact lenses? Does client have dry eyes? Infection with tuberculosis, syphilis, HIV? What is typical eye hygiene?
- **P**erception by the client of the problem. What does client think is wrong?
- Assessing the condition of conjunctiva, the condition of eyelids and eyelashes, the presence of exudate, whether tearing is occurring, any visible abscess on palpebral border, a palpable abscess in eyelid, opacity of the cornea, and visual acuity testing comparing unaffected and affected eyes.

Nursing Care Plan

Nursing Assessment

History (Subjective Data)
- Change in vision
- Pain, itching, burning
- Excessive watering
- Blurred vision, double vision (diplopia)
- Loss in field of vision, blind spots, floating spots
- Difficulty with vision at night
- Pain in bright light
- Frontal headache
- Halos around lights
- Frequent reddening of eye—conjunctivitis
- Discharge, eye crusted on awakening
- Eyes feel dry—wearing contact lenses, glasses
- Regular medication
- History of glaucoma in family
- History of diabetes, hypertension
- Date of last eye examination

Physical Assessment (Objective Data)
- Observing for redness of conjunctiva, swelling, secretions, excessive tearing
- Change in visual acuity
- Noting any squinting, tilting head
- Noting ability to move eyebrows and eyes

Nursing Diagnosis
- Pain related to inflammation or infection of the eye or surrounding tissues.
- Sensory-perceptual alteration (visual) related to blepharospasm, photophobia, diminished visual acuity, visual distortions
- Risk for injury related to visual impairment

- Risk for infection related to poor eye hygiene
- Knowledge deficit related to disease process, prevention, and treatment

Nursing Interventions

General Interventions for Visually Impaired
- Speaking as you enter the room and before touching patient
- Telling the patient when you are leaving
- Not moving objects without asking patient
- Giving special orientation to room on admission
- Setting up meal tray and orient patient to food

Preoperative
- Describing procedure—local anesthetic
- Discharge teaching—eye drops, activity restrictions
- Starting stool softeners to prevent constipation
- Washing face well with surgical soap
- Instilling eye drops as order

Postoperative
- Be gentle—no jarring movement
- Treat nausea immediately with antiemetics
- Monitoring for pain or visual changes (sign of bleeding)
- Eye patching with nonallergic tape
- Patching both eye if restricting movement of eye
- Metal eye shield at night for extra protection
- Physician orders for positioning instilling eye drops
- Washing hands, give patient tissue
- Removing eye patch, gently cleanse with wet gauze
- Patient supine or head lilted up, look up
- Pulling lower lid down
- Not touching dropper to patient's eye
- Putting pressure with finger over lacrimal duct to decrease systemic absorption
- Asking to close eye gently and rotate eyeball to distribute medication. Not squeezing eye shunt
- Applying new patch with nonallergic tape.

EYE BANKING AND CORNEAL TRANSPLANTATION

It is an organization that deals with the collection, storage, and distribution of donor eyes for the purpose of corneal grafting:
- Corned blindness is a major form of visual deprivation in developing countries. A high percentage of these individuals can be visually rehabilitated by corneal transplantation (keratoplasty), a procedure that has a very high rate of success among organ transplants. Quality of donor cornea, the nature of recipient pathology, and the availability of appropriate postoperative care are the factors that determine the final outcome of this procedure.
  In corneal grafting, this diseased and opaque cornea is replaced by a healthy transparent cornea taken from a donor eye.
- A corneal transplant can take one of the two forms: a full-thickness penetrating keratoplasty, involving excision and replacement of the entire cornea, or a lamellar keratoplasty, which removes and replaces a superficial layer of corneal tissue.

Functions of Eye Bank

Procurement and supply of donor cornea to the corneal surgeons is the primary goal of eye banks:

1. The eye bank collects the eyes of voluntary registered eye donors after their death of those deceased persons when enlightened relatives agree to donate the eyes as a service to humanity. From hospital deaths and from postmortem cases, after obtaining the consent from the next of kin.

2. These eyes are processed by the eye bank and are supplied to eye surgeons for corneal grafting and other sight restoring operations.

3. Before proceeding for recovery eye bank personnel should ascertain the following details: location, age of the donor, cause of death, and time of death.

Contraindications for Donation

- All eye banks have age limits both minimum and maximum
- Previous corneal graft
- Death of unknown cause
- Dementia
- Creutzfeldt–Jakob disease
- Subacute sclerosing panencephalitis
- Congenital rubella
- Reyes syndrome
- Active viral encephalitis or encephalitis of unknown origin
- Active septicemia
- Rabies
- Retinoblastomas, tumors of the anterior segment
- Active ocular infections
- Pterygium—other superficial disorders of the conjunctiva or corneal surface
- Certain intraocular or anterior segment surgeries
- Leukemia
- Active disseminated lymphomas
- Hepatitis B and C, HTLV-1 or 2, HIV, syphilis
- Behavioral and or social issues, that is, homosexual or other high-risk sexual behavior within the last 5 years
- Intravenous drug use for nonmedical reasons within the last 5 years
- Exposure to infectious disease within the last year by contact with an open wound, needle stick, or mucous membrane
- Tattooing or piercing within the last 12 months using shared instrument

Retrieval Procedure

- Retrieval procedure could be either enucleation or corneal scleral rim excision.
- Eye bank team should carry only validated sterile instruments for retrieval.
- Eye bank team on arrival at the location should locate the next of kin and convey condolence and obtain death certificate.
- In the absence of a death certificate, the registered medical practitioner should satisfy self that life is extinct.
- The eye bank team should obtain consent on a consent form from the legal custodian of the donor.

- After obtaining consent the donor should be identified either through a tag or through the next of kin.
- The eye bank team should then proceed to prepare the site.
- Gross physical examination should be conducted with utmost respect for observations regarding build: average, healthy or emaciated.
- Eye bank team should look out for needle marks on the arm, skin lesions, etc.
- Eye bank team should look out for ulcers or gangrene in exposed areas.
- Ocular examination should be conducted.
- Medical records and medical information should be obtained.
- Information for hemodilution should be obtained.
- Social history of the donor should be obtained wherever possible from the next of kin.

ROLE OF NURSE DURING CORNEAL TRANSPLANTATION

- Explaining the transplant procedure to the patient and answer any questions he may have.
- Advising him that healing will be slow and that his vision may not be completely restored until the sutures are removed, which may be in about a year.
- Telling the patient that most corneal transplants are performed under local anesthesia and that he can expect momentary burning during injection of the anesthetic.
- Explaining to him that the procedure will last for about an hour and that he must remain still until it has been completed.
- Telling the patient that analgesics will be available after surgery because he may experience a dull aching.
- Informing him that a bandage and protective shield will be placed over the eye.
- As ordered, administer a sedative or an osmotic agent to reduce IOP.
- Ensuring that the patient has signed a consent form.

After Surgery

- After the patient recovers from the anesthetic, assessing for and immediately report sudden, sharp, or excessive pain, bloody, purulent, or clear viscous drainage or fever.
- As ordered, instilling corticosteroid eyedrops or topical antibiotics to prevent inflammation and graft rejection.
- Instructing the patient to lie on his back or on his unaffected side, with the bed flat or slightly elevated as ordered. Also, have him avoid rapid head movements, hard coughing or sneezing, bending over, and other activities that could increase IOP; likewise, he should not squint or rub his eyes.
- Reminding the patient to ask for help in standing or walking until he adjusts to changes in his vision.
- Making sure that all his personal items are within his field of vision.

Home Care Instructions

- Teaching the patient and his family to recognize the signs of graft rejection (inflammation, cloudiness, drainage, and pain at the graft site).
- Instructing them to immediately notify the doctor if any of these signs occur.
- Emphasizing that rejection can occur many years after surgery; stressing the need for assessing the graft *daily* for the rest of the patient's life. Also, reminding the patient to keep regular appointments with his doctor.
- Telling the patient to avoid activities that increase IOP, including extreme exertion, sudden, jerky movements, lifting or pushing heavy objects and straining during defecation.

- Explaining that photophobia, a common adverse reaction, gradually decreases as healing progresses.
- Suggesting wearing dark glasses in bright light.
- Teaching the patient how to correctly instill prescribed eyedrops.
- Reminding the patient to wear an eye shield when sleeping.
- Telling the patient to consult with the surgeon before driving or participating in sports or other recreational activities.

MULTIPLE CHOICE QUESTIONS

1. **For a client having an episode of acute narrow-angle glaucoma, a nurse expects to give which of the following medications?**
   A. Acetazolamide (Diamox)
   B. Urokinase (Abbokinase)
   C. Atropine
   D. Furosemide (Lasix)

2. **After the nurse instills atropine drops into both eyes for a client undergoing ophthalmic examination, which of the following instructions would be given to the client?**
   A. Wear dark glasses in bright light because the pupils are dilated
   B. Avoid wearing your regular glasses when driving
   C. Be careful because the blink reflex is paralyzed
   D. Be aware that the pupils may be unusually small

3. **When developing a teaching session on glaucoma for the community, which of the following statements would the nurse stress?**
   A. White and Asian individuals are at the highest risk for glaucoma
   B. Glaucoma is easily corrected with eyeglasses
   C. Yearly screening for people ages 20–40 years is recommended
   D. Glaucoma can be painless and vision may be lost before the person is aware of a problem

4. **The nurse is caring for a client with a diagnosis of detached retina. Which assessment sign would indicate that bleeding has occurred as a result of the retinal detachment?**
   A. A sudden sharp pain in the eye
   B. A reddened conjunctiva
   C. Complaints of a burst of black spots or floaters
   D. Total loss of vision

5. **The nurse is developing a plan of care for the client scheduled for cataract surgery. The nurse documents which more appropriate nursing diagnosis in the plan of care?**
   A. Imbalanced nutrition
   B. Anxiety
   C. Self-care deficit
   D. Disturbed sensory perception

6. **During the early postoperative period, the client who had a cataract extraction complains of nausea and severe eye pain over the operative site. The initial nursing action is to:**
   A. Administer the ordered main medication and antiemetic
   B. Reassure the client that this is normal
   C. Turn the client on his or her operative side
   D. Call the physician

7. **In preparation for cataract surgery, the nurse is to administer prescribed eye drops. The nurse reviews the physician's orders, expecting which type of eye drops to be instilled?**
   A. An osmotic diuretic
   B. A mydriatic medication
   C. A miotic agent
   D. A thiazide diuretic

8. **The nurse is performing an admission assessment on a client with a diagnosis of detached retina. Which of the following is associated with this eye disorder?**
   A. A yellow discoloration of the sclera
   B. Total loss of vision
   C. Pain in the affected eye
   D. A sense of a curtain falling across the field of vision

9. **Which of the following symptoms would occur in a client with a detached retina?**
   A. Homonymous hemianopia
   B. Flashing lights and floaters
   C. Ptosis
   D. Loss of central vision

10. **The nurse is caring for a client following enucleation. The nurse notes the presence of bright red blood drainage on the dressing. Which nursing action is appropriate?**
    A. Mark the drainage on the dressing and monitor for any increase in bleeding
    B. Notify the physician
    C. Document the finding
    D. Continue to monitor the drainage

Answers

1. A   2. A   3. D   4. C   5. D   6. D   7. B   8. D   9. B   10. D

BIBLIOGRAPHY

1. Black JM, Hawks JH. Medical Surgical Nursing: Clinical Management for Positive Outcomes, vol 2, 8th edition. New Delhi: Elsevier; 2010. pp. 1704-15.
2. Bucher L, Lewis SL, Heitkemper MM, Dirksen SR. Lewis's Medical Surgical Nursing. New Delhi: Elsevier; 2011. pp. 416-23.
3. Clark A, Morlet N, Jonathan Q, Preen DB, Semmens JB. Whole population trends in complications of cataract surgery over 22 years in Western Australia. Ophthalmology. 2011;118(6):1055-61.
4. Kanski JJ. Clinical Ophthalmology: A Systematic Approach, 2nd edition. Hong Kong; 1989. pp. 1-12.
5. Nettina SM. Lippincott Manual of Nursing Practice, 9th edition. New Delhi: Wolters Kluwer; 2010. pp. 594-98.
6. Williams LS, Hopper PD. Understanding Medical Surgical Nursing, 7th edition. Philadelphia: Davis Company; 1999. pp. 1040-57.

Nursing Management of Patient with Neurological Disorders

> AT THE END OF THIS CHAPTER, THE STUDENTS WILL BE ABLE TO LEARN ABOUT THE MANAGEMENT OF:
>
> ➢ Headache
> ➢ Head injures
> ➢ Spinal injuries
> ➢ Paraplegia
> ➢ Hemiplegia
> ➢ Quadriplegia
> ➢ Spinal cord compression-hernia ion of intervertebral disk
> ➢ Tumors of the brain and spinal cord
> ➢ Intracranial and cerebral aneurysms abscess, neurocysticercosis
> ➢ Movement disorder
> ➢ Chorea
> ➢ Seizures
> ➢ Cerebrovascular accidents (CVA)
> ➢ Cranial, spinal neuropathies—Bell's palsy, trigeminal neuralgia (TN)
> ➢ Peripheral neuropathies; Barré syndrome
> ➢ Myasthenia gravis
> ➢ Multiple sclerosis (MS)
> ➢ Degenerative, delirium, dementia, Alzheimer's disease
> ➢ Parkinson's disease
> ➢ Management of unconscious patients and patients with stroke
> ➢ Role of the in communicating with patient having neurological deficit
> ➢ Rehabilitation of patients with neurological deficit
> ➢ Role of nurse in long-stay facility (institutions) and at home

REVIEW OF ANATOMY AND PHYSIOLOGY

The nervous system has been divided into two components: the central nervous system (CNS), which is composed of the brain and the spinal cord, and the peripheral nervous system, which is composed of ganglia and peripheral nerves that lie outside the brain and spinal cord.

Peripheral Nervous System

The peripheral nervous system has been, in turn, divided into two subsystems: somatic and autonomic.

Somatic subsystem includes sensory neurons of the dorsal root and cranial ganglia that innervate the skin, muscles, and joints and provide sensory information to the CNS about muscle and limb position and about the environment.

Autonomic subsystem includes the motor system for the viscera, the smooth muscles, and exocrine glands. It in turn consists of three segregated subdivisions: the sympathetic system that participates in the response of the body to stress. The parasympathetic system acts to conserve the body's resources and restore homeostasis. The enteric nervous system controls the function of smooth muscle of the gut.

Central Nervous System

The CNS consists of six main regions **(Fig. 19.1):**

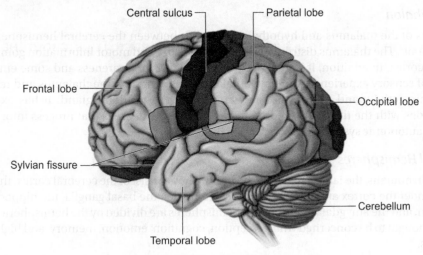

Fig. 19.1: Structure of brain.

Spinal Cord

It extends from the base of the skull through the first lumbar vertebra. The spinal cord receives sensory information from the skin, joints, and muscles of the trunk and limbs, and contains the motor neurons responsible for both voluntary and reflex movements. It also receives sensory information from the internal organs and control many visceral functions. Within the spinal cord there is an orderly arrangement of sensory cell groups that receive input from the periphery and motor cell groups that control specific muscle groups. In addition, the spinal cord contains ascending pathway through which sensory information reaches the brain and descending pathways that relay motor command from the brain to motor neurons.

Medulla

This structure is the direct rostral extension (this means toward the head and nose) of the spinal cord. Together with the pons, it participates in regulating blood pressure and respiration. It resembles the spinal cord in both organization and function.

Pons

It lies rostral to the medulla and contains a large number of neurons that relay information from the cerebral hemispheres to the cerebellum. The cerebellum lies dorsal to the pons and medulla. It has a distinctive corrugated surface. The cerebellum receives somatosensory input from the spinal cord, motor information from the cerebral cortex and balance information from the vestibular organs of the inner ear. The cerebellum integrates this information and coordinates the planning, timing, and patterning of skeletal muscle contractions during movement. The cerebellum plays a major role in the control of posture, head, and eye movements.

Midbrain

This is the smallest brainstem component which lies rostral to the pons. The midbrain contains essential relay nuclei of the auditory and visual system. Several regions of this structure play an important role in the direct control of eye movement, whereas others are involved in motor control of skeletal muscles.

Diencephalon

It consists of the thalamus and hypothalamus. It lies between the cerebral hemispheres and the midbrain. The thalamus distributes almost all sensory and motor information going to the cerebral cortex. In addition, it is thought to regulate levels of awareness and some emotional aspects of sensory experiences. The hypothalamus lies ventral to the thalamus and regulates autonomic activity and the hormonal secretion by the pituitary gland. It has extensive connections with the thalamus, midbrain and some cortical areas that process information from the autonomic system.

Cerebral Hemispheres

It forms, in humans, the largest region of the brain. They consist of the cerebral cortex, the white matter under the cortex and three deeply located nuclei: the basal ganglia, the hippocampus formation, and the amygdala. The cerebral hemispheres are divided by the hemispheric fissure and are thought to be concerned with perception, cognition, emotion, memory, and high motor functions.

Basal Ganglia

The major components of the basal ganglia are the caudate nucleus, the putamen, and the globus pallidus. The basal ganglia have an important role in regulation of movement and also contribute to cognitive functions.

Hippocampus and Amygdala

The hippocampus and amygdala are part of the so-called limbic system. The hippocampus is involved in memory storage. The amygdala coordinates the actions of the autonomic and endocrine systems and is involved in emotions.

NEUROLOGICAL ASSESSMENT

The neurological examination allows the examiner to evaluate various areas of the brain. Nurses observe for clinical manifestations that may be abnormal and relate them to general areas of the nervous system that may be causing the disturbance.

During Assessing the Nervous System

- Do you have any history of head injury?
- Do you have frequent or severe headaches?

Assessing for Syncope and Vertigo

- Investigating for dizziness or vertigo
- Inquiring about seizures

- Assessing for swallowing, speech, and coordination
- Inquiring about difficulty in swallowing
- Inquiring about coordination difficulties

Assessing for Neurological Deficits

- Investigating about numbness or tingling
- Inquiring about the patient's neurologic history
- Investigating about any mental health disorders

Mental Status: Appearance and Hygiene

- Presenting appearance: Overall appearance including apparent age, ethnicity, height, and weight
- Assessing for basic grooming and hygiene

Mental Status: Coordination, Behavior, and Speech

- Assessing the motor coordination
- Assessing the behavior such as unconcerned, evasive, negative, irritable, depressive, anxious
- Assessing the speech, normal rate, and volume, or is it pressured, slow, accented
- Assessing the gait. Gross gait abnormalities should be noted
- Assessing for mental status: Eye contact, comprehension, and memory and recall
- Assessing the comprehension
- Assessing the recall and memory
- Assessing the mental status: Orientation, attention, and thought processes
- Assessing the concentration and attention
- Assessing the thought processes

Mental Status: Hallucinations, Judgment, and Intellect

- Assessing the hallucinations and delusions
- Assessing the judgment and insight

Twelve Cranial Nerves

1. **Cranial nerve I—olfactory:**
   - Checking that air can move freely through each nostril by occluding one at a time
   - Using an alcohol pad to check sense of smell
2. **Cranial nerve II—optic:**
   - Checking visual acuity by using either a Snellen eye chart
   - Move your finger and begin bringing it in toward your nose
3. **Cranial nerve III—oculomotor; cranial nerve IV—trochlear; cranial nerve VI—abducens:** While client holds his head still, trace an "H" in the air, and have the patient follow your finger with only their eyes or not.
4. **Cranial nerve V—trigeminal:**
   - *Sensory:* Having the client close his eyes. Lightly touch temporal and on the jawbone, asking client to ask when he feels the touch and where
   - *Motor:* Having the client clench and grind his teeth.
5. **Cranial nerve VII—facial:** Observing for facial symmetry with the client's relaxed expression.
6. **Cranial nerve VIII—vestibulocochlear:** Rubbing your fingers together next to each ear. Asking client if the sound is the same on both sides.

7. **Cranial nerve IX—glossopharyngeal; cranial nerve X—vagus; cranial nerve XII—hypoglossal:** Having the client stick out his tongue and say "Ahhhhh." The uvula should be midline, and the palate and uvula should rise. The tongue should also be midline.

8. **Cranial nerve XI—spinal accessory:** Asking client to turn his head to the left, while place some resistance against their face with the right hand. Repeating this with the patient turning to the right with resistance. The strength should be equal bilaterally.

Assessment of Cerebellar Function

- **Gait:** Having the client walk heel to toe in a straight line.
- **The heel to shin test:** The heel to shin test is a measure of coordination and may be abnormal if there is loss of motor strength, proprioception or a cerebellar lesion. If motor and sensory systems are intact, an abnormal, asymmetric heel to shin test is highly suggestive of an ipsilateral cerebellar lesion.

Glasgow Coma Scale

The Glasgow coma scale **Table 19.1** assesses how the brain functions as whole. The scale assesses three major brain functions: eye opening, motor response, and verbal response.

- A completely normal person will score 15 on the scale overall.
- Scores of <7 reflect coma

TABLE 19.1: The Glasgow coma scale.

Response	Scale	Score
Eye opening response	Eyes open spontaneously	4 Points
	Eyes open to verbal command, speech or shout	3 points
	Eyes open to pain (not applied to face)	2 points
	No eye opening	1 points
Verbal response	Oriented	5 points
	Confused conversation, but able to answer questions	4 points
	Inappropriate responses, words discernible	3 points
	Incomprehensible sounds or speech	2 points
	No verbal response	1 points
Motor response	Obeys commands for movement	6 points
	Purposeful movement to painful stimulus	5 points
	Withdraws from pain	4 points
	Abnormal (spastic) flexion, decorticate posture	3 points
	Extensor (rigid) response, decerebrate posture	2 points
	No motor response	1 point

DISORDERS OF THE NERVOUS SYSTEM

BELL'S PALSY

Bell's palsy is a paralysis or weakness of the muscles on one side of face. Damage to the facial nerve that controls muscles on one side of the face causes that side of face to droop. The nerve damage may also affect sense of taste. The weakness usually affects one side of the face. Rarely, both sides are affected (**Fig. 19.2**).

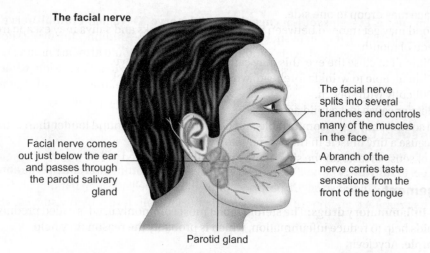

The facial nerve

The facial nerve splits into several branches and controls many of the muscles in the face

Facial nerve comes out just below the ear and passes through the parotid salivary gland

A branch of the nerve carries taste sensations from the front of the tongue

Parotid gland

Fig. 19.2: Bell's palsy.

Etiology

It is thought that inflammation develops around the facial nerve as it passes through the skull from the brain. The inflammation may squash (compress) the nerve as it passes through the skull. The nerve then partly, or fully, stops working until the inflammation goes. If the nerve stops working, the muscles that the nerve supplies also stop working.

- Cold sore (herpes simplex) virus
- Chickenpox (varicella-zoster) virus

Signs and Symptoms

- Weakness of the face which is usually one sided. The weakness normally develops quickly **(Fig. 19.3)**.

Bell's palsy

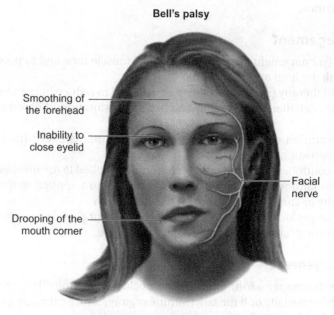

Smoothing of the forehead

Inability to close eyelid

Facial nerve

Drooping of the mouth corner

Fig. 19.3: Clinical manifestations of Bell's palsy.

- Face may droop to one side.
- Food may get trapped between gum and cheek. Drinks and saliva may escape from the side of mouth.
- Difficult to close the eye, this may cause a watery or dry eye.
- Difficult able to wrinkle forehead, whistle or blow out cheek.
- Difficulty with speech.
- Painless or cause just a mild ache.
- Loud sounds may be uncomfortable and normal noises may sound louder than usual. This is because a tiny muscle in the ear may stop working.
- Loss of sense of taste on the side of the tongue that is affected.

Management

- **Anti-inflammatory drugs:** The steroid tablet most commonly used is called prednisolone. Steroids help to reduce inflammation, which is probably the reason they help.
- **Example:** Acyclovir
- **Eye protection:** Acyclovir
  - An eye pad or goggles to protect the eye.
  - Eye drops to lubricate the eye during the day.
  - Eye ointment to lubricate the eye overnight.
  - Tape the upper and lower lid together when you are asleep. Other procedures are sometimes done to keep the eye shut until the eyelids recover.
- **Physiotherapy:** A treatment called, "facial retraining" with facial exercises may help.
- **Injections of botulism toxin** (Botox) may help if spasm develops in the facial muscles.
- Various surgical techniques can help with the cosmetic appearance.

Complications

- Corneal ulcers
- Blindness
- Impaired nutrition

Medical Management

The objectives of management are to maintain facial muscle tone and to prevent or minimize complication with the help of the following:

- Corticosteroid therapy (prednisone) may be initiated to reduce inflammation and edema, which reduces vascular compression and permits restoration of blood circulation to the nerve.
- Early administration of corticosteroids appears to diminish severity, relieve pain, and minimize denervation.
- Facial pain is controlled with analgesic agents or heat applied to the involved side of the face.
- Additional modalities may include electrical stimulation applied to the face to prevent muscle atrophy or surgical exploration of the facial nerve.
- Surgery may be performed if a tumor is suspected, for surgical decompression of the facial nerve, and for surgical rehabilitation of a paralyzed face.

Surgical Management

- **Facial nerve decompression:** The surgeon decides if the maxillary segment should be decompressed externally or if the labyrinthine segment and geniculate ganglion should be decompressed with a middle fossa craniotomy.

- **Suborbicularis oculi fat (SOOF) lift:** The SOOF is deep to the orbicularis oculi muscle and superficial to the periosteum below the inferior orbital rim. An SOOF lift is designed to lift and suspend the midfacial musculature. The procedure may also elevate the upper lip and the angle of the mouth to improve facial symmetry.
- **Lateral tarsal strip procedure:** An SOOF lift is commonly performed in conjunction with a lateral tarsal strip procedure to correct horizontal lower-lid laxity and to improve apposition of the lid to the globe. First, lateral canthotomy and cantholysis are performed. Then, the anterior lamella is removed, and the lateral tarsal strip is shortened and attached to the periosteum at the lateral orbital rim.
- **Implants in eyelid:** Implantable devices have been used to restore dynamic lid closure in cases of severe, symptomatic lagophthalmos. These procedures are best for patients with poor Bell phenomenon and decreased corneal sensation. Gold or platinum weights, a weight-adjustable magnet, or palpebral springs can be inserted into the eyelids. Pretarsal gold-weight implantation is most commonly performed. The implants are easily removed if nerve function returns.
- **Tarsorrhaphy:** Tarsorrhaphy decreases horizontal lid opening by fusing the eyelid margins together, increasing support of the precorneal lake of tears and improving coverage of the eye during sleep. The procedure can be done in the office and is particularly suitable for patients who are unable or unwilling to undergo other surgery. It can be completed as either a temporary or a permanent measure. Permanent tarsorrhaphy is performed if nerve recovery is not expected.

Tarsorrhaphy can be performed laterally, centrally, or medially. The lateral procedure is the most common; however, it can restrict the monocular temporal visual field. Central tarsorrhaphy offers good corneal protection, but it occludes vision and can be cosmetically unacceptable. Medial or paracentral tarsorrhaphy is performed lateral to the lacrimal puncta and can offer good lid closure without substantially affecting the visual field.

Other Surgeries

Muscle transposition, nerve grafting, and brow lift
1. **Transposition of temporalis:** Transposition of the temporalis muscle can be used to reanimate the face and to provide lid closure by using the fifth cranial nerve. Strips from the muscle and fascia are placed in the upper and lower lids as an encircling sling. Patients initiate movement by chewing or clenching their teeth.
2. **Facial nerve grafting or hypoglossal–facial nerve anastomosis:** Reinnervation of the facial nerve by means of facial nerve grafting or hypoglossal–facial nerve anastomosis can be used in cases of clinically significant permanent paralysis to help restore relatively normal function to the orbicularis oculi muscle or eyelids.
3. **Direct brow lift:** Brow ptosis is repaired with a direct brow lift. Care should be taken in the presence of corneal decompensation because lifting the brow can cause worsening of lagophthalmos, especially if lid closure is poor. A gold-weight implant can be placed or lower-lid resuspension can be performed simultaneously to prevent this complication.

Nursing Management

Teaching patients with Bell's palsy to care for them at home is an important nursing priority.

Teaching Eye Care

Because the eye usually does not close completely, the blink reflex is diminished, so the eye is vulnerable to injury from dust and foreign particles. Corneal irritation and ulceration may occur. Distortion of the lower lid alters the proper drainage of tears. Encouraging the client for the following:

- Covering the eye with a protective shield at night
- Applying eye ointment to keep eyelids closed during sleep
- Closing the paralyzed eyelid manually before going to sleep
- Wearing wraparound sunglasses or goggles to decrease normal evaporation from the eye

Teaching about Maintaining Muscle Tone

- Showing patient how to perform facial massage with gentle
- Upward motion several times daily when the patient can tolerate the massage
- Demonstrating facial exercises, such as wrinkling the forehead
- Blowing out the cheeks, and whistling, in an effort to prevent muscle atrophy
- Instructing patient to avoid exposing the face to cold and drafts

Diet and Nutrition

- Instructing patient to chew on the unaffected side of his mouth
- Providing soft and nutritionally balanced diet. Eliminating hot fluids and foods.
- Giving frequent mouth care, being particularly careful to remove residues of food that collects between the cheeks and gums.

TRIGEMINAL NEURALGIA (TIC DOULOUREUX)

The trigeminal nerve (TN) (also called the fifth cranial nerve) is one of the main nerves of the face. It comes through the skull from the brain in front of the ear. It is called *tri*geminal as it splits into three main branches. Each branch divides into many smaller nerves. The nerves from the first branch go to scalp, forehead and around eye. The nerves from second branch go to the area around cheek. The nerves from the third branch go to the area around jaw.

The branches of the trigeminal nerve take sensations of touch and pain to the brain from face, teeth, and mouth. The trigeminal nerve also controls the muscles used in chewing and the production of saliva and tears.

In TN sudden pains that come from one or more branches of the trigeminal nerve. The pains are usually severe. The second and third branches are the most commonly affected. Therefore the pain is usually around the cheek or jaw or both. The first branch is less commonly affected, so pain over forehead and around eye is less common. TN usually affects one side of the face **(Fig. 19.4)**.

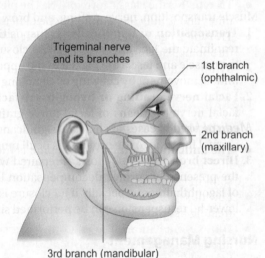

Trigeminal nerve and its branches

1st branch (ophthalmic)

2nd branch (maxillary)

3rd branch (mandibular)

Fig. 19.4: Trigeminal neuralgia.

Etiology

- Tumor
- Multiple sclerosis (MS)
- Abnormality of the base of the skull

Signs and Symptoms

Triggers of Pain Attacks

- Chewing, talking, or smiling
- Drinking cold or hot fluids
- Touching, shaving, brushing teeth, blowing the nose
- Encountering cold air from an open automobile window

Pain Localization

- Patients can localize their pain precisely.
- The pain commonly runs along the line dividing either the mandibular and maxillary nerves or the mandibular and ophthalmic portions of the nerve.
- The pain shoots from the corner of the mouth to the angle of the jaw
- Pain jolts from the upper lip or canine teeth to the eye and eyebrow
- Pain involves the ophthalmic branch of the facial nerve.

Qualities of Pain

- Characteristically severe, paroxysmal, and lancinating
- Commences with a sensation of electrical shocks in the affected area
- Begins to fade within seconds, only to give way to a burning ache lasting seconds to minutes.
- Painfully abates between attacks, even when they are severe and frequent
- Attacks may provoke patients to grimace, wince, or make an aversive head movement, as if trying to escape the pain, thus producing an obvious movement, or tic, hence called "tic douloureux."

Types of "Tic Douloureux"

Trigeminal neuralgia (TN) can be split into different categories depending on the type of pain:
- **TN type 1** is the classic form of TN. The piercing and stabbing pain only happens at certain times and is not constant. This type of neuralgia is known as idiopathic.
- **TN type 2** can be referred to as atypical TN. Pain is more constant and involves aching, throbbing, and burning sensations.
- **Symptomatic TN** is when pain results from an underlying cause, such as MS.

Management

Medical Management

- The **anticonvulsant** carbamazepine is the first-line treatment, second-line medications include baclofen, lamotrigine, oxcarbazepine, phenytoin, gabapentin, pregabalin, and sodium valproate.
- Low doses of some **antidepressants** such as amitriptyline are thought to be effective in treating neuropathic pain.
- **Duloxetine** can also be used in some cases of neuropathic pain, and as it is also an antidepressant, it can be particularly helpful where neuropathic pain and depression are combined.
- **Opiates** such as morphine and oxycodone can be prescribed, and there is evidence of their effectiveness on neuropathic pain, especially if combined with gabapentin.
- **Gallium maltolate** in a cream or ointment base has been reported to relieve refractory postherpetic TN.

Deep Brain Stimulation

It involves delivering an electrical pulse to a part of the brain using a probe. A scanning technique (usually MRI or CT) is used to make sure the probe is in the right place.

Surgical Management

An operation is an option if medication does not work or causes troublesome side effects. Basically, surgery for TN falls into two categories:

- **Decompression surgery:** This means an operation to relieve the pressure on the trigeminal nerve. As TN is due to a blood vessel in the brain pressing on the trigeminal nerve, it leaves the skull. An operation can ease the pressure from the blood vessel (decompress the nerve) and therefore ease symptoms. This operation has the best chance of long-term relief of symptoms. However, it is a major operation involving a general anesthetic and brain surgery to get to the root of the nerve within the brain. Although usually successful, there is a small risk of serious complications, such as a stroke or deafness, following this operation.
- **Ablative surgical treatments:** Ablative means to destroy. There are various procedures that can be used to destroy the root of the trigeminal nerve and thus ease symptoms. For example, one procedure is called stereotactic radiosurgery (Gamma knife surgery). This uses radiation targeted at the trigeminal nerve root to destroy the nerve root. The advantage of these ablative procedures is that they can be done much more easily than decompression surgery as they do not involve formal brain surgery. So, there is much less risk of serious complications or death than there is with decompression surgery.
- **Balloon compression:** It works by injuring the insulation on nerves that are involved with the sensation of light touch on the face. The procedure is performed in an operating room under general anesthesia. A tube called a cannula is inserted through the cheek and guided to where one branch of the trigeminal nerve passes through the base of the skull. A soft catheter with a balloon tip is threaded through the cannula and the balloon is inflated to squeeze part of the nerve against the hard edge of the brain covering and the skull. After about a minute, the balloon is deflated and removed, along with the catheter and cannula. Balloon compression is generally an outpatient procedure, although sometimes the patient may be kept in the hospital overnight. Pain relief usually lasts 1–2 years.
- **Glycerol injection:** It is also generally an outpatient procedure in which the individual is sedated with intravenous (IV) medication. A thin needle is passed through the cheek, next to the mouth, and guided through the opening in the base of the skull where the third division of the trigeminal nerve (mandibular) exits. The needle is moved into the pocket of spinal fluid that surrounds the trigeminal nerve center. The procedure is performed with the person sitting up, since glycerol is heavier than spinal fluid and will then remain in the spinal fluid around the ganglion. The glycerol injection bathes the ganglion and damages the insulation of trigeminal nerve fibers. This form of rhizotomy is likely to result in recurrence of pain within a year to 2 years. However, the procedure can be repeated multiple times.
- **Radiofrequency thermal lesioning** (also known as "RF ablation" or "RF lesion") is most often performed on an outpatient basis. The individual is anesthetized and a hollow needle is passed through the cheek through the same opening at the base of the skull where the balloon compression and glycerol injections are performed. The individual is briefly awakened and a small electrical current is passed through the needle, causing tingling in the area of the nerve where the needle tips rests. When the needle is positioned so that the tingling occurs in the area of TN pain, the person is then sedated and the nerve area is gradually heated with an electrode, injuring the nerve fibers. The electrode and needle are then removed and the person is awakened. The procedure can be repeated until the

desired amount of sensory loss is obtained—usually a blunting of sharp sensation, with preservation of touch.

- **Stereotactic radiosurgery** (Gamma knife, CyberKnife) uses computer imaging to direct highly focused beams of radiation at the site where the trigeminal nerve exits the brain stem. This causes the slow formation of a lesion on the nerve that disrupts the transmission of sensory signals to the brain.
- **Microvascular decompression** (MVD) is not only the most invasive of all surgeries for TN but also offers the lowest probability that pain will return. About half of the individuals undergoing MVD for TN will experience recurrent pain within 12–15 years. This inpatient procedure, which is performed under general anesthesia, requires that a small opening be made through the mastoid bone behind the ear. While viewing the trigeminal nerve through a microscope or endoscope, the surgeon moves away the vessel (usually an artery) that is compressing the nerve and places a soft cushion between the nerve and the vessel. Unlike rhizotomies, the goal is not to produce numbness in the face after this surgery. Individuals generally recuperate for several days in the hospital following the procedure and will generally need to recover for several weeks after the procedure.
- **Neurectomy** (also called partial nerve section), which involves cutting part of the nerve, may be performed near the entrance point of the nerve at the brain stem during an attempted MVD if no vessel is found to be pressing on the trigeminal nerve. Neurectomies also may be performed by cutting superficial branches of the trigeminal nerve in the face. When done during MVD, a neurectomy will cause more long-lasting numbness in the area of the face that is supplied by the nerve or nerve branch that is cut. However, when the operation is performed in the face, the nerve may grow back and in time sensation may return. With neurectomy, there is a risk of creating anesthesia dolorosa.

Nursing Management

- Instructing the client to avoid factors that can trigger the attack and result in exhaustion and fatigue.
- Avoiding foods that are too cold or too hot.
- Chewing foods in the affected side.
- Using cotton pads gently, wash face and for oral hygiene.
- Providing teaching to clients who have sensory loss as a result of a treatment.
- Inspection of the eye for foreign bodies, which the client will not be able to feel, should be done several times a day.
- Warm normal saline irrigation of the affected eye two to three times a day is helpful in preventing corneal infection.
- Dental check-ups every 6 months are encouraged, since dental caries will not produce pain.
- Explaining to the client and his family the disease and its treatments.

EPILEPSY

Refer page 680 under Emergency and Disaster Nursing.

PARKINSONISM

Parkinson's disease is a neurodegenerative disorder that leads to progressive deterioration of motor function due to loss of dopamine-producing brain cells and is characterized by progressive loss of muscle control, which leads to trembling of the limbs and head while at rest, stiffness, slowness, and impaired balance.

Etiology and Risk Factors

- Age is the largest risk factor for the development and progression of Parkinson's disease. Most people who develop Parkinson's disease are older than 60 years of age.
- Men are affected about 1.5–2 times more often than women.
- A small number of individuals are at increased risk because of a family history of the disorder.
- Head trauma, illness, or exposure to environmental toxins such as pesticides and herbicides may be a risk factor.

Signs and Symptoms

- **Tremors:** Trembling in fingers, hands, arms, feet, legs, jaw, or head. Tremors most often occur while the individual is resting, but not while involved in a task. Tremors may worsen when an individual is excited, tired, or stressed.
- **Rigidity:** Stiffness of the limbs and trunk, which may increase during movement. Rigidity may produce muscle aches and pain. Loss of fine hand movements can lead to cramped handwriting (micrographia) and may make eating difficult.
- **Bradykinesia:** Slowness of voluntary movement. Over time, it may become difficult to initiate movement and to complete movement. Bradykinesia together with stiffness can also affect the facial muscles and result in an expressionless, "mask-like" appearance.
- **Postural instability:** Impaired or lost reflexes can make it difficult to adjust posture to maintain balance. Postural instability may lead to falls.
- **Parkinsonian gait:** Individuals with more progressive Parkinson's disease develop a distinctive shuffling walk with a stooped position and a diminished or absent arm swing. It may become difficult to start walking and to make turns. Individuals may freeze in mid-stride and appear to fall forward while walking **(Fig. 19.5)**.

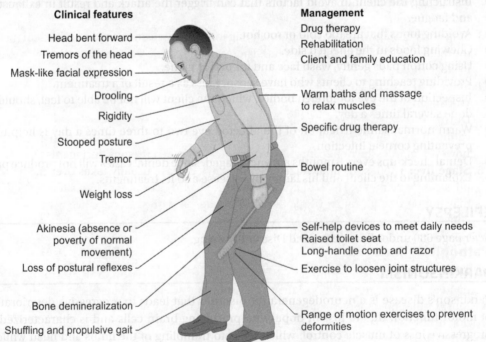

Clinical features

- Head bent forward
- Tremors of the head
- Mask-like facial expression
- Drooling
- Rigidity
- Stooped posture
- Tremor
- Weight loss
- Akinesia (absence or poverty of normal movement)
- Loss of postural reflexes
- Bone demineralization
- Shuffling and propulsive gait

Management

Drug therapy
Rehabilitation
Client and family education

- Warm baths and massage to relax muscles
- Specific drug therapy
- Bowel routine
- Self-help devices to meet daily needs
- Raised toilet seat
- Long-handle comb and razor
- Exercise to loosen joint structures
- Range of motion exercises to prevent deformities

Fig. 19.5: Clinical manifestations.

Secondary Symptoms of Parkinson's Disease

While the main symptoms of Parkinson's disease are movement-related, progressive loss of muscle control and continued damage to the brain can lead to secondary symptoms. Some of the secondary symptoms include:

- Anxiety, insecurity, and stress
- Confusion, memory loss, and dementia
- Constipation
- Depression
- Difficulty swallowing and excessive salivation
- Diminished sense of smell
- Increased sweating
- Male erectile dysfunction
- Skin problems
- Slowed, quieter speech, and monotone voice
- Urinary frequency/urgency
- Slow blinking
- Stooped position

Parkinson's Disease Stages

1. **Stage one:** During this initial phase of the disease, a patient usually experiences mild symptoms. These symptoms may inconvenience the day-to-day tasks the patient would otherwise complete with ease. Typically, these symptoms will include the presence of tremors or experiencing shaking in one of the limbs.
2. **Stage two:** In the second stage of Parkinson's disease, the patient's symptoms are bilateral, affecting both limbs and both sides of the body. The patient usually encounters problems walking or maintaining balance and the inability to complete normal physical tasks becomes more apparent.
3. **Stage three:** Stage three symptoms of Parkinson's disease can be rather severe and include the inability to walk straight or to stand. There is a noticeable slowing of physical movements in stage three.
4. **Stage four:** This stage of the disease is accompanied by severe symptoms of Parkinson's. Walking may still occur, but it is often limited and rigidity and bradykinesia are often visible. During this stage, most patients are unable to complete day-to-day tasks, and usually cannot live on their own. The tremors or shakiness that takes over during the earlier stages, however, may lessen or become nonexistent for unknown reasons during this time.
5. **Stage five:** The last or final stage of Parkinson's disease usually takes over the patients' physical movements. The patient is usually unable to take care of himself or herself and may not be able to stand or walk during this stage. A patient at stage five usually requires constant one-on-one nursing care.

Pathophysiology

- A substance called dopamine acts as a messenger between two brain areas—the substantia nigra and the corpus striatum—to produce smooth, controlled movements.
- Most of the movement-related symptoms of Parkinson's disease are caused by a lack of dopamine due to the loss of dopamine-producing cells in the substantia nigra.
- When the amount of dopamine is too low, communication between the substantia nigra and corpus striatum becomes ineffective, and movement becomes impaired.

- The greater the loss of dopamine, the worse the movement-related symptoms. Other cells in the brain also degenerate to some degree and may contribute to nonmovement related symptoms of Parkinson's disease.

Diagnostic Evaluation

- At least two of the three major symptoms are present (tremor at rest, muscle rigidity, and slowness).
- The onset of symptoms started on one side of the body.
- Symptoms are not due to secondary causes such as medication or strokes in the area controlling movement.
- Symptoms are significantly improved with levodopa.

Management

Medical Management

- Levodopa, Sinemet, levodopa, and carbidopa
- Pramipexole, ropinirole, bromocriptine
- Selegiline, rasagiline
- Amantadine or anticholinergic medications to reduce early or mild tremors
- Entacapone

Other Medications

- Memantine, rivastigmine, galantamine for cognitive difficulties
- Antidepressants for mood disorders
- Gabapentin, duloxetine for pain
- Fludrocortisone, midodrine, Botox, sildenafil for autonomic dysfunction
- Armodafinil, clonazepam, zolpidem for sleep disorders

Nursing Care Plan

Nursing Diagnosis

- Impaired physical mobility related to stiffness and muscle weakness
- Self-care deficits related to neuromuscular weakness, decreased strength, loss of muscle control/coordination
- Impaired bowel elimination: Constipation related to medication and decreased activity
- Imbalanced nutrition: Less than body requirements related to tremor, slowing the process of eating, difficulty chewing and swallowing
- Impaired verbal communication related to the decrease in the volume of speech, delayed speech, inability to move facial muscles
- Ineffective individual coping related to depression and dysfunction due to disease progression
- Knowledge deficit related to information resources inadequate maintenance procedures.

Interventions

- Examining existing mobility and observation of an increase in damage
- Doing exercise program increases muscle strength
- Encouraging bath and massage the muscle
- Helping clients perform range of motion (ROM) exercises, self-care according to tolerance

- Collaborating physiotherapists for physical exercise
- Assessing the ability and the rate of decline and the scale of 0–4 to perform activities of daily living (ADL)
- Avoiding what not to do the client and help if needed
- Collaborative provision of laxatives and consulting a doctor of occupational therapy
- Teaching and supporting the client during the client's activities
- Environmental modifications
- Referring speech therapy
- Teaching clients to use facial exercises and breathing methods to correct the words, volume, and intonation
- Breathing deeply before speaking to increase the volume and number of words in sentences of each breath
- Practicing speaking in short sentences, reading aloud in front of the glass or into a voice recorder (tape recorder) to monitor progress.

MYASTHENIA GRAVIS

Myasthenia gravis is a chronic autoimmune neuromuscular disease characterized by varying degrees of weakness of the skeletal (voluntary) muscles of the body. The name myasthenia gravis, which is Latin and Greek in origin, literally means "grave muscle weakness."

Etiology

1. **Autoimmunity:** In myasthenia gravis, the immune system produces antibodies that block or destroy muscles' receptor sites for a neurotransmitter called acetylcholine. Antibodies may also block the function of a protein called a muscle-**specific receptor tyrosine kinase. This protein is involved in forming the nerve-muscular junction. When antibodies block the function of this protein, it may lead to myasthenia gravis.**
2. **Thymus gland:** Tumors of the thymus (thymomas). Usually, thymomas are not cancerous. In some people, myasthenia gravis is not caused by antibodies blocking acetylcholine or the muscle-specific receptor tyrosine kinase. This type of myasthenia gravis is called antibody-negative myasthenia gravis. Antibodies against another protein, called lipoprotein-related protein 4, may play a part in the development of this condition.
3. **Genetic factors:** Rarely, mothers with myasthenia gravis have children who are born with myasthenia gravis (neonatal myasthenia gravis). If treated promptly, children generally recover within 2 months after birth.

Factors that can worsen myasthenia gravis
- Fatigue
- Illness
- Stress
- Extreme heat
- Some medications—such as beta blockers, quinidine gluconate, quinidine sulfate, quinine (qualaquin), phenytoin (dilantin), certain anesthetics, and some antibiotics.

Signs and Symptoms

1. **Eye muscles:** In more than half the people who develop myasthenia gravis, their first signs and symptoms involve eye problems, such as:
   - Drooping of one or both eyelids (ptosis)
   - Double vision (diplopia), which may be horizontal or vertical, and improves or resolves when one eye is closed.

2. **Face and throat muscles:** In about 15% of people with myasthenia gravis, the first symptoms involve face and throat muscles, which can cause:
   - Altered speaking
   - Difficulty swallowing
   - Problems chewing
   - Limited facial expressions
3. **Neck and limb muscles:** Myasthenia gravis can cause weakness in neck, arms, and legs, but this usually happens along with muscle weakness in other parts of body, such as eyes, face, or throat.

   The disorder usually affects arms more often than legs. However, if it affects legs, patient may waddle while walking. If neck is weak, it may be hard to hold up head.

   Patient may have difficulty in:
   - Breathing
   - Seeing
   - Swallowing
   - Chewing
   - Walking
   - Using arms or hands
   - Holding up head

Diagnostic Evaluation

Diagnosis may be made on the basis of neurological health by testing:
- Reflexes
- Muscle strength
- Muscle tone
- Senses of touch and sight
- Coordination
- Balance
- The key sign that points to the possibility of myasthenia gravis is muscle weakness that improves with rest. Tests to help confirm the diagnosis may include:
  - **Edrophonium test:** Injection of the chemical edrophonium chloride (Tensilon) may result in a sudden, although temporary, improvement in muscle strength. This is an indication that the patient may have myasthenia gravis. Edrophonium chloride blocks an enzyme that breaks down acetylcholine, the chemical that transmits signals from nerve endings to muscle receptor sites.
  - **Ice pack test:** In this test, a bag **filled with ice is placed on eyelid. After 2 minutes, doctor removes the bag and analyzes droopy eyelid for signs of improvement.**
  - **Blood analysis:** A blood test may reveal the presence of abnormal antibodies that disrupt the receptor sites where nerve impulses signal muscles to move.
  - **Repetitive nerve stimulation:** In this nerve conduction study, **electrodes are attached to skin over the muscles to be tested.**
  - **Single-fiber electromyography (EMG):** EMG measures the electrical activity traveling between brain and muscle. It involves inserting a fine wire electrode through skin and into a muscle.
  - **Imaging scans:** CT scan or an MRI to check if there's a tumor or other abnormality in thymus.
  - **Pulmonary function tests:** To evaluate whether condition is affecting breathing.

Management

Medical Management

- **Cholinesterase inhibitors:** Medications such as pyridostigmine enhance communication between nerves and muscles. These medications do not cure the underlying condition, but they may improve muscle contraction and muscle strength.
- **Corticosteroids:** Corticosteroids such as prednisone inhibit the immune system, limiting antibody production.
  Prolonged use of corticosteroids, however, can lead to serious side effects, such as bone thinning, weight gain, diabetes, and increased risk of some infections.
- **Immunosuppressants:** Such as azathioprine, mycophenolate mofetil, cyclosporine, or tacrolimus. Side effects of immunosuppressants can be serious and may include nausea, vomiting, gastrointestinal upset, increased risk of infection, liver damage, and kidney damage.
- **Plasmapheresis:** This procedure uses a filtering process similar to dialysis. Blood is routed through a machine that removes the antibodies that block transmission of signals from nerve endings to muscles' receptor sites.
  Other risks associated with plasmapheresis include a drop in blood pressure, bleeding, heart rhythm problems or muscle cramps. Some people may also develop an allergic reaction to the solutions used to replace the plasma.
- **IV immunoglobulin (IVIg):** This therapy provides normal antibodies, which alters the immune system response. IVIg has a lower risk of side effects than do plasmapheresis and immune-suppressing therapy. Side effects, which usually are mild, may include chills, dizziness, headaches, and fluid retention.

Surgical Management

About 15% of the people with myasthenia gravis have a tumor in their thymus gland, a gland under the breastbone that is involved with the immune system. If patient is having a tumor, called a thymoma, thymectomy may be performed as an open surgery or as a minimally invasive surgery.

Minimally invasive thymectomy may include:
- **Video-assisted thymectomy:** In one form of this surgery, surgeons make a small incision in neck and use a long thin camera (video endoscope) and small instruments to visualize and remove the thymus gland through neck.
- **Robot-assisted thymectomy:** In a robot-assisted thymectomy, surgeons make several small incisions in the side of chest. Surgeons conduct the procedure to remove the thymus gland using a robotic system, which includes a camera arm and mechanical arms.

Nursing Care Plan

Nursing Diagnosis

- Ineffective breathing pattern related to respiratory muscle weakness
- Impaired physical mobility related to weakness of voluntary muscles
- Risk for aspiration related to the weakness of bulbar muscles
- Self-care deficit related to muscle weakness, general fatigue
- Imbalanced nutrition: less than body requirements related to dysphagia, intubation, or muscle paralysis.

Interventions

- Assessing the breathing pattern
- Administering oxygen in case of emergency arrest
- Encouraging deep breathing exercise to strengthen the respiratory muscle tone
- Installing grab bars or railings in places
- Keeping floors clean, and move any loose rugs out of areas
- Using electric appliances and power tools
- Trying to use an electric toothbrush, electric can openers and other electrical tools to perform tasks when possible to save the energy
- Wearing an eye patch if having a double vision, as this can help relieve the problem
- Trying wearing the eye patch while you write, read or watch television. Periodically switch the eye patch to the other eye to help reduce eyestrain
- Encouraging to eat when patient has good muscle strength
- Taking time chewing the food and taking a break between bites of food
- Encouraging to eat small meals several times a day may be easier to handle
- Encouraging to eat mainly soft foods and avoiding foods that require more chewing, such as raw fruits or vegetables

GUILLAIN–BARRÉ SYNDROME OR INFECTIOUS POLYNEURITIS

Guillain–Barré syndrome is an acute condition that involves progressive muscle weakness or paralysis. It is an autoimmune disorder in which the body's immune system attacks its own nervous system, causing inflammation that damages the myelin sheath of the nerve. This damage (demyelination) slows or stops the conduction of impulses through the nerve. The impairment of nerve impulses to the muscles leads to symptoms that may include muscle weakness, paralysis, spasms, numbness, tingling or pins-and-needle sensations, and tenderness.

Etiology

- *Campylobacter jejuni* infection: Campylobacter infection is also the most common risk factor for Guillain–Barré. It is often found in undercooked food, especially poultry.
- Influenza
- Cytomegalovirus
- Epstein–Barr virus infection
- *Mycoplasma pneumonia*
- HIV or AIDS

Pathophysiology

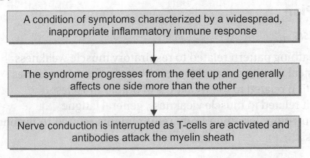

A condition of symptoms characterized by a widespread, inappropriate inflammatory immune response

↓

The syndrome progresses from the feet up and generally affects one side more than the other

↓

Nerve conduction is interrupted as T-cells are activated and antibodies attack the myelin sheath

Contd...

Contd...

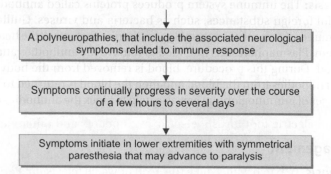

A polyneuropathies, that include the associated neurological symptoms related to immune response

Symptoms continually progress in severity over the course of a few hours to several days

Symptoms initiate in lower extremities with symmetrical paresthesia that may advance to paralysis

Signs and Symptoms

- Loss of tendon reflexes in the arms and legs
- Tingling or numbness (mild loss of sensation)
- Muscle tenderness or pain (may be a cramp-like pain)
- Uncoordinated movement (cannot walk without help)
- Low blood pressure or poor blood pressure control
- Abnormal heart rate
- Blurred vision and double vision
- Clumsiness and falling
- Difficulty moving face muscles
- Muscle contractions
- Feeling the heartbeat

Emergency Symptoms

- Breathing temporarily stops
- Cannot take a deep breath
- Difficulty breathing
- Difficulty swallowing
- Drooling
- Fainting
- Feeling light-headed when standing

Diagnostic Evaluation

- **Spinal tap:** This test is also referred to as a lumbar puncture. A spinal tap involves taking a small amount of fluid from the spine in the lower back. The fluid is then tested to detect protein levels. People with Guillain–Barré typically have higher-than-normal levels of protein in their cerebrospinal fluid (CSF).
- **EMG:** An EMG is a nerve function test. It reads electrical activity from the muscles and helps to learn if the muscle weakness is caused by nerve damage or muscle damage.

Management

- **Physical therapy:** Before recovery, a caregiver may need to manually move the arms and legs. This will help keep the muscles strong and mobile. After recovery, physical therapy will help to strengthen and flex the muscles again. Therapy includes massages, exercises, and frequent position changes.

- **Plasmapheresis:** The immune system produces proteins called antibodies that normally attack harmful foreign substances, such as bacteria and viruses. Guillain–Barré occurs when the immune system mistakenly makes antibodies that attack the healthy nerves of the nervous system. Plasmapheresis is intended to remove the antibodies attacking the nerves from the blood. During this procedure, blood is removed from the body by machine that removes the antibodies from the blood and then the blood is returned to the body.
- **IVIg:** High doses of immunoglobulin can also help to block the antibodies causing Guillain–Barré.

Nursing Management

Nursing Diagnosis

- Ineffective breathing pattern and airway clearance related to respiratory muscle weakness or paralysis, decreased cough reflex, immobilization
- Impaired physical mobility related to paralysis, ataxia
- Risk for impaired skin integrity, pressure sores related to muscle weakness, paralysis, impaired sensation, changes in nutrition, incontinence
- Imbalanced nutrition, less than body requirements related to difficulty chewing, swallowing, fatigue, limb paralysis
- **Impaired elimination:** Constipation, diarrhea, related to inadequate food intake, immobilization
- Impaired verbal communication related to the VII cranial nerve paralysis, tracheostomy
- Ineffective coping related to the patient's disease state

Interventions

- Monitoring respiratory status through vital capacity measurements, rate and depth of respirations, and breath sounds.
- Monitoring level of muscle weakness as it ascends toward respiratory muscles. Watching breathlessness while talking which is a sign of respiratory fatigue.
- Monitoring the patient for signs of impending respiratory failure.
- Monitoring gag reflex and swallowing ability.
- Positioning patient with the head of bed elevated to provide for maximum chest excursion.
- Avoiding giving opioids and sedatives that may depress respirations.
- Positioning patient correctly and provide range-of-motion exercises.
- Providing good body alignment, range-of-motion exercises, and change of position to prevent complications such as contractures, pressure sores, and dependent edema.
- Ensuring adequate nutrition without the risk of aspiration.
- Encouraging physical and occupational therapy exercises to help the patient regain strength during rehabilitation phase.
- Providing assistive devices as needed (cane or wheelchair) to maximize independence and activity.
- If verbal communication is possible, discussing the patient's fears and concerns.
- Providing choices in care to give the patient a sense of control.
- Teaching patient about breathing exercises or using of an incentive spirometer to re-establish normal breathing patterns.
- Instructing patient to wear good supportive and protective shoes while out of bed to prevent injuries due to weakness and paresthesia.
- Instructing patient to check feet routinely for injuries because trauma may go unnoticed due to sensory changes.

- Urging the patient to maintain normal weight because additional weight will further stress monitor function.
- Encouraging scheduled rest periods to avoid fatigue.

MULTIPLE SCLEROSIS

Multiple sclerosis (MS) is a disease in which immune system attacks the protective sheath (myelin) that covers nerves. Myelin damage disrupts communication between brain and the rest of body. Ultimately, the nerves themselves may deteriorate a process that's currently irreversible.

Etiology and Risk Factors

These factors may increase risk of developing MS:
- **Age:** MS can occur at any age, but most commonly affects people between the ages of 15 and 60.
- **Sex:** Women are about twice as likely as men are to develop MS.
- **Family history:** If one of the parents or siblings has had MS, you are at a higher risk of developing the disease.
- **Certain infections:** A variety of viruses have been linked to MS, including Epstein–Barr, the virus that causes infectious mononucleosis.
- **Race:** White people are at the highest risk of developing MS.
- **Climate:** MS is far more common in countries with temperate climates.
- **Certain autoimmune diseases:** Like thyroid disease, type 1 diabetes or inflammatory bowel disease.
- **Smoking:** Smokers who experience an initial event of symptoms that may signal MS are more likely than nonsmokers to develop a second event that confirms relapsing–remitting MS.

Pathophysiology

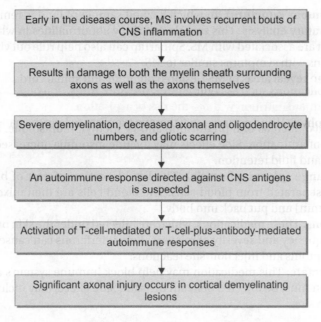

Early in the disease course, MS involves recurrent bouts of CNS inflammation

↓

Results in damage to both the myelin sheath surrounding axons as well as the axons themselves

↓

Severe demyelination, decreased axonal and oligodendrocyte numbers, and gliotic scarring

↓

An autoimmune response directed against CNS antigens is suspected

↓

Activation of T-cell-mediated or T-cell-plus-antibody-mediated autoimmune responses

↓

Significant axonal injury occurs in cortical demyelinating lesions

Signs and Symptoms

Signs and symptoms of MS vary, depending on the location of affected nerve fibers. MS signs and symptoms may include:

- Numbness or weakness in one or more limbs that typically occurs on one side of the body at a time, or the legs and trunk
- Partial or complete loss of vision, usually in one eye at a time, often with pain during eye movement
- Double vision or blurring of vision
- Tingling or pain in parts of body
- Electric-shock sensations that occur with certain neck movements, especially bending the neck forward
- Tremor, lack of coordination, or unsteady gait
- Slurred speech
- Fatigue
- Dizziness
- Problems with bowel and bladder function

Complications

People with MS also may develop:

- Muscle stiffness or spasms
- Paralysis, typically in the legs
- Problems with bladder, bowel, or sexual function
- Mental changes, such as forgetfulness or mood swings
- Depression
- Epilepsy

Diagnostic Evaluation

- **Blood tests:** It helps to rule out infectious or inflammatory diseases with symptoms similar to MS.
- **Spinal tap (lumbar puncture):** In which a small sample of fluid is removed from spinal canal for laboratory analysis. This sample can show abnormalities in white blood cells or antibodies that are associated with MS. Spinal tap can also help rule out viral infections and other conditions with symptoms similar to MS.
- **MRI:** Which can reveal areas of MS (lesions) on brain and spinal cord.

Management

- **Corticosteroids:** Such as oral prednisone and IV methylprednisolone, are prescribed to reduce nerve inflammation. Side effects may include insomnia, increased blood pressure, mood swings, and fluid retention.
- **Plasma exchange (plasmapheresis):** The liquid portion of part of blood (plasma) is removed and separated from blood cells. The blood cells are then mixed with a protein solution (albumin) and put back into body.
- **Beta interferons:** These medications, which are injected under the skin or into muscle, can reduce the frequency and severity of relapses. Beta interferons can cause side effects such as flu-like symptoms and injection-site reactions.
- **Glatiramer acetate:** This medication may help block immune system's attack on myelin. The medication must be injected beneath the skin. Side effects may include skin irritation at the injection site.

- **Dimethyl fumarate:** This twice-daily oral medication can reduce relapses. Side effects may include flushing, diarrhea, nausea, and lowered white blood cell count.
- **Fingolimod:** This once-daily oral medication reduces relapse rate. Heart rate must be monitored for 6 hours after the first dose because heartbeat may be slowed. Other side effects include high blood pressure and blurred vision.
- **Teriflunomide:** This once-daily medication can reduce relapse rate. Teriflunomide can cause liver damage, hair loss, and other side effects. It is also known to be harmful to a developing fetus.
- **Natalizumab:** This medication is designed to block the movement of potentially damaging immune cells from bloodstream to brain and spinal cord. The medication increases the risk of a viral infection of the brain called progressive multifocal leukoencephalopathy. It is generally given to people who have more severe or active MS, or who do not respond to or cannot tolerate other treatments.
- **Mitoxantrone:** This immunosuppressant drug can be harmful to the heart and is associated with development of blood cancers. Mitoxantrone is usually used only to treat advance **multiple sclerosis**.
- **Physical therapy:** A physical or occupational therapist can teach like stretching and strengthening exercises.
- **Muscle relaxants:** Muscle relaxants such as baclofen and tizanidine may help.
- Medications to reduce fatigue.
- **Other medications:** Medications may also be prescribed for depression, pain, and bladder or bowel control problems that are associated with MS.

Nursing Care Plan

Nursing Diagnosis

Fatigue related to decreased energy production, increased energy requirements to perform activities

Interventions

- Noting and accepting presence of fatigue.
- Identifying and reviewing factors affecting ability to be active: Temperature extremes, inadequate food intake, insomnia, use of medications, time of day.
- Scheduling ADLs in the morning if appropriate.
- Determining need for walking aids. Providing braces, walkers, or wheelchairs. Reviewing safety considerations.
- Accepting when patient is unable to do activities.
- Planning care consistent rest periods between activities. Encouraging afternoon nap.
- Assisting with physical therapy. Increasing patient comfort with massages and relaxing baths.
- Stressing the need for stopping exercise or activity just short of fatigue.
- Investigating appropriateness of obtaining a service dog.
- Recommending participation in groups involved in fitness or exercise.

Self-care deficit related to neuromuscular, perceptual impairment

Interventions

- Determining current activity level and physical condition. Assessing degree of functional impairment using 0–4 scale.
- Encouraging patient to perform self-care to the maximum of ability as defined by patient. Do not rush patient.
- Assisting according to degree of disability; allowing as much autonomy as possible.
- Encouraging patient input in planning schedule.

- Allotting sufficient time to perform tasks and displaying patience when movements are slow.
- Encouraging scheduling activities early in the day or during the time when energy level is best.
- Noting presence of fatigue.
- Anticipating hygienic needs and calmly assisting as necessary with care of nails, skin, and hair; mouth care; and shaving.
- Providing assistive devices and aids as indicated: Shower chair, elevated toilet seat with arm supports.
- Providing massage and active or passive ROM exercises on a regular schedule. Encouraging the use of splints or footboards as indicated.
- Repositioning frequently when patient is immobile. Providing skin care to pressure points, such as sacrum, ankles, and elbows. Positioning properly and encourage to sleep prone as tolerated.
- Consulting with physical and occupational therapist.
- Problem-solving ways to meet nutritional and fluid needs.
- Encouraging stretching and toning exercises and the use of medications, cold packs, and splints and maintenance of proper body alignment, when indicated.

Low self-esteem related to change in structure and function
Interventions
- Establishing and maintaining a therapeutic nurse–patient relationship, discussing fears and concerns.
- Acknowledging reality of grieving process related to actual or perceived changes. Helping patient deal realistically with feelings of anger and sadness.
- Supporting the use of defense mechanisms, allowing patient to deal with information in own time and way.
- Noting withdrawn behaviors and the use of denial or over concern with body and disease process.
- Reviewing information about course of disease, possibility of remissions, prognosis.
- Providing accurate verbal and written information about what is happening and discuss with patient.
- Explaining that labile emotions are not unusual. Problem-solving ways to deal with these feelings.
- Assessing interaction between patients. Noting changes in relationship.
- Noting presence of depression and impaired thought processes and expressions of suicidal ideation.
- Discussing the use of medications and adjuncts to improve sexual function.
- Providing open environment for patient to discuss concerns about sexuality, including management of fatigue, spasticity, arousal, and changes in sensation.

Powerlessness and hopelessness related to illness-related regimen, unpredictability of disease
Intervention
- Noting behaviors indicative of powerlessness or hopelessness. Patient may say statements of despair.
- Discussing plans for the future. Suggesting visiting alternative care facilities, taking a look at the possibilities for care as condition changes.
- Encouraging and assist patient to identify activities he or she would like to be involved in within the limits of his or her abilities.
- Acknowledging reality of situation, at the same time expressing hope for patient.
- Assisting patient to identify factors that are under own control. Listing things that can or cannot be controlled.

- Encouraging patient to assume control over as much of own care as possible.
- Discussing needs openly with patient, setting up agreed-on routines for meeting identified needs.
- Incorporating patient's daily routine into home care schedule or hospital stay, as possible.
- Referring vocational rehabilitation as indicated.

Risk for ineffective coping related to physiological changes, psychological conflicts, and impaired judgment

Intervention

- Assessing current functional capacity and limitations; note presence of distorted thinking processes, labile emotions, cognitive dissonance.
- Determining patient's understanding of current situation and previous methods of dealing with life's problems.
- Discussing the ability to make decisions, care for children or dependent adults, handle finances.
- Maintaining an honest, reality-oriented relationship.
- Encouraging verbalization of feelings and fears, accepting what patient says in a nonjudgmental manner.
- Encouraging patient to tape-record important information and listen to the recording periodically.
- Providing clues for orientation: Calendars, clocks, notecards, and organizers.
- Observing nonverbal communication: Posture, eye contact, movements, gestures, and use of touch. Comparing with verbal content and verify meaning with patient as appropriate.

CEREBROVASCULAR ACCIDENT (STROKE)

A cerebrovascular accident is also called a CVA, brain attack, or stroke. It occurs when blood flow to a part of the brain is suddenly stopped and oxygen cannot get to that part. This lack of oxygen may damage or kill the brain cells. Death of a part of the brain may lead to loss of certain body functions controlled by that affected part and it lasts longer than 24 hours.

A transient ischemic attack (TIA)—also called a ministroke—is a brief episode of symptoms similar to those having a stroke. A TIA is caused by a temporary decrease in blood supply to part of brain. It lasts less than 5 minutes.

Etiology and Types

- **Ischemic stroke:** An ischemic stroke occurs when a blood clot blocks a blood vessel, preventing blood and oxygen from getting to a part of the brain. When a clot forms somewhere else in the body and gets lodged in a brain blood vessel, it is called an embolic stroke. When the clot forms in the brain blood vessel, it is called a thrombotic stroke.
- **Hemorrhagic stroke:** A hemorrhagic stroke occurs when a blood vessel ruptures, or hemorrhages, which then prevents blood from getting to part of the brain. The hemorrhage may occur in a blood vessel in the brain, or in the membrane that surrounds the brain. It may be of following type:
  - **Intracerebral hemorrhage:** In an intracerebral hemorrhage, a blood vessel in the brain bursts and spills into the surrounding brain tissue, damaging brain cells. Brain cells beyond the leak are deprived of blood and damaged. High blood pressure, trauma, vascular malformations, use of blood-thinning medications, and other conditions may cause intracerebral hemorrhage.
  - **Subarachnoid hemorrhage:** In a subarachnoid hemorrhage, an artery on or near the surface of brain bursts and spills into the space between the surface of brain and skull. This bleeding is often signaled by a sudden, severe headache. A subarachnoid

hemorrhage is commonly caused by the rupture of an aneurysm, a small sack-shaped or berry-shaped outpouching on an artery in the brain.

Risk Factors

- High blood pressure
- Cigarette smoking or exposure to second-hand smoke
- High cholesterol level
- Diabetes
- Overweight or obese
- Physical inactivity
- Obstructive sleep apnea
- Cardiovascular disease, including heart failure, heart defects, heart infection or abnormal heart rhythm
- Using some birth control pills or hormone therapies that include estrogen
- Heavy drinking
- Using drugs such as cocaine and methamphetamines
- Having regular checkups after being diagnosed with pre-eclampsia
- Personal or family history of stroke, heart attack or TIA
- Being age 55 or older.
- Race: Black has a higher risk of stroke than people of other races.
- Gender: Stroke is more common in women than men, and more deaths from stroke occur in women.

Pathophysiology

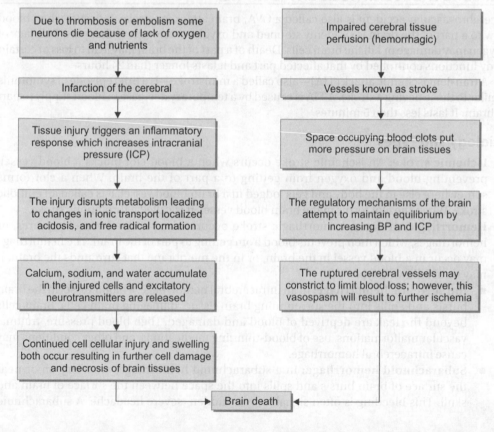

Signs and Symptoms

- Difficulty walking
- Dizziness
- Loss of balance and coordination
- Difficulty speaking or understanding others who are speaking
- Numbness or paralysis in the face, leg, or arm, most likely on just one side of the body
- Blurred or darkened vision
- A sudden headache, especially when accompanied by nausea, vomiting, or dizziness **(Fig. 19.6).**

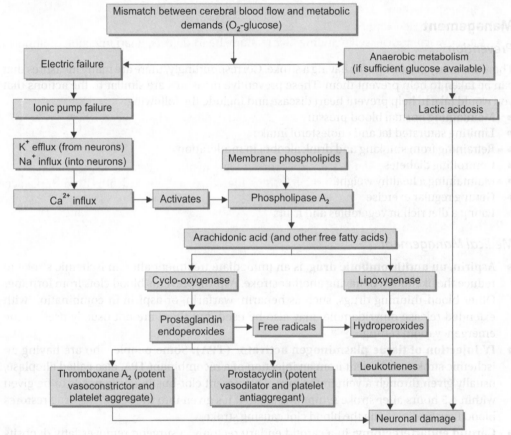

Fig. 19.6: Biochemical changes during stroke.

Diagnostic Evaluation

- Physical examination
- **Personal and family history of heart disease,** TIA or stroke.
- **Blood tests:** To evaluate the clotting time, bleeding time, etc.
- **Computerized tomography scan:** Brain imaging plays a key role in determining a stroke and what type of stroke may be experiencing. A CT scan uses a series of X-rays to create a detailed image of brain. A CT scan can show a brain hemorrhage, tumors, strokes, and other conditions. A dye is injected into blood vessels to view blood vessels in neck and brain in greater detail.
- **Magnetic resonance imaging:** An MRI uses powerful radio waves and magnets to create a detailed view of brain. An MRI can detect brain tissue damaged by an ischemic stroke and brain hemorrhages.

- **Carotid ultrasound:** In this test, sound waves create detailed images of the inside of the carotid arteries in neck. This test shows buildup of fatty deposits (plaques) and blood flow in carotid arteries.
- **Cerebral angiogram:** In this test, a thin, flexible tube (catheter) is inserted through a small incision, usually in groin, and guides it through major arteries and into carotid or vertebral artery. A dye is injected into blood vessels to make them visible under X-ray imaging. This procedure gives a detailed view of arteries in brain and neck.
- **Echocardiogram:** This imaging technique uses sound waves to create a picture of heart. It can help to find the source of blood clots.

Management

Prevention

There are many risk factors for having a stroke. Correspondingly, there are many measures that can be taken to help prevent them. These preventive measures are similar to the actions that you would take to help prevent heart disease and include the following:
- Maintaining normal blood pressure
- Limiting saturated fat and cholesterol intake
- Refraining from smoking and drink alcohol in moderation
- Controlling diabetes
- Maintaining a healthy weight
- Getting regular exercise
- Eating a diet rich in vegetables and fruits

Medical Management

- **Aspirin, an antithrombotic drug**, is an immediate treatment after an ischemic stroke to reduce the likelihood of having another stroke. Aspirin prevents blood clots from forming. Other blood-thinning drugs, such as heparin, warfarin, or aspirin in combination with extended release dipyridamole, may also be used, but these are not usually used in the emergency room setting.
- **IV injection of tissue plasminogen activator (TPA):** Some people who are having an ischemic stroke can benefit from an injection of a recombinant TPA, also called alteplase, usually given through a vein in the arm. This potent clot-busting drug needs to be given within 4.5 hours after stroke symptoms begin if it's given into the vein. This drug restores blood flow by dissolving the blood clot causing stroke.
- **Carotid endarterectomy:** In a carotid endarterectomy, a surgeon removes fatty deposits (plaques) from carotid arteries. In this procedure, a small incision along the front of neck opens carotid artery and removes fatty deposits that block the carotid artery.
- **Angioplasty and stents:** In an angioplasty, a surgeon inserts a catheter with a mesh tube and balloon on the tip into an artery in groin and guides it to the blocked carotid artery in neck. Surgeon inflates the balloon in the narrowed artery and inserts a mesh tube into the opening to keep artery from becoming narrowed after the procedure.
- **Surgical clipping:** A surgeon places a tiny clamp at the base of the aneurysm, to stop blood flow to it. This can keep the aneurysm from bursting.
- **Coiling (endovascular embolization):** In this procedure, a surgeon inserts a catheter into an artery in groin and guides it to brain using X-ray imaging. Then guides tiny detachable coils into the aneurysm (aneurysm coiling). The coils fill the aneurysm, which blocks blood flow into the aneurysm and causes the blood to clot.

Nursing Care Plan

Nursing Diagnosis

Ineffective cerebral tissue perfusion related to interruption of blood flow

Interventions

- Determining factors related to individual situation, cause for coma, decreased cerebral perfusion and potential for increased ICP.
- Monitoring and documenting neurological status frequently and compare with baseline.
- Monitoring vital signs, that is, hypertension/hypotension, comparing BP readings in both arms, heart rate, and rhythm; auscultating for murmurs, respirations; noting patterns and rhythm, e.g., periods of apnea after hyperventilation, Cheyne–Stokes respiration.
- Evaluating pupils, noting size, shape, equality, light reactivity.
- Documenting changes in vision, e.g., reports of blurred vision, alterations in visual field and perception.
- Assessing higher functions, including speech, if patient is alert.
- Positioning with head slightly elevated and in neutral position.
- Maintaining bedrest, providing a quiet environment, and restricting visitors as indicated. Providing rest periods between care activities, limiting duration of procedures.
- Preventing straining at stool, holding breath.
- Assessing for nuchal rigidity, twitching, increased restlessness, irritability, onset of seizure activity.
- Administering supplemental oxygen as indicated.
- Administering medications as indicated: Alteplase, anticoagulants, (e.g., warfarin sodium, low-molecular-weight heparin, antiplatelet agents, aspirin, dipyridamole, ticlopidine). Antihypertensives, peripheral vasodilators, (e.g., cyclandelate, papaverine, isoxsuprine), steroids, (e.g., dexamethasone).
- Preparing for surgery, as appropriate, (e.g., endarterectomy, microvascular bypass, cerebral angioplasty).
- Monitoring laboratory studies as indicated, [e.g., prothrombin time (PT), activated partial thromboplastin time (aPTT), Dilantin level].

Impaired physical mobility related to neuromuscular abnormality

Interventions

- Assessing functional ability of impairment initially and on a regular basis.
- Changing positions at least every 2 hours (supine, side lying) and possibly more often if placed on affected side.
- Positioning in prone position once or twice a day if patient can tolerate.
- Propping extremities in functional position, using footboard during the period of flaccid paralysis. Maintaining neutral position of head.
- Using arm sling when patient is in upright position, as indicated.
- Evaluating the use and need for positional aids and splints during spastic paralysis, placing pillow under axillae to abduct arm, elevating arm and hand.
- Observing affected side for color, edema, or other signs of compromised circulation.
- Inspecting skin regularly, particularly over bony prominences. Gently massaging any reddened areas and provide aids such as sheepskin pads as necessary.
- It is necessary to begin active/passive range of motion exercise to all extremities.
- Assisting to develop sitting balance (e.g., raise head of bed, assist to sit on edge of bed, having patient use the strong arm to support body weight and strong leg to move affected leg, increase sitting time) and standing balance (e.g., put flat walking shoes on patient, support patient's lower back with hands while positioning own knees outside patient's knees, assist in using parallel bars/walkers).

- Getting patient up in chair as soon as vital signs are stable, except following the cerebral hemorrhage.
- Padding chair seat with foam or water-filled cushion and assist patient to shift weight at frequent intervals.
- Providing egg-crate mattress, water bed, flotation device, or specialized beds (e.g., kinetic), as indicated.

Disturbed sensory perceptions related to disturbed sensory reception and neuromuscular dysfunction

Interventions

- Observing behavioral responses, (e.g., hostility, crying, inappropriate affect, agitation, hallucination).
- Eliminating extraneous noise and stimuli as necessary.
- Speaking in calm, quiet voice, using short sentences. Maintaining eye contact.
- Reorienting patient frequently to environment, staff, and procedures.
- Evaluating for visual deficits. Noting loss of visual field, changes in depth perception (horizontal/vertical planes), and presence of diplopia.
- Approaching patient from visually intact side. Leaving light on, position objects to take advantage of intact visual fields. Patching affected eye if indicated.
- Assessing sensory awareness, (e.g., differentiation of hot/cold, dull/sharp, position of body parts/muscle, joint sense).
- Stimulating sense of touch, (e.g., giving patient objects to touch, grasp).
- Protecting from temperature extremes, assess environment for hazards. Recommending testing warm water with unaffected hand.

Ineffective coping related to situational crisis and cognitive–perceptual changes

Interventions

- Assessing the extent of altered perception and related degree of disability. Determining functional independence measure score.
- Identifying meaning of the loss, dysfunction, and change to patient. Noting ability to understand events, provide realistic appraisal of situation.
- Determining outside stressors, (e.g., family, work, social, future nursing/healthcare needs).
- Encouraging patient to express feelings, including hostility or anger, denial, depression, sense of disconnectedness.
- Noting whether patient refers to the affected side as "it" or denies affected side and says it is "dead."
- Identifying previous methods of dealing with life problems. Determining presence and quality of support systems.
- Emphasizing small gains either in recovery of function or independence.
- Supporting behaviors and efforts such as increased interest, participation in rehabilitation activities.
- Monitoring for sleep disturbance, increased difficulty concentrating, and statements of inability to cope, lethargy, and withdrawal.
- Referring neuropsychological evaluation and/or counseling if indicated.

Self-care deficit related to neuromuscular impairment and decreases strength and endurance

Interventions

- Assessing abilities and level of deficit (0–4 scale) for performing ADLs.
- Avoiding doing things for patient that patient can do for self but providing assistance as necessary.
- Be aware of impulsive behavior and actions suggestive of impaired judgment.
- Maintaining a supportive, firm attitude. Allowing patient sufficient time to accomplish tasks.
- Providing positive feedback for efforts and accomplishments.

- Creating a plan for visual deficits that are present, (e.g., place food and utensils on the tray related to patient's unaffected side, situating the bed so that patient's unaffected side is facing the room with the affected side to the wall, positioning furniture against wall and out of travel path).
- Providing self-help devices, (e.g., button/zipper hook, knife–fork combinations, long-handled brushes, extensions for picking things up from floor, toilet riser, leg bag for catheter, shower chair).
- Assisting and encourage good grooming and makeup habits.
- Encouraging family member to allow patient to do as much as possible for self.
- Assessing patient's ability to communicate the need to void and ability to use urinal, bedpan. Taking patient to the bathroom at frequent and periodic intervals for voiding if appropriate.
- Identifying previous bowel habits and re-establish normal regimen. Increasing bulk in diet, encourage fluid intake, increased activity.

Risk for impaired swallowing related to neuromuscular dysfunction
Intervention

- Reviewing individual pathology and ability to swallow, noting extent of paralysis, clarity of speech, facial, tongue involvement, ability to protect airway and episodes of coughing or choking, presence of adventitious breath sounds, amount and character of oral secretions.
- Having suction equipment available at bedside, especially during early feeding efforts.
- Promoting effective swallowing, (e.g., schedule activities, medications to provide a minimum of 30 minutes rest before eating, providing pleasant environment free of distractions, assisting patient with head control and support, and positioning based on specific dysfunction).
- Placing patient in upright position during and after feeding as appropriate.
- Providing oral care based on individual need prior to meal.
- Season food with herbs, spices, lemon juice, etc., according to patient's preference, within dietary restrictions.
- Placing food of appropriate consistency in unaffected side of mouth.
- Touching parts of the cheek with tongue blade and apply ice to weak tongue.
- Feeding slowly, allowing 30–45 minutes for meals.
- Offering solid foods and liquids at different times.
- Maintaining upright position for 45–60 minutes after eating.
- Maintaining accurate intake output, record calorie count.
- Encouraging participation in exercise.
- Administering IV fluids and or tube feedings.
- Coordinating multidisciplinary approach to develop treatment plan that meets individual needs.

Knowledge deficit related to lack of exposure and cognitive limitation
Interventions

- Evaluating type and degree of sensory–perceptual involvement.
- Including family in discussions and teaching.
- Discussing specific pathology and individual potentials.
- Identifying signs and symptoms requiring further follow-up, (e.g., changes or decline in visual, motor, sensory functions, alteration in mentation or behavioral responses, severe headache).
- Reviewing current restrictions or limitations and discuss planned resumption of activities (including sexual relations).
- Providing written instructions and schedules for activity, medication, important facts.
- Encouraging patient to refer to list communications or notes instead of depending on memory.
- Discussing plans for meeting self-care needs.
- Referring discharge planner, home care supervisor, visiting nurse.

- Suggesting patient reduce or limit environmental stimuli, especially during cognitive activities.
- Recommending patient seeks assistance in problem-solving process and validate decisions, as indicated.
- Reviewing importance of balanced diet, low in cholesterol and sodium if indicated. Discussing the role of vitamins and other supplements.
- Referring to reinforce importance of follow-up care by rehabilitation team, e.g., physical, occupational, speech, vocational therapists.

MENINGITIS

Meningitis is an inflammation of the meninges the layer that surrounds the brain and spinal cord and characterized by headache, fever, a stiff neck, etc.

Etiology and Types

1. **Bacterial meningitis:** Bacteria such as *Streptococcus pneumonia*, *Neisseria meningitidis*, **and** *Haemophilus influenzae* enter the bloodstream and cause acute bacterial meningitis.
2. **Viral meningitis:** Viruses such as herpes simplex virus, HIV, and mumps also can cause viral meningitis.
3. **Chronic meningitis:** Chronic meningitis develops over 2 weeks or more and characterized by headache, fever, vomiting, and mental cloudiness.

Pathophysiology

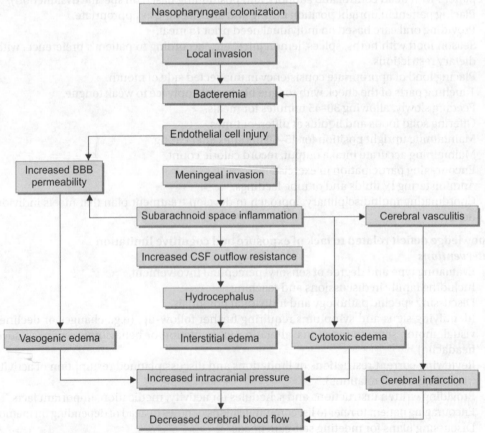

(BBB: blood-brain barrier; CF: cerebrospinal fluid)

Clinical Manifestations

- Sudden high fever
- Stiff neck
- Severe headache
- Headache with nausea or vomiting
- Confusion or difficulty concentrating
- Seizures
- Sleepiness or difficulty waking
- Sensitivity to light
- No appetite or thirst.

Kernig's sign: Patient is kept in supine position, hip, and knee are flexed to a right angle, and then knee is slowly extended by the examiner. The appearance of resistance or pain during extension of the patient's knees beyond 135° constitutes a positive Kernig's sign.

Brudzinski sign: The examiner keeps one hand behind the patient's head and the other on chest in order to prevent the patient from rising. Reflex flexion of the patient's hips and knees after passive flexion of the neck constitutes a positive Brudzinski sign **(Figs. 19.7A and B)**.

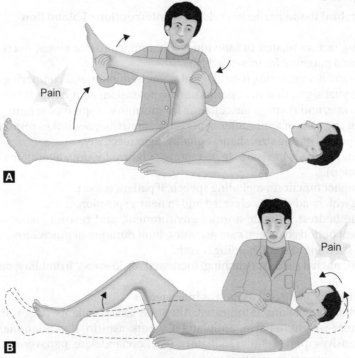

Figs. 19.7A and B: (A) Kernig's sign; (B) Brudzinski's sign.

Complications

Meningitis complications can be severe like

- Hearing loss
- Memory difficulty
- Learning disabilities
- Brain damage

- Gait problems
- Seizures
- Kidney failure
- Shock
- Death

Management

Age	Antibiotic
0–4 weeks	Ampicillin plus either cefotaxime or an aminoglycoside
1 month–50 years	Vancomycin plus cefotaxime or ceftriaxone
>50 years	Vancomycin plus ampicillin plus ceftriaxone or cefotaxime plus vancomycin
Impaired cellular immunity	Vancomycin plus ampicillin plus either cefepime or meropenem
Recurrent meningitis	Vancomycin plus cefotaxime
Basilar skull fracture	Vancomycin plus cefotaxime
Head trauma, neurosurgery, or CSF shunt	Vancomycin plus ceftazidime, cefepime, or meropenem

Nursing Care Plan

Nursing Diagnosis

Ineffective cerebral tissue perfusion related to interruption of blood flow

Interventions

- Determining factors related to individual situation, cause for coma, decreased cerebral perfusion, and potential for increased ICP.
- Monitoring and documenting neurological status frequently and comparing with baseline.
- Monitoring vital signs, that is, hypertension/hypotension; comparing BP readings in both arms, heart rate, and rhythm; auscultating for murmurs, respirations; noting patterns and rhythm, (e.g., periods of apnea after hyperventilation, Cheyne–Stokes respiration).
- Evaluating pupils, noting size, shape, equality, light reactivity.
- Documenting changes in vision, (e.g., reports of blurred vision, alterations in visual field and perception).
- Assessing higher functions, including speech, if patient is alert.
- Positioning with head slightly elevated and in neutral position.
- Maintaining bedrest, provide a quiet environment, and restrict visitors as indicated. Providing rest periods between care activities, limit duration of procedures.
- Preventing straining at stool, holding breath.
- Assessing for nuchal rigidity, twitching, increased restlessness, irritability, onset of seizure activity.
- Administering supplemental oxygen as indicated.
- Administering medications as indicated: Alteplase, anticoagulants, (e.g., warfarin sodium, low-molecular-weight heparin, antiplatelet agents, aspirin, dipyridamole, ticlopidine). Antihypertensives, peripheral vasodilators, (e.g., cyclandelate, papaverine, isoxsuprine), steroids, (e.g., dexamethasone).
- Preparing for surgery, as appropriate, (e.g., endarterectomy, microvascular bypass, cerebral angioplasty).
- Monitoring laboratory studies as indicated, (e.g., PT, aPTT, Dilantin level).

Impaired physical mobility related to neuromuscular abnormality

Interventions

- Assessing functional ability of impairment initially and on a regular basis.
- Changing positions at least every 2 hours (supine, side lying) and possibly more often if placed on affected side.

- Positioning in prone position once or twice a day if patient can tolerate.
- Propping extremities in functional position, using footboard during the period of flaccid paralysis. Maintaining neutral position of head.
- Using arm sling when patient is in upright position, as indicated.
- Evaluating use and need for positional aids and splints during spastic paralysis, placing pillow under axillae to abduct arm, elevating arm and hand.
- Observing affected side for color, edema, or other signs of compromised circulation.
- Inspecting skin regularly, particularly over bony prominences. Gently massaging any reddened areas and provide aids such as sheepskin pads as necessary.
- It is necessary to begin active/passive range of motion exercise to all extremities.
- Assisting to develop sitting balance (e.g., raise head of bed, assist to sit on edge of bed, having patient use the strong arm to support body weight and strong leg to move affected leg, increase sitting time) and standing balance (e.g., put flat walking shoes on patient, support patient's lower back with hands while positioning own knees outside patient's knees, assist in using parallel bars/walkers).
- Getting patient up in chair as soon as vital signs are stable, except following cerebral hemorrhage.
- Padding chair seat with foam or water-filled cushion, and assisting patient to shift weight at frequent intervals.
- Providing egg-crate mattress, water bed, flotation device, or specialized beds (e.g., kinetic), as indicated.

Disturbed sensory perceptions related to disturbed sensory reception and neuromuscular dysfunction
Interventions
- Observing behavioral responses, (e.g., hostility, crying, inappropriate affect, agitation, hallucination).
- Eliminating extraneous noise and stimuli as necessary.
- Speaking in calm, quiet voice, using short sentences. Maintaining eye contact.
- Reorienting patient frequently to environment, staff, and procedures.
- Evaluating for visual deficits. Noting loss of visual field, changes in depth perception (horizontal/vertical planes), and presence of diplopia.
- Approaching patient from visually intact side. Leaving light on, position objects to take advantage of intact visual fields. Patching affected eye if indicated.
- Assessing sensory awareness, (e.g., differentiation of hot/cold, dull/sharp, position of body parts/muscle, joint sense).
- Stimulating sense of touch, (e.g., give patient objects to touch, grasp).
- Protecting from temperature extremes, assess environment for hazards. Recommending testing warm water with unaffected hand.

Ineffective coping related to situational crisis and cognitive–perceptual changes
Interventions
- Assessing the extent of altered perception and related degree of disability. Determining functional independence measure score.
- Identifying meaning of the loss, dysfunction and change to patient. Noting ability to understand events, provide realistic appraisal of situation.
- Determining outside stressors, (e.g., family, work, social, future nursing/health-care needs).
- Encouraging patient to express feelings, including hostility or anger, denial, depression, sense of disconnectedness.

- Noting whether patient refers to the affected side as "it" or denies affected side and says it is "dead."
- Identifying previous methods of dealing with life problems. Determining presence and quality of support systems.
- Emphasizing small gains either in recovery of function or independence.
- Supporting behaviors and efforts such as increased interest, participation in rehabilitation activities.
- Monitoring for sleep disturbance, increased difficulty concentrating, and statements of inability to cope, lethargy, and withdrawal.
- Referring neuropsychological evaluation and/or counseling if indicated.

ENCEPHALITIS

Encephalitis is an inflammation of the brain tissue. It is caused by viral or bacterial infections.
- **Primary encephalitis:** It occurs when a virus directly infects the brain and spinal cord.
- **Secondary encephalitis:** It occurs when an infection enters in brain through some other organ or tissue.

Etiology

Viral infections such as mumps, Epstein–Barr virus, HIV, cytomegalovirus.

Pathophysiology

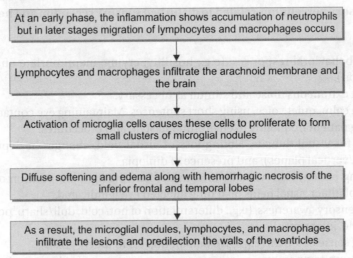

At an early phase, the inflammation shows accumulation of neutrophils but in later stages migration of lymphocytes and macrophages occurs

↓

Lymphocytes and macrophages infiltrate the arachnoid membrane and the brain

↓

Activation of microglia cells causes these cells to proliferate to form small clusters of microglial nodules

↓

Diffuse softening and edema along with hemorrhagic necrosis of the inferior frontal and temporal lobes

↓

As a result, the microglial nodules, lymphocytes, and macrophages infiltrate the lesions and predilection the walls of the ventricles

Clinical Manifestations

- Fever
- Headache
- Vomiting
- Stiffness of neck
- Lethargy
- Confusion
- Drowsiness
- Hallucinations
- Slow gait

- Coma
- Seizures
- Photophobia

Diagnostic Evaluation

- **Spinal tap or lumbar puncture:** In this test, the CSF is tested for viral or bacterial infection.
- **Brain imaging with CT scan or MRI:** These tests detect changes in brain structure. They can rule out other possible explanations for symptoms, such as a tumor or stroke.
- **Electroencephalograph (EEG):** An EEG uses electrodes (small metal disks with wires) attached to the scalp to record brain activity.
- **Blood tests:** A blood test can reveal signs of a viral infection.
- **Brain biopsy:** It includes removal of small samples of brain tissue to test for infection. This procedure is rarely performed because there's a high risk of complications.

Management

- Bed rest
- Nonsteroidal anti-inflammatory drugs (NSAIDs)
- Corticosteroids
- Mechanical ventilation
- Lukewarm sponge baths
- Anticonvulsants
- Sedatives (for restlessness, aggressiveness, and irritability)
- IV fluids

Complications

- Amnesia
- Personality changes
- Epilepsy
- Fatigue
- Physical weakness
- Intellectual disability
- Lack of muscle coordination
- Vision problems
- Hearing problems
- Speaking issues
- Coma
- Death

Nursing Management

Nursing Diagnosis

Ineffective cerebral tissue perfusion related to interruption of blood flow
Interventions
- Determining factors related to individual situation, cause for coma, decreased cerebral perfusion and potential for increased ICP.
- Monitoring and documenting neurological status frequently and comparing with baseline.
- Monitoring vital signs, that is, hypertension/hypotension; comparing BP readings in both arms, heart rate and rhythm, auscultating for murmurs, respirations; noting patterns and rhythm, (e.g., periods of apnea after hyperventilation, Cheyne–Stokes respiration).

- Evaluating pupils, noting size, shape, equality, light reactivity.
- Documenting changes in vision, (e.g., reports of blurred vision, alterations in visual field and perception).
- Assessing higher functions, including speech, if patient is alert.
- Positioning with head slightly elevated and in neutral position.
- Maintaining bedrest, providing a quiet environment, and restricting visitors as indicated. Providing rest periods between care activities, limiting duration of procedures.
- Preventing straining at stool, holding breath.
- Assessing for nuchal rigidity, twitching, increased restlessness, irritability, onset of seizure activity.
- Administering supplemental oxygen as indicated.
- Administering medications as indicated: Alteplase, anticoagulants, (e.g., warfarin sodium, low-molecular-weight heparin, antiplatelet agents, aspirin, dipyridamole, ticlopidine). Antihypertensives, peripheral vasodilators, (e.g., cyclandelate, papaverine, isoxsuprine), steroids, (e.g., dexamethasone).
- Preparing for surgery, as appropriate, e.g., endarterectomy, microvascular bypass, cerebral angioplasty.
- Monitoring laboratory studies as indicated, (e.g., PT, aPTT, Dilantin level).

Impaired physical mobility related to neuromuscular abnormality
Interventions
- Assessing functional ability of impairment initially and on a regular basis.
- Changing positions at least every 2 hours (supine, side lying) and possibly more often if placed on affected side.
- Positioning in prone position once or twice a day if patient can tolerate.
- Propping extremities in functional position, using footboard during the period of flaccid paralysis. Maintaining neutral position of head.
- Using arm sling when patient is in upright position, as indicated.
- Evaluating use and need for positional aids and splints during spastic paralysis, placing pillow under axillae to abduct arm, elevating arm and hand.
- Observing affected side for color, edema, or other signs of compromised circulation.
- Inspecting skin regularly, particularly over bony prominences. Gently massage any reddened areas and provide aids such as sheepskin pads as necessary.
- It is necessary to begin active/passive range of motion exercise to all extremities.
- Assisting to develop sitting balance (e.g., raising head of bed, assisting to sit on edge of bed, having patient use the strong arm to support body weight and strong leg to move affected leg, increase sitting time) and standing balance (e.g., putting flat walking shoes on patient, supporting patient's lower back with hands while positioning own knees outside patient's knees, assisting in using parallel bars/walkers).
- Getting patient up in chair as soon as vital signs are stable, except following cerebral hemorrhage.
- Padding chair seat with foam or water-filled cushion and assisting patient to shift weight at frequent intervals.
- Providing egg-crate mattress, water bed, flotation device, or specialized beds (e.g., kinetic), as indicated.

Disturbed sensory perceptions related to disturbed sensory reception and neuromuscular dysfunction
Interventions
- Observing behavioral responses, (e.g., hostility, crying, inappropriate affect, agitation, hallucination).

- Eliminating extraneous noise and stimuli as necessary.
- Speaking in calm, quiet voice, using short sentences. Maintaining eye contact.
- Reorienting patient frequently to environment, staff, and procedures.
- Evaluating for visual deficits. Noting loss of visual field, changes in depth perception (horizontal/vertical planes), and presence of diplopia.
- Approaching patient from visually intact side. Leaving light on, position objects to take advantage of intact visual fields. Patching affected eye if indicated.
- Assessing sensory awareness, (e.g., differentiation of hot/cold, dull/sharp, position of body parts/muscle, joint sense).
- Stimulating sense of touch, (e.g., giving patient objects to touch, grasp).
- Protecting from temperature extremes, assessing environment for hazards. Recommending testing warm water with unaffected hand.

Ineffective coping related to situational crisis and cognitive–perceptual changes
Interventions
- Assessing the extent of altered perception and related degree of disability. Determining functional independence measure score.
- Identifying meaning of the loss, dysfunction and change to patient. Noting ability to understand events, provide realistic appraisal of situation.
- Determining outside stressors, (e.g., family, work, social, future nursing/health-care needs).
- Encouraging patient to express feelings, including hostility or anger, denial, depression, sense of disconnectedness.
- Noting whether patient refers to the affected side as "it" or denies affected side and says it is "dead."
- Identifying previous methods of dealing with life problems. Determining the presence and quality of support systems.
- Emphasizing small gains either in recovery of function or independence.
- Supporting behaviors and efforts such as increased interest, participation in rehabilitation activities.
- Monitoring for sleep disturbance, increased difficulty concentrating, and statements of inability to cope, lethargy, and withdrawal.
- Referring neuropsychological evaluation and/or counseling if indicated.

HYDROCEPHALUS

Hydrocephalus is a congenital condition in which the CSF builds up in the skull and makes the skull swell and large. This condition can result in brain damage, developmental delay, physical, and intellectual impairments.

Etiology
- Blockage in the flow of CSF
- Poor absorption of CSF
- Excess production of CSF
- Birth defect to spinal cord
- Genetic abnormality
- Maternal infections during pregnancy
- Meningitis
- Bleeding disorder in the brain during or shortly after delivery
- Injuries during or after delivery
- Head trauma
- CNS tumors

Clinical Manifestations

- Bulging fontanel
- Increasing head circumference
- Fixed and downward
- Seizures
- Extreme fussiness
- Vomiting
- Excessive sleepiness
- Poor feeding
- Low muscle tone and strength
- High-pitched cries
- Changes in personality
- Changes in facial gesture
- Crossed eyes
- Delayed growth
- Trouble eating
- Poor coordination
- Loss of bladder control

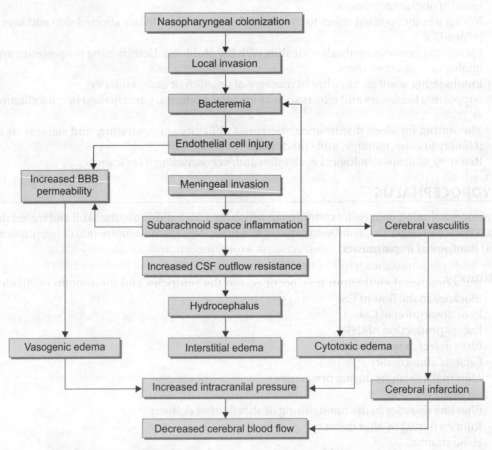

(BBB: blood-brain barrier; CF: cerebrospinal fluid)

Pathophysiology of Hydrocephalus

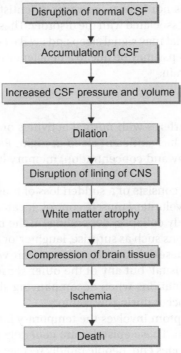

Disruption of normal CSF

↓

Accumulation of CSF

↓

Increased CSF pressure and volume

↓

Dilation

↓

Disruption of lining of CNS

↓

White matter atrophy

↓

Compression of brain tissue

↓

Ischemia

↓

Death

(CSF: cerebrospinal fluid; CNS: central nervous system)

Histopathology

1. **Obstruction of the basal cisterns:** There is inability of CSF to reach the arachnoid villi with a delay in emptying from the ventricles.
2. **Occlusion of the arachnoid villi:** Obstruction of the terminal CSF pathways results in a failure of the absorption of CSF into the venous sinuses.
3. **Increased sagittal sinus pressure:** Increased pressure in the venous sinuses and superior sagittal sinus, effects the ICP and CSF absorption. The pressure in the intracranial compartment rises up to 5 mm Hg or above the sinuses pressure; as a result, no absorption of CSF will occur.
4. **Atrophy of white matter:** Destruction of axons, myelin, and chronic astrogliosis.
5. **Multiple anomalies within ventricles:** Fibrosis of the choroid plexuses and stretching of the ependymal epithelium may occur within the ventricles and the septum pellucidum becomes fenestrated.
6. **Anomalies in surrounding brain:** Cerebral edema builds up in the brain and these can results in thinning and elongation of the interhemispheric commissures.

NARCOLEPSY

Narcolepsy is a neurological disorder that affects the control of sleep and wakefulness. People with narcolepsy experience excessive daytime sleepiness (EDS) and intermittent, uncontrollable episodes of falling asleep during the daytime. These sudden sleep attacks may occur during any type of activity at any time of the day.

Etiology

- The cause of narcolepsy is not known; however, scientists have made progress toward identifying genes strongly associated with the disorder. These genes control the production of chemicals in the brain that may signal sleep and awake cycles.
- Some experts think narcolepsy may be due to a deficiency in the production of a chemical called hypocretin by the brain.

Signs and Symptoms

- **EDS:** In general, EDS interferes with normal activities on a daily basis, whether or not a person with narcolepsy has sufficient sleep at night. People with EDS report mental cloudiness, a lack of energy and concentration, memory lapses, a depressed mood, and extreme exhaustion.
- **Cataplexy:** This symptom consists of a sudden loss of muscle tone that leads to feelings of weakness and a loss of voluntary muscle control. It can cause symptoms ranging from slurred speech to total body collapse, depending on the muscles involved, and is often triggered by intense emotions such as surprise, laughter, or anger.
- **Hallucinations:** Usually, these delusional experiences are vivid and frequently frightening. The content is primarily visual, but any of the other senses can be involved. These are called hypnagogic hallucinations when accompanying sleep onset and hypnopompic hallucinations when they occur during awakening.
- **Sleep paralysis:** This symptom involves the temporary inability to move or speak while falling asleep or waking up. These episodes are generally brief, lasting a few seconds to several minutes. After episodes end, people rapidly recover their full capacity to move and speak.
- **Microsleep** is a very brief sleep episode during which the patient continues to function (talk, put things away, etc.) and then awaken with no memory of the activities.

Diagnostic Evaluation

A physical examination and exhaustive medical history are essential for proper diagnosis of narcolepsy. Two tests that are considered essential in confirming a diagnosis of narcolepsy are the polysomnogram (PSG) and the multiple sleep latency test (MSLT).

- **Nocturnal PSG:** This overnight test measures the electrical activity of brain and heart, and the movement of muscles and eyes.
- **MSLT:** This test measures how long it takes to fall asleep during the day.
- **Spinal fluid analysis:** The lack of hypocretin in the CSF may be a marker for narcolepsy. Examining spinal fluid is a new diagnostic test for narcolepsy.

The Epworth Sleepiness Scale measures daytime sleepiness. Using the following scale to choose the most appropriate number for each situation:

0 = would *never* sleep
1 = *slight* chance of dozing or sleeping
2 = *moderate* chance of dozing or sleeping
3 = *high* chance of dozing or sleeping

Situation	Chance of dozing or sleeping
Sitting and reading	–
Watching TV	–
Sitting inactive in a public place	–

Contd...

Contd...

Situation	Chance of dozing or sleeping
Being a passenger in a motor vehicle for an hour or more	–
Lying down in the afternoon	–
Sitting and talking to someone	–
Sitting quietly after lunch (no alcohol)	–
Stopped for a few minutes in traffic while driving	–
Total score (add the scores up)	–

A total score of 10 or more is considered sleepy. A score of 18 or more is very sleepy.

Management

- **Scheduling sleep periods:** Taking a few brief, scheduled naps during the daytime (10–15 minutes each). Trying to get a good night's sleep during the same hours each night. Planned naps can prevent unplanned lapses into sleep.
- **Avoiding caffeine, alcohol, and nicotine:** These substances interfere with sleep.
- **Avoiding over-the-counter drugs that cause drowsiness:** Some allergy and cold medications can cause drowsiness, so should be avoided.
- **Involving employers, coworkers, and friends:** Alert others so that they can help when needed.
- **Carrying a tape recorder:** Record important conversations and meetings, in case you fall asleep.
- **Breaking up of larger tasks into small pieces:** Focus on one small thing at a time.
- **Exercise on a regular basis:** Exercise can make you feel more awake during the day and stimulate sleep at night. For example, take several short walks during the day.
- **Avoiding activities that would be dangerous if you had a sudden sleep attack:** If possible, do not drive, climb ladders, or use dangerous machinery. Taking a nap before driving may help you to manage any possible sleepiness.
- **Wearing a medical alert bracelet or necklace:** A bracelet or necklace will alert others if you suddenly fall asleep or become unable to move or speak.
- **Eating a healthy diet:** Aim for a diet rich in whole grains, vegetables, fruits, low-fat dairy, and lean sources of protein. Eating light or vegetarian meals during the day and avoid heavy meals before important activities.
- **Relaxing and managing emotions:** Narcolepsy symptoms can be triggered by intense emotions, so you may benefit from practicing relaxation techniques, such as breathing exercises, yoga, or massage.

Medical Management

Common medications use d to treat narcolepsy symptoms include:

- **Stimulants:** Stimulants are the mainstay of drug treatment for narcolepsy. These include modafinil, a stimulant used during the day to promote wakefulness and alertness.
- **Sodium oxybate:** This strong drug may be prescribed if one has severe cataplexy. Sodium oxybate is also known as gamma-hydroxybutyrate (GHB), or the "date rape drug" but is considered safe for treating narcolepsy when used responsibly to promote sound sleep, diminish daytime sleepiness, and reduce incidences of cataplexy.
- **Antidepressants:** Selective serotonin reuptake inhibitors used to treat depression may also be used to help suppress rapid eye movement (REM) sleep, and alleviate symptoms of cataplexy, hallucinations, and sleep paralysis.

Nursing Management

- Instructing patient to follow as consistent a daily schedule for retiring and arising as possible. This promotes regulation of the circadian rhythm and reduces the energy required for adaptation to changes.
- Instructing to avoid heavy meals, alcohol, caffeine, or smoking before retiring.
  Though hunger can also keep one awake, gastric digestion and stimulation from caffeine and nicotine can disturb sleep.
- Instructing to avoid large fluid intake before bedtime. For patients may need to void during the night.
- Increasing daytime physical activities as indicated, to reduce stress and promote sleep.
- Instructing to avoid strenuous activity before bedtime. Overfatigue may cause insomnia.
- Discourage pattern of daytime naps unless deemed necessary to meet sleep requirements or if part of one's usual pattern. Napping can disrupt normal sleep patterns. However, the elderly do better with frequent naps during the day to counter their shorter night-time sleep schedule.
- Suggesting the use of soporifics such as milk, which contains L-tryptophan that facilitates sleep.
- Recommending an environment conducive to sleep or rest (e.g., quiet, comfortable temperature, ventilation, darkness, closed door). Suggesting the use of earplugs or eye shades as appropriate.
- Suggesting engaging in a relaxing activity before retiring, such as warm bath, calm music, reading an enjoyable book, relaxation exercises.
- Explaining the need to avoid concentrating on the next day's activities or on one's problems at bedtime.
- Suggesting using hypnotics or sedatives as ordered.
- If unable to fall asleep after about 30–45 minutes, suggesting getting out of bed and engaging in a relaxing activity.
- Providing nursing aids (e.g., back rub, bedtime care, pain relief, comfortable position, relaxation techniques).
- Organize nursing care: Eliminating nonessential nursing activities. Preparing patient for necessary anticipated interruptions/disruptions.
- Attempting to allow for sleep cycles of at least 90 minutes.
- Moving patient to room farther from the nursing station if noise is a contributing factor.
- Posting a "Do not disturb" sign on the door.

HEADACHE

Headache is a pain in any region of the head. Headaches may occur on one or both sides of the head, be isolated to a certain location, radiate across the head from one point, or have a vise-like quality. A headache may be a sharp pain, throbbing sensation or dull ache. Headaches may appear gradually or suddenly, and they may last less than an hour or for several days.

Types of Headache

Chronic Tension Headache

Chronic tension-type headaches may be the result of stress or fatigue, but more than likely, they can be attributed to physical problems, psychological issues, or depression. A pattern of chronic tension-type headaches generally begins between the ages of 20 and 40 years, and every personality type can experience them.

Symptoms
The muscles between head and neck contract for hours or days.
- A tightness around neck or even feel as if head and neck were in a cast and only certain positions seem to provide relief.
- Feeling of soreness, a tightening band around head (a "vice-like" ache), a pulling, or pressure sensations.
- The pain is continuous, annoying, but not throbbing.

Headache primarily occurs in forehead, temples, or the back of head and neck.
- Changes in sleep patterns if headaches are related to anxiety, then you may have trouble falling asleep or may suffer from insomnia. If headaches are associated with depression, then you may awaken frequently during the night, awaken before you wanted to in the morning, or you may be sleeping excessively (hypersomnia).
- Shortness of breath
- Constipation
- Nausea
- Weight loss
- Ongoing fatigue
- Decreased sexual drive
- Palpitations
- Dizziness
- Unexpected crying
- Menstrual changes

Etiology and Risk Factors
- Poor posture, close work under poor lighting conditions, or cramps from assuming an unnatural head or neck position for long periods
- Arthritis, particularly cervical arthritis
- Abnormalities in neck muscles, bones or disks
- Eye straining caused when one eye is compensating for another eye's weakness
- Misalignment of teeth or jaws
- Noise or lighting
- Job conflicts and family relationships
- Grief
- Depression

Management
- There are two goals when treating any type of headache: prevent future attacks, abort or relieve current pain.
- Prevention includes taking prescribed medications, avoiding or minimizing the causes, and learning self-help measures, such as biofeedback or relaxation exercises.
- **NSAIDs**, fenoprofen, flurbiprofen, ketoprofen.
- **Antidepressants: Tricyclics (nonsedating)**, protriptyline, desipramine.
- **Antidepressants: Tricyclics (sedating)**, amitriptyline, doxepin.

Migraine Headache

Migraines deserve the attention they receive, one headache can put the life "on hold" for a few hours or several days. Migraine is responsible for more job absenteeism and disrupted family life than any other headache type.

Symptoms

Migraine often begins as a dull ache and then develops into a constant, throbbing and pulsating pain at the temples, as well as the front or back of one side of the head. The pain is usually accompanied by nausea and vomiting, and sensitivity to light and noise.

The two most prevalent types of migraine are migraine with aura (formerly referred to as classic migraine) and migraine without aura (formerly referred to as common migraine).

Etiology

Physical and environmental causes

- Stress
- Fatigue
- Oversleeping or lack of sleep
- Fasting or missing a meal
- Food or medication that affects the diameter of blood vessels
- Caffeine
- Chocolate
- Alcohol
- Menses
- Hormonal changes
- Changes in barometric pressure
- Changes in altitude

Foods and diet

Specific foods are suspected of triggering at least 30% of the migraine headaches. Foods that contain: additives such as nitrates and nitrites (usually in processed meats), yellow (annatto) food coloring, and MSG (monosodium glutamate). Canned or processed foods, Chinese foods, tenderizer, and seasonings such as soy sauce may contain MSG.

Tyramine

Red wines and most alcoholic beverages, aged cheeses and processed meats (including pizza and hot dogs), peanuts, chicken livers, pickled foods, sourdough bread, bread and crackers containing cheese, broad beans, peas, lentils. Foods to eat in moderation include avocados, bananas, citrus fruits, figs, raisins, red plums, raspberries, and chocolates.

Management

- There are two goals when treating migraine, or any other headache: to relieve the pain and prevent future attacks.
- Once migraine has been diagnosed, treatment will begin by identifying those circumstances or factors that trigger it.
- Keeping a daily calendar of activities, foods, beverages, prescription and over-the-counter medications, physical and environmental factors, stressful situations, sleep patterns, and characteristics of the headache itself.
- Beta blockers, propranolol, timolol.
- Calcium channel blockers, verapamil, diltiazem.
- Antiepilepsy medication, divalproex sodium, neurontin.
- NSAIDs, fenoprofen, flurbiprofen.
- Antidepressants: Tricyclics (nonsedating), protriptyline, desipramine.

Self-help treatments for migraine and tension-type headaches

- Counseling and psychotherapy
- Relaxation training

- Progressive muscle relaxation
- Guided imagery
- Biofeedback
- Acupuncture
- Physical and massage therapy

Cluster Headache

In this, the attacks come in groups. The pain arrives with little, if any, warning, and it has been described as the most severe and intense of any headache type. It generally lasts from 30 to 45 minutes, although it might persist for several hours before it disappears. Cluster headaches frequently surface during the morning or late at night, the cluster cycle can last weeks or months and then can disappear for months or years.

Symptoms
- The headache is usually unilateral and rarely switches sides from one attack to another.
- One might feel the pain begin around one eye, "like a nail or knife stabbing or piercing" the eye, or as if someone "were pulling out" eye, it may be accompanied by a tearing or bloodshot eye and a runny nose on the side of the headache.
- It can radiate from the eye to the forehead, temple and cheek on the same side.
- The pain of a cluster headache has been described as piercing, burning, throbbing, and pulsating.

Etiology
Unlike migraine headaches, cluster headaches are not the result of heredity. Sufferers, however, usually do have a history of chronic smoking, and alcohol frequently triggers a cluster headache. Because the level of histamine increases in a person's blood and urine during a cluster headache, which dilate or expand blood vessels, influence a cluster headache.

Management
Verapamil, prednisone, ergotamine tartrate, lithium carbonate, divalproex sodium, histamine acid phosphate.

HEAD INJURIES

Head injuries are dangerous. They can lead to permanent disability, mental impairment, and even death. To most people, head injuries are considered an acceptable risk when engaging in sports and other types of recreational activities.

Head injuries are injuries to the scalp, skull, or brain caused by trauma. Concussions are the most common type of sports-related brain injury. A concussion is a type of traumatic brain injury that happens when the brain is jarred or shaken hard enough to bounce against the skull.

Types of Head Injuries

There are three common types of traumatic head injury:
1. **Closed injury:** A closed injury does not break or open the skull or penetrate brain tissue. However, it can still cause bruising or swelling of the brain.
2. **Open injury:** An open injury is any damage that penetrates the skull. The damage may cause bleeding within the brain's tissues. It may also produce skull fractures or cause the skull bones to press into brain tissue.

3. **Concussion:** A concussion occurs when brain is shaken. It may lead to loss of consciousness and headache.

Causes of Head Injury

Many types of trauma can cause a head injury.

- **Gunshot wounds** can cause head injuries when the bullet penetrates the skull and enters the brain. This can damage the blood vessels and cause bleeding.
- **Vehicle accidents** are common causes of traumatic head injuries.
- **Violent shaking** is a common cause of brain trauma in infants and young children.
- **Falling and hitting head** can damage the skull, scalp, or brain. Falls may cause any type of head injury.
- **Assault** can lead to a head injury. Being kicked, punched, or struck in the head can cause a concussion, closed or open brain injury.

Management

- Checking the person's level of response using the AVPU code:
  - **A**—is the person alert, eyes open and responding to questions
  - **V**—does the person respond to voice, obey simple commands
  - **P**—does the person respond to pain (e.g., eyes open or movement in response to being pinched)
  - **U**—is the person unresponsive.
- Regularly monitor and record vital signs—level of response, breathing and pulse. Even if the person appears to recover fully, watch them for any deterioration in their level of response.
- When the person has recovered, place them in the care of a responsible person. If a person has been injured on the sports field, never allow them to 'play on' without first obtaining medical advice.
- Advise the person to go to hospital if, following a blow to the head, they develop symptoms such as headache, vomiting, confusion, drowsiness, or double vision.

Treatment of Acute Head Injury

- Cervical collar
- Craniotomy, surgical incision into cranium (may be necessary to evacuate a hematoma or evacuate contents to make room for swelling to prevent herniation)
- Oxygen therapy, intubation, and mechanical ventilation (to provide controlled hyperventilation to decrease elevate ICP)
- Restricted oral intake for 24–48 hours
- Ventriculostomy, insertion of a drain into the ventricles (to drain CSF in the presence of hydrocephalus, which may occur as a result of head injury; can also be used to monitor ICP).

Pharmacological Management

Following are the list of pharmacological management:

- Analgesic: codeine phosphate
- Anesthetic: lidocaine
- Anticonvulsant: phenytoin
- Barbiturate: pentobarbital

- Diuretic: mannitol, furosemide to combat cerebral edema
- Dopamine (intropin) to maintain cerebral perfusion pressure (CPP) above 50 mm Hg (if blood pressure is low and ICP is elevated)
- Glucocorticoid: dexamethasone to reduce cerebral edema
- Histamin-2 (H2) receptor antagonist such as cimetidine, ranitidine, famotidine
- Mucosal barrier fortifier: sucralfate
- Posterior pituitary: vasopressin if client develops diabetes insipidus.

Nursing Care Plan

Assessment

- Assessing neurologic status as follows: level of consciousness as per Glasgow coma scale, pupil size, symmetry, and reaction to light, extraocular movement, gaze preference, speech and thought processes, memory, motor-sensory signs and drift, increased tone, increased reflexes, Babinski reflex, deteriorating neurological signs indicate increased cerebral ischemia.
- Evaluating the presence or absence of protective reflexes (e.g., swallowing, gagging, blinking, coughing).
- Monitoring vital signs.
- Monitoring arterial blood gases and pulse oximetry. Recommended parameters of PaO_2 >80 mm Hg and $PaCO_2$ <35 mm Hg with normal ICP. If patient's lungs are being hyperventilated to decrease ICP, $PaCO_2$ should be between 25 and 30 mm Hg.
- Monitoring input and output with urine-specific gravity. Reporting urine-specific gravity >1.025 or urine output <1.50 mL/kg/h, may indicate decreased renal perfusion and possible associated decrease in CPP.
- Monitoring ICP if measurement device is in place. Reporting ICP >15 mm Hg for 5 minutes.
- Calculating CPP, should be approximately 90–100 mm Hg and not <50 mm Hg to ensure blood flow to brain.
- Monitoring serum electrolytes, blood urea nitrogen, creatinine, glucose, osmolality, hemoglobin, and hematocrit as indicated, to detect treatment complications such as hypovolemia.
- Monitoring closely when treatment of increased ICP begins to taper, *ICP* may increase as treatment is tapered.

Nursing Diagnosis

- Ineffective airway clearance and impaired gas exchange related to brain injury
- Ineffective cerebral tissue perfusion related to increased ICP, decreased CPP, and possible seizures
- Deficient fluid volume related to decreased level of consciousness (LOC) and hormonal dysfunction
- Imbalanced nutrition, less than body requirements, related to increased metabolic demands, fluid restriction, and inadequate intake
- Risk for injury related to seizures, disorientation, restlessness, or brain damage
- Risk for imbalanced body temperature related to damaged temperature-regulating mechanisms in the brain

- Risk for impaired skin integrity related to bed rest, hemiparesis, hemiplegia, immobility, or restlessness
- Disturbed thought processes (deficits in intellectual function, communication, memory, information processing) related to brain injury
- Disturbed sleep pattern related to brain injury and frequent neurologic checks
- Interrupted family processes related to unresponsiveness of patient, unpredictability of outcome, prolonged recovery period, and the patient's residual physical disability and emotional deficit
- Deficient knowledge about brain injury, recovery, and the rehabilitation process.

Interventions

- Assessing neurologic and respiratory status to monitor for sign of increased ICP and respiratory distress.
- Monitoring and recording vital sign and intake and output, hemodynamic variables, ICP, CPP, specific gravity, laboratory studies, and pulse oximetry to detect early sign of compromise.
- Observing for sign of increasing ICP to avoid treatment delay and prevent neurologic compromise.
- Assessing for CSF leak as evidenced by otorrhea or rhinorrhea. CSF leak could leave the patient at risk for infection.
- Assessing for pain. Pain may cause anxiety and increase ICP.
- Checking cough and gag reflex to prevent aspiration.
- Checking for sign of diabetes insipidus (low urine specific gravity, high urine output) to maintain hydration.
- Administering IV fluids to maintain hydration.
- Administering oxygen to maintain position and patency of endotracheal tube if present, to maintain airway and hyperventilate the patient and to lower ICP.
- Providing suctioning; if patient is able, assist with turning, coughing, and deep breathing to prevent pooling of secretions.
- Maintaining position, patency and low suction of nasogastric tube (NGT) to prevent vomiting.
- Maintaining seizure precautions to maintain patient safety.
- Administering medication as prescription to decrease ICP and pain.
- Allowing a rest period between nursing activities to avoid increase in ICP.
- Encouraging the patient to express feeling about changes in body image.
- Providing appropriate sensory input and stimuli with frequent reorientation to foster awareness of the environment.
- Providing means of communication, such as a communication board to prevent anxiety.
- Providing eye, skin, and mouth care to prevent tissue damage.
- Turning the patient every 2 hours or maintain in a rotating bed if condition allows preventing skin breakdown.
- Monitoring patient's neurologic status, ICP and vital signs at least every hour.
- Notifying physician for collaborative management or institute a protocol to respond to a sustained ICP greater than 20.
- Maintaining patient's head of the bed at 30° elevation or higher and patient's body in a neutral position. Not allowing pronounced neck or hip flexion.

- Monitoring the patient's temperature and maintain it within designated parameters, aggressively treat hyperthermia.
- Monitoring patient's blood gases; collaborate with physician and respiratory therapist to resolve hypercarbia, hypocarbia, or hypoxia.
- Suction only after preoxygenating the patient and for less than 10 seconds at a time.
- Spread nursing activities out, not clustering them.

SPINAL INJURY

A spinal cord injury is a damage to any part of the spinal cord or nerves at the end of the spinal canal, often causes permanent changes in strength, sensation, and other body functions below the site of the injury.

Types of Spinal Injuries

Following are the list of types of spinal injuries:
- **Cervical spinal cord injury C1–C8—quadriplegia also known as tetraplegia:** Cervical level injuries cause paralysis or weakness in both arms and legs (quadriplegia). All regions of the body below the level of injury or top of the back may be affected. Sometimes, this type of injury is accompanied by loss of physical sensation, respiratory issues, bowel, bladder, and sexual dysfunction. This area of the spinal cord controls signals to the back of the head, neck and shoulders, arms and hands, and diaphragm. Since the neck region is so flexible, it is difficult to stabilize cervical spinal cord injuries. Patients with cervical level injuries may be placed in a brace or stabilizing device.
- **Thoracic spinal cord injury T1–T12:** Thoracic level injuries are less common because of the protection given by the rib cage. Thoracic injuries can cause paralysis or weakness of the legs (paraplegia) along with loss of physical sensation, bowel, bladder, and sexual dysfunction. In most cases, arms and hands are not affected. This area of the spinal cord controls signals to some of the muscles of the back and part of the abdomen. With these types of injuries, most patients initially wear a brace on the trunk to provide extra stability.
- **Lumbar spinal cord injury L1–L5:** Lumbar level injuries result in paralysis or weakness of the legs (paraplegia). Loss of physical sensation, bowel, bladder, and sexual dysfunction can occur. The shoulders, arms, and hand function are usually unaffected. This area of the spinal cord controls signals to the lower parts of the abdomen and the back, the buttocks, some parts of the external genital organs, and parts of the leg. These injuries often require surgery and external stabilization.
- **Sacral spinal cord injury S1–S5:** Sacral level injuries primarily cause loss of bowel and bladder function as well as sexual dysfunction. These types of injuries can cause weakness or paralysis of the hips and legs. This area of the spinal cord controls signals to the thighs and lower parts of the legs, the feet, and genital organs.
- **Complete and incomplete:** An incomplete injury means that the ability of the spinal cord to convey messages to or from the brain is not completely lost, some sensation and movement are possible below the level of injury. A complete injury is indicated by a total lack of sensory and motor function below the level of injury. But the absence of motor and sensory function below the injury site does not necessarily mean that there are no remaining intact axons or nerves crossing the injury site, just that they do not function appropriately following the injury.

Types of Paralysis

Following are the list of types of paralysis:

- **Complete paraplegia:** Complete paraplegia is a condition that results in permanent loss of movement and sensation at the T1 level or below. At the T1 level, there is normal hand function, and as the levels moved down, the spinal column improved abdominal control, respiratory function, and sitting balance may occur.
- **Complete tetraplegia:** Complete tetraplegia is a condition that results in permanent loss of movement and sensation in all four limbs. Spinal cord injuries that result in complete tetraplegia most often occur at levels C1 through C8. The degree of functionality is a direct result of where the injury to the spine occurred.
- **Anterior cord syndrome:** The injury occurs at the front of the spinal cord, leaving the person with partial or complete loss of ability to sense pain, temperature, and touch below the level of injury. Some people with this type of injury later recover some movement.
- **Central cord syndrome:** The injury occurs at the center of the spinal cord, and usually results in the loss of arm function. Some leg, bowel, and bladder control may be preserved. Some recovery from this injury may start in the legs, and then move upward.
- **Posterior cord syndrome:** The injury occurs toward the back of the spinal cord. Usually, muscle power, pain, and temperature sensation are preserved. However, the person may have trouble with limb coordination.
- **Brown–Sequard syndrome:** This injury occurs on one side of the spinal cord. Pain and temperature sensation will be present on the injured side, but impairment or loss of movement will also result. The opposite side of the injury will have normal movement, but pain and temperature sensation will be affected or lost.
- **Cauda equine lesion:** Damage to the nerves that fan out of the spinal cord at the first and second lumbar region of the spine can cause partial or complete loss of movement and feeling. Depending upon the extent of initial damage, sometimes these nerves can grow back and resume functionality.
- **Hemiplegia** is a term used to describe paralysis, severe weakness, or rigid movement on either the right or left side of the body. Hemiplegia can also be associated with limited use of the hand, balance issues, speech issues, and visual field problems.

Etiology

The main causes of hemiplegia are as follows:

- Brain damage as the result of disrupted blood flow
- Stroke
- Cerebral palsy
- Perinatal strokes in infants, and traumatic brain injury

Types of Hemiplegia

There are several different types of hemiplegia, which include the following:

a. **Facial hemiplegia:** Paralysis occurs on one side of the face.
b. **Cerebral hemiplegia:** A brain lesion disrupts the flow of blood to the brain.
c. **Spastic hemiplegia:** Characterized by paralysis and spastic movements on the affected side.
d. **Spinal hemiplegia:** Caused by lesions that have formed on the spine.

Pathophysiology

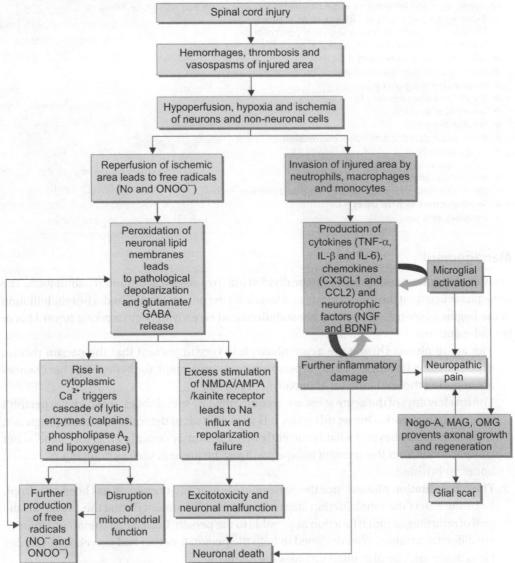

Signs and Symptoms

- Loss of movement
- Loss of sensation, including the ability to feel heat, cold, and touch
- Loss of bowel or bladder control
- Exaggerated reflex activities or spasms
- Changes in sexual function, sexual sensitivity, and fertility
- Pain or an intense stinging sensation caused by damage to the nerve fibers in spinal cord
- Difficulty breathing, coughing or clearing secretions from lungs

Emergency Signs and Symptoms

Emergency signs and symptoms of spinal cord injury after an accident may include the following:

❖ Extreme back pain or pressure in neck, head, or back
❖ Weakness, in coordination or paralysis in any part of body
❖ Numbness, tingling or loss of sensation in hands, fingers, feet, or toes
❖ Loss of bladder or bowel control
❖ Difficulty with balance and walking
❖ Impaired breathing after injury
❖ An oddly positioned or twisted neck or back
❖ Loss of consciousness
❖ Low breathing rate
❖ Restlessness, clumsiness, or lack of coordination
❖ Severe headache
❖ Slurred speech or blurred vision
❖ Stiff neck or vomiting
❖ Sudden worsening of symptoms after initial improvement
❖ Swelling at the site of the injury
❖ Persistent vomiting

Management

Treatment for spinal cord injuries can be divided into two stages: acute and rehabilitation. The acute phase begins at the time of injury and lasts until the person is stabilized. The rehabilitation phase begins as soon as the person has stabilized and is ready to begin working toward his or her independence.

1. **The acute phase:** During the acute phase, it is very important that the person receive prompt medical care. The faster the person accesses treatment, the better his or her chances are at having the least amount of impairment possible.

   The first few days of the acute stage are accompanied by spinal shock, in which the person's reflexes do not work. During this stage, it is very difficult to determine an exact prognosis, as some function beyond what is currently being seen may occur later. At this stage, other complications from the accident or injury will also be present, such as brain injury, broken bones, or bruising.

2. **The rehabilitation phase:** Once the acute phase is over and the person has been stabilized, he or she enters the rehabilitation stage of treatment. Treatment during this phase has the goal of returning as much function as possible to the person. Because all spinal cord injuries are different, a unique plan designed to help the person function and succeed in everyday life is designed. The plan often includes the following:

   ▪ Helping the person understand his or her injuries.
   ▪ Helping the person understand the details regarding his or her care.
   ▪ Helping the person become as independent as possible in everyday activities such as bathing, eating, dressing, grooming, and wheelchair use.
   ▪ Helping the person learn to accept a new lifestyle, especially pertaining to sexual, recreational, and housing options.
   ▪ Helping the person learn how to instruct caregivers in how to assist them.
   ▪ Preparing them for vocational rehabilitation.
   ▪ In most cases, rehabilitation occurs at an approved and accredited spinal cord injury treatment center.

Specific Level of Spinal Cord Injury and Rehabilitation Potential

- **C2 or C3:** Patient is completely dependent for all care.
- **C4:** Dependent for all cares and usually needs a ventilator.
- **C5:** Patient may be able to feed himself using assistive devices, usually needs a type of respiratory support but may be able to break without a ventilator.
- **C6:** Patient may be able to push himself on wheelchair indoors and may be able to perform daily living tasks such as eating, grooming, and dressing.
- **C7:** Patient may be able to drive a car with special adaptations or can propel a wheelchair outside.
- **C8:** Same as C7.
- **T1–T6:** Patient may be able to become independent with self-care and use of a wheelchair.
- **T6–T12:** Patient may improve sitting balance and be able to participate in athletic activities with the use of a wheelchair.
- **L1–L5:** Patient may be able to walk short distances with assistive devices.

Nursing Intervention

- Assessing functional ability of impairment initially and on a regular basis.
- Changing positions at least every 2 hours (supine, side lying) and possibly more often if placed on affected side.
- Positioning in prone position once or twice a day if patient can tolerate.
- Propping extremities in functional position, using footboard during the period of flaccid paralysis. Maintaining neutral position of head.
- Using arm sling when patient is in upright position, as indicated.
- Evaluating use and need for positional aids and splints during spastic paralysis, placing pillow under axillae to abduct arm, elevating arm and hand.
- Observing affected side for color, edema, or other signs of compromised circulation.
- Inspecting skin regularly, particularly over bony prominences. Gently massaging any reddened areas and provide aids such as sheepskin pads as necessary.
- It is necessary to begin active/passive range of motion exercise to all extremities.
- Assisting to develop sitting balance (e.g., raise head of bed, assist to sit on edge of bed, having patient use the strong arm to support body weight and strong leg to move affected leg, increase sitting time) and standing balance (e.g., put flat walking shoes on patient, support patient's lower back with hands while positioning own knees outside patient's knees, assist in using parallel bars/walkers).
- Getting patient up in chair as soon as vital signs are stable, except following cerebral hemorrhage.
- Padding chair seat with foam or water-filled cushion and assisting patient to shift weight at frequent intervals.
- Providing egg-crate mattress, water bed, flotation device, or specialized beds (e.g., kinetic), as indicated.
- Assessing abilities and level of deficit (0–4 scale) for performing ADLs.
- Avoiding doing things for patient that patient can do for self, but providing assistance as necessary.
- Be aware of impulsive behavior and actions suggestive of impaired judgment.
- Maintaining a supportive, firm attitude. Allowing patient sufficient time to accomplish tasks.
- Providing positive feedback for efforts and accomplishments.

- Creating a plan for visual deficits that are present, e.g., place food and utensils on the tray related to patient's unaffected side, situating the bed so that patient's unaffected side is facing the room with the affected side to the wall, positioning furniture against wall and out of travel path.
- Providing self-help devices, e.g., button/zipper hook, knife–fork combinations, long-handled brushes, extensions for picking things up from floor, toilet riser, leg bag for catheter, shower chair.
- Assisting and encourage good grooming and makeup habits.
- Encouraging family member to allow patient to do as much as possible for self.
- Assessing patient's ability to communicate the need to void and ability to use urinal, bedpan. Taking patient to the bathroom at frequent and periodic intervals for voiding if appropriate.
- Identifying previous bowel habits and re-establish normal regimen. Increasing bulk in diet, encourage fluid intake, increased activity.

MULTIPLE CHOICE QUESTIONS

1. **Amyloid plaques and neurofibrillary tangles are the hallmarks of:**
   A. Alzheimer's disease
   B. Amyotrophic lateral sclerosis
   C. Ataxia telangiectasia
   D. Autism

2. **Difficulty speaking and understanding speech is termed:**
   A. Apnea
   B. Ataxia
   C. Aphasia
   D. Dyslexia

3. **The most common form of transient facial paralysis is:**
   A. Alzheimer's disease
   B. Transient ischemic attack
   C. Bell's palsy
   D. Erb's palsy

4. **Gradually increasing pain and weakness and numbness in the hand or wrist that radiates up the arm suggest:**
   A. Amyotrophic lateral sclerosis
   B. Carpal tunnel syndrome
   C. Bloch–Sulzberger syndrome
   D. Dystonia

5. **All of the following may be associated with Guillain–Barré syndrome, *except*:**
   A. Weakening or tingling sensation in the legs
   B. Weakness in the arms and upper body
   C. Nearly complete paralysis
   D. First symptom is altered mental status

6. **Which of the following statement about herpes zoster is not true?**
   A. It is caused by the varicella-zoster virus
   B. It causes burning, tingling pain and lesions, generally on one side of the body
   C. Anyone who has had chickenpox is at risk of postherpetic neuralgia
   D. It is a sexually transmitted disease

7. **Diagnostic tests for epilepsy include all of the following, *except*:**
   A. Simple blood tests
   B. EEG
   C. Brain scan
   D. Wada test

8. **Treatment for epilepsy to eliminate or sharply reduce the frequency of seizures may involve all of the following, *except*:**
   A. Cognitive-behavioral therapy
   B. Narrow-spectrum and broad-spectrum antiepileptic drugs
   C. Vagus-nerve stimulation
   D. Surgery

9. **The most common inherited neurological disorder is:**
   A. Bloch–Sulzberger Syndrome
   B. Charcot–Marie–Tooth disease
   C. Alpers' disease
   D. Asperger syndrome

10. **A severe form of epilepsy that appears during the first year of life is called:**
   A. Dandy–Walker syndrome
   B. Devic's syndrome
   C. Dravet syndrome
   D. Fabry disease

11. **Lack of ceramide trihexosidase, also known as alpha-galactoside-A causes:**
   A. Fahr's syndrome
   B. Fabry disease
   C. Fisher syndrome
   D. Gaucher's disease

12. **Symptoms of trigeminal neuralgia may include all of the following, *except*:**
   A. Extreme, intermittent facial pain in the jaw or cheek
   B. Tingling or numbness on one side of the face
   C. Pain triggered by contact with the face or facial movements
   D. Inability to swallow

13. **All of the following are true about Tourette syndrome, *except*:**
   A. Drug treatment completely eliminates symptoms
   B. It is involuntary and may be a chronic condition
   C. Symptoms are generally most severe during adolescence
   D. Symptoms are generally detected in children

14. **Huntington's disease is a heritable disorder that involves:**
   A. Sudden paralysis
   B. Chorea, loss of cognitive abilities, and emotional disturbance
   C. Uncontrollable swearing and repetitive actions
   D. Inability to recognize faces

15. **All of the following statements about amyotrophic lateral sclerosis are true, *except*:**
   A. It causes degeneration and death of upper and lower motor neurons
   B. Patients lose strength and control of voluntary muscles
   C. It impairs cognition and senses
   D. It progresses rapidly and is fatal

16. **Children with Angelman syndrome generally display all of the following, *except*:**
   A. Developmental delays and speech impairment
   B. Feeding problems
   C. Seizures
   D. Loss of hearing and sense of smell

17. **All of the following are true about autism, *except*:**
   A. Affected persons have communication, interpersonal, and behavioral problems
   B. Affected persons display obsessive or repetitive behaviors and interests
   C. It is the direct result of immunization with thimerosal-containing vaccines
   D. Early intervention is associated with improved outcomes

18. **Brain and spinal tumors may be treated with any or all of the following modalities, *except*:**
   A. Surgery
   B. Radiation
   C. Chemotherapy
   D. Positron emission tomography

19. **Symptoms of Parkinson's disease include all of the following,** *except*:
    A. Tremors of the hands, arms, legs, jaw, and face
    B. Stiff limbs
    C. Bradykinesia and impaired balance
    D. Impaired cognition

20. **Narcolepsy is a disorder characterized by:**
    A. Narcotic abuse
    B. Grand mal seizures
    C. Reliance on soporific drugs
    D. Inability to regulate sleep–wake cycles

Answers

1. A	2. C	3. C	4. B	5. D	6. D	7. A	8. A	9. B	10. C
11. B	12. D	13. A	14. B	15. C	16. D	17. C	18. D	19. D	20. D

BIBLIOGRAPHY

1. Agid Y, Cervera P, Hirsch E, et al. Biochemistry of Parkinson's disease 28 years later: A critical review. Mov Disord. 1989;4:126-44.
2. Calne DB. Treatment of Parkinson's disease. N Engl J Med. 1993;329:1021-27.
3. Cottrell DA, Kremenchutzky M, Rice GP, et al. The natural history of multiple sclerosis: a geographically based study. 5. The clinical features and natural history of primary progressive multiple sclerosis. Brain. 1999;122:625-39.
4. Fearnley JM, Lees AJ. Aging and Parkinson's disease: Substantia nigra regional selectivity. Brain. 1991;114:2283-2301.
5. Gerfen CR, Engber TM, Mahan LC, et al. D1 and D2 dopamine receptor regulated gene expression of striatonigral and striatopallidal neurons. Science. 1990;250:1429-32.
6. Gibb WRG, Lees AJ. Pathological clues to the cause of Parkinson's disease. In: Marsden CD, Fahn S (Eds). Movement Disorders. Oxford: Butterworth-Heinemann; 1994. pp. 147-66.
7. Gibb WRG. Functional neuropathology in Parkinson's disease. Eur Neurol. 1997;38:21-5.
8. Gibb WRG. Neuropathology of the substantia nigra. Eur Neurol. 1991;31:48-59.
9. Goldstein M, Lieberman A. The role of the regulatory enzymes of catecholamine synthesis in Parkinson's disease. Neurology. 1992;42:8-12.
10. Graybiel AM, Hirsch EC, Agid Y. The nigrostriatal system in Parkinson's disease. Adv Neurol. 1990;53:17-29.
11. Greenberg DA. Glutamate and Parkinson's disease. Ann Neurol. 1994;35:639.
12. Lennon VA, Kryzer TJ, Pittock SJ, Verkman AS, Hinson SR. IgG marker of optic-spinal multiple sclerosis binds to the aquaporin-4 water channel. J Exp Med. 2005;202:473-7.
13. Lennon VA, Wingerchuk DM, Kryzer TJ, et al. A serum autoantibody marker of neuromyelitis optica: Distinction from multiple sclerosis. Lancet. 2004;364:2106-12.
14. Lucchinetti C, Scheithauer B, Rodriguez M, Lassman H. Heterogeneity of multiple sclerosis lesions: implications for the pathogenesis of demyelination. Ann Neurol. 2000;47:707-17.
15. Lucchinetti CF, Popescu BF, Bunyan RF, et al. Inflammatory cortical demyelination in early multiple sclerosis. N Engl J Med. 2011;365:2188-97.
16. Wichmann T. Physiology of the basal ganglia and pathophysiology of movement disorders of basal ganglia origin. In: Watts RL, Koller WC (Eds). Movement Disorders – Neurological Principles and Practice. New York: McGraw-Hill; 1997. pp. 87-97.
17. Wingerchuk DM, Lennon VA, Pittock SJ, Lucchinetti CF, Weinshenker BG. Revised diagnostic criteria for neuromyelitis optica. Neurology. 2006;66:1485-89.

Burn and Cosmetics Surgeries

AT THE END OF THIS CHAPTER, THE STUDENTS WILL BE ABLE TO LEARN ABOUT:
- Burn
- Pathophysiology of burn
- Management of burn
- Role of nurse
- Legal aspects
- Rehabilitation
- Special therapies
- Psychosocial aspects
- Types of wound care in burn
- Fluid therapy during burn
- Skin grafting

INTRODUCTION

Burns may be treated with first aid, in an out-of-hospital setting, or may require more specialized treatment such as those available at specialized burn centers. Managing burn injuries properly is important because they are common, painful and can result in disfiguring and disabling scarring, amputation of affected parts or death in severe cases. Complications such as shock, infection, multiple organ dysfunction syndrome, electrolyte imbalance, and respiratory distress may occur. The treatment of burns may include the removal of dead tissue (debridement), applying dressings to the wound, fluid resuscitation, administering antibiotics, and skin grafting.

ASSESSMENT OF BURN AND SKIN (REFER INTEGUMENTARY SYSTEM)

BURNS

Definition

A **burn** is a type of injury to flesh or skin caused by heat, electricity, chemicals, light, radiation, or friction. Most burns affect only the skin (epidermal tissue). Rarely, deeper tissues, such as muscle, bone, and blood vessels, can also be injured.

Cause

Burns are caused by a wide variety of substances and external sources such as exposure to chemicals, friction, electricity, radiation, and heat **(Fig. 20.1)**.

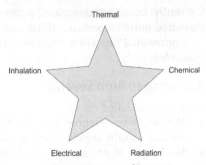

Fig. 20.1: Causes of burn.

Chemical

Most chemicals that cause chemical burns are strong acids or bases. Chemical burns can be caused by corrosive chemical compounds such as sulfuric acid and sodium hydroxide. Hydrofluoric acid can cause damage down to the bone and its burns are sometimes not immediately evident. Chemical burns can be either first, second, or third-degree burns, depending on the duration of contact, strength of the substance, and other factors.

Electrical

Electrical burns are caused by either an electric shock or an uncontrolled short circuit (a burn from a hot, electrified heating element is *not* considered an electrical burn).

The true incidence of electrical burn injury is unknown. This is sufficient to cause cardiac arrest and ventricular fibrillation but generates relatively low heat energy deposit into skin, thus producing few or no burn marks at all. High voltage electricity, on the other hand, is a common cause of third- and fourth-degree burns due to the extreme heat yielded by high temperature arcs and flashover associated with voltages over 1,000 V.

Radiation

Radiation burns are caused by protracted exposure to UV light (as from the sun), radiation therapy (in people undergoing cancer therapy), sunlamps, and X-rays. By far the most common burn associated with radiation is sun exposure.

Scalding

Scalding is caused by hot liquids (water or oil) or gases (steam), most commonly occurring from exposure to high temperature tap water in baths or showers or spilled hot drinks. A so-called immersion scald is created when an extremity is held under the surface of hot water. A blister is a "bubble" in the skin filled with serous fluid as part of the body's reaction to the heat and the subsequent inflammatory reaction. The blister "roof" is dead, and the blister fluid contains toxic inflammatory mediators. Generally scald burns are first- or second-degree burns, but third-degree burns can result, especially with prolonged contact.

Inhalational Injury

Steam, smoke, and high temperatures can cause inhalational injury to the airway and/or lungs.

Types of Burns

Burns can be classified by mechanism of injury, depth, extent, and associated injuries and comorbidities.

According to Depth

Currently, burns are described according to the depth of injury to the dermis and are loosely classified into first, second, third, and fourth degrees.

Figure 20.2 describes degrees of burn injury under this system as well as provide pictorial examples.

According to Burn Severity

Burns are classified as:
- **Minor:** All first-degree burns as well as second-degree burns that involve <10% of the body surface usually are classified as minor.
- **Moderate:** Burns involve the hands, feet, face, or genitals. Second-degree burns involve >10% of body surface area.

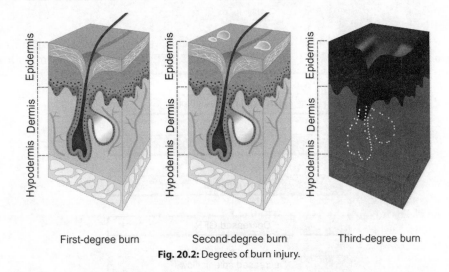

First-degree burn   Second-degree burn   Third-degree burn

Fig. 20.2: Degrees of burn injury.

- **Severe:** Burn surface involvement of 25% body surface area. All third-degree burns are classified as severe burn.

According to the Extent of Body Surface Area

Burns can also be assessed in terms of total body surface area (BSA) (TBSA), which is the percentage affected by partial-thickness or full-thickness burns. The rule of 9s is used as a quick and useful way to estimate the affected area.

The rule of 9s: It was introduced by Alexander Wallace. The rule of 9s is the quick way to calculate the extent of burn.

Pathophysiology

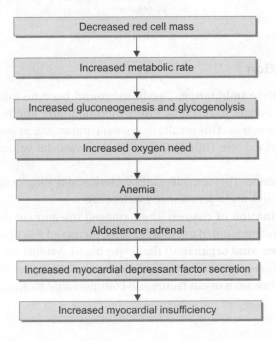

Decreased red cell mass

↓

Increased metabolic rate

↓

Increased gluconeogenesis and glycogenolysis

↓

Increased oxygen need

↓

Anemia

↓

Aldosterone adrenal

↓

Increased myocardial depressant factor secretion

↓

Increased myocardial insufficiency

Contd...

Contd...

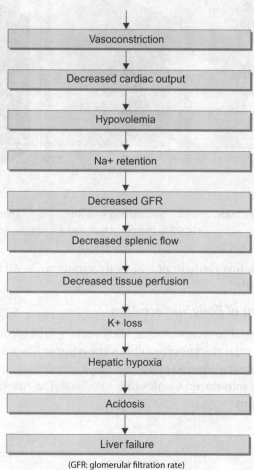

(GFR: glomerular filtration rate)

Clinical Manifestation

- **Fluid and electrolyte imbalance:** The burn wound become rapidly edematous due to microvascular changes induced by direct thermal injury and by release of chemical mediators of inflammation. This results in systemic intravascular losses of water, sodium, albumin, and red blood cells (RBCs). Unless the intravascular volume is rapidly restored, shock develops.
- **Metabolic disturbance:** This is evidenced by increased resting oxygen consumption, an excessive nitrogen loss, and a pronounced weight loss.
- **Bacterial contamination of tissues:** The damaged integument creates a vast area for surface infection and invasion of microorganisms. Increased risk of septic shock.
- **Complications from vital organs:** All the major organ systems are affected by the burn injury. Renal insufficiency can result from nephron obstruction with myoglobulin and hemoglobulin. Multisystem organ failure is a common final pathway leading to late burn mortality.

Diagnostic Studies in Burn

- **Complete blood count:** Initial increased hematocrit (Hct) suggests hemoconcentration due to fluid shift/loss. Later decreased Hct and RBCs may occur because of heat damage to vascular endothelium. Leukocytosis can occur because of loss of cells at wound site and inflammatory response to injury.
- **Arterial blood gases:** Reduced PaO_2 and increased $PaCO_2$ may be seen with carbon monoxide retention. Acidosis may occur because of reduced renal function and loss of respiratory compensatory mechanism.
- **Carboxyhemoglobin:** Elevation of >15% indicates carbon monoxide poisoning.
- **Alkaline phosphate:** Elevated because of interstitial fluid shift.
- **Serum glucose:** Elevated
- **Blood urea nitrogen:** Elevated
- **Urine:** Reddish-black color of urine is due to presence of myoglobin.
- **ECG:** Sign of myocardial ischemia/dysrhythmias may occur with electrical burn.
- **Electrolyte imbalance**

Burn Management and Plastic Surgeries

The burn patients have the same priorities as all other trauma patients.

Assess

- Airway
- Breathing: It is necessary to be aware of inhalation and rapid airway compromise
- Circulation: Fluid replacement
- Disability: Compartment syndrome
- Exposure: Percentage area of burn

Essential Management Points

- The burning should be stopped.
- ABCDE.
- The percentage area of burn should be determined (the rule of 9s).
- Good IV access and early fluid replacement

Determination of Severity of the Burn

- Burned surface area
- Depth of burn
- Other considerations
- Morbidity and mortality rise with increasing burned surface area
- It also rises with increasing age so that even small burns may be fatal in elderly people.

Burn Management in Adults

- The "rule of 9s" is commonly used to estimate the burned surface area in adults **(Fig. 20.3)**.
- The body is divided into anatomical regions that represent 9% (or multiples of 9%) of the total body surface. The outstretched palm and fingers approximate to 1% of the body surface area.

- If the burned area is small, it should be assessed how many times patient's hand covers the area.
- Morbidity and mortality rise with increasing burned surface area. It also rises with increasing age so that even small burns may be fatal in elderly people.

Anatomic surface	Percentage of total body surface
Head and neck	9
Anterior trunk	18
Posterior trunk	18
Arms, including hands	9 each
Legs, including feet	18 each
Genitalia	1

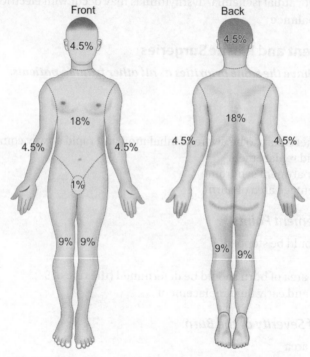

Fig. 20.3: Rule of 9s for establishing extent of body surface burned.

Burn Management in Children

Burn management in children is as follows:

- The "rule of 9s" method is to imprecise for estimating the burned surface area in children because the infant or child's head and lower extremities represent different proportions of surface area than in an adult.
- Burns greater than 15% in an adult, greater than 10% in a child to elderly are serious **(Fig. 20.4)**.

Depth of burn	Characteristics	Cause
First-degree burn	➢ Erythema ➢ Pain ➢ Absence of blisters	Sunburn
Second-degree (partial thickness)	➢ Red or mottled ➢ Flash burns	Contact with hot liquids
Third-degree (full thickness)	➢ Dark and leathery ➢ Dry	➢ Fire ➢ Electricity or lightning ➢ Prolonged exposure to hot liquids/objects

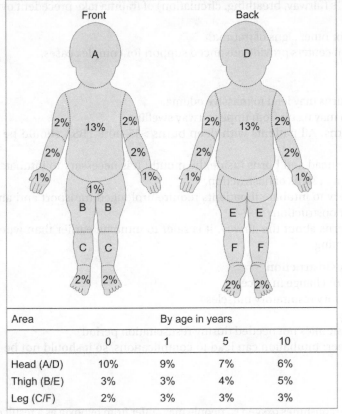

Area	By age in years			
	0	1	5	10
Head (A/D)	10%	9%	7%	6%
Thigh (B/E)	3%	3%	4%	5%
Leg (C/F)	2%	3%	3%	3%

Fig. 20.4: Estimating the burned surface area in children.

Depth of Burn

It is important to estimate the depth of the burn to assess its severity and to plan future wound care. Burns can be divided into three types, as shown below.

It is common to find all three types within the same burn wound and the depth may change with time, especially if infection occurs. Any full-thickness burn is considered serious.

Serious Burn Requiring Hospitalization

- Greater than 15% burns in an adult
- Greater than 10% burns in a child
- Any burn in the very the elderly or the infirm

- Any full-thickness burn
- Burns of special regions: face, hands, feet, perineum
- Circumferential burns
- Inhalation injury
- Associated trauma or significant preburn illness, for example, diabetes.

Treatment

- General information: All burn patients should initially be treated with the principles of advanced burn and/or trauma life support.
  - The ABC's (airway, breathing, circulation) of trauma take precedent over caring for the burn.
  - Search for other signs of trauma.
- Verified burn centers provide advanced support for complex cases.

Airway

- Extensive burns may lead to massive edema.
- Obstruction may result from upper airway swelling.
- Massive burns: All patients with deep burns >35–40% TBSA should be endotracheally intubated.
- Burns to the head and burns inside the mouth: It is necessary to intubate early if there is massive burn or signs of obstruction.
- It is necessary to intubate if patients require prolonged transport and any concern with potential for obstruction.
- If any concerns about the airway, it is safer to intubate earlier than when the patient is decompensating.

Signs of Airway Obstruction
- Hoarseness or change in voice
- Use of accessory respiratory muscles
- High anxiety
  - Tracheostomies not needed during resuscitation period
  - Remember: Intubation can lead to complications, so it should not be intubated if not needed.

Breathing

- Hypoxia: Fire consumes oxygen so people may suffer from hypoxia as a result of flame injuries.
- Carbon monoxide (CO).
  - Byproduct of incomplete combustion
  - Binds hemoglobin with 200 times the affinity of oxygen
  - Leads to inadequate oxygenation
  - Diagnosis of CO poisoning

Nondiagnostic
- PaO_2 (partial pressure of O_2 dissolved in serum)
- Oximeter (difference in oxy- and deoxyhemoglobin)
- Patient color ("cherry red" with poisoning)

Diagnostic
- Carboxyhemoglobin levels
- <10% is normal
- >40% is severe intoxication

Circulation

- Obtaining IV access anywhere possible
- Unburned areas preferred
- Burned areas acceptable
- Central access more reliable if proficient
- Cutdowns are the last resort

Resuscitation in Burn Shock (First 24 Hours)

- Massive capillary leak occurs after major burns.
- Fluids shift from intravascular space to interstitial space.
- Fluid requirements increase with greater severity of burn (larger percentage of TBSA, increase depth, inhalation injury, associate injuries—see above).
- Fluid requirements decrease with less severe burn (may be less than calculated rate).
- IV fluid rate dependent on physiologic response.
- Foley catheter should be placed to monitor urine output.
- Goal for adults: urine output of 0.5 mL/kg/h.
- Goal for children: urine output of 1 mL/kg/h.
- If urine output below these levels, fluid rate increases.
- Preferred fluid: lactated Ringer's solution.
- Isotonic
- Cheap
- Easily stored
- Resuscitation formulas are just a guide for initiating resuscitation.

Resuscitation Formulas

Parkland formula most commonly used.

- IV fluid—lactated Ringer's solution.
- Fluid calculation: 4 × weight in kg × % TBSA burn.
- 1/2 of that volume in the first 8 hours should be given.
- Other 1/2 in next 16 hours should be given.
- Warning: Despite the formula suggesting of cutting the fluid rate in half at 8 hours, the fluid rate should be gradually reduced throughout the resuscitation to maintain the targeted urine output, that is, not following the second part of the formula that says to reduce the rate at 8 hours, by adjusting the rate based on the urine output.

Example

- 100-kg man with 80% TBSA burn.
- Parkland formula: 4 × 100 × 80 = 32,000 mL, giving 1/2 in first 8 hours = 16,000 mL in first 8 hours, starting rate = 2,000 mL/h.
- Adjusting fluid rate to maintain urine output of 50 mL/h.
- Albumin may be added toward end of 24 hours if not adequate response.

Resuscitation endpoint

- When maintenance rate is reached (approximately 24 hours), fluids should be changed to D50.5NS with 20 mEq KCl at maintenance level.
- Maintenance fluid rate = basal requirements + evaporative losses.
- Basal fluid rate: Adult basal fluid rate = 1,500 × BSA (for 24 hours), pediatric basal fluid rate (<20 kg) = 2,000 × BSA (for 24 hours).
- Evaporative fluid loss: adult: (25+% TBSA burn) × BSA = mL/h, pediatric (<20 kg): (35+% TBSA burn) × BSA = mL/h.

WOUND CARE

First Aid

- If the patient arrives at the health facility without first aid having been given, the burn should be drenched thoroughly with cool water to prevent further damage and all burned clothing should be removed.
- If the burn area is limited, the site should be immersed in cold water for 30 minutes to reduce pain and edema and to minimize tissue damage.
- If the area of the burn is large, after it has been doused with cool water, clean wraps should be applied about the burned area (or the whole patient) to prevent systemic heat loss and hypothermia.
- Hypothermia is a particular risk.
- First 6 hours following injury are critical; the patient should be transported with severe burns to a hospital as soon as possible.

Initial Treatment

- Initially, burns are sterile. The treatment should be focused on speedy healing and prevention of infection.
- In all cases, tetanus prophylaxis should be administered.
- Except in very small burns, all bullae should be debrided. Adherent necrotic (dead) tissue should be excised initially, and all necrotic tissue over the first several days should be debrided.
- After debridement, the burn should be cleansed with 0.25% (2.5 g/L) chlorhexidine solution, 0.1% (1 g/L) cetrimide solution, or another mild water-based antiseptic.
- Alcohol-based solutions should not be used.
- Gentle scrubbing will remove the loose necrotic tissue. A thin layer of antibiotic cream (silver sulfadiazine) should be applied.
- The burn should be dressed with petroleum gauze and dry gauze thick enough to prevent seepage to the outer layers.

Daily Treatment

- The dressing should be changed daily (twice daily if possible) or as often as necessary to prevent seepage through the dressing. On each dressing, any loose tissue should be changed and removed.
- The wounds for discoloration or hemorrhage should be inspected, which indicate developing infection.
- Fever is not a useful sign as it may persist until the burn wound is closed.
- Cellulitis in the surrounding tissue is a better indicator of infection.
- Systemic antibiotics should be given in cases of hemolytic streptococcal wound infection or septicemia.
- *Pseudomonas aeruginosa* infection often results in septicemia and death. It should be treated with systemic aminoglycosides.
- Topical antibiotic chemotherapy should be administered daily. Silver nitrate (0.5% aqueous) is the cheapest, which is applied with occlusive dressings but does not penetrate eschar. It depletes electrolytes and stains the local environment.
- Silver sulfadiazine (1% miscible ointment) with a single layer dressing. It has limited eschar penetration and may cause neutropenia.
- Mafenide acetate (11% in a miscible ointment) is used without dressings. It penetrates eschar but causes acidosis. Alternating these agents is an appropriate strategy.

Treating Burned Hands with Special Care to Preserve Function

- The hands should be covered with silver sulfadiazine and placed in loose polythene gloves or bags secured at the wrist with a crepe bandage.
- The hands should be elevated for the first 48 hours, and then hand exercises should be started.
- At least once a day, the gloves should be removed, the hands are to be bathed, the burn should be inspected and then silver sulfadiazine and the gloves should be reapplied.
- If skin grafting is necessary, treatment should be considered by a specialist after healthy granulation tissue appears.

Healing Phase

- The depth of the burn and the surface involved influence the duration of the healing phase. The superficial burns heal rapidly without infection.
- Split thickness skin grafts should be applied to full-thickness burns after wound excision or the appearance of healthy granulation tissue.
- It is necessary to plan to provide long-term care to the patient.
- Burn scars undergo maturation, at first being red, raised, and uncomfortable. They frequently become hypertrophic and form keloids. They flatten, soften, and fade with time, but the process is unpredictable and can take up to 2 years.

In Children

- The scars cannot expand to keep pace with the growth of the child and may lead to contractures.
- It is necessary to arrange for early surgical release of contractures before they interfere with growth.
- Burnt scars on the face lead to cosmetic deformity, ectropion, and contractures about the lips. Ectropion can lead to exposure keratitis and blindness and lip deformity restricts eating and mouth care.
- It is necessary to consider specialized care for these patients as skin grafting is often not sufficient to correct facial deformity.

OTHER WOUND CARE METHODS

1. **Exposure method:** Leaving a burn open is a poor option but where dressings are not possible it may be the only option. The patients are washed daily and kept of clean dry sheets with another sheet or mosquito net draped over a frame to reduce the pain from air currents and to reduce contamination from the environment. Ambient temperature control is important to maintain normothermia. Exposure is less painful for full-thickness burns than for partial-thickness burns but has little else to recommend it.
2. **Tubbing:** Most modern burn units avoid the regular immersion of patients in water both because they practice early excision and grafting and because of the high risks developing resistant strains of bacteria in the tub environment and of patient cross infection. It is said that tubbing can be helpful to clean the wounds that gently removes eschar as it separates. When early wound infections develop the tub should be suspected. It is necessary to avoid the routine immersion of infected patients in filthy bathtubs of cold water on the basis of ignorance and tradition.
3. **Bland dressings:** These provide a clean, moist wound healing environment, absorb exudates, protect from contamination, and provide comfort at a fraction of the cost of

antibiotic dressings. Where antibiotic dressings are scarce bland dressings are a very acceptable solution for burns. Expensive topical antibiotic dressings may be reserved for infected wounds. Paraffin gauze is widely available and can be manufactured locally. Honey and ghee dressings were first advocated in Ayurvedic texts 2,000 years ago and remain an excellent choice for bland burn dressings. Two parts honey is mixed with one part ghee (clarified butter), and a stack of gauze dressings is poured over in a tray. It should be covered and stored. Vegetable oil or mineral oil may be substituted for ghee. Gauze sheets can be applied directly to the wound in a single layer and covered with plain dry gauze to absorb exudates, then wrapped. Dressings should be changed at least ever second day, or when soiled.

4. **Antimicrobial dressing:** There exist numerous topical antimicrobial agents that are effective in delaying the onset of invasive wound infections, but none prevent them entirely. This is why they must be used in conjunction with a goal of early surgical wound closure when possible. A brief review of the agents most likely to be available to low- and middle-income countries will follow. There are also alternative synthetic wound coverings and newer silver-ionized agents that can be used; however, they are often very costly and inaccessible in low-income countries. A more detailed review, as well as instructions for preparation, can be found in these references.

BURN WOUND DRESSINGS

ANTIMICROBIAL SALVES	
Silver sulfadiazine (Flamazine, Silvadene)	Broad-spectrum antimicrobial, painless and easy to use, does not penetrate eschar, deeply may leave black tattoos from silver ion; mild inhibition of epithelialization
Mafenide acetate (Sulfamylon)	Broad-spectrum antimicrobial; penetrates eschar well; may cause pain in sensate skin; wide application causes metabolic acidosis, therefore only suitable for small areas; mild inhibition of epithelialization
Bacitracin	Ease of application; painless; antimicrobial spectrum not as wide as above agents
Neomycin	Ease of application; painless; antimicrobial spectrum not as wide
Polymyxin B	Ease of application; painless; antimicrobial spectrum not as wide
Nystatin (Mycostatin)	Effective in inhibiting most fungal growth; cannot be used in combination with mafenide acetate
Mupirocin (Bactroban)	More effective staphylococcal coverage; does not inhibit epithelialization; expensive
Antimicrobial soaks	
0.5% silver nitrate	Effective against all microorganisms; stains contacted areas; leaches sodium from wounds; may cause methemoglobinemia
5% mafenide acetate	Wide antibacterial coverage; no fungal coverage; painful on application to sensate wound; wide application associated with metabolic acidosis, and therefore generally used for small high-risk areas such as cartilage coverage in nose and ears
0.025% sodium hypochlorite (Dakin's solution)	Effective against almost all microbes, particularly gram-positive organisms; mildly inhibits epithelialization
0.25% acetic acid	Effective against most organisms, particularly gram-negative ones; mildly inhibits epithelialization
Synthetic coverings	
Opsite	Provides a moisture barrier; inexpensive; decreased wound pain; use complicated by accumulation of transudate and exudate requiring removal; no antimicrobial properties
Biobrane	Provides a wound barrier; associated with decreased pain; use complicated by accumulation of exudate risking invasive wound infection; no antimicrobial properties
TransCyte	Provides a wound barrier; decreased pain; accelerated wound healing; use complicated by accumulation of exudate; no antimicrobial properties

Contd...

Contd...

Integra	Provides complete wound closure and leaves a dermal equivalent; sporadic take rates; no antimicrobial properties. Allows for coverage with a very thin skin graft with no dermis. Very expensive product
Biologic coverings	
Xenograft (pig skin)	Completely closes the wound; provides some immunologic benefits; must be removed or allowed to slough
Allograft (homograft, cadaver skin)	Provides all the normal functions of skin; can leave a dermal equivalent; epithelium must be removed or allowed to slough

Essentials of Burn Reconstruction

❖ Strong patient–surgeon relationship
❖ Psychological support
❖ Clarify expectations
❖ Explain priorities
❖ Note all available donor sites
❖ Start with a "winner" (easy and quick operation)
❖ As many surgeries as possible in preschool years
❖ Offer multiple, simultaneous procedures
❖ Reassure and support patient

Escharotomy

An escharotomy is defined as a surgical incision through burn eschar (necrotic skin). This procedure is usually performed within the first 24 hours of burn injury. Burn eschar has an unyielding, leathery consistency and is characterized by denatured proteins and coagulated vessels in the skin, which are the result of thermal, chemical or electrical injury.

Technique: Escharotomy (incision through the eschar) releases the constricting tissue allowing the body tissues and organs to maintain their normal perfusion and function. In most cases a single incision is inadequate to provide release of the constricting burn eschar. Escharotomy incisions are routinely performed on both sides of the torso or the medial and lateral sides of each affected limb. For the abdomen and chest, transverse incisions are often required to permit restoration of respiratory movement. The escharotomy procedure is most commonly performed using conscious sedation at bedside, in emergency room, hydrotherapy room, or ICU but may be done in operating room if general anesthesia is required.

Escharotomies release the constriction caused by burn eschar but do not remove the eschar. Once the patient is stable enough to be taken to the operating room, generally between the second to seventh days postburn, the burn eschar is excised to the level of viable underlying tissue. In some cases, escharotomies are performed through partial-thickness burns (second-degree burns), which will eventually heal without the need for excision and grafting. Delayed primary closure of escharotomy incisions may produce better functional and cosmetic results than those achieved if the escharotomies are allowed to close by secondary intention.

Debridement of Burn Wounds

Debridement is the removal of loose, devitalized, necrotic, and/or contaminated tissue, foreign bodies, and other debris on the wound using mechanical or sharp techniques (such as curetting, scraping, rongeuring, or cutting). The level of debridement is defined by the level of the tissue removed, not the level exposed by the debridement process.

Purpose: Debridement cleans the wound and allows it to heal more rapidly with reduced risk of infection.

Technique: Debridement can be accomplished in a number of ways using same surgical instruments used for excision.

Excision of Burn Wounds

Excision is a surgical procedure requiring incision through the deep dermis (including subcutaneous and deeper tissues) of open wounds, burn eschar, or burn scars. This entails surgical removal of all necrotic tissue. Burn scars can also be excised in preparation for surgical reconstruction.

Purpose: Excision is typically performed on deep burns that would not heal on their own. The goal is to remove all necrotic and nonviable tissue and to prepare the wound for immediate or delayed wound closure. The skin and subcutaneous tissues are removed followed by wound care (such as application of topical antimicrobials, temporary biologic or synthetic wound covers), immediate or later grafting, flap closure, and other reconstructive procedures. Unlike debridement, excisional techniques create a wound surface that is fully vascularized and ready for application of temporary or permanent skin replacement or substitute.

Technique: Burn debridement (cleaning) and excision (escharectomy) are routinely performed by experienced burn surgeons. Though the techniques and instruments used for debridement and excision are often similar, burn excision is significantly more difficult and requires greater time and physical effort to achieve meticulous burn wound preparation for subsequent grafting with synthetic or biological materials.

The excisional technique may vary but is typically performed in one of two ways: tangential excision (which is usually performed on deep partial-thickness burns) and full-thickness excision.

- **Tangential excision** involves surgical removal of successive layers of the burn wound down to viable dermis.
- **Full-thickness excision**—often using electrocautery—involves removal of the burn wound down to viable subcutaneous tissue or to fascia.

Skin Grafting

This is often used for burn patients; skin is removed from one area of the body and transplanted to another. There are two types of skin graft: split-thickness grafts, in which just a few layers of outer skin are transplanted, and full-thickness grafts, which involve all of the dermis. There is usually permanent scarring that is noticeable.

During a skin graft, a special skin-cutting instrument known as a dermatome removes the skin from an area (the donor site) usually hidden by clothing such as the buttocks or inner thigh. Once removed, the graft is placed on the area in need of covering and held in place by a dressing and a few stitches. The donor site is also covered with a dressing to prevent infection from occurring. Recovery time from a split-thickness skin graft is generally fairly rapid, often <3 weeks. For full-thickness skin graft patients, the recovery time is a few weeks longer. Aside from burn patients, skin grafts can also be used during breast or nose reconstruction.

Single- and Multiple-Stage Excision and Grafting

Single-stage Excision and Grafting

Surgical closure of burn wounds achieves two goals. The first is to facilitate optimal and rapid healing of the wound, minimizing deleterious consequences such as scar contracture while maximizing the best functional and cosmetic outcomes. The second is to ameliorate the adverse influence of the burn wounds on the body's systemic responses, especially the immune and metabolic systems. Meticulous-wound preparation and application of skin grafts lead to excellent functional and cosmetic results, but this becomes progressively more difficult in patients with more extensive burn injuries. In life-threatening burns, procedures which improve patient survival by reducing wound infection, hypermetabolism, and immunosuppression assume priority over those which may optimize later functional and cosmetic results.

The single-stage approach to excision and grafting of burn wounds includes **seven intraoperative components:**

- Initial decision-making—which is modified as necessary throughout the procedure—including:
  - Area(s) to be excised usually based on the patient's physiologic state as well as the degree to which the anticipated blood loss will be tolerated.
  - Depth of the excision, a complex decision involving the anticipated blood loss, the ability of the patient's excised wounds to support the growth of a newly transplanted skin graft, and considerations regarding long-term cosmetic results.
  - Location of donor sites, including the thickness of the skin to be harvested, the ease of dressing application, and the degree to which the donor site scar will remain masked by clothing in the future.
- Excision of the burn wound, with close monitoring of the patient's vital signs because of intraoperative blood loss.
- Achieving hemostasis with electrocautery and topical application of solutions containing vasoconstrictive agents (such as epinephrine or phenylephrine) and/or procoagulants (such as thrombin).
- Harvesting the donor skin (which may be preceded by subcutaneous injection of an electrolyte solution containing vasoconstrictive agents to reduce blood loss, as well as local anesthetics to reduce postoperative pain).
- Modification/expansion of the skin graft by meshing. Expansion is often necessary for patients with extensive burns and/or limited skin graft donor sites.
- Applying and securing the skin graft to the excised wound bed with some combination of absorbable or nonabsorbable sutures, staples, fibrin glue, synthetic adhesives, and/or tapes.
- Placement of dressings and splints to avoid mechanical shear of the grafts and to maintain proper positioning.
- It is clear that single-stage excision and grafting is a complex, time-consuming process, which is often physiologically stressful on the patient and may be poorly tolerated in patients with large burn injuries. It is ideal treatment for small burns in healthy patients.

Multiple-stage Excision and Grafting

The alternative to single-stage excision and grafting is to perform the necessary steps in a planned sequence where part of the burn wound is excised initially and the remainder is removed in one or more subsequent operations. This is often done with cosmetically important areas such as the face, as well as with more extensive burns or burns in physiologically less stable patients.

For patients with small burns that are located in functionally and cosmetically important areas, the excision is done on the initial operative day and the freshly excised wound bed is protected with a temporary covering to prevent desiccation and infection. This is followed in 1–2 days by harvesting and placement of the skin autografts. Staged skin grafting of face burns allows inspection for hematomas or inadequately excised areas that would lead to graft loss and can result in nearly 100% graft take.

- For patients with physiological challenges that increase the risk of complications with excision, concluding the initial operation after obtaining hemostasis reduces the chance of hypotensive complications. Temporary wound coverings can be expeditiously applied because they are prepackaged to simplify placement and because there is less need for careful placement of temporary coverings that will be removed within a few days.

- For patients with burns too extensive to be completely excised and grafted in one stage, multiple procedures allow safe removal of the eschar with improved graft take. Most often, the burn eschar is excised on the first few visits to the operating room, and the goal is for complete eschar removal within the first 5-7 days after injury. At the next operative procedure, the results of the first excision can be viewed, with further excision being performed and temporary dressings, skin substitutes, or skin replacements applied if needed. Sometimes by the time the last areas of burn are being excised on the third or fourth visit to the OR, the first areas of excision are ready for permanent autografting. The other advantage of staging the excision and grafting procedures is that donor sites are given time to re-epithelialize between harvesting sessions.

Burn Wound Coverage

Burn wound coverage is a unique surgical process. Simple, small burn wounds are excised and covered by either a full-thickness skin graft, in which the donor site is primarily closed, or by a split-thickness skin graft. Even though it seems a simple procedure, the surgeon must first choose the thickness to harvest the graft. He will then decide whether to mesh the graft (which would allow the drainage of fluid from beneath) or apply it as a sheet graft without perforations. The thicker the graft, the less it will contract, yet the more difficult it is to obtain 100% engraftment and the more difficult it is for the donor site to heal.

As the extent of the burn increases, the operative procedures and decision making become more complex. Early excision of burn wounds improves patient survival. However, excision alone without grafting leaves an open wound that must be covered in order to prevent infection, decrease fluid losses, and reduce the risk of scar contractures.

Skin Substitutes and Skin Replacements

Skin substitutes and skin replacements include:

- *Skin substitute:* A biomaterial, engineered tissue or combination of materials and cells or tissues that can be substituted for skin autograft or allograft in a clinical procedure.
- *Skin replacement:* A tissue or graft that permanently replaces lost skin with healthy skin.

Temporary Wound Coverage

Temporary skin substitutes are used when the wound is too extensive to be closed in one stage because there is not enough donor skin available, because the patient is too ill to undergo the creation of another wound that results when skin is harvested from a donor site, because there is a question regarding the viability of the recipient bed, or because of a concern regarding potential infectious complications. The gold standard temporary skin substitute is cadaver **allograft.**

- **Allograft:** Allograft is obtained from skin banks to ensure quality and safety. Allograft may be used as fresh, refrigerated tissue or as frozen tissue, which is thawed immediately prior to use will. Allograft adheres and induces vascularization on an appropriately prepared wound bed. It will decrease the loss of fluids, proteins, and electrolytes and drying of the recipient bed. It also decreases bacterial contamination, diminishes pain, improves the patient's ability to participate in all types of therapy, is a marker for the ability of the wound to accept an autograft, and promotes wound healing in partial-thickness wounds. In some patients, cultured keratinocytes can be applied onto the vascularized allodermis once the alloepidermis has been removed. Other temporary skin substitutes are used to provide transient wound coverage and to create a physiologically homeostatic environment. **Skin xenografts**—also termed heterografts.

- **Xenograft** (pigskin) is used at many institutions in the same manner as allograft. The application of xenograft on a debrided mid-dermal burn might prevent/obviate the need for excision and autografting.

Permanent Wound Coverage

Permanent wound coverage is as follows:

- A **full-thickness skin graft** contains all components of the skin: epidermis, dermis, hair follicles and nerve endings. The most important advantage of full-thickness grafts is decreased scar formation; however, because there is no dermis to regenerate epithelial coverage, the donor site of a full-thickness skin graft must be closed either with primary direct closure or with a split-thickness skin graft; local advancement of skin flaps is a rarely used option. Full-thickness grafts are thus usually used to cover small, functionally and cosmetically important areas (such as eyelids and digits).

- The **split-thickness skin graft** is the most common method used to achieve permanent wound coverage. It includes the entire epidermis but the dermal layer is split by the dermatome blade. With thicker split-thickness grafts, more dermis is transferred with the skin graft (such as 15/1,000 of inch or greater). This reduces the risk of scar formation at the recipient site, but it takes longer for the donor site to heal. Furthermore, the thicker the graft, the more likely the donor site will heal with a scar and the less likely the donor site may be reharvested for further grafts. There are a number of commercially available products to facilitate permanent wound coverage.

- **Acellular human dermal allograft** is devoid of epidermis and must be covered by a thin-split-thickness autograft at the time of the initial operation; however, it replaces a portion of the missing dermis on the newly covered wound, thus reducing postoperative scarring. Another permanent wound coverage product is a **dermal regenerative template** constructed with bovine collagen and shark chondroitin sulfate with a silicone surface layer. This is applied to an excised wound bed that is well vascularized and free from infection and provides wound coverage much like other skin substitutes; however, after the template becomes vascularized, it forms a neodermis (usually within 10 days to 3 weeks) and when the silicone layer is removed, an epidermal autograft (<0.008 inches thickness) can be applied. This intermingling of autograft on a biosynthetic neodermis is permanent, unlike the wound coverage provided by temporary skin substitutes. This approach may be lifesaving and provides quality skin coverage.

- Cultured epidermal autograph (CEA), also referred to as "test tube" skin, was introduced to provide permanent skin coverage for patients with extensive burns. This product has limitations, including sensitivity to infection and the lack of a dermis, which leads to fragility of the healed skin and severe scarring. However, the short- and long-term results of CEA application can be improved by the use of a sandwich technique, in which CEA is applied over a vascularized allogeneic dermis or alloderm. If the CEA is applied to a well-vascularized dermal bed, the dermis is created by using allograft that is allowed to engraft and remove the epidermis after the dermis is vascularized.

Others

- **Microsurgery:** Have patient lost a finger, toe, ear, or even a lip? Microsurgery may allow for those to be reattached. Simply stated, it is a procedure in which the surgeon uses a microscope for surgical assistance in reconstructive procedures. By using a microscope, the surgeon can actually sew tiny blood vessels or nerves, allowing him or her to repair damaged nerves and arteries. This may also be a method to relieve facial paralysis or reconstruct breasts. Microsurgery is frequently used with other surgical procedures such as the free flap procedure.

- **Free flap procedure:** A free flap procedure is often performed during breast reconstruction or following surgery to remove head or neck cancer. During the procedure, muscle, skin, or bone is transferred along with the original blood supply from one area of the body (donor site) to the surgical site in order to reconstruct the area. The procedure often involves the use of microsurgery. Healing of the surgical site can be slow and require frequent wound care. Total recovery may take 6–8 weeks or longer.

- **Tissue expansion:** Tissue expansion is a medical procedure that enables patient's body to "grow" extra skin for use in reconstructive procedures. This is accomplished by inserting an instrument known as a "balloon expander" under the skin near the area in need of repair. Over time, this balloon will be gradually filled with saline solution (salt water), slowly causing the skin to stretch and grow, and much the same way a woman's skin stretches during pregnancy. Once enough extra skin has been grown, it is then used to correct or reconstruct a damaged body part. This procedure is especially common for breast reconstruction.

Tissue expansion has many advantages; in that, the skin color and texture are a near perfect match for the area in which it is needed, and there is little scarring since there is no removal of skin from one area to another. The major drawback to tissue expansion is the length of the procedure, which can be as long as 4 months. During this period, as the balloon expander grows, the bulge under the skin grows with it. This bulge may be desirable for a breast reconstruction patient; however, for patients undergoing this procedure for scalp repair, the bulge may be uncomfortably noticeable.

Dealing with Deficiency of Tissue

At this point, the burn injury must be assessed for deficiency in tissue. If there is no deficiency and local tissues can be easily mobilized, excision and direct closure or Z-plasties can be performed.

Traditional Z-plasty to release a burn scar contracture. (1) The burn scar, showing the skin tension lines. (2) Z-plasty is performed by rotating two transposition flaps with an angle of 60° with the middle limb of the Z on the scar. (3) Final appearance after insetting of flaps. The lengthening of the tissue and the change of scar pattern should be noted. Z-plasties can be combined with other flaps (five-limb Z-plasty, seven-limb Z-plasty, etc.).

Skin Changes after Cosmetic Surgery

As patient continues to heal, patient will notice changes in the color, appearance, and feeling of patient's skin at the surgical site. Patient also may notice numbness, a tingling sensation, or minimal feeling around patient's incisions. This is normal. These sensations will continue to improve over the next few months.

Perfusion and Circulation after Cosmetic Surgery

After patient's cosmetic surgery, it is important to monitor perfusion (passage of fluid) and circulation of the wound site. Wearing clothing that constricts or applies pressure around patient's wound should be avoided. Also, patient's doctor may give patient additional instructions to help with circulation to the wound.

Signs of Infection at the Surgical Site

The following are signs indicating that there may be an infection at the surgical site. Patient's doctor should be notified right away if patient experiences any of the following symptoms:

- White pimples or blisters around incision lines.
- An increase in redness, tenderness, or swelling of the surgical site.
- Drainage from the incision line. Occasionally, a small amount of bloody or clear yellow-tinged fluid may drain. The patient's doctor should be notified if it persists or if it changes in consistency.
- A marked or sudden increase in pain not relieved by the pain medication.

Patient may experience some other, more general signs of infection that will require medical treatment. If the patient notices any of the following symptoms of infection, it is important that patient should call patient's health care provider as soon as possible:

- A persistent elevation of body temperature greater than 100.5°F (The patient's temperature should be taken daily, at the same time each day).
- Sweats or chills
- Skin rash
- Sore or scratchy throat or pain when swallowing
- Sinus drainage, nasal congestion, headaches, or tenderness along the upper cheekbones
- Persistent, dry or moist cough that lasts more than 2 days
- White patches in patient's mouth or on patient's tongue
- Nausea, vomiting, or diarrhea
- Trouble urinating: pain or burning, constant urge or frequent urination
- Bloody, cloudy, or foul-smelling urine

POSTOPERATIVE DAILY EVALUATION AND MANAGEMENT

Operated Burn Wounds

Despite the most attentive precautions in the operating room, many patients will return to the burn intensive care unit with hypothermia, which is treated by increasing the ambient temperature of the patient's room and positioning portable heating units over the patient's bed. As the patient's body temperature begins to rise toward normal, vasoconstriction in the periphery abates and the patient becomes tachycardiac, hypovolemic, and oliguric. The hypovolemia of rewarming can be anticipated and treated with the infusion of additional crystalloid fluids run through a fluid warmer.

In most cases, the postoperative care of burn patients following excision and grafting is uncomplicated. Any fluid and electrolyte replacements are corrected and adequate nutritional intake is assured. Many patients can begin a regular diet the morning following surgery unless they are ventilator dependent. Continuation and/or resumption of enteral feedings begins in critically ill patients as soon as there is evidence of bowel function. Combinations of short- and long-acting narcotics and benzodiazepines are used for pain relief and sedation.

The dressings and splints are typically removed on the fourth or fifth day following skin grafting; they may, however, be reapplied for a more lengthy period of time in order to maintain proper positioning. Physical and occupational therapy resumes at this time, and patients are encouraged to resume as much independent activity as possible. For patients with smaller burns, discharge typically occurs within 48 hours of removing the dressings.

Many options are available for postoperative care of skin grafts. Grafts and donor sites should be kept clean, moist and covered. After discharge, patients return weekly to the outpatient clinic until all wounds, including donor sites, have re-epithelialized and satisfactory progress is being made in therapy. Monthly or bimonthly visits for up to 6 months are necessary to ensure that patients achieve optimal restoration of functional capabilities, including range of motion, strength and endurance, and return to their preinjury work status.

Care of Burn Wounds Unrelated to Previously Operated Wounds

Not all burn wounds require surgical intervention. Superficial second-degree burns will close within 2 weeks and require only moist antimicrobial dressings. These second-degree burns need to be monitored closely by experienced nurses and burn doctors since infections such as cellulitis are common and can result in extension of the depth of the burn. In addition, the progress of patients in physical and occupational therapy must be monitored, and pain medications frequently adjusted. For these reasons, daily evaluation and management of nonoperatively treated burn wounds merit recognition in the reimbursement process.

Unrelated Conditions

Thermal injuries result in perturbation of many systemic processes. Metabolic rate is increased, sometimes to double that of the uninjured healthy person. Because of increased metabolism, carbon dioxide production is greatly increased, resulting in the need for augmented minute ventilation. The immune system is impaired, and bacterial and fungal infections are common. Management of pain and anxiety are challenging because of the magnitude of physical discomfort and emotional distress.

Many patients with extensive thermal injuries, inhalation injuries or multiple comorbid conditions require intensive care in specialized units. ICU care includes management of fluids and electrolytes, assessment of airway, management of mechanical ventilators, establishment and evaluation of nutritional supplementation, and monitoring and treatment of infectious processes. The physician skills required for the management of these complex patients come only with residency and fellowship training programs that emphasize critical care. The surgical skills needed to treat burn patients in the perioperative period are related but not identical to the requisite critical care skills. For this reason, billing for critical care services during the 90-day global period for skin grafting is a legitimate and well-recognized service for the treatment of medical conditions unrelated to the management of the postoperative burn wound.

POSTDISCHARGE BURN WOUND MANAGEMENT

Discharge and Follow-Up

Following discharge from the hospital, the condition of the burn patient ranges from fully independent at home to completely dependent in a skilled nursing facility. At the point of discharge, the patient is typically breathing without continuous ventilatory support, is hemodynamically stable, and is showing no signs of sepsis. However, there may be resolving conditions still requiring treatment, such as infections, open wounds, and the need for nutritional support. Some patients are discharged on intravenous antibiotics; others finish their prescribed courses with oral agents. Most burn patients still have open wounds or donor sites at the time of discharge; more discussion follows later. Some are still receiving enteral feedings through feeding tubes, often because they have not successfully passed a swallowing evaluation. The resolution of these issues may require 3 months or more, and progress is monitored in the outpatient clinic or at the rehabilitation/skilled nursing facility.

Open wounds are present in nearly all patients discharged from burn centers. These may be second-degree burns which are being allowed to epithelialize on their own without surgery. There may also be unhealed donor sites that were created for split-thickness autografting. In addition, many third-degree burns that have been grafted do not have 100% graft take (adherence and vascularity leading to viable incorporation of the graft), and there may be areas of granulation tissue that eventually heal by secondary intention (horizontal migration of epithelial cells and contraction of the wound). These open areas of third-degree burns may be small (1-2 mm) or much larger. Most wounds require daily care which may range from one–three dressing changes daily.

Follow-Up

Scar Prevention

For burns that take longer than 3 weeks to heal or for wounds that have been grafted, hypertrophic scarring can be minimized with the use of compression therapy with custom-made garments that apply 25–30 mm Hg pressure to all wounds. Gel pads can be added underneath or sewn into the garments to apply extra compression. Compression therapy is continued throughout the wound healing process (approximately 12–18 months). Lotion application with massage therapy is used to keep the healed or grafted areas soft and supple.

Contracture Prevention

Contractures refer to hypertrophic scar formation over joints that result in decreased range of motion. Aggressive attention to occupational and physical therapy, with appropriate consultation, is necessary to ensure optimal results. Active and passive ranges of motion exercises are instituted and splints are worn at night and between exercise periods. Patients with burns are at risk for contractures and are followed for years to monitor for the development of these complications.

Psychological Sequelae

Burn scarring can lead to significant psychological sequelae and the assistance of a trained psychologist or psychiatrist can be an important addition to the overall care of these patients.

NUTRITIONAL MANAGEMENT

Assessment

All inpatients with a deep burn injury are assessed by a dietician, in order to establish whether a need exists for nutritional intervention.

Goals of Nutritional Management

- To promote optimal wound healing and rapid recovery from burn injuries
- To minimize risk of complications, including infections during the treatment period
- To attain and maintain normal nutritional status
- To minimize metabolic disturbances during the treatment process

Objectives of Nutritional Management

- Providing nutrition via enteral route within 6–18 hours postburn injury
- Maintaining weight within 5–10% of preburn weight
- Preventing signs and symptoms of micronutrient deficiency
- Minimizing hyperglycemia
- Minimizing hypertriglyceridemia

Nutritional Management

Enteral Feeding should be Commenced Early

Appropriate nutritional management of the severely burned patient is necessary to ensure optimal outcome. Initiation of early enteral feeding, within 6–18 hours postburn injury, is recognized as beneficial and has been shown to be safe in children and in adults. Advantages of utilizing the enteral route, as opposed to the parenteral route, include improved nitrogen balance, reduced hypermetabolic response, and reduced immunological complications and mortality.

Aggressive Nutritional Support is Often Required

Although oral nutrition is encouraged, young children with severe burn injuries often require nasogastric feeding as they tend to have difficulty meeting their nutritional goals with oral intake alone.

Energy Requirements are Elevated by the Burn Injury

The hypermetabolic response associated with severe burn injury results in high-calorie requirements to allow optimal healing and outcome. Several predictive equations exist which enable estimations of energy requirements. Changes in management of these patients in the past decade have resulted in some reduction in the metabolic response and care must be taken to avoid overfeeding. Variation in energy is needed between individuals, as well as with time, means that indirect calorimetry is recommended where practical to aid in determining energy expenditure.

Protein Requirements are Substantially Increased

Aggressive protein delivery, providing approximately 20% of calories from protein, has been associated with improved mortality and morbidity.

An increased requirement exists for nutrients associated with healing and immune function. Provision of those nutrients known to be associated with healing and immune function, particularly vitamins A, C, E, some B vitamins and zinc, is especially important. Recent studies have indicated that benefits may also be achieved by supplementation with various additives, including fish oil and arginine.

COMPLICATIONS OF SURGERIES FOR BURN MANAGEMENT

Complications to surgery in patients with burns include bleeding, infection, or graft loss. If infection is suspected, dressings can be changed to include broad-spectrum aqueous Sulfamylon solution.

Outcome and prognosis: With the exception of infants, the prognosis for survival in children and adolescents is quite good. In the past decade, the size of a survivable injury has increased from 70% BSA burned to more than 95% BSA burned in children younger than 15 years.

NURSING MANAGEMENT

Assessment

- Obtaining thorough history, including causative agent, duration of exposure, circumstances of injury, age, initial treatment taken, pre-existing medical problems, allergies, tetanus immunization, height, and weight
- Performing ongoing assessment of hemodynamic and respiratory status, condition of wounds, and signs of infection.

Nursing Diagnosis

Ineffective Gas Exchange Related to Inhalation Injury

Goal: Achieving adequate oxygenation and respiratory functions

Interventions:
- Providing humidified 100% oxygen until CO level is known
- Assessing for signs of hypoxemia
- Noting character and amount of respiratory secretions
- Providing mechanical ventilation when required

Decreased Cardiac Output Related to Fluid Shift and Hypovolemic Shock

Goal: Supporting cardiac output

Interventions:
- Positioning the patient to increase venous return
- Giving fluids as prescribed
- Monitoring vital signs
- Checking level of conscious

Ineffective Peripheral Tissue Perfusion Related to Edema

Goal: Promoting peripheral circulation

Interventions:
- Removing all jewelry and clothing
- Elevating extremities
- Monitoring peripheral pulses hourly
- Monitoring tissue pressure

Risk for Infection Related to Reconstructive Surgeries

Goal: Preventing risk for infections.

Interventions:
- Checking vital signs
- Assessing signs of wound infection—redness and discharge
- Changing dressing as prescribed
- Applying antibiotic topically and also administer through IV route

Other Nursing Diagnosis

- Risk for excess fluid volume related to fluid resuscitation
- Impaired skin integrity related to burn injury and surgical intervention
- Impaired urinary elimination related to indwelling catheter
- Ineffective thermoregulation related to loss of skin surface
- Impaired physical mobility related to edema, pain, skin, and joint contractures
- Impaired nutrition less than body requirement related to hypermetabolic response to burn injury
- Risk for injury related to decreased gastric mobility and stress response
- Acute pain related to injured nerves in burn wound and skin tightness
- Ineffective coping related to fear and anxiety
- Disturbed body image related to cosmetic and functional sequelae of burn wound

MULTIPLE CHOICE QUESTIONS

1. **A 65-year-old man patient has experienced full-thickness electrical burns on the legs and arms. As a nurse you know this patient is at a risk for the following: Select all that apply:**
   A. Acute kidney injury   B. Dysrhythmia
   C. Iceberg effect   D. Hypernatremia
   E. Bone fractures   F. Fluid volume overload

2. **A patient who experiences an alkali chemical burn is easier to treat because the skin will neutralize the chemical rather than with an acidic chemical burn. True or False**
   A. True   B. False

3. **As a nurse providing care to a patient who experienced a full-thickness electrical burn, you know to monitor the patient's urine for:**
   A. Hemoglobin and myoglobin
   B. Free iron and white blood cells
   C. Protein and red blood cells
   D. Potassium and urea

4. **Select the patient below who is at most risk for complications following a burn:**
   A. A 42-year-old man with partial-thickness burns on the front of the right and left arms and legs.
   B. A 25-year-old woman with partial-thickness burns on the front of the head and neck and front and back of the torso.
   C. A 36-year-old man with full-thickness burns on the front of the left arm.
   D. A 10-year-old with superficial burns on the right leg.

5. **The _____ layer of the skin helps regulate our body temperature.**
   A. Epidermis   B. Dermis
   C. Hypodermis   D. Fascia

6. **You receive a patient who has experienced a burn on the right leg. You note the burn contains small blisters and is extremely pinkish red and shiny/moist. The patient reports severe pain. You document this burn as:**
   A. First degree (superficial)
   B. Second degree (partial thickness)
   C. Third degree (full thickness)
   D. Fourth degree (deep-full thickness)

7. **Based on the depth of the burn in figure 1 (picture is above), you would expect to find:**
   A. Report of sensation to only pressure
   B. Blanching
   C. Anesthetization to feeling
   D. Extreme pain

8. **A 58-year-old woman patient has superficial partial-thickness burns to the anterior head and neck, front and back of the left arm, front of the right arm, posterior trunk, front and back of the right leg, and back of the left leg. Using the rule of 9s, calculate the total body surface area percentage that is burned?**
   A. 63   B. 81
   C. 72   D. 54

9. **A 30-year-old woman patient has deep partial-thickness burns on the front and back of the right and left leg, front of right arm, and anterior trunk. The patient weighs 63 kg. Use the Parkland burn formula: What is the flow rate during the first 8 hours (mL/h) based on the total you calculated?**
   A. 921 mL/h
   B. 938 mL/h
   C. 158 mL/h
   D. 789 mL/h

10. **A patient has a burn on the back of the torso that is extremely red and painful but no blisters are present. When you pressed on the skin it blanches. You document this as a:**
   A. First-degree (superficial) burn
   B. Second-degree (partial-thickness) burn
   C. Third-degree (full-thickness) burn
   D. Fourth-degree (deep full-thickness) burn

Answers

1. A   2. A   3. D   4. C   5. D   6. D   7. B   8. D   9. B   10. D

BIBLIOGRAPHY

1. Achauer BM. Burn Reconstruction. New York: Thiene; 1991.
2. Barret JP, Herndon DN. Color Atlas of Burn Care. London: WB Saunders; 2001.
3. Brou JA, Robson MC, McCauley RL. Inventory of potential reconstructive needs in the patient with burns. J Burn Care Rehabil. 1989;10:555-60.
4. Brunner SA. Textbook of Medical Surgical Nursing, 5th edition. Philadelphia: Lippincott Company; 1982.
5. Engrav LH, Donelan MB. Operative Techniques in Plastic and Reconstructive Surgery. Face Burns: Acute Care and Reconstruction. London: WB Saunders; 1997.
6. Greenwood JE. Burn Injury and Explosions: An Australian Perspective. Eplasty. 2009;9:e40.
7. Holmes JH, 4th. Critical issues in burn care. J Burn Care Res. 2008;29(6 Suppl 2):S180-7.
8. Orgill DP. Excision and skin grafting of thermal burns. N Engl J Med. 2009;360(9):893-901.

Oncological Disorders

AT THE END OF THIS CHAPTER, THE STUDENTS WILL BE ABLE TO LEARN ABOUT THE
FOLLOWING NURSING MANAGEMENTS FOR PATIENTS WITH ONCOLOGICAL CONDITIONS

➤ Structure and characteristics of normal and cancer cells
➤ Nursing assessment—history and physical assessment
➤ Prevention screening, early detection, warning signs of cancer
➤ Epidemiology, etiology, classification
➤ Oncological emergencies
➤ Modalities of treatment
➤ Immunotherapy
➤ Chemotherapy
➤ Radiotherapy
➤ Surgical intervention
➤ Stem cell
➤ Bone marrow transplant
➤ Gene therapy
➤ Psychosocial aspect of cancer
➤ Rehabilitation
➤ Palliative care
➤ Home care
➤ Hospice care
➤ Stomal therapy
➤ Psychosocial aspects

CANCER

Cancer is an important public health concern in India and throughout the world. Body is composed of many millions of tiny cells, each a self-contained living unit. Normally, each cell coordinates with others that compose tissues and organs of your body. One way that this coordination occurs is reflected in how cells reproduce themselves. Normal cells in the body grow and divide for a period of time and then stop growing and dividing. Thereafter, they only reproduce themselves as necessary to replace defective or dying cells.

Cancer occurs when this cellular reproduction process goes out of control. In other words, cancer is a disease characterized by uncontrolled, uncoordinated, and undesirable cell division. Unlike normal cells, cancer cells continue to grow and divide for their whole lives, replicating into more and more harmful cells. Neoplasm means new growth that extends beyond the normal tissue boundaries.

The abnormal growth and division observed in cancer cells are caused by damage in these cells' DNA (genetic material inside cells that determines cellular characteristics and functioning). There are a variety of ways by which cellular DNA can become damaged and defective. For example, environmental factors (such as exposure to tobacco smoke) can initiate a chain of events that results in cellular DNA defects that lead to cancer. Alternatively, defective DNA can be inherited from your parents. As cancer cells divide and replicate themselves, they often form into a clump of cancer cells known as a tumor. Tumors cause many of the symptoms of cancer by pressuring, crushing, and destroying surrounding noncancerous cells and tissues.

The scope, responsibilities, and goals of cancer nursing, also called oncology nursing, are as diverse and complex as those of any nursing specialties.

Terminology Related to Cancer

- **Hypertrophy:** Hypertrophy is the increase in the volume of an organ or tissue due to the enlargement of its component cells.
- **Atrophy:** It is shrinkage in cell size leading to the decrease in organ size. The decrease in cell size is due to less blood supply, nutrition, etc. It is mostly associated with ageing.
- **Hyperplasia:** It is an increase in the number of the new cells in an organ or tissue, as cells multiply volume also increases. It is a mitotic response, but it is reversible when the stimulus is removed. This distinguishes it from malignant growth, which continues after the stimulus is removed. Hyperplasia may be hormonally induced. Example is breast changes of a girl in puberty or of a pregnant woman.
- **Metaplasia:** It is a cell transformation in which a highly specialized cell changes to a less specialized cell.
- **Differentiation:** It is the processes by which immature cells become mature cells with specific functions. In cancer, this describes how much or how little tumor tissue looks like the normal tissue it came from. Well-differentiated cancer cells look more like normal cells and tend to grow and spread more slowly than poorly differentiated or undifferentiated cancer cells. Differentiation is used in tumor grading systems, which are different for each type of cancer.

Characteristics of Cancer Cells

- **Pleomorphism:** Refers to variability in size and shape of cells and their nuclei.
- **Hyperchromatism:** It refers to the development of excess chromatin or of excessive nuclear staining.
- **Polymorphism:** The nucleus is large and varies in shape.
- **Aneuploidy:** It is a term used to describe a chromosome problem that is caused by an extra or missing chromosome.
- **Abnormal chromosome arrangements**
- **Loss of proliferative control:** In normal cell, cell production stops when stimulus is gone, producing a balance between cells growing and dying. But in cancer, proliferation continues once the stimulus initiates the process and progress to uncontrolled growth.
- **Loss of capacity to differentiate:** It is the processes by which immature cells become mature cells and acquire specific structural and functional characteristics. In cancer, this describes how much or how little tumor tissue looks like the normal tissue it came from. Well-differentiated cancer cells look more like normal cells and tend to grow and spread more slowly than poorly differentiated or undifferentiated cancer cells.
- **Chromosomal insatiability:** Cancer cells are genetically less stable than normal cells because of the development of abnormal chromosome arrangement.
- **Capacity of metastasis**: It is the capacity of cancer cells that they may spread from a primary site to distant sites, and it is aided by production of enzymes on the surface of the cancer cell.

Classification of Cancer

1. Tumors according to behavior come in two forms: benign and malignant

Characteristics	Benign	Malignant
Cell characteristics	Well-differentiated cell	Undifferentiated
Mode of growth	Does not infiltrate the surrounding tissues; usually encapsulated	Infiltrate and destroy the surrounding tissues
Rate of growth	Slow	Fast
Metastasis	Does not spread by metastasis	Metastasis occurs
General effects	Local effects	Generalized effects
Ability to cause death	Usually not cause death	Usually cause death
Reoccurrence	Rarely occur after removal	may occur after removal
Shape	Regular in shape	Irregular
Vascularity	Slight	Moderate to marked
Encapsulated	Usually	Rarely

2. Tumors according to histological analysis (appearance of cell and degree of differentiation)
   - **Grade I:** Cell differs slightly from parent cells.
   - **Grade II:** Cells are more abnormal and less differentiated.
   - **Grade III:** Very abnormal cells and poorly differentiated.
   - **Grade IV:** Cells will immature and undifferentiated.

Clinical Staging

- **Stage 0:** Carcinoma in situ
- **Stage 1:** Tumor is limited to the tissue of origin
- **Stage 2:** Limited local spread
- **Stage 3:** Extensive local and regional spread
- **Stage 4:** Metastasis

Etiology of Cancer

The etiology of cancer can be viewed from two perspectives: its molecular origins within individual cells and its external causes in terms of personal and community risks. Together, these perspectives form a multidimensional web of causation by which cancers arise from the interplay of casual events occurring in over time.

Host Factors

1. **Genetic factors:** About 5–10% of adult cancers arise in hereditary setting. Genes underlying hereditary cancer are involved in control of cell growth and differentiation or in DNA repair and maintenance of genomic integrity. They are oncogenes, tumor suppressor genes, and DNA repair genes. Characteristics of hereditary cancers also include early age onset, family history, and evidence of autosomal dominant transmission of cancer susceptibility.

2. **Hormones:** Endogenous hormones have received considerable research attention with respect to cancers of breast, ovary, and endometrium in women and those of prostate and testis in men. Neoplasia is a consequence of prolonged hormonal stimulation of the particular target organ, the normal growth, and function of which is controlled by one or more steroid or polypeptide hormones.

3. Female cancer sites demonstrate a clear etiologic role for endogenous estrogen (estradiol) in both breast and endometrial cancers and probable role for gonadotropin in ovarian cancer. In breast cancer, association of increased cancer risk with low parity, late age at

first birth, early menarche, late menopause, all of which are due to heightened exposure to endogenous estrogen. In endometrial cancer, the etiological role of estrogen is supported strongly by the fact that postmenopausal risk has increased greatly by estrogen replacement therapy in the absence of progesterone replacement. For ovarian cancers, estrogens do not appear to increase risk with oral contraceptive use suggest a role for gonadotropin.

4. **Immune mechanisms:** The occurrence of particular types of cancer under various conditions of immunological impairment supports the general concept that normal mechanism of immune-surveillance is important for the control of carcinogenesis. Certain cancers, especially non-Hodgkin's lymphoma, occur with increased frequency in persons treated with immune-suppression for tissue transplantation, etc.

Environmental Factors

- **Chemical factors:** Chemical origin of human malignancies—observation of unusual cancer incidences in certain occupational groups. Chemical carcinogens are organ specific and target epithelial cells. They are genotoxic or nongenotoxic. Genotoxic carcinogens have high chemical reactivity, can be metabolized to reactive intermediate by the host, and target DNA in nucleus and mitochondria. Mechanism action of nongenotoxic carcinogens is controversial.

    Known chemical carcinogens in humans
    - Lung—tobacco smoke, arsenic, asbestos
    - Pleura—asbestos
    - Oral cavity—tobacco smoke, alcohol, nickel compounds
    - Esophagus—tobacco, alcohol, smoke, salted, pickled foods
    - Colon—heterocyclic amines
    - Liver—aflatoxin, vinyl chloride, tobacco, alcohol
    - Kidney—tobacco smoke, phenacetin
    - Prostate—cadmium
    - Skin—arsenic, coal tar, soot, PUVA
    - Bone marrow—benzene, tobacco smoke, antineoplastic agents
- **Physical factors:** Radiation is of two types:
    - **Ionizing radiation**—X-rays, electrons, protons
    - **Nonionizing radiation**—Ultraviolet (UV) rays
- **Diet:** Major role of diet and nutrition in influencing cancer risk is well established.
    - Naturally occurring dietary carcinogens
        - **Natural pesticides:** Allyl isothiocyanate in cabbage, cauliflower, etc., hydrazine in mushrooms and pyrrolidine in herbal tea
        - **Mycotoxins:** Aflatoxins in corn, peanut, and ochratoxins in grains.
    - **Products of food preparation and processing:** Urethane in all fermented foods, heterocyclic aromatic amines in barbecued chicken, etc., and nitroso-compounds in cured meat and dairy cheese products.
    - **Synthetic carcinogens in diet (synthetic derivatives):**
        - Intentional: colorants, flavorants, sweetness
        - Unintentional: pesticides, solvents, and packaging derived chemicals.

Detection and Prevention of Cancer

Cancer develops in the body very silently until it becomes to certain stage, patient lead a normal life without any complaints. Initially, it produces mild symptoms as found in other ailments. Disease detected at an early stage produces better results on treatment and even cure, whereas advanced disease shows poor results on treatment.

Primary Prevention

The goal is to protect healthy people from developing a disease to reduce the impact of carcinogens:
- Reducing the risk of cancer
- Lifestyle modification to reduce the exposure to suspected carcinogens and promoting agents
- Eating balanced diet especially green-yellow (cabbage family) whole grains, fresh fruits
- Adequate fiber diet
- Regular exercise regime
- Adequate rest period in between work periods
- Having health examination regularly after 30 years
- Reducing the stress
- Enjoy consistent period of relaxation and leisure
- Increasing intake of vitamin A and vitamin C
- Reducing dietary fat, alcohol consumption, and smoking

Caution

As the word "caution" describes:

C—Changes in bathroom habits. This can be anything from changes in the bowel movements (watery or too hard) to frequency (going more often or infrequently). Any long-term changes in bathroom habits should be informed to your doctor.

A—A sore that does not heal. This can also be a sign of diabetes, but sores that do not heal within a usual amount of time need to be checked.

U—Unusual discharge and bleeding. Moles and freckles should not bleed or drain. Other unusual draining issues should be checked out as well.

T—Thickness or lumps in the breast or other places. Breast lumps can be cysts that are normal in the course of your menstrual cycle, or they can be the beginnings of breast tumors. If you notice a lump, have a mammogram to see if there is something there other than fluid.

I—Indigestion and difficulty in swallowing. Indigestion can come from many things; even very frequent indigestion can be a sign of acid reflux or other normal conditions. However, it can also be a sign of some cancers.

O—Obvious changes in moles or warts. Warts and moles should not change shapes or colors or thickness. Any of these changes can signal a chance of skin cancer.

N—Nagging cough and hoarseness. This can go along with the difficulty in swallowing. It can also be a sign of lung and other cancers.

Secondary Prevention (Early Detection and Screening of Cancer)

Secondary prevention is an approach to detect the abnormal changes at the beginning of the development of malignancy. It involves screening and early detection methods such as mammogram and pap test. This can help us to identify any abnormal changes in our body before they become cancerous. Therefore, it is effective to prevent cancer from fully developing. Sometimes, secondary cancer prevention can involve the treatment of precancerous lesions in an attempt to reverse carcinogenesis so that the lesion can regress.

Diagnostic Tests
- Blood tests (CBC, RFT, LFT, electrolytes)
- Radioimmunology assay
- Tumor markers

- Stool test (colon and rectal cancer)
- Cytological tests
- Pap smear
- Endometrial tissue sampling
- Monoclonal antibodies
- Radiographic and imaging studies
- Positron emission tomography (PET), SPET
- Biopsy
- Sigmoidoscopy
- Proctoscopy
- Bone marrow examination

Cancer-related check-up: A cancer-related check-up is recommended every 3 years for people aged 20–40 years and every year for people aged 40 years and older. This examination should include health counseling and depending on a person's age, might include examination for cancer of the thyroid, oral cavity, skin, lymph nodes, testes, and ovaries.

- **Breast:** Women aged 40 years and older should have an annual mammogram, an annual clinical breast examination (CBE) by a health care professional, and should perform monthly breast self-examination (BSE). Women aged 20–39 years should have a CBE by a health-care professional every 3 years and should perform monthly BSE.
- **Colon and rectum:** Beginning at age 50, men and women should follow one of the examination schedules below:
  - A fecal occult blood test every year and a flexible sigmoidoscopy every 5 years
  - A colonoscopy every 10 years
  - A double-contrast barium enema every 5–10 years
- **Prostate:** The ACS recommends that both the prostate-specific antigen blood test and the digital rectal examination be offered annually, beginning at the age of 50. Men in high-risk groups, such as those with a strong familial predisposition or African-Americans may begin at a younger age (45 years).
- **Uterus:** All women who are or have been sexually active or who are 18 and older should have an annual pap test and pelvic examination. After three or more consecutive satisfactory examinations with normal findings, the pap test may be performed less frequently.
- **Endometrium:** Women at high risk for cancer of the uterus should have a sample of endometrial tissue examined when menopause begins.

Tertiary Prevention

Tertiary prevention is an approach to control the cancer and prevention of disease-related complications. It involves a variety of aspects of patient care such as quality of life, adjuvant therapies, surgical intervention, and palliative care.

VARIOUS TREATMENT MODALITIES OF CANCER

There are various cancers in the body and all cancer had various and different treatment modalities to treat them. Although various modalities are present but common are chemotherapy, radiation therapy, surgeries, and palliative therapy.

Chemotherapy

Chemotherapy is the use of chemical agents to kill cells. In conversational usage, the term chemotherapy refers to the chemical treatment of cancer.

Mechanism of Action of Chemotherapeutic Drugs

Chemotherapeutic drugs inhibit the process of mitosis, or cell division. Since malignant (cancer) cells divide without control or order, these drugs effectively target cancerous growths. Some chemo drugs cause cancer cells to die altogether by stimulating a process known as apoptosis (programed cell-death). Although chemotherapeutic drugs are designed to target fast-dividing cancer cells, they inadvertently damage healthy cells. The faster a healthy cell divides, the more likely it is to be affected by chemotherapy. Chemotherapeutic drugs have been developed to target various rates of mitosis (cell division), but the slower the rate of division, the greater the risk of healthy cell damage.

The Focus of Chemotherapy Treatment

- **Curative:** Curative chemotherapy is intended to kill all the cancer cells in the body, curing the patient of cancer.
- **Palliative:** This approach involves prolonging the patient's life by controlling cancer growth, spread, and invasion into other tissues. Palliative treatments are also used to help relieve cancer-related symptoms, improving the patient's quality of life.
- **Adjuvant:** This treatment strategy involves using chemotherapy alongside other cancer treatment options. Adjuvant chemotherapy is usually administered after surgery or radiotherapy to kill any remaining cancer cells in the body.
- **Neoadjuvant chemotherapy:** The focus of neoadjuvant chemotherapy is to reduce the size of a tumor preceding surgery or other treatment options.

Classification of Chemotherapeutic Drugs

Chemotherapy drugs can be divided into several groups based on factors such as how they work, their chemical structure, and their relationship to another drug.

1. **Alkylating agents**: These chemical agents utilize the cellular property of electronegativity to add alkyl groups to cells. Electronegativity is a cell's ability to attract electrons. When a cell inadvertently attracts alkyl groups, the alkyl alters the cell's DNA, resulting in cell death or impaired mitosis.

    Alkylating agents directly damage DNA to prevent the cancer cell from reproducing. As a class of drugs, these agents are not phase specific; in other words, they work in all phases of the cell cycle. Alkylating agents are used to treat many different cancers, including leukemia, lymphoma, Hodgkin disease, multiple myeloma, sarcoma, as well as cancers of the lung, breast, and ovary.

    Because these drugs damage DNA, they can cause long-term damage to the bone marrow. In rare cases, this can eventually lead to acute leukemia. The risk of leukemia from alkylating agents is "dose dependent," meaning that the risk is small with lower doses, but goes up as the total amount of the drug used gets higher. The risk of leukemia after getting alkylating agents is highest about 5–10 years after treatment.

    There are different classes of alkylating agents, including:

    - **Nitrogen mustards:** Mechlorethamine (nitrogen mustard), chlorambucil, cyclophosphamide, ifosfamide, and melphalan
    - **Nitrosoureas:** Streptozocin, carmustine, and lomustine
    - **Alkyl sulfonates:** Busulfan
    - **Triazines:** Dacarbazine and temozolomide (Temodar)
    - **Ethylenimines:** Thiotepa and altretamine (hexamethylmelamine)

2. **Antimetabolite:** These chemical agents mask themselves as purine (one of the building blocks of DNA). When a cell accepts the masked antimetabolites, it becomes unable to

incorporate genuine purine into its DNA. This results in cellular DNA damage. These agents damage cells during the S phase. They are commonly used to treat leukemias, cancers of the breast, ovary, and the intestinal tract, as well as other types of cancer.

Examples of antimetabolites:

- 5-Fluorouracil (5-FU)
- 6-Mercaptopurine (6-MP)
- Capecitabine (Xeloda)
- Cladribine
- Clofarabine
- Cytarabine (Ara-C)
- Floxuridine
- Fludarabine
- Gemcitabine (Gemzar)
- Hydroxyurea
- Methotrexate
- Pemetrexed (Alimta)
- Pentostatin

3. **Antitumor antibiotics**

   Anthracyclines: Anthracyclines are antitumor antibiotics that interfere with enzymes involved in DNA replication. These drugs work in all phases of the cell cycle. They are widely used for a variety of cancers. A major consideration when giving these drugs is that they can permanently damage the heart if given in high doses. For this reason, lifetime dose limits are often placed on these drugs.

   Examples of anthracyclines:

   - Daunorubicin
   - Doxorubicin (Adriamycin)
   - Epirubicin
   - Idarubicin

   Other antitumor antibiotics

   Antitumor antibiotics that are not anthracyclines include:

   - Actinomycin-D
   - Bleomycin
   - Mitomycin-C

   Mitoxantrone is an antitumor antibiotic that is similar to doxorubicin in many ways, including the potential for damaging the heart. This drug also acts as a topoisomerase II inhibitor and can lead to treatment-related leukemia. Mitoxantrone is used to treat prostate cancer, breast cancer, lymphoma, and leukemia.

4. **Topoisomerase inhibitors:** These drugs interfere with enzymes called topoisomerases, which help separate the strands of DNA so they can be copied. They are used to treat certain leukemias, as well as lung, ovarian, gastrointestinal, and other cancers.

   - Examples of topoisomerase I inhibitors include topotecan and irinotecan (CPT-11).
   - Examples of topoisomerase II inhibitors include etoposide (VP-16) and teniposide. Mitoxantrone also inhibits topoisomerase II.

   Treatment with topoisomerase II inhibitors increases the risk of a second cancer—acute myelogenous leukemia. With this type of drug, a secondary leukemia can be seen as early as 2–3 years after the drug is given.

5. **Mitotic inhibitors:** Mitotic inhibitors are often plant alkaloids and other compounds derived from natural products. They can stop mitosis or inhibit enzymes from making proteins needed for cell reproduction.

These drugs work during the M phase of the cell cycle but can damage cells in all phases. They are used to treat many different types of cancer including breast, lung, myelomas, lymphomas, and leukemias. These drugs are known for their potential to cause peripheral nerve damage, which can be a dose-limiting side effect.

Examples of mitotic inhibitors include:

- Taxanes: paclitaxel and docetaxel
- Epothilones: ixabepilone
- Vinca alkaloids: vinblastine, vincristine
- Estramustine (emcyt)

6. **Corticosteroids:** Steroids are natural hormones and hormone-like drugs that are useful in treating some types of cancer (lymphoma, leukemias, and multiple myeloma), as well as other illnesses. When these drugs are used to kill cancer cells or slow their growth, they are considered chemotherapy drugs.

Corticosteroids are also commonly used as *antiemetics* to help prevent nausea and vomiting caused by chemotherapy. They are used before chemotherapy to help prevent severe allergic reactions (hypersensitivity reactions), too. When a corticosteroid is used to prevent vomiting or allergic reactions, it is not considered chemotherapy. Examples include prednisone, methylprednisolone (solumedrol), and dexamethasone (decadron).

Miscellaneous Chemotherapy Drugs

Some chemotherapy drugs act in slightly different ways and do not fit well into any of the other categories. Examples include drugs such as L-asparaginase, which is an enzyme, and the proteosome inhibitor bortezomib (Velcade).

Hormone Therapy

Drugs in this category are sex hormones, or hormone-like drugs, that change the action or production of female or male hormones. They are used to slow the growth of breast, prostate, and endometrial (uterine) cancers, which normally grow in response to natural hormones in the body. These cancer treatment hormones do not work in the same ways as standard chemotherapy drugs, but rather by preventing the cancer cell from using the hormone it needs to grow or by preventing the body from making the hormones.

Examples:

- The antiestrogens: Fulvestrant, tamoxifen, and toremifene
- Aromatase inhibitors: Anastrozole (arimidex), exemestane (aromasin), and letrozole (femara)
- Progestins: Megestrol acetate
- Estrogens
- Antiandrogens: Bicalutamide, flutamide, and nilutamide
- Gonadotropin-releasing hormone, also known as luteinizing hormone-releasing hormone agonists.

Side Effects of Chemotherapy

Although side effect management has come a long way in recent years, chemotherapy drugs still affect healthy cells. Sometimes, the effects of cell damage are temporary, but sometimes they are long term or even permanent.

Short-term Side Effects

- Hair loss
- Bleeding

- Fatigue
- Infertility
- Cognitive impairment
- Sensory abnormalities: Food tastes different, odors are perceived differently, etc.
- Lung damage
- Nervous tissue damage
- Liver damage

Temporary Effects

- Nausea
- Vomiting
- Diarrhea
- Dry mouth
- Constipation
- Mouth sores
- Difficulty swallowing
- Loss of appetite

Most of these side effects will diminish or disappear completely after chemo treatment stops.

Long-term Side Effects

Long-term chemo effects are rare. As cancer patients live longer and longer lives, doctors are uncovering side effects that do not show until many years after treatment ends.

- **Nervous tissue damage:** This may result in sensory abnormalities and impaired cognitive function. This is rare.
- **Hematuria:** Blood in the urine
- **Organ damage:** This typically involves heart, lung, or kidney impairment.

Role of Nurse in Chemotherapy

- **Prior to chemotherapy administration**
  - **Review:**
    - The chemotherapy drugs prescription which should have, name of antineoplastic agent, dosage, route of administration, date and time that each agent to be administered
    - Accurately identify the client
    - Medications to be administered in conjunction with the chemotherapy, e.g., antiemetic, sedatives, etc.
  - **Assessing the clients' condition including:**
    - Most recent report of blood counts including hemoglobin (Hb), hematocrit, white blood cells and platelets
    - Presence of any complicating condition which could contraindicate chemotherapeutic agent administration, i.e., infection, severe stomatitis, decreased deep tendon reflexes, or bleeding.
    - Physical status, level of anxiety, and psychological status
  - **Preparing for potential complications:**
    - Reviewing the policy and have medication and supplies available for immediate intervention the event of extravasation.
    - Reviewing the procedure and have medication available for possible anaphylaxis.
  - **Assuring accurate preparation of the agent:**
    - Accuracy of dosage calculation
    - Expiry date of the drug to be checked

♦ Procedure for correct reconstitution
♦ Recommended procedures for administration
♦ Assessing the patients' understanding of the chemotherapeutic agents and administration procedures.

- **Calculation of drug dosage:** It is calculated based on the body surface area.
- **Drug reconstitution/preparation:** Pharmacy staff should reconstitute all drugs preprime the intravenous tubing under a class II biologic safety cabinet (BSC). In certain conditions, nurses may be required to reconstitute medications. When preparing and reconstituting safe handling guidelines to be followed:
  - Aseptic technique should be followed.
  - Personal protective equipment include disposable surgical gloves, long sleeves gown, and elastic cuffs.
  - Protective eye goggles if no BSC
  - To minimize exposure
  - Wash hands before and after drug handling
  - Limiting access to drug preparation area
  - Keep labeled drug spill kit near preparation area
  - Opening drug vials/ampoules away from body
  - Placing absorbent pad on work surface
  - Wrapping alcohol wipe around neck of ampoule before opening
  - Labeling all chemotherapeutic drugs

  The following guidelines to be kept in mind:
  - Inspecting the solution, container and tubing for signs of contamination including particles, discoloration, cloudiness, and cracks or tears in bottle or bag.
  - Aseptic technique to be followed.
  - Preparing medicines according to manufacturer's directions.
  - Selecting a suitable vein
  - Large veins on the forearm are the preferred site.
  - Using distal veins first, and choosing a vein above areas of flexion.
  - For nonvesicant drugs, the distal veins of the hands (metacarpal veins) should be used: then the veins of the forearms (basilic and cephalic veins).
  - For vesicants, use only the veins of the forearms. Avoiding the use of metacarpal and radial areas.
  - Avoiding the antecubital fossa and the wrist because an extravasation in these areas can destroy nerves and tendons, resulting in loss of function.
  - Peripheral sites should be changed daily before administration of vesicants.
  - Avoiding the use of small lumen veins to prevent damage due to friction and the decreased ability to dilute acidic drugs and solutions.
  - Selecting the shortest catheter with the smallest gauge appropriate for the type and duration of the infusion.
  - Applying a small amount of iodine-based antiseptic ointment over the insertion site and covering the area with sterile gauze.
- **Documentation:** Chemotherapeutic drugs, dose, route, and time, premedications, postmedications, prehydration, and other infusions and supplies used for chemotherapy regimen. Any complaints by the patient of discomfort and symptoms experienced before, during, and after chemotherapeutic infusion.
- **Disposal of supplies and unused drugs:**
  - Not clipping or recapping needles or breaking syringes
  - Placing all supplies used intact in a leak proof, puncture proof, appropriate labeled container

- Placing all unused drugs in containers in a leak proof, puncture proof, appropriately labeled container
- Disposing containers filled with chemotherapeutic supplies and unused drugs in accordance with regulations of hazardous wastes.
- **Management of chemotherapeutic spills:**
  - Chemotherapy spills should be cleaned up immediately by properly protected personnel trained in the appropriate procedure.
  - A spill should be identified with a warning sign so that other person will not be contaminated.
- **Staff education:**
  - All personnel involved in the care should receive an orientation to chemo.
  - Drugs including their known risk, relevant techniques and procedures for handling, the proper use of protective equipment and materials, spill procedures, and medical policies covering personnel handling chemo agents.
  - Personnel handling blood, vomits, or excreta from patients who have received chemotherapy should wear disposable gloves and gowns to be appropriately discarded after use.
- **Extravasation management:** Extravasation is the accidental infiltration of vesicant or irritant chemotherapeutic drugs from the vein into the surrounding tissues at the IV site. A vesicant is an agent that can produce a blister or tissue destruction. An irritant is an agent that is capable of producing venous pain at the site of and along the vein with/without an inflammatory reaction. Injuries that may occur as a result of extravasations include sloughing of tissue, infection, pain, and loss of mobility of an extremity.

Prevention of extravasation: Nursing responsibilities for the prevention of extravasation include the following:
- Knowledge of drugs with vesicant potential
- Skill in drug administration
- Identification of risk factors, e.g., multiple venepunctures
- Anticipation of extravasation and knowledge of management protocol
- New venepuncture site daily if peripheral access is used
- Administration of drug in a quiet, unhurried environment
- Testing vein patency without using chemotherapeutic agents
- Providing adequate drug dilution
- Careful observation of access site and extremity throughout the procedure
- Ensuring blood return from IV site before, during, and after vesicant drug infusion
- Educating patients regarding symptoms of drug infiltration, e.g., pain, burning, stinging sensation at IV site.

Extravasation management at peripheral site
According to agency policy and approved antidote should be readily available.
The following procedure should be initiated:
- The use of the drug should be stopped.
- Leaving the needle or catheter in place.
- Aspirating any residual drug and blood in the IV tubing, needle, or catheter, and suspected infiltration site.
- Instilling the IV antidote
- Removing the needle
- If unable to aspirate the residual drug from the IV tubing, needle or catheter should be removed.

- Injecting the antidote subcutaneously clockwise into the infiltrated site using 25 G needle; changing the needle with each new injection.
- Avoiding to apply pressure on the suspected infiltration site
- Applying topical ointment if ordered
- Cover lightly with an occlusive sterile dressing
- Applying cold or warm compresses as indicated
- Elevating the extremity
- Observing regularly for pain, erythema, indurations, and necrosis
- Documentation of extravasations management
- All nursing personnel should be alerted and prepared for the possible complication of anaphylaxis.

Radiation Therapy

Radiation therapy is the medical use of ionizing radiation, generally as part of cancer treatment to control or kill malignant cells. Radiation therapy may be curative in a number of types of cancer if they are localized to one area of the body. It may also be used as part of curative therapy, to prevent tumor recurrence after surgery to remove a primary malignant tumor (e.g., early stages of breast cancer). Radiation therapy is synergistic with chemotherapy and has been used before, during, and after chemotherapy in susceptible cancers.

Radiotherapy may be used for curative or adjuvant cancer treatment. It is used as palliative treatment (where cure is not possible and the aim is for local disease control or symptomatic relief) or as therapeutic treatment (where the therapy has survival benefit and it can be curative). Total body irradiation is a radiotherapy technique used to prepare the body to receive a bone marrow transplant.

Types of Radiation Therapy

Radiation has a wide range of energies that form the electromagnetic spectrum. The spectrum has two major divisions:
1. Nonionizing radiation
2. Ionizing radiation.

Nonionizing radiation: It ranges from extremely low-frequency radiation. These are indirectly ionizing. They do not themselves produce chemical and biological damage, but when absorbed in the medium through which they pass, they give up their energy to produce fast-moving electrons by either the Compton, photoelectric or pair production processes.

Ionizing radiation: Higher frequency UV radiation begins to have enough energy to break chemical bonds. X-ray and gamma-ray radiation, which are at the upper end of magnetic radiation, have very high frequencies (in the range of 100 billion Hertz) and very short wavelengths of about 1 PM. Ionization is the process in which a charged portion of a molecule is given enough energy to break away from the atom. This process results in the formation of two charged particles or ions: The molecule with a net positive charge and the free electron with a negative charge.

There are three main kinds of ionizing radiation:
1. Alpha particles, which include two protons and two neutrons.
2. Beta particles, which are essentially high-speed electrons.
3. Gamma rays and X-rays, which are pure energy (photons).

Alpha radiation: Alpha radiation is a heavy, very short-range particle and is actually an ejected helium nucleus. Some characteristics of alpha radiation are as follows:

- Most alpha radiation is not able to penetrate human skin.
- Alpha-emitting materials can be harmful to humans if the materials are inhaled, swallowed, or absorbed through open wounds.
- Alpha radiation travels only a short distance (a few inches) in air but is not an external hazard.
- Alpha radiation is not able to penetrate clothing.
- Examples of some alpha emitters: Radium, radon, uranium, and thorium.

Beta radiation: Beta radiation is a light, short-range particle and is actually an ejected electron. Some characteristics of beta radiation are:
- Beta radiation may travel several feet in air and is moderately penetrating.
- Beta radiation can penetrate human skin to the "germinal layer," where new skin cells are produced. If high levels of beta-emitting contaminants are allowed to remain on the skin for a prolonged period of time, they may cause skin injury.
- Beta-emitting contaminants may be harmful if deposited internally.
- Clothing provides some protection against beta radiation.
- Examples of some pure beta emitters: strontium-90, carbon-14, tritium, and sulfur-35.

Gamma and X-radiation: Gamma radiation and X-rays are highly penetrating electromagnetic radiation. Some characteristics of these radiations are:
- Gamma radiation or X-rays are able to travel many feet in air and many inches in human tissue. They readily penetrate most materials and are sometimes called "penetrating" radiation.
- X-rays are like gamma rays. X-rays, too, are penetrating radiation. Sealed radioactive sources and machines that emit gamma radiation and X-rays, respectively, constitute mainly an external hazard to humans.
- Gamma radiation and X-rays are electromagnetic radiation, such as visible light, radio waves, and UV light. These electromagnetic radiations differ only in the amount of energy they have. Gamma rays and X-rays are the most energetic of these.
- Dense materials are needed for shielding from gamma radiation. Clothing provides little shielding from penetrating radiation but will prevent contamination of the skin by gamma-emitting radioactive materials.
- Gamma radiation is easily detected by survey meters with a sodium iodide detector probe.
- Gamma radiation and characteristic X-rays frequently accompany the emission of alpha and beta radiation during radioactive decay.
- Examples of some gamma emitters: iodine-131, cesium-137, cobalt-60, radium-226, and technetium-99m.

Treatment

Radiation is used to treat a carefully defined area of the body to achieve local control of disease. As radiation has an effect on tissues only within the treatment field, it is not appropriate as an independent modality for patients with systemic disease. However, radiation may be used, independently or in combination with chemotherapy, to treat primary tumors or for palliative control of metastatic lesions. Radiation can be delivered externally (teletherapy) or internally (brachytherapy). As with other cancer therapies, the goals of radiation therapy are cure, control, or palliation. There are multiple settings in which radiation may be used, including:
- **Definitive or primary therapy:** Used an independent treatment modality with curative intent (e.g., for the cancers of the lung, prostate, bladder, head/neck, Hodgkin's lymphoma).
- **Neoadjuvant therapy:** Given (with/without chemotherapy) preoperatively to minimize the tumor burden and improve the likelihood of complete surgical resection, making a previously inoperable tumor.

- **Adjuvant therapy:** Administered following surgery or chemotherapy to improve local control of disease and reduce the risk of local disease recurrence.
- **Prophylaxis:** Administered to high-risk areas to prevent future cancer development (such as prophylactic cranial irradiation to prevent brain metastasis secondary to small cell lung cancer).
- **Disease control:** Limiting tumor growth to extend the symptom-free period as much as possible.
- **Palliation:** Given to prevent or relieve distressing symptoms, such as pain (bone metastasis) or shortness of breath (obstructing bronchial tumor), and for prevention of neurologic function (brain metastasis or spinal cord compression).

External radiation: Teletherapy (external beam radiation) is the most common form of radiation treatment delivery. With this technique, the patient is exposed to radiation from a megavoltage treatment machine. Machines that used to deliver treatment may include the cobalt-60 machine, which emits gamma rays from a radioactive source, which produces neutrons or protons, linear accelerator, which generates ionizing radiation from electricity and can have multiple energies.

Internal radiation: Brachytherapy which means "close." It consists of the implantation or insertion of radioactive materials directly into the tumor or in close proximity adjacent to the tumor (intracavitary or intraluminal). This allows for direct dose delivery to the target with minimal exposure to the surrounding health tissues. Brachytherapy is commonly used in combination with external radiation as a supplemental "boost" treatment.

Sources of brachytherapy include temporarily sealed sources, such as iridium-192 and cesium-137 and permanent sealed sources, such as iodine-125, gold-198, and palladium-103. These are supplied in the form of seeds or ribbons. With a temporary implant, the source may be placed into a special catheter or metal tube that has been inserted into the tumor area. This method is commonly used for tumors of the head and neck cancer, lung, and gynecologic malignancies.

New ways of radiation therapy: New ways of delivering radiation therapy are making it safer and more effective. Some of these methods are already being used, while others need more study before they can be approved for widespread use. And scientists around the world continue to look for better and different ways to use radiation to treat cancer. Here are just a few areas of current research interest:

- **Hyperthermia** is the use of heat to treat cancer. Heat has been found to kill cancer cells, but when used alone it does not destroy enough cells to cure the cancer. Heat created by microwaves and ultrasound is being studied in combination with radiation and appears to improve the effect of the radiation.
- **Radiosensitizers** are drugs that make cancer cells more sensitive to radiation. Some chemotherapy drugs already in use (such as 5-fluorouracil or 5-FU) are known to be radiosensitizers.
- **Radioprotectors** are substances that protect normal cells from radiation. These types of drugs are useful in areas where its hard not to expose vital normal tissues to radiation when treating a tumor, such as the head and neck area. Some radioprotectors, such as amifostine (Ethyol), are already in use, while others are being studied in clinical trials.

Side Effects of Radiation Therapy

- **Radio dermatitis:** Radiation may cause an acute or chronic inflammatory condition of the skin. The first symptom, erythema, may appear a few days after administration of a sufficient single dose or days later after administration of repeated small doses. When the injury is severe, the patient experiences pain and itching. Areas of necrosis develop, and subcutaneous and deeper tissues are involved. If hairy surfaces are involved, permanent baldness may result.

- **Cancer of the skin:** Exposure to X-ray and radium has induced cancer of the skin in many research workers in the specialty, especially in the early or pioneer years when the need for protection for workers was not known.
- **Growth retardation and bone lesions:** The growing fetus may be injured by radiation of the mother's pelvis, especially during the early months of pregnancy. Serious deformity of the skeletal and nervous systems of the unborn child.
- **Gastrointestinal response to radiation-induced damage:** Particularly where RT is directed at any patient of the gastrointestinal tract, it may have marked effects on an individual's ability to ingest, digest, or absorb nutrients.
- Radiation cystitis
- Urethritis
- Permanent infertility in child-bearing age

Nursing Care Plan

1. Anxiety related to the prescribed radiation therapy and insufficient knowledge of treatments and self-care measures

Intervention

- Encouraging the client to share fears and beliefs regarding radiation. Delaying the teaching if the client is experiencing severe anxiety.
- Reviewing general principles of RT as necessary. Providing written materials, such as client education booklets.
- Reinforcing the treatment plan covering the following items: area to be administered, marking and tattoos, shielding of vital organs.
- Explaining the fatigue that accompanies RT
- Explaining skin reactions and precautions
- Encouraging family to share concerns

2. High risk for altered oral mucous membrane related to dry mouth or inadequate oral hygiene or radiation tooth decay

Intervention

- Explaining the signs and symptoms of mucositis and stomatitis
- Stressing the need to have caries filled and bad or loose teeth extracted before initiation of RT to head and neck.
- Emphasizing the need for regular oral hygiene during and after therapy
- Brushing with fluoridated toothpaste after meals
- Using a soft toothbrush
- Rinsing mouth with topical fluoride solutions after brushing
- Encouraging oral fluid intake, moistening lips
- Avoiding commercial mouthwashes, very spicy or hot drinks, alcoholic beverages, tobacco, highly seasoned food and acidic foods, such as oranges, grapes, and tomatoes.
- Offering topical relief of pain with lidocaine ointment or ice chips.
- Explaining the need for dental examinations during and after the course of treatment.

3. Impaired skin integrity related to effects of radiation on the epithelial and basal cells

Intervention

- Explaining the effects of radiation of skin (redness, tanning, peeling, and itching, hairless, decreased perspiration) and monitoring skin in the irradiated areas.

- **For alopecia:** Helping patient plan for a wig or scarf or hat before hair loss. Having patient gently wash and gently combing the remaining hair, reassuring that hair will grow back after therapy.
- **For dermatitis:** Observing irradiated area daily, teaching them not to wash the treated area until therapist tells. Avoiding hard soap, ointments, creams, cosmetics, and deodorants on treated skin unless approved by therapist.
- **For moist desquamation:** Showering or irradiating the area frequently, using moist wound healing dressing. Avoiding the use of adhesive tapes; assisting patient with bathing to maintain marking; having patient avoid excessive heat, sunlight, tight restrictive clothing, and soap. Providing skincare to special skin folds, such as buttocks, perineum, groin, and axilla.
- Using an electric razor only—no blades—to shave the irradiated area
- Instructing the client to report any skin changes promptly
- After the skin is properly healed, precautions in sun should be taught, a sunscreen lotion should be used. Increasing exposure time very slowly, discontinuing sun exposure if redness occurs. Protecting treated skin with hats, etc.

4. Altered comfort related to stimulation of vomiting center and damage to the gastrointestinal tract (GIT) mucosa cells secondary to radiation
Intervention
- Promoting a positive attitude about radiotherapy and reinforce its killing effects.
- Explaining the possible reasons for nausea and vomiting.
- Encouraging to have small, frequent meals.
- Instructing to avoid hot/cold liquids, high fat, high-fiber diet, spicy food, and caffeine.
- Teaching stress reduction techniques, such as relaxation techniques and guided imagery.

5. Impaired mobility related to fatigue and altered motor function
Intervention
- Planning frequent rest periods
- Avoiding injury
- Using assistive devices for ambulation as required
- Assessing reflexes, tactile sensation, and movement in extremities and report abnormal findings
- Observing for Lhermitte's sign (sensation of electric shock-running down back and over extremities), which shows cervical cord compression.

6. Altered nutrition, less than body requirements related to decreased oral intake, reduced salivation, dysphasia, nausea, and vomiting, increase BUN and diarrhea
Intervention
- Helping the client identify reasons for inadequate nutrition and explain possible causes
- Stressing the need to increase calorie intake
- Encouraging resting before meals
- Offering small frequent meals
- Maintaining good oral hygiene before and after meals
- Instructing the client to avoid high fatty and oily foods
- Considering clients' likes and dislikes pertaining food intake

7. Grieving related to changes in lifestyle, role, finances, functional capacity, body image, and health lose
Intervention
- Providing opportunity to ventilate feelings, discuss loss openly
- Encouraging to use positive coping strategies

- Encouraging to express feeling to worth
- Promoting grief at each stage
- Maintaining safe and secure environment
- Exploring reasons for and meaning of fears
- Reducing environmental stimuli and provide safe environment

8. Altered family process related to imposed changes in family roles, responsibly, and relationship

Intervention

- Conveying an understanding of the situation and its impact on the family
- Exploring the family's perception of the situation
- Trying to promote family bonding by involving family in client's care, encouraging humor
- Preparing the family members for signs of stress, depression, anxiety, anger, and dependency in the client
- Encouraging family to call on its social network for emotional and other support
- Directing toward community agencies and other sources of assistance as needed

Surgical Therapy

Surgical removal of the entire cancer remains the ideal and most frequently used treatment method. Surgical treatment is used in oncology nursing for diagnosis of disease, reconstruction, prevention of disease, type, extent of the disease, etc.

- **Primary treatment:** It involves removal of a malignant tumor and a margin of adjacent normal tissue. The main goal of primary treatment is to reduce the total body tumor burden.
- **Adjuvant treatment:** It is also called debulking. It is the removal of large portion of tumor and remaining cancer cells are destroyed by other systemic treatments.
- **Salvage treatment:** It involves the use of an extensive surgical approach to treat local recurrence after a less extensive approach has been implemented. For example, mastectomy after lumpectomy and radiation therapy.
- **Palliative treatment:** It is used to minimize disease or cancer-related symptoms without trying to surgically cure the cancer. The goal of palliative treatment is to just relieve the symptoms and make the patient more comfortable.
- **Combination treatment:** In this, surgery is combined with other treatment modalities to improve the treatment outcome. Example includes preoperative and postoperative chemotherapy and radiation therapy.

Surgical Techniques

Several techniques are used in the treatment of cancer, which include:

- **Electrosurgery:** In this type of surgery, cancer cells are destroyed by high-frequency electrical current applied by electrodes, needle, etc. It is used in cancer of skin, oral cavity, etc.
- **Cryosurgery:** Cryosurgery technique is used for the destruction of cancer cells by producing temperature below $-166.2°F$ ($-200°C$). It causes freezing in cells, as freezing continues, cell membranes rupture. Carbon dioxide, nitrous oxide, and Freon are the three common gases used as freezing agents in cryosurgery.
- **Lasers:** In this technique, laser light is used for destruction. In this process, photons are emitted that causes various interactions in tissues or cells, which include photocoagulation, vaporization, photochemical reactions, and ablation.

- **Photodynamic therapy (PDT):** It involves intravenous injection of a photosensitizing drug, followed by exposure to a laser light within 24–48 hours of injection, which results in fluorescence of cancer cells and cell death.

Nursing Management

- Disturbed body image related to surgical procedure
- Ineffective family coping related to diagnosis of cancer
- Ineffective individual coping related to diagnosis of cancer
- Risk of fluid volume deficit related to extensive surgery
- Risk for infection related to immunocompromised status from disease condition
- Knowledge deficit related to areas of self-care activities

Preoperative Care

- Reducing anxiety
- Enhancing physical well-being
- Health education

Postoperative Care

- **Palliative therapy:** Palliative care is care given to improve the quality of life of patients who have a serious or life-threatening disease, such as cancer. The goal of palliative care is to prevent or treat, as early as possible, the symptoms and side effects of the disease and its treatment, in addition to the related psychological, social, and spiritual problems. The goal is not to cure. Palliative care is also called *comfort care*, *supportive care*, and *symptom management*.
- Palliative care is given throughout a patient's experience with cancer. It should begin at diagnosis and continue through treatment, follow-up care, and the end of life. Any medical professional may provide palliative care by addressing the side effects and emotional issues of cancer; some have a particular focus on this type of care. A palliative care specialist is a health professional who specializes in treating the symptoms, side effects, and emotional problems experienced by patients. The goal is to maintain the best possible quality of life.
- Often, palliative care specialists work as part of a multidisciplinary team to coordinate care. This palliative care team may consist of doctors, nurses, registered dieticians, pharmacists, and social workers. Palliative care specialists may also make recommendations to primary care physicians about the management of pain and other symptoms. People do not give up their primary care physician to receive palliative care.
- Palliative care can address a broad range of issues, integrating an individual's specific needs into care. The physical and emotional effects of cancer and its treatment may be very different from person to person. For example, differences in age, cultural background, or support systems may result in very different palliative care needs.

Comprehensive palliative care will take the following issues into account for each patient:

- **Physical:** Common physical symptoms include pain, fatigue, loss of appetite, nausea, vomiting, shortness of breath, and insomnia. Many of these can be relieved with medicines or by using other methods, such as nutrition therapy, physical therapy, or deep breathing techniques. Also, chemotherapy, radiation therapy, or surgery may be used to shrink tumors that are causing pain and other problems.
- **Emotional and coping:** Palliative care specialists can provide resources to help patients and families deal with the emotions that come with a cancer diagnosis and cancer treatment.

Depression, anxiety, and fear are only a few of the concerns that can be addressed through palliative care. Experts may provide counseling, recommend support groups, hold family meetings, or make referrals to mental health professionals.

- **Practical:** Cancer patients may have financial and legal worries, insurance questions, employment concerns, and concerns about completing advance directives. For many patients and families, the technical language and specific details of laws and forms are hard to understand. To ease the burden, the palliative care team may assist in coordinating the appropriate services. For example, the team may direct patients and families to resources that can help with financial counseling, understanding medical forms or legal advice, or identifying local and national resources, such as transportation or housing agencies.
- **Spiritual:** With a cancer diagnosis, patients and families often look more deeply for meaning in their lives. Some find the disease brings them more faith, whereas others question their faith as they struggle to understand why cancer happened to them. An expert in palliative care can help people explore their beliefs and values so that they can find a sense of peace or reach a point of acceptance that is appropriate for their situation.

COLORECTAL CANCER

Colorectal cancer, commonly known as colon cancer or bowel cancer, is a cancer from uncontrolled cell growth in the colon or rectum (parts of the large intestine), or in the appendix. Colorectal cancer refers to the malignancies of colon and rectum.

Causes

- High intake of fat
- Alcohol
- Red meat
- Obesity
- Smoking
- Lack of physical exercise
- Older age
- Male gender
- Family history of colorectal cancer and polyps
- Presence of polyps in the large intestine
- Inflammatory bowel diseases
- Chronic ulcerative colitis

Stages of Colorectal Cancer

Colon and rectal cancer are staged according to how far they have spread through the walls of the colon and rectum and whether they have spread to other parts of the body.

Staging Colon Cancer

1. **Stage 0:** Stage 0 cancer of the colon is very early cancer. The cancer is found only in the innermost lining of the colon.
2. **Stage I:** The cancer has spread beyond the innermost lining of the colon to the second and third layers and involves the inside wall of the colon. The cancer has not spread to the outer wall of the colon or outside the colon.
3. **Stage II:** The tumor extends through the muscular wall of the colon, but there is no cancer in the lymph nodes (small structures that are found throughout the body that produce and store cells that fight infection).

4. **Stage III:** The cancer has spread outside the colon to one or more lymph nodes (small structures that are found throughout the body that produce and store cells that fight infection).
5. **Stage IV:** The cancer has spread outside the colon to other parts of the body, such as the liver or the lungs. The tumor can be of any size and may/may not include affected lymph nodes (small structures that are found throughout the body that produce and store cells that fight infection).

Staging of Rectal Cancer

Rectal cancer is staged much the same way as colon cancer, but because the tumor is much lower down in the colon, the treatment options may vary.

1. **Stage 0:** In stage 0 rectal cancer, the tumor is located only on the inner lining of the rectum. To treat this early-stage cancer, surgery can be performed to remove the tumor or a small section of the rectum where the cancer is located can be removed.
2. **Stage I:** This is an early form or limited form of cancer. The tumor has broken through the inner lining of the rectum but has not made it past the muscular wall.
3. **Stage II:** This cancer is a little more advanced. The tumor has penetrated all the way through the bowel wall and may have invaded other organs, such as the bladder, uterus, or prostate gland.
4. **Stage III:** The tumor has spread to the lymph nodes (small structures that are found throughout the body that produce and store cells that fight infection).
5. **Stage IV:** The tumor has spread to distant parts of the body (metastasized). The tumor can be any size and sometimes is not that large. The liver and lung are two favored places for rectal cancer to spread.

Pathophysiology

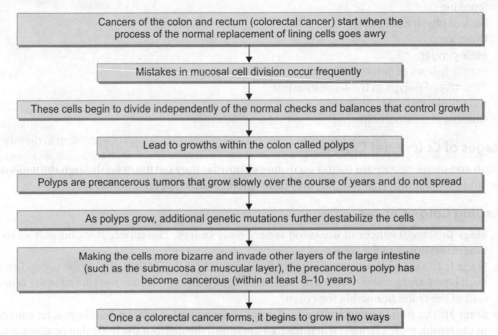

Cancers of the colon and rectum (colorectal cancer) start when the process of the normal replacement of lining cells goes awry

↓

Mistakes in mucosal cell division occur frequently

↓

These cells begin to divide independently of the normal checks and balances that control growth

↓

Lead to growths within the colon called polyps

↓

Polyps are precancerous tumors that grow slowly over the course of years and do not spread

↓

As polyps grow, additional genetic mutations further destabilize the cells

↓

Making the cells more bizarre and invade other layers of the large intestine (such as the submucosa or muscular layer), the precancerous polyp has become cancerous (within at least 8–10 years)

↓

Once a colorectal cancer forms, it begins to grow in two ways

Contd...

Contd...

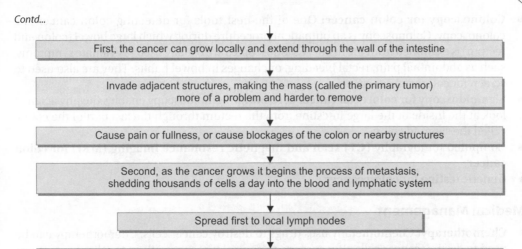

First, the cancer can grow locally and extend through the wall of the intestine

Invade adjacent structures, making the mass (called the primary tumor)
more of a problem and harder to remove

Cause pain or fullness, or cause blockages of the colon or nearby structures

Second, as the cancer grows it begins the process of metastasis,
shedding thousands of cells a day into the blood and lymphatic system

Spread first to local lymph nodes

Spread to the liver, the abdominal cavity, and the lung are the
next most common destinations of metastatic spread

Signs and Symptoms

The symptoms and signs of colorectal cancer depend on the location of tumor in the bowel, and whether it has spread elsewhere in the body (metastasis). The classic warning signs include:

- Worsening constipation
- Blood in the stool
- Weight loss, fever
- Loss of appetite
- Nausea and vomiting in someone over 50 years old
- Rectal bleeding
- Anemia
- Weight loss
- Change in bowel habits

Diagnostic Tests

- **Stool test for colon cancer:** Finding colon cancer early is key to beating it. That is why doctors recommend a yearly fecal occult blood test, which tests for invisible blood in the stool, an early sign of colon cancer.
- **Fecal occult blood test:** Fecal occult blood is tested for the presence of microscopic or invisible blood in the stool, or feces. Fecal occult blood can be a sign of a problem in digestive system, such as a growth, or polyp, or cancer in the colon or rectum. If microscopic blood is detected, it is important for doctor to determine the source of bleeding to properly diagnose and treat the problem.

What causes blood to appear in stool?
Blood may appear in the stool because of one or more of the following conditions:
1. Benign (noncancerous) or malignant (cancerous) growths or polyps of the colon
2. Hemorrhoids (swollen blood vessels near the anus and lower rectum that can rupture causing bleeding)
3. Anal fissures (splits or cracks in the lining of the anal opening)
4. Intestinal infections that cause inflammation
5. Ulcers
6. Ulcerative colitis
7. Crohn's disease
8. Diverticular disease, caused by outpouchings of the colon wall
9. Abnormalities of the blood vessels in the large intestine

- **Colonoscopy for colon cancer:** One of the best tools for detecting colon cancer is a colonoscopy. Colonoscopy is an outpatient procedure during which large bowel (colon and rectum) is examined from the inside. Colonoscopies are usually used to evaluate symptoms, such as abdominal pain, rectal bleeding, or changes in bowel habits. They are also used to screen for colorectal cancer.
- **Sigmoidoscopy for colorectal cancer screening:** Sigmoidoscopy enables the physician to look at the inside of the large intestine from the rectum through the last part of the colon, called the sigmoid colon.
- Computed tomography **(CT) scan and magnetic resonance imaging (MRI) for colon cancer**.
- **Genetic testing for colon cancer**

Medical Management

- **Chemotherapy:** Chemotherapy uses drugs to destroy cancer cells. Chemotherapy can be used to destroy cancer cells after surgery, to control tumor growth or to relieve symptoms of colon cancer.
- **Radiation therapy:** Radiation therapy uses powerful energy sources, such as X-rays, to kill any cancer cells that might remain after surgery, to shrink large tumors before an operation so that they can be removed more easily, or to relieve symptoms of colon cancer and rectal cancer. Radiation therapy is rarely used in early-stage colon cancer but is a routine part of treating rectal cancer, especially if the cancer has penetrated through the wall of the rectum or traveled to nearby lymph nodes. Radiation therapy, usually combined with chemotherapy, may be used after surgery to reduce the risk that the cancer may recur in the area of the rectum where it began.
- **Targeted drug therapy:** Drugs that target specific defects that allow cancer cells to proliferate are available to people with advanced colon cancer, including bevacizumab (Avastin), cetuximab (Erbitux) and panitumumab (Vectibix). Targeted drugs can be given along with chemotherapy or alone. Targeted drugs are typically reserved for people with advanced colon cancer.
- **Alternative treatment:** Alternative treatments may help you cope with a diagnosis of colon cancer. Nearly, all people with cancer experience some distress. Common signs and symptoms of distress after diagnosis might include sadness, anger, difficulty concentrating, difficulty sleeping and loss of appetite. Alternative treatments may help redirect thoughts away from your fears, at least temporarily, to give some relief.

> **Alternative treatments that may help relieve distress include:**
> ❖ Art therapy
> ❖ Dance or movement therapy
> ❖ Exercise
> ❖ Meditation
> ❖ Music therapy
> ❖ Relaxation exercises

Surgery for Colorectal Cancer

The types of surgery used to treat colon and rectal cancers are slightly different, so they are described separately.

1. **Opening colectomy:** A colectomy (sometimes called a *hemicolectomy*, *partial colectomy*, or *segmental resection*) removes part of the colon, as well as nearby lymph nodes. The surgery is referred to as an *open colectomy* if it is done through a single incision in the abdomen.

The day before surgery, patient will most likely be told to completely empty his/her bowel. This is done with a bowel preparation, which may consist of laxatives and enemas. Just before the surgery, patient will be given general anesthesia, which puts patient into a deep sleep.

During the surgery, surgeon will make an incision in his/her abdomen and remove the part of the colon with the cancer and a small segment of normal colon on either side of the cancer. Usually, about one-fourth to one-third of colon is removed, but more or less may be removed depending on the exact size and location of the cancer. The remaining sections of colon are then reattached. Nearby lymph nodes are removed at this time as well. Most experts feel that taking out as many nearby lymph nodes as possible is important, but at least 12 should be removed.

When patient wake up after surgery, patient will have some pain and probably will need pain medicines for 2 or 3 days. For the first couple of days, patient will be given intravenous (IV) fluids. During this time, patient may not be able to eat or patient may be allowed limited liquids, as the colon needs some time to recover. But a colon resection rarely causes any major problems with digestive functions, and patient should be able to eat solid food again in a few days.

It is important that patient is as healthy as possible for this type of major surgery, but in some cases, an operation may be needed right away. If the tumor is large and has blocked the colon, it may be possible for the doctor to use a colonoscope to put a stent (a hollow metal or plastic tube) inside the colon to keep it open and relieve the blockage for a short time and help prepare for surgery a few days later.

2. **Laparoscopic-assisted colectomy:** This newer approach to removing part of the colon and nearby lymph nodes may be an option for some earlier stage cancers. Instead of making one long incision in the abdomen, the surgeon makes several smaller incisions. Special long instruments are inserted through these incisions to remove part of the colon and lymph nodes. One of the instruments, called a *laparoscope*, has a small video camera on the end, which allows the surgeon to see inside the abdomen. Once the diseased part of the colon has been freed, one of the incisions is made larger to allow for its removal. This type of operation requires the same type of preparation before surgery and the same type of anesthesia during surgery as an open colectomy. Because the incisions are smaller than with an open colectomy, patients may recover slightly faster and have less pain than they do after standard colon surgery.

3. **Polypectomy and local excision:** Some early colon cancers (stage 0 and some early–stage I tumors) or polyps can be removed by surgery through a colonoscope. When this is done, the surgeon does not have to cut into the abdomen. For a polypectomy, the cancer is removed as part of the polyp, which is cut at its stalk (the area that resembles the stem of a mushroom). Local excision removes superficial cancers and a small amount of nearby tissue.

Rectal Surgery

Surgery is usually the main treatment for rectal cancer, although radiation and chemotherapy will often be given before or after surgery. Several surgical methods can be used for removing or destroying rectal cancers.

- **Polypectomy and local excision:** These procedures, described in the colon surgery section, can be used to remove superficial cancers or polyps. They are done with instruments inserted through the anus, without making a surgical opening in the skin of the abdomen.

- **Local transanal resection (full-thickness resection):** As with polypectomy and local excision, local transanal resection (also known as *transanal excision*) is done with instruments inserted through the anus, without making an opening in the skin of the abdomen. This operation cuts through all layers of the rectum to remove cancer as well as some surrounding normal rectal tissue and then closes the hole in the rectal wall. This procedure can be used to remove some stage I rectal cancers that are relatively small and not too far from the anus. It is usually done with local anesthesia (numbing medicine)—patient is not asleep during the operation.

- **Transanal endoscopic microsurgery:** This operation can sometimes be used for stage I cancers that are higher in the rectum than could be reached using the standard transanal resection. An especially designed magnifying scope is inserted through the anus and into the rectum, allowing the surgeon to do a transanal resection with great precision and accuracy. This operation is only done at certain centers, as it requires special equipment and surgeons with special training and experience.

- **Low anterior resection:** Some stage I rectal cancers and most stage II or III cancers in the upper third of the rectum (close to where it connects with the colon) can be removed by low anterior resection. In this operation, the part of the rectum containing the tumor is removed without affecting the anus. The colon is then attached to the remaining part of the rectum so that after the surgery, patient will move his/her bowels in the usual way.

- **Proctectomy with coloanal anastomosis:** Some stage I and most stage II and III rectal cancers in the middle and lower third of the rectum require removing the entire rectum (proctectomy). The colon is then connected to the anus (coloanal anastomosis). The rectum has to be removed to do a total mesorectal excision, which is required to remove all of the lymph nodes near the rectum. This is a harder procedure to do, but modern techniques have made it possible. Sometimes, when a coloanal anastomosis is done, a small pouch is made by doubling back a short segment of colon (colonic J-pouch) or by enlarging a segment (coloplasty). This small reservoir of colon then functions as a storage space for fecal matter like the rectum did before surgery.

- **Abdominoperineal (AP) resection:** This operation is more involved than a low anterior resection. It can be used to treat some stage I cancers and many stage II or III rectal cancers in the lower third of the rectum (the part nearest to the anus), especially if the cancer is growing into the sphincter muscle (the muscle that keeps the anus closed and prevents stool leakage). Here, the surgeon makes one incision in the abdomen, and another in the perineal area around the anus. This incision allows the surgeon to remove the anus and the tissues surrounding it, including the sphincter muscle. Because the anus is removed, patient will need a permanent colostomy to allow stool a path out of the body.

- **Pelvic exenteration:** If the rectal cancer is growing into nearby organs, a pelvic exenteration may be recommended. This is an extensive operation. Not only will the surgeon remove the rectum, but also nearby organs, such as the bladder, prostate (in men), or uterus (in women) if the cancer has spread to these organs. Patient will need a colostomy after pelvic exenteration. If the bladder is removed, patient will also need a urostomy (opening where urine exits the front of the abdomen and is held in a portable pouch).

Side Effects of Colorectal Surgery

Potential side effects of surgery depend on several factors, including the extent of the operation and a person's general health before surgery. Most people will have at least some pain after the operation, but it usually can be controlled with medicines if needed. Eating problems usually resolve within a few days of surgery.

Other problems may include bleeding from the surgery, blood clots in the legs, and damage to nearby organs during the operation. Rarely, the new connections between the ends of the intestine may not hold together completely and may leak, which can lead to infection. It is also possible that the abdominal incision might open up, becoming an open wound. After the surgery, patient might develop scar tissue in the abdomen that can cause organs or tissues to stick together. These are called *adhesions*. In some cases, adhesions can block the bowel, requiring further surgery.

- **Colostomy or ileostomy:** Some people may need a temporary or permanent colostomy (or ileostomy) after surgery. This may take some time to get used to and may require some lifestyle adjustments. If a patient has a colostomy or ileostomy, he/she will need help in learning how to manage it. Especially trained ostomy nurses or enterostomal therapists can do this. They will usually see patient in the hospital before his/her operation to discuss the ostomy and to mark a site for the opening. After the operation, they may come to his or her house or an outpatient setting to give the patient more training.
- **Sexual function and fertility after colorectal surgery:** If the patient is a man, an AP resection may stop his erections or ability to reach orgasm. In other cases, the pleasure at orgasm may become less intense. Normal aging may cause some of these changes, but they may be made worse by the surgery.

Surgery and Other Local Treatments for Colorectal Cancer Metastases

Sometimes, surgery for cancer that has spread (metastasized) to other organs can help the patient to live longer or, depending on the extent of the disease, may even cure the patient. If only a small number of metastases are present in the liver or lungs (and nowhere else), they can sometimes be removed by surgery. This will depend on their size, number, and location.

In some cases, if it is not possible to remove the tumors with surgery, nonsurgical treatments may be used to destroy (ablate) tumors in the liver. But these methods are less likely to be curative. Several different techniques may be used.

- **Radiofrequency ablation (RFA):** RFA uses high-energy radio waves to kill tumors. A thin, needle-like probe is placed through the skin and into the tumor under CT or ultrasound guidance. An electric current is then run through the tip of the probe, releasing high-frequency radio waves that heat the tumor and destroy the cancer cells.
- **Ethanol (alcohol) ablation:** Also known as *percutaneous ethanol injection*, this procedure injects concentrated alcohol directly into the tumor to kill cancer cells. This is usually done through the skin using a needle, which is guided by ultrasound or CT scans.
- **Cryosurgery (cryotherapy):** Cryosurgery destroys a tumor by freezing it with a metal probe. The probe is guided through the skin and into the tumor using ultrasound. Then very cold gasses are passed through the probe to freeze the tumor, killing the cancer cells. This method can treat larger tumors than either of the other ablation techniques, but it sometimes requires general anesthesia.
- **Nursing assessment:**
  - Interviewing patient regarding dietary habits and family and medical history to identify risk factors
  - Questioning the patient regarding symptoms of colorectal cancer, changes in bowel habits, rectal bleeding tarry stools, abdominal discomfort, weight loss, anemia, etc.
  - Palpating abdomen for tenderness and presence of mass
  - Testing stool for occult blood

Nursing Care Plan

Nursing Diagnosis

1. Chronic pain related to malignancy, inflammation and possible intestinal obstruction
Intervention
- Assessing type and severity of pain
- Administering prescribed analgesics

- Evaluating effectiveness of analgesics
- Using alternative therapies to relieve pain, such as relaxation therapy.

2. Imbalance nutrition less than body requirements related to malignancy effects and weight loss

Intervention

- Serving high-calorie, low-residue diet
- Observing and recording fluid losses
- Maintaining hydration through IV therapy
- Checking the weight of patient

3. Constipation or diarrhea related to change in bowel lumen and disease process

Intervention

- Monitoring amount, consistency, frequency, and color of stool.
- For constipation, using laxatives or enema as needed and encouraging exercise and adequate fluids and fibers.
- For diarrhea, encouraging adequate fluid intake to prevent fluid volume deficit and electrolyte imbalance.
- Administering antidiarrheal drugs to treat diarrhea related to radiation and chemotherapy

4. Fatigue related to anemia, radiation, and chemotherapy

Interventions

- Assessing the patient's ability to perform activities
- Making an activity plan to reduce workload
- Allowing frequent rest periods to regain energy
- Administering blood products to combat anemia

5. Risk for complications related to metastatic nature of disease

Interventions

- Checking for signs of complications, such as acute pain in any other organ, breathing difficulty
- Educating patient for MRI or CT scan of chest, liver, etc.
- Checking the lab values of carcinoembryonic antigen (CEA)
- Educating for follow-up care

6. High risk for infection related to colostomy

Interventions

- Checking vital signs especially temperature
- Checking stoma for appearance and discharge
- Providing stoma care
- Changing and clearing the pouch at proper timings.

ESOPHAGEAL CANCER

Esophageal cancer is malignancy of the esophagus. Esophageal tumors usually lead to dysphagia (difficulty swallowing), pain and other symptoms. Small and localized tumors are treated surgically with curative intent. Larger tumors tend not to be operable and hence are treated with palliative care; their growth can still be delayed with chemotherapy, radiotherapy or a combination of the two. In some cases, chemo- and radiotherapy can render these larger tumors operable. Prognosis depends on the extent of the disease and other medical problems but is generally fairly poor.

Definition

Cancer that forms in tissues lining the esophagus. Two types of esophageal cancer are squamous cell carcinoma (cancer that begins in flat cells lining the esophagus) and adenocarcinoma (cancer that begins in cells that make and release mucus and other fluids).

Causes and Risk Factors

- Smoking
- Heavy drinking
- Damaging from acid reflux

Acid Reflux Raises Risk

This sphincter also prevents stomach contents from refluxing back into the esophagus. If stomach juices with acid and bile come into the esophagus, it causes indigestion or heartburn. For example, reflux and gastroesophageal reflux disease.

- A medical history of other head and neck cancers increases the chance of developing a second cancer in the head and neck area, including esophageal cancer.
- Plummer–Vinson syndrome (anemia and esophageal webbing)
- Radiation therapy
- Coeliac disease predisposes toward squamous cell carcinoma
- Obesity
- Thermal injury as a result of drinking hot beverages

Esophageal Cancer Types

- **Adenocarcinoma** is the most common type, especially in white males. It starts in gland cells in the tissue, most often in the lower part of the esophagus near the stomach. The major risk factors include reflux and Barrett's esophagus.
- **Squamous cell carcinoma or cancer**, also called epidermoid carcinoma, begins in the tissue that lines the esophagus, particularly in the middle and upper parts. Risk factors include smoking and drinking alcohol.

Stages of Cancer

1. **Stage 0 (carcinoma in situ):** In stage 0, abnormal cells are found in the innermost layer of tissue lining the esophagus. These abnormal cells may become cancer and spread into nearby normal tissue. Stage 0 is also called carcinoma in situ.
2. **Stage I:** In stage I, cancer has formed and spread beyond the innermost layer of tissue to the next layer of tissue in the wall of the esophagus.
3. **Stage II:** Stage II esophageal cancer is divided into stage IIA and stage IIB, depending on where the cancer has spread.
   a. **Stage IIA:** Cancer has spread to the layer of esophageal muscle or to the outer wall of the esophagus.
   b. **Stage IIB:** Cancer may have spread to any of the first three layers of the esophagus and to nearby lymph nodes.
4. **Stage III:** In stage III, cancer has spread to the outer wall of the esophagus and may have spread to tissues or lymph nodes near the esophagus.
5. **Stage IV:** Stage IV esophageal cancer is divided into two stages, IVA and IVB, depending on where the cancer has spread.
   - **Stage IVA:** Cancer has spread to nearby or distant lymph nodes.
   - **Stage IVB:** Cancer has spread to distant lymph nodes in other parts of the body.

Signs and Symptoms

- Dysphagia
- Odynophagia (painful swallowing)
- Pain behind the sternum or in the epigastrium, often of a burning, heartburn
- Hoarse-sounding cough, a result of the tumor affecting the recurrent laryngeal nerve
- Nausea and vomiting, regurgitation of food, coughing
- Cough, fever
- If the disease has spread elsewhere, this may lead to symptoms related to this—liver metastasis could cause jaundice and ascites, lung metastasis could cause shortness of breath, pleural effusions, etc.
- Hemoptysis

Diagnostic Evaluation

- **Esophagoscopy:** A procedure to look inside the esophagus to check for abnormal areas. An esophagoscope is inserted through the mouth or nose and down the throat into the esophagus. An esophagoscope is a thin, tube-like instrument with a light and a lens for viewing.
- **Endoscopic ultrasound:** A procedure in which an endoscope is inserted into the body, usually through the mouth or rectum. A probe at the end of the endoscope is used to bounce high-energy sound waves off internal tissues or organs and make echoes. The echoes form a picture of body tissues called a sonogram. This procedure is also called endosonography.
- **CT scan**
- **Esophagogastroduodenoscopy (endoscopy):** This involves the passing of a flexible tube down the esophagus and examining the wall.
- **Biopsies** taken of suspicious lesions are then examined histologically for signs of malignancy.
- **PET scan:** A procedure to find malignant tumor cells in the body. A small amount of radionuclide glucose (sugar) is injected into a vein. The PET scanner rotates around the body and makes a picture of where glucose is being used in the body. Malignant tumor cells show up brighter in the picture because they are more active and take up more glucose than normal cells do.
- **Barium swallow:** A series of X-rays of the esophagus and stomach. The patient drinks a liquid that contains barium (a silver-white metallic compound). The liquid coats the esophagus and stomach, and X-rays are taken. This procedure is also called an upper GI series.

Management

Esophageal Stent

If the patient cannot swallow at all, an esophageal stent may be inserted to keep the esophagus patent; stents may also assist in occluding fistulas.

- **Laser therapy** is the use of high-intensity light to destroy tumor cells; it affects only the treated area. This is typically done if the cancer cannot be removed by surgery. The relief of a blockage can help to reduce dysphagia and pain.
- **PDT:** A type of laser therapy, involves the use of drugs that are absorbed by cancer cells. When exposed to a special light, the drugs become active and destroy the cancer cells.
- **Chemotherapy**
- **Radiotherapy** is given before, during, or after chemotherapy or surgery.

Surgical Management

Esophagectomy: Surgery to remove some or most of the esophagus is called an esophagectomy. Often, a small part of the stomach is removed as well. The upper part of the esophagus is then connected to the remaining part of the stomach. Part of the stomach is pulled up into the chest or neck to become the new esophagus. It may be done by two approaches:

1. **Opening esophagectomy:** Many different approaches can be used in operating on esophageal cancer. For a transthoracic esophagectomy, the esophagus is removed with the main incisions in the abdomen and the chest. If the main incisions are in the abdomen and neck, it is called a transhiatal esophagectomy. Some approaches use incisions in the neck, chest, and abdomen.

2. **Minimally invasive esophagectomy:** For some early cancers, the esophagus can be removed through several small incisions instead of one or two large incisions. The surgeon puts a scope (like a tiny telescope) through one of the incisions to see everything during the operation.

Nursing Management

Nursing Diagnosis

- Altered nutrition less than body requirement difficulty in swallowing secondary to disease condition
- Pain related to disease condition or surgery
- Anxiety related to disease condition, its treatment and prognosis
- Knowledge deficit related to treatment and prognosis

1. Altered nutrition less than body requirement difficulty in swallowing secondary to disease condition

Interventions

- Assessing the level of daily nutrition
- Assessing the likes and dislikes of the patients
- Providing small and frequent diet to the patient
- If needed, providing the food through nasogastric tube
- Maintaining intake output chart

2. Pain related to disease condition or surgery

Interventions

- Assessing the level of pain
- Providing a comfortable position to the patient
- Providing diversional therapy to the patient
- Administering analgesic as per the doctor's order

3. Anxiety related to disease condition, its treatment, and prognosis

Interventions

- Assessing the level of anxiety
- Diversional therapy provided to the patient
- Comfortable environment provided to the patient
- Answering each question of the patient
- Administering antianxiety drug as prescribed by the doctor

4. Knowledge deficit related to treatment and prognosis.

Interventions

- Assessing the level of knowledge related to disease condition
- Answering each question of the patient

- Clarifying all doubts of the patient
- Giving information regarding the disease and its treatment

GASTRIC CANCER

Gastric cancer was once the second most common cancer in the world. In most developed countries, however, rates of stomach cancer have declined dramatically over the past half century. Men have a higher incidence of gastric cancer than women. Most of these deaths occur in people older than 40 years of age.

Tumors in the stomach can be benign or malignant. Gastric cancer is a disease in which tumors are found in the stomach. Stomach cancer is common throughout the world and affects all races, it is more common in men than women and has its peak age range between 40 and 60 years old. If it is not diagnosed quickly, it may spread to other parts of your stomach as well as to other organs. There are twice as many males with this disease than females.

Stomach cancer usually begins in cells in the inner layer of the stomach. Over time, the cancer may invade more deeply into the stomach wall. A stomach tumor can grow through the stomach's outer layer into nearby organs, such as the liver, pancreas, esophagus, or intestine.

Causes/Risk Factors of Gastric Cancer

- ***Helicobacter pylori* infection:** *H. pylori* is a bacterium that commonly infects the inner lining (the mucosa) of the stomach. Infection with *H. pylori* can cause stomach inflammation and peptic ulcers.
- **Long-term inflammation of the stomach:** People who have conditions associated with long-term stomach inflammation (such as the blood disease pernicious anemia) are at increased risk of stomach cancer.
- **Smoking:** Smokers are more likely than nonsmokers to develop stomach cancer. Heavy smokers are most at risk.
- **Family history:** Close relatives (parents, brothers, sisters, or children) of a person with a history of stomach cancer are somewhat more likely to develop the disease themselves. If many close relatives have a history of stomach cancer, the risk is even greater.
- **Poor diet, lack of physical activity**.
- **Obesity** people who eat a diet high in foods that are smoked, salted, or pickled have an increased risk for stomach cancer.
- A lack of physical activity may increase the risk of stomach cancer.

Pathophysiology

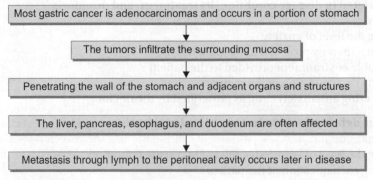

Signs and Symptoms

Stomach cancer is often either asymptomatic or it may cause only nonspecific symptoms. By the time symptoms occur, the cancer has often reached an advanced stage and may have also metastasized. Stomach cancer can cause the following signs and symptoms:

Stage 1 (Early)

- Indigestion or a burning sensation (heartburn)
- Loss of appetite, especially for meat
- Abdominal discomfort or irritation

Stage 2 (Middle)

- Weakness and fatigue
- Bloating of the stomach, usually after meals

Stage 3 (Late)

- Abdominal pain in the upper abdomen
- Nausea and occasional vomiting
- Diarrhea or constipation
- Weight loss
- Bleeding (vomiting blood or having blood in the stool) which will appear as black. This can lead to anemia.
- **Dysphagia:** This feature suggests a tumor in the cardiac or extension of the gastric tumor into the esophagus.

Diagnostic Evaluations

- **Physical examination:** Abdomen for fluid, swelling, or other changes. Also will check for swollen lymph nodes.
- **Endoscopy:** Uses a thin, lighted tube (endoscope) to look into your stomach.
- **Biopsy:** An endoscope has a tool for removing tissue.
- **CT** scanning of the abdomen may reveal gastric cancer but is more useful to determine invasion into adjacent tissues, or the presence of spread to local lymph nodes.
- **Gastroscopic examination:** This involves insertion of a fiberoptic camera into the stomach to visualize it.

Management

Treatment for stomach cancer may include surgery, chemotherapy, and radiation therapy.

Surgery

Surgery is the most common treatment. The surgeon removes part or all of the stomach, as well as the surrounding lymph nodes, with the basic goal of removing all cancer and a margin of normal tissue.

- **Endoscopic mucosal resection** is a treatment for early gastric cancer (tumor only involves the mucosa. In this procedure, the tumor, together with the inner lining of stomach (mucosa), is removed from the wall of the stomach using an electrical wire loop through the endoscope. The advantage is that it is a much smaller operation than removing the stomach.
- **Endoscopic submucosal dissection** is a similar technique used to resect a large area of mucosa in one piece. If the pathologic examination of the resected specimen shows incomplete resection or deep invasion by tumor, the patient would need a formal stomach resection.

- Surgery to remove stomach cancer the types of operation have to remove stomach cancer will depend on which part of the stomach the cancer is in. If cancer is near the area where stomach joins food pipe (esophagus) may need part of food pipe removed as well.
- **Gastric bypass procedures:** In this, the stomach is divided into a small upper pouch and a much larger lower "remnant" pouch and then rearranges the small intestine to connect to both.

Radiation Therapy

This is the use of high-energy rays to damage cancer cells and stop them from growing. When used, it is generally in combination with surgery and chemotherapy or used only with chemotherapy in cases where the individual is unable to undergo surgery.

Complications of Abdominal Surgery

- **Infection:** Infection of the incisions or of the inside of the abdomen (peritonitis, abscess) may occur due to release of bacteria from the bowel during the operation.
- **Venous thromboembolism:** Any injury, such as a surgical operation, causes the body to increase the coagulation of the blood.
- **Hemorrhage:** Many blood vessels must be cut in order to divide the stomach and to move the bowel. Any of these may later begin bleeding, either into the abdomen (intra-abdominal hemorrhage), or into the bowel itself (gastrointestinal hemorrhage).
- **Hernia:** A hernia is an abnormal opening, either within the abdomen or through the abdominal wall muscles. An internal hernia may result from surgery and rearrangement of the bowel, and is a cause of bowel obstruction.
- **Bowel obstruction:** Abdominal surgery always results in some scarring of the bowel, called adhesions. A hernia, either internal or through the abdominal wall, may also result.

Preoperative Management

- **Preoperative assessment:** The patient's preoperative physiological status is a major factor in determining outcome after major surgery. Although scoring systems including a variety of parameters have been evaluated, the previous medical history and concurrent morbidity remain the strongest predictors.
- **Medical history:** A detailed medical history and physical examination is a prerequisite to the assessment of any anesthetic and operative risk. Cardiorespiratory disease has been identified as the commonest coexisting disease in patients presenting for esophagectomy. Preexisting ischemic heart disease, poorly controlled hypertension, and pulmonary dysfunction are all associated with increased operative morbidity, particularly in the elderly and following upper abdominal and thoracic surgery. The efficacy of any medication prescribed for cardiorespiratory conditions should be evaluated at an early stage.
- **Social habits:** Smoking is a significant etiological factor in preoperative morbidity. All patients must be encouraged to stop smoking preoperatively.
- **Preoperative investigations:** The minimum preoperative investigations for all patients undergoing gastric or esophageal surgery should include baseline hematological and biochemical profiles, arterial blood gases on air, pulmonary functions tests, a resting electrocardiogram, and a chest X-ray.
- **Nutritional status:** Obesity is associated with increased operative risk.
- **Psychological preparation:** All patients should be counseled about treatment options, paying particular attention to the results and limitations of surgery. A clear description of the preoperative period should be given. An assessment of pretreatment symptoms

on quality of life of the patient should be carefully undertaken as there is accumulating evidence of quality of life scores having an independent effect on outcome.

- **Thromboembolic prophylaxis:** Appropriate measures should be taken against the risk of Thromboembolic complications. Antithromboembolic stockings, low molecular weight heparin, and preoperative calf compression should be employed.
- **Antibiotic prophylaxis:** Broad-spectrum antibiotic prophylaxis should be administered preoperatively.
- **Blood crossmatch:** Four units of blood should be crossmatched prior to surgery. Transfusion however should be avoided if at all possible as the immunological suppressive effect can adversely affect survival.

Postoperative Management

- Meticulous attention to the maintenance of fluid balance and respiratory care is essential in the immediate postoperative period.
- Pain control
- Pulmonary physiotherapy
- Early mobilization is important in the prevention of venous thrombosis and pulmonary embolism.
- Promoting pulmonary ventilation
- Providing adequate analgesic during its few days
- Encouraging ambulation
- Promoting nutrition and family education
- Adding food in a small amount at a frequent interval until well tolerated
- Monitoring weight regularly

Stomach Cancer Prevention

Gastric cancer can sometimes be associated with known risk factors for the disease. Many risk factors are modifiable though not all can be avoided.

- **Diet and lifestyle:** Excessive salt intake has been identified as a possible risk factor for gastric cancer. Having a high intake of fresh fruits and vegetables may be associated with a decreased risk of gastric cancer. Studies have suggested that eating foods that contain beta-carotene and vitamin C may decrease the risk of gastric cancer, especially if the intake of micronutrients is inadequate.
- **Preexisting conditions:** Infection with a certain bacteria, *H. pylori*, is associated with an increased risk of gastric cancer. Long-standing reflux of gastric contents and the development of an abnormal cellular lining are also associated with an increased risk of cancer at the junction of the stomach and esophagus.
- **Example:** Berries, walnuts, etc.
- **Citrus fruits:** It is no secret that oranges, tangerines, and clementines bring us vitamin C; they are among the richest sources of this critical vitamin.

Nursing Care Plan

Nursing Assessment

Careful selection of the varying therapeutic modalities is essential. Such selection should consider not only the nature of the symptoms to be relieved but also the general medical and psychological status of the patient. Decisions should be taken in the context of the predicted prognosis and the effect of any treatment intervention on quality of life.

Nursing Diagnosis

Preoperative

- Acute pain related to the growth of cancer cells
- Anxiety related to plan surgery
- Imbalanced nutrition less than body requirements related to nausea, vomiting, and no appetite
- Activity intolerance related to physical weakness.

Postoperative

- Ineffective breathing pattern related to the influence of anesthesia
- Acute pains related to interruption of the body secondary to invasive procedures or surgical intervention.
- Imbalanced nutrition less than body requirements related to fasting status
- Risk for infection related to an increased susceptibility secondary to the procedure.

Intervention

- Encouraging the patient to eat small and frequent portions of nonirritating foods to decrease gastric irritation.
- Food supplements should be high in calories as well as vitamin A and C *and* iron to enhance tissue repair.
- The nurse administers analgesic as prescribed.
- A continuous infusion of an opioid may be necessary for severe pain.
- The nurse helps the patient express fears, concern grief and diagnosis.
- Encouraging the patient to participate in treatment decisions.

LIVER CANCER

Liver cancer or hepatic cancer is a cancer that originates in the liver. Liver cancers are malignant tumors that grow on the surface or inside the liver.

Classification

1. **Primary liver cancer:** It can be benign and malignant.

Origin	Benign	Malignant
Hepatocytes	Adenoma	Hepatocellular carcinoma
Connective tissues	Fibroma	Sarcoma
Blood vessels	Hemangioma	Hemangioendothelioma
Bile ducts	Cholangioma	Carcinoma

2. **Secondary (metastatic) liver cancer:** Secondary (metastatic) cancer reaches the liver by spreading through the blood system from a primary tumor at a separate site.
3. **Mixed tumors:** Rarer forms of liver cancer include:
   - Mesenchymal tissue
   - Sarcoma
   - Hepatoblastoma, a rare malignant tumor, primarily developing in children. Most of these tumors form in the right lobe.
   - Cholangiocarcinoma
   - Angiosarcoma and hemangiosarcoma
   - Lymphoma of liver

Etiology and Risk Factors

- Younger population mainly females
- Chronic liver disease—cirrhosis, HBV, and HCV
- Chemical toxins such as vinyl chloride
- Carcinogens in herbal medicines
- Mycotoxins such as aflatoxins
- Oral contraceptives
- Metastasis

Signs and Symptoms of Primary Liver Cancer

Cholangiocarcinoma

- Sweating
- Jaundice
- Abdominal pain
- Weight loss
- Hepatomegaly

Hepatocellular carcinoma

- Abdominal mass
- Abdominal pain
- Emesis
- Anemia
- Back pain
- Jaundice
- Itching
- Weight loss

Signs and Symptoms of Secondary Liver Cancer

- Tiredness
- Loss of appetite
- Nausea
- A dragging sensation or heaviness felt up under the lower ribs on the right-hand side of the body.
- Pain in the upper part of the belly, particularly on bending forward.

Diagnostic Tests

- **Physical examination and history**: The first symptom is usually a pain in the right side. Weight loss is common and sometimes patients have episodes of severe pain, fever, and nausea. Rapidly deteriorating health, weakness, swelling, and jaundice.
- **Blood tests**: Most useful is AFP (alpha-fetoprotein). AFP is a protein produced by the liver, and an elevated level can indicate tumor growth, though some patients with liver cancer have normal AFP levels.
- **CEA test.**
- **Diagnostic imaging:** Ultrasound scan, CT, and MRI scans are required—liver imaging may include a four-phase CT, including spiral CT scans obtained during hepatic arterial and portal venous phases following intravenous contrast administration, or MRI. These techniques can accurately demonstrate the number of primary tumors within the liver and their relationship to vascular structures.

- An **image-guided biopsy** consists of the placement of a biopsy needle through the patients skin into an organ of interest using imaging for guidance. The most commonly used imaging modality are ultrasonography, and computer thermography (CT).

Management

The correct treatment of liver cancer can mean the difference between life and death. Not all patients with cancers in the liver are potentially curable. These are some of the treatments available—surgery, chemotherapy, immunotherapy, PDT, hyperthermia, radiation therapy, and radiosurgery.

Hepatocellular Carcinoma

- Partial hepatectomy to resect the entire tumor
- Liver transplantation
- Cryoablation
- Chemoembolization
- Radiotherapy
- Sorafenib
- RFA

Cholangiocarcinoma

- PDT
- Brachytherapy
- Radiotherapy
- Liver transplantation

Hepatoblastoma

- Chemotherapy, including vincristine, cyclophosphamide, and doxorubicin
- Radiotherapy
- Liver transplantation
- Surgical resection

Photodynamic Therapy

It is a form of phototherapy using nontoxic light-sensitive compounds that are exposed selectively to light, whereupon they become toxic to targeted malignant and other diseased cells. It is used clinically to treat a wide range of medical conditions, including wet age-related macular degeneration and malignant cancers, and is recognized as a treatment strategy that is both minimally invasive and minimally toxic.

Transarterial Therapy

Patients with hepatocellular carcinoma (HCC) and cirrhosis are frequently treated with transarterial therapy, a technique that delivers treatments directly into the liver. To gain access to the liver, physicians first make a small incision in the patient's leg and then place a long catheter into the femoral artery. Guided by fluoroscopy, the physician then moves the catheter up through the blood vessels to the hepatic artery, one of the two blood vessels that feed the liver. These procedures are usually performed in a hospital's radiology suite, and patients remain conscious but sedated throughout the procedures.

Types of transarterial therapy include:

- **Transarterial chemoembolization (TACE) with Lipiodol:** TACE involves delivery of chemotherapy directly to the liver, followed by a process to "lock in" (embolize) the chemotherapy. In this therapy, Lipiodol—a thick, oily substance—is mixed with chemotherapy (platinol, mitomycin-C, and adriamycin) and injected under radiological guidance directly into the artery supplying the tumor. The Lipiodol acts to contain the chemotherapy within the tumor and blocks further blood flow to the tumor. Blocking the flow of blood to the cancer helps to kill the cancer cells, as it cuts off the tumor's food and oxygen supply.

- **TACE with doxorubicin-filled beads:** Doxorubicin is a chemotherapeutic agent that helps stop the growth of tumor cells. In this therapy, doxorubicin-filled beads are delivered directly to the liver, which releases chemotherapy slowly over time and also blocks the blood flow to the tumor. With doxorubicin-filled beads, the delivery of chemotherapy-filled beads prolongs the dwell time of the chemotherapeutic agent and enhances drug delivery to liver tumors.
- **Radioactive yttrium beads:** This therapy uses radioactive yttrium beads delivered via a catheter into the hepatic artery. The beads precisely deliver radiation to the tumor, which kills the tumor cells. The beads are quite small and do not occlude the blood flow, which allows access to the tumor again if further treatment is needed. This therapy can be used in larger tumors than the above therapies and may also be used if the portal vein is occluded since the arterial flow to the liver is not occluded.

Surgical Interventions for Liver Cancer

- **Surgical resection (tumor removal):** If patients can withstand surgery and have sufficient liver function, resection offers an excellent 5-year survival rate of more than 50%. Liver cancer can recur after resection, and close surveillance is required. Surgical resection involves the removal of one or more sections of the liver in which a tumor(s) exists. Typically, surgeons can remove up to 70% of a cancerous liver (if there is no or mild fibrosis), and it will regenerate in about 2–6 weeks following surgery. Unfortunately, less than 10% of patients are candidates for liver resection.
- **Liver transplantation:** While a liver transplant represents an excellent cure for most patients with HCC, the limited organ supply makes this option unattainable for some. Patients who may benefit from liver transplantation include those with small and cirrhosis.

Nursing Care Plan

Nursing Management

For nonoperative patients

Assessment
Assessing the client for:
- Metabolic malfunctions
- Pain
- Bleeding problems
- Ascites
- Edema
- Hypoproteinemia
- Jaundice
- Endocrine complications
- Complications of chemotherapy

Common Interventions
- Taking time to prepare client in the diagnostic stage for various procedures
- Intervening postprocedure complications

- Administering analgesics for pain as per prescription
- Assisting client and family to gain knowledge about the conditions and to offer necessary support to cope with the condition.

Nursing Diagnosis

1. Activity intolerance related to anemia from poor nutrition and bleeding

Intervention

- Alternate rest and activity
- Assisting in ADL
- Monitoring Hb and hematocrit levels
- Administering blood transfusion and iron supplements if prescribed

2. Imbalanced nutrition; less than body requirement related to impaired liver functions

Intervention

- Weighing daily
- Monitoring nutritional intake
- Providing oral hygiene before meals
- Providing small and frequent diet
- Serving meal in attractive manner considering likes and dislikes of client

3. Risk for complications related to chemotherapy

Intervention

- Monitoring for ulcers in mouth, alopecia, photophobia, etc.
- Weighing daily
- Providing oral hygiene
- Advising to wear sunglasses when going out
- Checking for the signs of bleeding
- Giving psychological support and clear doubts of the client

Other Nursing Diagnosis

1. Acute pain related to tumor
2. Imbalanced fluid and electrolytes related to bleeding and ascites.

Nursing Management for Client Undergone Surgery

Following are the information about nursing management for client undergone surgery:

Preoperative care:

- Do complete physical and psychological assessment
- Conducting varies laboratory tests
- Matching donor and recipient blood and tissues reports
- Assessing clients' health needs

Postoperative care:

- Monitoring for signs of rejection, infection, and occlusion of blood vessels
- Administering prescribed immunosuppressive drugs
- **Monitoring vital signs:** Respiration, cardiovascular, neurological, and hemodynamic status also
- Assessing reports of liver function tests
- Monitoring fluid and electrolyte status
- Monitoring wound drains and bile drains for patency
- Noting bile characteristics—amount, color, and consistency
- Assessing the needs of family

BREAST CANCER

Breast cancer is a very common cancer after cervical cancer. Breast cancer begins when the cells in the breast start growing in an uncontrolled manner. These uncontrolled cells form the lump in breast that can be felt during breast self-examination. The breast cancer can be malignant if it grows in surrounding tissues. Breast cancer spreads through the lymph nodes, lymph vessels, and lymph fluid. As the lymph node drains into the axillary nodes of breast and around the collar bone.

Pathophysiology

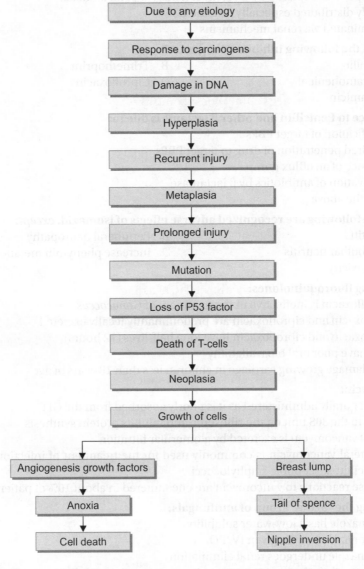

Due to any etiology
↓
Response to carcinogens
↓
Damage in DNA
↓
Hyperplasia
↓
Recurrent injury
↓
Metaplasia
↓
Prolonged injury
↓
Mutation
↓
Loss of P53 factor
↓
Death of T-cells
↓
Neoplasia
↓
Growth of cells
↓

Angiogenesis growth factors → Breast lump

Anoxia → Tail of spence

Cell death → Nipple inversion

Treatments and management are the same as described above in this chapter "Radiation and chemotherapy".

MULTIPLE CHOICE QUESTIONS

1. **All of the following antibiotics bind to the 50S subunit of the ribosome thereby inhibiting protein synthesis,** *except***:**
   - A. Chloramphenicol
   - B. Erythromycin
   - C. Linezolid
   - D. Doxycycline
   - E. Clindamycin

2. **Pharmacokinetics of doxycycline:**
   - A. 20% bound by serum proteins
   - B. 60–70% absorption after oral administration
   - C. Absorption is impaired by divalent cations, Al^{3+}, and antacids
   - D. Widely distributed especially into the CSF
   - E. Is eliminated via renal mechanisms

3. **Which of the following inhibits DNA gyrase?**
   - A. Penicillin
   - B. Trimethoprim
   - C. Chloramphenicol
   - D. Ciprofloxacin
   - E. Gentamicin

4. **Resistance to Penicillin and other β lactams is due to:**
   - A. Modification of target PBPs
   - B. Impaired penetration of drug to target PBPs
   - C. Presence of an efflux pump
   - D. Inactivation of antibiotics by β lactamase
   - E. All of the above

5. **All of the following are recognized adverse effects of isoniazid,** *except***:**
   - A. Hepatitis
   - B. Peripheral neuropathy
   - C. Retrobulbar neuritis
   - D. Increase phenytoin metabolism
   - E. CNS toxicity

6. **Regarding fluoroquinolones:**
   - A. Ciprofloxacin is ineffective in the treatment of *Gonococcus*
   - B. Norfloxacin and ciprofloxacin are predominantly fecally excreted
   - C. Norfloxacin and ciprofloxacin have long half-lives (12 hours)
   - D. They have poor oral bioavailability
   - E. May damage growing cartilage in children less than 18 years of age

7. **Vancomycin:**
   - A. Is never orally administered as it is poorly absorbed from the GIT
   - B. Binds to the 30S unit on the ribosome and inhibits protein synthesis
   - C. 60% of vancomycin is excreted by glomerular filtration
   - D. Parenteral vancomycin is commonly used for the treatment of infections caused by methicillin-susceptible staphylococci
   - E. Adverse reactions to vancomycin are encountered in about 10% of patients

8. **Regarding the "azole" group of antifungals:**
   - A. Fluconazole has a low-water solubility
   - B. Ketoconazole may be given IV/PO
   - C. Itraconazole undergoes renal elimination
   - D. Clotrimazole is the treatment of choice for systemic candidiasis—given orally
   - E. They work by reduction of ergosterol synthesis by inhibition of fungal cytochrome P450 enzymes

9. The fluoroquinolones:
   A. May be administered to patients with severe *Campylobacter* infection
   B. Work by inhibiting dihydrofolate reductase
   C. Have little effect against gram-positive organisms
   D. Are heavily metabolized in the liver
   E. Are safe to give to breastfeeding mothers

10. Clindamycin:
   A. Inhibits bacterial cell wall synthesis
   B. Is often used for prophylaxis of endocarditis in patients with valvular disease who are undergoing dental procedures
   C. Penetrates through BBB into CSF well
   D. Works well against enterococci and gram-negative aerobic organisms
   E. Is 10% protein bound

11. Which of the following is a second-generation cephalosporin?
   A. Ceftazidime   B. Cephalothin
   C. Cefotaxime   D. Cefaclor
   E. Cephalexin

12. The cephalosporin with the highest activity against gram-positive cocci is:
   A. Cefaclor   B. Cephalothin
   C. Cefuroxime   D. Cefepime
   E. Cefotaxime

13. Regarding the penicillin:
   A. Penicillin ix excreted into breast milk to levels 3–15% of those present in the serum
   B. Absorption of amoxil is impaired by food
   C. Benzathine penicillin is given PO
   D. Penicillins are 90% excreted by glomerular filtration
   E. Dosage of nafcillin should be adjusted in the presence of renal failure

14. Rifampicin:
   A. Inhibits hepatic microsomal enzymes
   B. Inhibits DNA synthesis
   C. Is bactericidal for mycobacteria
   D. Is not appreciably protein bound
   E. Is predominantly excreted unchanged in the urine

15. Regarding resistance to antibiotics:
   A. Penicillinases cannot inactivate cephalosporins
   B. Macrolides can be inactivated by transferases
   C. Mutation of aminoglycoside binding site is its main mechanism of resistance
   D. Tetracycline resistance is a marker for multidrug resistance
   E. Resistance to antibiotics is rarely plasmid encoded

16. Concerning toxicity of antibiotics:
   A. Enamel dysplasia is common with aminoglycosides
   B. Gray baby syndrome occurs with rifampicin use
   C. A disulfiram-like reaction can occur with macrolides
   D. Hemolytic anemias can occur with sulfonamide use
   E. Nephritis is the most common adverse reaction with isoniazid

17. **Which of the following is considered to be bacteriostatic?**
   A. Penicillin
   B. Chloramphenicol
   C. Ciprofloxacin
   D. Cefoxitin
   E. Tobramycin

18. **Half-life of amphotericin B is:**
   A. 2 seconds
   B. 20 minutes
   C. 2 hours
   D. 2 weeks
   E. 2 months

19. **Regarding antiseptic agents—all of the following are true, *except*:**
   A. Sodium hypochlorite is an effective antiseptic for intact skin
   B. Potassium permanganate is an effective bactericidal agent
   C. Formaldehyde may be used to disinfect instruments
   D. Chlorhexidine is active against gram-positive cocci
   E. Ethanol is an effective skin antiseptic because it denatures microbial proteins

20. **Ciprofloxacin:**
   A. Is a defluorinated analog of nalidixic acid
   B. Inhibits topoisomerases
   C. Has no gram-positive cover
   D. Has bioavailability of 30%
   E. May cause an arthropathy

21. **Flucloxacillin:**
   A. Is ineffective against streptococci
   B. Is active against enterococci and anaerobes
   C. Blocks transpeptidation and inhibits peptidoglycan synthesis
   D. Is poorly absorbed orally
   E. Has excellent penetration into CNS and prostate

22. **Aminoglycosides:**
   A. Have a β lactam ring
   B. Can produce neuromuscular blockade
   C. Are DNA gyrase inhibitors
   D. Normally reach high CSF concentrations
   E. Have good oral absorption but high first-pass metabolism

23. **Ribosomal resistance occurs with:**
   A. Sulfonamides
   B. Penicillin
   C. Fluoroquinolones
   D. Macrolides
   E. Trimethoprim

24. **Regarding antivirals:**
   A. Delvindine is a nucleoside reverse transcriptase inhibitor (NRTI)
   B. Zidovudine (AZT) is a nonnucleoside reverse transcriptase inhibitor (NNRTI)
   C. NRTIs activate HIV-1 reverse transcriptase
   D. Abacavir is a protease inhibitor
   E. NRTIs require intracytoplasmic activation to the triphosphate form

25. **All of the following are true regarding metronidazole, *except*:**
   A. It is used to treat giardia
   B. It causes a metallic taste in the mouth
   C. It inhibits alcohol dehydrogenase
   D. It is used to treat *Gardnerella*
   E. It is useful against *Trichomonas vaginalis*

Answers

1. D	2. C	3. D	4. E	5. C	6. E	7. E	8. E	9. A	10. B
11. D	12. B	13. A	14. C	15. C	16. D	17. B	18. D	19. A	20. D
21. C	22. B	23. D	24. E	25. C					

BIBLIOGRAPHY

1. Astin M, Griffin T, Neal RD, Rose P, Hamilton W. The diagnostic value of symptoms for colorectal cancer in primary care: A systematic review. Br J Gen Pract. 2011;61(586):231-43. doi:10.3399/bjgp11X572427. PMC 3080228. PMID 21619747.
2. Black MA. Textbook of Medical Surgical Nursing, 8th edition. Noida: Elsevier.
3. Brunner SA. Textbook of Medical Surgical Nursing, 5th edition. Philadelphia: Lippincott Company; 1982.
4. Cancer Genome Atlas Network. Comprehensive molecular characterization of human colon and rectal cancer. Nature. 2012;487:330-37.
5. Colorectal cancer incidence, mortality and prevalence worldwide in 2008—Summary.
6. Ferlay J, Shin HR, Bray F, Forman D, Mathers C, Parkin DM. GLOBOCAN 2008 v2.0, Cancer incidence and mortality worldwide: IARC CancerBase no. 10. Lyon, France: International Agency for Research on Cancer; 2010. [Accessed October 11, 2012].
7. Lippincot. Manual or Nursing Practice, 8th edition. Lippincott Williams and Wilkins. Jaypee Brothers. pp. 664-67.
8. Yamada T (Ed), David HA, et al. Principles of Clinical Gastroenterology, Chichester, West Sussex: Wiley-Blackwell; 2008. p. 381.

Emergency and Disaster Nursing

INTRODUCTION

Disaster

A disaster can be defined as any occurrence that causes damage, ecological disruption, loss of human life, deterioration of health and health services on a scale sufficient to warrant as extraordinary response from outside the affected community or area.

—WHO

An occurrence of a severity and magnitude that normally results in death, injuries and property damage that cannot be managed through the routine procedure and resources of government.

—Federal Emergency Management Agency

A disaster can be defined as an occurrence either nature or manmade that causes human suffering and creates human needs that victims cannot alleviate without assistance.

—American Red Cross

United Nations defines disaster is the occurrence of a sudden or major misfortune which disrupts the basic fabric and normal functioning of a society or community.

DISASTER NURSING

Disaster nursing can be defined as the adaptation of professional nursing skills in recognizing and meeting the nursing physical and emotional needs resulting from a disaster. The overall goal of disaster nursing is to achieve the best possible level of health for the people and the community involved in the disaster.

"Disaster nursing is nursing practiced in a situation where professional supplies, equipment, physical facilities, and utilities are limited or not available."

DISASTER alphabetically means

D—Destructions

I—Incidents

S—Sufferings

A—Administrative, financial failures

S—Sentiments

T—Tragedies

E—Eruption of communicable diseases

R—Research program and its implementation

Types of Disaster

- **Natural:** These are primarily natural events. It is possible that certain human activities could maybe aid in some of these events, but, by and large, these are mostly natural events.
  - Earthquakes
  - Volcanoes
  - Floods
  - Tornado, typhoons, cyclones
- **Man-made:** These are mostly caused due to certain human activities. The disasters themselves could be unintentional, but are caused due to some intentional activity. Most of these are due to certain accidents that could have been prevented, if sufficient precautionary measures were put in place:
  - Nuclear leaks
  - Chemical leaks/spillover
  - Terrorist activities
  - Structural collapse

Principles of Disaster Nursing

Following are the principles of disaster nursing:
1. Making most efficient use of hand, brain, energy, and time.
2. Making sure that every moment should be counted.
3. Expecting the unexpected.
4. Be economical in use of supply.
5. Applying three cardinal rules: Assess respiration, stop hemorrhage, and care of shock.
6. Following the principle of saving the life, preserving the function, and providing comfort.
7. Speeding in the disaster is important but do not be hasty.
8. Those who care for themselves but not for others should be removed from the group.

Factors Affecting Disaster

- **Host factors:** In the epidemiological framework as applied to disaster the host is human-kind. Host factors are those characteristics of humans that influence the severity of the disaster effect. Host factors include:
  - Age
  - Immunization status
  - Degree of mobility
  - Emotional stability
- **Environmental factors:**
  - **Physical factors:** Weather conditions, the availability of food, time when the disaster occurs, the availability of water, and the functioning of utilities, such as electricity and telephone service.
  - **Chemical factors:** Influencing disaster outcome include leakage of stored chemicals into the air, soil, groundwater, or food supplies. For example, Bhopal Gas Tragedy.
  - **Biological factors:** Are those that occur or increase as a result of contaminated water, improper waste disposal, insect or rodent proliferations, improper food storage or lack of refrigeration due to interrupted electrical services. Bioterrorism: Releasing viruses, bacteria, or other agents caused illness or death.
  - **Social factors:** Are those that contribute to the individual social support systems. Loss of family members, changes in roles, and the questioning of religious beliefs are social factors to be examined after a disaster.
  - **Psychological factors:** Psychological factors are closely related to agents, host, and environmental conditions. The nature and severity of the disaster affect the psychological distress experienced by the victims.

Phases of Disaster

- **Preimpact phase:** Occurs prior to the onset of the disaster. Includes the period of threat and warning.
- **Impact phase:** Period of time when disaster occurs, continuing to immediately following disaster. It involves inventory and rescues period, assessment of the extent of losses, identification of remaining sources, planning for use of resource, rescue of victims, minimizing further injuries, and property damage. May be brief when disasters strike suddenly and are over in minutes (airplane crash, building collapse) or lengthy as incident continues (earthquake, flood, tsunami, etc.)
- **Postimpact phase:** Occurs when majority of rescue operations are completed. It involves remedy and recovery period; honeymoon phase—feeling of euphoria; appearances of little effect by disaster; disillusionment phase—feeling of anger, disappointment, and resentment. Reconstruction phase—acceptance of loss, coping with stereo, and rebuilding.
- **Rehabilitation:** The final phase in a disaster should lead to the restoration of the predisaster conditions. The pattern of healthy needs with change rapidly, moving from casualty treatment to more primary health care **(Fig. 22.1)**.

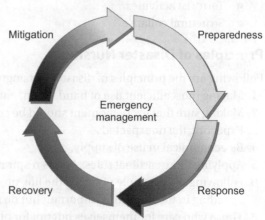

Fig. 22.1: Disaster cycle.

Disaster Cycle and Management

There are three fundamental aspects of disaster management:
1. Disaster response
2. Disaster preparedness
3. Disaster mitigation

These three aspects of disaster management correspond to different phases in the so-called disaster cycle.
- Disaster impact
- Mitigation
- Preparedness
- Reconstruction
- Rehabilitation
- Response
- Risk reduction phase before a disaster
- Recovery phase after a disaster.

Phases of emergency department:

The four phases of emergency management.

Phases	Details
Mitigation: Preventing future emergencies or minimizing their effects	➢ Includes any activities that prevent an emergency, reduce the chance of an emergency happening, or reduce the damaging effects of unavoidable emergencies ➢ Buying flood- and fire insurance for home is a mitigation activity ➢ Mitigation activities take place before and after emergencies
Preparedness: Preparing to handle an emergency	➢ Includes plans or preparations made to save lives and to help response and rescue operations ➢ Evacuation plans and stocking food and water are both examples of preparedness ➢ Preparedness activities take place before an emergency occurs
Response: Responding safely to an emergency	➢ Includes actions taken to save lives and prevent further property damage in an emergency situation. Response is putting preparedness plans into action ➢ Seeking shelter from a tornado or turning off gas valves in an earthquake are both response activities ➢ Response activities take place during an emergency
Recovery: Recovering from an emergency	➢ Includes actions taken to return to a normal or an even safer situation following an emergency ➢ Recovery includes getting financial assistance to help pay for the repairs ➢ Recovery activities take place after an emergency

Phases of Disaster

Mitigation	This phase includes any activities that prevent an emergency, reduce the likelihood of occurrence, or reduce the damaging effects of unavoidable hazards. Mitigation activities should be considered long before an emergency. For example, to mitigate fire in home, follow safety standards in selecting building materials, wiring, and appliances. But an accident involving fire could happen. To protect yourself and animals from the costly burden of rebuilding after a fire, one should buy fire insurance. These actions reduce the danger and damaging effects of fire
Preparedness	This phase includes developing plans for what to do, where to go, or who to call for help before an event occurs, actions that will improve the chances of successfully dealing with an emergency. For instance, posting emergency telephone numbers, holding disaster drills, and installing smoke detectors are all preparedness measures. Other examples include identifying where you would be able to shelter your animals in a disaster. You should also consider preparing a disaster kit with essential supplies for your family and animals

Contd...

Contd...

Response	Your safety and well-being in an emergency depend on how prepared you are and on how you respond to a crisis. By being able to act responsibly and safely, you will be able to protect yourself, your family, others around you and your animals. Taking cover and holding tight in an earthquake, moving to the basement with your pets in a tornado, and safely leading horses away from a wildfire are examples of safe response. These actions can save lives
Recovery	After an emergency and once the immediate danger is over, your continued safety and well-being will depend on your ability to cope with rearranging your life and environment. During the recovery period, you must take care of yourself and your animals to prevent stress-related illnesses and excessive financial burdens. During recovery, you should also consider things to do that would lessen the effects of future disasters

Responsibilities of Various Agencies in Emergency and Disaster Management

Emergency management works when local, state, and federal governments fulfill emergency management responsibilities. Voluntary organizations also have important responsibilities during disasters.

Personal responsibilities	Animal owners have the ultimate responsibility for their animals. Community disaster preparedness plans try to incorporate the care of animals and their owners in their plans, but plans can only coordinate care they cannot always provide it. The best way to be prepared is to create a personal emergency plan that includes provisions to care for animals. You can learn how to prepare such a plan from your local Red Cross office, local emergency management agency, and numerous other groups. Be prepared to deal with the four phases of most emergencies
Local government responsibilities	Local governments make plans and provide resources to protect their citizens from the hazards that threaten their communities. This is done through mitigation activities, preparedness plans, response to emergencies, and recovery operations. Wherever you live within the United States, a county or municipal agency has been designated as local emergency management agency. The local government level is the most important at which to develop emergency management plans because local governments serve as the link between you and the State and Federal agencies in the emergency management network. It includes the following responsibilities: ➤ Identifying hazards and assessing their potential risk to the community ➤ Determining the community's capability to mitigate against, prepare for, respond to, and recover from major emergencies ➤ Identifying and employing methods to improve the community's emergency management capability through efficient use of resources, improved coordination, and cooperation with other communities and with the State and Federal governments ➤ Establishing mitigation measures, such as building codes, zoning ordinances, or land-use management programs ➤ Developing and coordinating preparedness plans ➤ Establishing warning systems ➤ Stocking emergency supplies and equipment ➤ Educating the public and training emergency personnel ➤ Assessing damage caused by the emergency
	➤ Activating response plans and rescue operations ➤ Ensuring that shelter and medical assistance are provided ➤ Recovering from the emergency and helping citizens return to normal life as soon as possible

Contd...

Contd...

State government responsibilities	The state emergency management office is responsible for protecting communities and citizens within the state. The state office carries out statewide emergency management activities, helps coordinate emergency management activities involving more than one community, or assists individual communities when they need help. If any community lacks the resources needed to protect itself or to recover from a disaster, the state may help with money, personnel, or other resources
Federal government responsibilities	At the federal level of government, the FEMA is involved in mitigation, preparedness, response, and recovery activities. FEMA helps the states in several ways. FEMA provides the following programs: ➢ Training programs and research information on the latest mitigation measures ➢ Review and coordination of state emergency plans ➢ Financial assistance ➢ Flood insurance to individuals and businesses in communities that join the NFIP ➢ Subsidies to state and local offices of emergency management for maintaining emergency management programs ➢ Guidance and coordination for plans to warn and protect the nation in national security emergencies ➢ Coordination of services for disaster response and recovery activities
Voluntary agencies and organizations	One of the most important voluntary organizations in terms of disasters is the Red Cross Society. The Red Cross provides relief to victims of disasters. Each local agency is responsible for providing disaster relief services in the community. In large scale disasters, volunteers from across the country may respond. The Red Cross provides individuals and families with food, shelter, first aid, clothing, bedding, medicines, and other services

(FEMA: Federal Emergency Management Agency; NFIP: National Flood Insurance Programme)

Nursing Responsibilities During Disaster

The nursing management of mass casualties can be divided into search and rescue, first aid, triage and stabilization of victims, hospital treatment and redistribution of patients to other hospitals if necessary.

Search, Rescue, and First Aid

After a major disaster, the need for search, rescue, and first aid is likely to be so great that organized relief services will be able to meet only a small fraction of the demand. Most immediate help comes from the uninjured survivors.

Field Care

Most injured persons converge spontaneously to health facilities, using whatever transport is available, regardless of the facilities, operating status. Providing proper care to casualties requires that the health service resources be redirected to this new priority. Bed availability and surgical services should be maximized. Provisions should be made for food and shelter. A center should be established to respond to inquiries from patient's relatives and friends. Priority should be given to victim's identification and adequate mortuary space should be provided.

Triage

When the quantity and severity of injuries overwhelm, the operative capacity of health facilities, a different approach to medical treatment must be adopted. The principle of "first come, first treated" is not followed in mass emergencies. Triage consists of rapidly classifying the injured on the basis of the severity of their injuries and the likelihood of their survival with prompt medical intervention. It must be adopted to locally available skills. Higher priority is granted to victims whose immediate or long-term prognosis can be dramatically affected by simple intensive care. Patients who require a great deal of attention with questionable benefits have the lowest priority. Triage is the only approach that can provide maximum benefit to the greatest number of injured in a major disaster situation.

Although different triage systems have been adopted and are still in use in some countries, the most common classification uses the internationally accepted four-color code system. Red indicates high priority treatment or transfer, yellow signals medium priority, green indicates ambulatory patients, and black for dead patients.

Triage should be carried out at the site of disaster, in order to determine transportation priority, and admission to the hospital or treatment center where the patient's needs and priority of medical care will be reassessed. Ideally, local health workers should be taught the principles of triage as part of disaster training.

Persons with minor or moderate injuries should be treated at their own homes to avoid social dislocation and the added drain on resources of transporting them to central facilities. The seriously injured should be transported to hospitals with specialized treatment facilities.

Tagging

All patients should be identified with tags stating their name, age, place of origin, triage category, diagnosis, and initial treatment.

Identification of dead

Taking care of the dead is an essential part of the disaster management. A large number of dead can also impede the efficiency of the rescue activities at the site of the disaster. Care of the dead includes: (1) removal of the dead from the disaster scene, (2) shifting to the mortuary, (3) identification, and (4) reception of bereaved relatives. Proper respect for the dead is of great importance.

Relief Phase

This phase begins when assistance from outside starts to reach the disaster area. The type and quantity of humanitarian relief supplies are usually determined by two main factors: (1) the type of disaster, and (2) the type and quantity of supplies available locally.

Immediately following a disaster, the most critical health supplies are those needed for treating casualties and preventing the spread of communicable diseases. Following the initial emergency phase, needed supplies will include food, blankets, clothing, shelter, sanitary engineering equipment and construction material. A rapid damage assessment must be carried out in order to identify needs and resources. Disaster managers must be prepared to receive large quantities of donations. There are four principal components in managing humanitarian supplies: (1) acquisition of supplies, (2) transportation, (3) storage, and (4) distribution.

Epidemiologic Surveillance and Disease Control

Disasters can increase the transmission of communicable diseases through the following mechanisms:
- Overcrowding and poor sanitation in temporary resettlements. This accounts in part for the reported increase in acute respiratory infections, etc.
- Population displacement may lead to the introduction of communicable diseases to which either the migrant or indigenous populations are susceptible.

- Disruption and the contamination of water supply, damage to sewerage system, and power systems are common in natural disasters.
- Disruption of routine control programs as funds and personnel are usually diverted to relief work.
- Ecological changes may favor breeding of vectors and increase the vector population density.
- Displacement of domestic and wild animals, who carry with them zoonoses that can be transmitted to humans as well as to other animals. Leptospirosis cases have been reported following large floods (as in Orissa, India, after the super cyclone in 1999). Anthrax has been reported occasionally.
- Provision of emergency food, water, and shelter in a disaster situation from different or new source may itself be a source of infectious disease.

The principles of preventing and controlling communicable diseases after a disaster are to:
- Implement as soon as possible all public health measures, to reduce the risk of disease transmission
- Organize a reliable disease reporting system to identify outbreaks and to promptly initiate control measures
- Investigate all reports of disease outbreaks rapidly.

Vaccination

- Health authorities are often under considerable public and political pressure to begin mass vaccination programs, usually against typhoid, cholera, and tetanus.
- The WHO does not recommend typhoid and cholera vaccines in routine use in endemic areas. The newer typhoid and cholera vaccines have increased efficacy, but because they are multidose vaccines, compliance is likely to be poor.
- Significant increases in tetanus incidence have not occurred after natural disasters. Mass vaccination of population against tetanus is usually unnecessary. The best protection is maintenance of a high level of immunity in the general population by routine vaccination before the disaster occurs, and adequate wound cleaning and treatment.
- If tetanus immunization was received >5 years ago in a patient who has sustained an open wound, a tetanus toxoid booster is an effective preventive measure.
- If cold-chain facilities are inadequate, they should be requested at the same time as vaccines.

Nutrition

Natural disaster may affect the nutritional status of the population by affecting one or more components of food chain depending on the type, duration, and extent of the disaster, as well as the food and nutritional conditions existing in the area before the catastrophe. Infants, children, pregnant women, nursing mothers, and sick persons are more prone to nutritional problems after prolonged drought or after certain types of disasters, such as hurricanes, floods, land or mudslides, volcanic eruptions, and sea surges involving damage to crops, to stocks, or to food distribution systems.

The immediate steps for ensuring that the food relief program will be effective include:
  a. Assessing the food supplies after the disaster
  b. Gauging the nutritional needs of the affected population
  c. Calculating daily food rations and need for large population groups
  d. Monitoring the nutritional status of the affected population.

Rehabilitation

The final phase in a disaster should lead to restoration of the predisaster conditions. Rehabilitation starts from the very first moment of a disaster. A provision by external agencies of sophisticated medical care for a temporary period has negative effects. On the withdrawal of such care, the population is left with a new level of expectation which simply cannot be fulfilled.

In first weeks after disaster, the pattern of health needs will change rapidly, moving from casualty treatment to more routine primary health care. Services should be reorganized and restructured. Priorities also will shift from health care toward environmental health measures. **Some of them are as follows:**

Water Supply

A survey of all public water supplies should be made. This includes distribution system and water source. It is essential to determine physical integrity of system components, the remaining capacities, and bacteriological and chemical quality of water supplied.

The main public safety aspect of water quality is microbial contamination. The first priority of ensuring water quality in emergency situations is chlorination. It is the best way of disinfecting water. It is advisable to increase residual chlorine level to about 0.2–0.5 mg/L. Low water pressure increases the risk of infiltration of pollutants into water mains. Repaired mains, reservoirs, and other units require cleaning and disinfection.

The existing and new water sources require the following protection measures:
1. Restricting access to people and animals; if possible, erecting a fence and appointing a guard.
2. Ensuring adequate excreta disposal at a safe distance from water source.
3. Prohibiting bathing, washing, and animal husbandry, upstream of intake points in rivers and streams.
4. Upgrading wells to ensure that they are protected from contamination.
5. Estimating the maximum yield of wells and if necessary. In many emergency situations, water has to be trucked to disaster site or camps. All water tankers should be inspected to determine fitness and should be cleaned and disinfected before transporting water.

Food Safety

Poor hygiene is the major cause of food-borne diseases in disaster situations. Where feeding programs are used (as in shelters or camps) kitchen sanitation is of utmost importance. Personal hygiene should be monitored in individuals involved in food preparation.

Basic Sanitation and Personal Hygiene

Many communicable diseases are spread through fecal contamination of drinking water and food. Hence, every effort should be made to ensure the sanitary disposal of excreta. Emergency latrines should be made available to the displaced, where toilet facilities have been destroyed. Washing, cleaning, and bathing facilities should be provided to the displaced persons.

Vector Control

Control program for vector-borne diseases should be intensified in the emergency and rehabilitation period, especially in areas where such diseases are known to be endemic. Of special concern are dengue fever and malaria, leptospirosis and rat-bite fever, typhus, and plague. Flood water provides ample breeding opportunities for mosquitoes.

POST-TRAUMATIC STRESS DISORDER AND REHABILITATION OF DISASTER VICTIMS

Post-traumatic stress disorders (PTSD) is a set of reactions to an extreme stressor, such as intense fear, helplessness, or horror that leads individuals to relieve the trauma.

Signs and Symptoms

- Episodes of repeated relieving of the trauma in intensive memories (flashbacks) or dreams.
- Flashbacks occurring—against the persisting background of a sense of "numbers" and emotional blunting.
- Detachment from other people.
- Unresponsiveness to surroundings.
- Anhedonia is the inability to experience pleasure.
- Avoidance of activities and situations reminiscent of the trauma.
- Fear and avoidance of cues that remind the sufferer of the original trauma.
- May be dramatic, acute bursts of fear, panic or aggression, triggered by stimuli arousing a sudden recollection and re-enactment of the trauma or the original reaction to it.

Predisposing Factors

- Personality traits—compulsive, asthenic
- History of neurotic illness, childhood abuse, who then suffer subsequent trauma.

Etiology

- Military combat
- Bombing or war
- Kidnapping
- Robbery
- Abuse—physical, sexual (e.g., rape), or psychological
- Terrorist attack
- Prisoner of war
- Torture
- Natural or man-made disasters
- Witnessing violence (domestic, criminal)
- Severe automobile accidents
- Seeing dead body or body parts
- Serious injury or death of family member or a close friend
- Diagnosis of life-threatening disease in self or child
- Unexpected death of family member or a close friend

High-Risk Group

- Children
- Disabled
- Elderly
- Women—young, single, widowed, orphaned, disabled—have lost children.
- Orphans from orphanages.
- Having the history of childhood abuse

Principles of Nursing Care in PTSD

- Consistent empathic approach to help the clients tolerate the intense memories and emotional pain.
- Simple reorienting, reassuring statements to prevent suicidal ideation.
- Trusting relationship to convey a sense of respect, acceptance of their distress, and belief in the client's reactions.
- Reconnecting the individuals with the existing support system.
- Restarting activities that provide a sense of mastery.
- Promoting independence and the client's highest level of functioning.
- Managing countertransference reactions.
- Group therapies to decrease isolation, to discuss the effect of trauma and develop alternative coping mechanisms.
- Encouraging the client to write/verbalize to manage reactions and feelings.
- Helping the client identify community resources.
- Teaching anxiety management strategies, such as relaxation, breaking techniques, and diverting the individuals' mind through involvement in activities.
- Changes in lifestyle, such as following a healthy diet, avoiding stimulants, intoxicants, regular exercise, and adequate sleep. Using medication as recommended.

Rehabilitation of Disaster Victims

In the postdisaster period, along with relief, rehabilitation and the care of physical health and injuries, mental health issues need to be given importance. Apart from material and logistic help, the suffering human beings will require human interventions.

Challenges of Rehabilitation

- Ensuring that people living in the relief camps have access to regular food supplies, additional sets of clothes, sanitation drinking, water, public health intervention—immunization, preventive health care, heat and rainproof shelters, child care and education facilities and support.
- Ensuring access to basic entitlements in terms of their compensation, government schemes, and credit institutions so that they can rebuild their homes and livelihood back to the same levels as before the disaster.
- Ensuring livelihood reintegration.
- Ensuring legal right and social justice to the disaster victims including filing of FIRs, investigation and contesting cases in the court.
- Providing psychosocial counseling and support for dealing with loss, betrayal, and anger.
- Community-based rehabilitation for widow's orphans, elderly, children and physically disabled.
- Actively rebuilding a culture of communal harmony and trust.

Kinds of Reactions Shown by Disaster Victims

- **Physical impact**—stomach aches, diarrhea, headaches, and body aches, physical impairments (limbs, sight, voice, hearing), injuries, fever, cough, cold, miscarriage, etc.
- **Emotional reactions**—anger, betrayal, irritability, revenge seeking, fear, anxiety, depression, withdrawal, grief, addiction to pan masala, cigarette, beedi, drug abuse (flaskbacks, numbness, depression)
- **Socioeconomic impact**—loss of trust between communities, lack of privacy, single-parent families, widows, orphan state with loss of both parents, discontinuity in educational plans

(e.g., loss of employment, homelessness migration, disorganization of life routines, material loss).

Psychosocial Interventions

Principles

- Ventilation
- Empathy
- Active listening
- Social support
- Externalization of interest
- Lifestyle choice
- Relaxation and recreation
- Spirituality
- Health care
- Work with individuals (willing to talk immediately and unwilling to talk)
    - For people who are willing to talk immediately:
        - Listen attentively
        - Do not interrupt
        - Acknowledge that you understand the pain and distress by learning forward
        - Look into the eyes
        - Console them by patting on the shoulders or touching or holding their hand as they cry
        - Respect the silence during interaction, do not try to fill it in by talking.
        - Keep reminding them "I am with you. It is good you are trying to release your distress by crying. It will make you feel better."
        - Do not ask them to stop crying.
    - For those unwilling to talk (angry, or remain mute and silent):
        - Do not get anxious or feel rejected, remain calm
        - Maintain regular contact and greet them
        - Maintain interaction
        - Acknowledge that you understand they are not to blame
        - Tell them you will return the next day or in a couple of days
        - Tell them you are not upset or angry because he/she did not talk.
    - Once the person starts talking, maintain a conversation using the following queries, such as:
        - How are you?
        - How are your other family members?
        - What can individuals do to recover?

Work with Families

- Sharing their experience of loss as a family.
- Contacting relatives to mobilize support and facilitate reconvey.
- Participating in rituals, such as prayers, keeping the dead persons' photographs.
- Making time for recreation.
- Resuming normal activities of the predisaster days with the family.
- Trying and doing things together as a writ and support one another.
- Be together as a family member. Not sending women and children and the aged too far off places for the sake of safety.

- Restarting activities that are special to your family, such as having meals together, praying, playing games, etc.
- Keep touching and comforting your parents, children, spouse, and the aged in your family.
- Keeping in constant touch with the family member who is hospitalized.

Work with the Community

- Group mourning
- Group meetings
- Supporting group initiatives
- Cultural aspects
- Rally
- Group participation for rebuilding efforts
- Sensitization process.

Rehabilitation of Special Groups

Aged people:
- Keeping them with their near and dear ones
- Visiting them regularly and spending time with them
- Touching them and allowing them to cry
- Re-establishing their daily routines
- Making them feel responsible by giving them some work to carry out which is not too difficult
- Getting them involved in relief work by requesting for their suggestion and advice, etc.
- Keeping them informed of positive news
- Attending to their medical ailments
- Organizing small group prayer meetings.

Disabled people:
- Removing them to places of safety
- Keeping them informed what is happening
- Getting them involved in activities
- Integrate them in group discussions
- Attend to their specific needs (wheelchairs, hearing aids)
- Helping them to overcome their feeling of insecurity
- Taking cognizance of the fact that mentally challenged people especially the women and children are vulnerable to sexual abuse, and help them.

Women:
- Helping them to be with their families
- Keep informing them what is happening
- Involving them in activities
- Involving them in relief and rehabilitation activities
- Initiating self-help formation
- Involving them in recreation
- Making them to spend time with young widows or people who have lost their children and supporting them.

Children:
- Letting him or her to be close to adults who are loved and familiar.
- Re-establishing some sort of a routine for them, such as eating, sleeping, going for programs
- Actions, such as touching, hugging, reassuring them verbally
- Allowing them to take about the event
- Encouraging them to play

- Involving them in activities, such as painting and drawing where they can express their emotions
- Organizing storytelling sessions, singing, songs, and games
- Praising coping behavior
- Providing referral if required
- Spending time on their studies once they return to school.

Policies Related to Emergency and Disaster Management

This policy aims at:
- Promoting a culture of prevention, preparedness, and resilience at all levels through knowledge, innovation, and education
- Encouraging mitigation measures based on technology, traditional wisdom, and environmental sustainability
- Mainstreaming disaster management into the developmental planning process
- Establishing institutional and technolegal frameworks to create an enabling regulatory environment and a compliance regime
- Ensuring efficient mechanism for identification, assessment, and monitoring of disaster risks
- Developing contemporary forecasting and early warning systems backed by responsive and fail-safe communication with information technology support
- Ensuring efficient response and relief with a caring approach toward the needs of the vulnerable sections of the society
- Undertaking reconstruction as an opportunity to build disaster-resilient structures and habitat for ensuring safer living
- Promoting a productive and proactive partnership with the media for disaster management.

Policy statement: To develop and implement an integrated action plan that will create an effective disaster management system at local, national and international levels.

Focus Areas and Strategies for Intervention

- **Making disaster risk reduction a development priority:** To incorporate disaster risk principles in the development agenda and other country programs, to enhance institutional capacity in disaster risk reduction, to develop national platforms for disaster risk reduction.
- **Improving early warning systems:** To monitor continuously the hazard and vulnerability threats, to develop standard risk and monitoring instruments, do a risk and hazard mapping, to foster an understanding of disaster management mechanisms through dissemination of information and advocacy.
- **Addressing priority development concerns to reduce underlying risk factors:** To integrate disaster risk reduction in poverty reduction strategy paper, to address sources of vulnerability especially outbreak of diseases and pests (HIV/AIDS, avian flu, locusts, etc.), to sensitize both local and traditional authorities with a view to understanding disaster prevention as a development challenge, mainstream gender, and youth policies in the development agenda.
- **Effective disaster response through disaster preparedness:** To promote contingency planning in all government departments and all other sectors to ensure alignment of national, local, and district disaster management plans, to review and periodically rehearse national preparedness and contingency plans for major hazards, to ensure that operational capacity exists within disaster management systems to enhance community resilience.

Policy Implementation Agencies and Structures

The policy will adopt various approaches to ensure that risk reduction in particular and disaster management in general is a national and local priority with strong involvement of local actors, the victims of disaster and institutional basis for implementation.

Agencies

I. National government organizations (NGOs)
II. Civil society organizations
III. Government agencies
IV. UN agencies
V. Private sector

Functions

a. Identifying, assessing, and monitoring disaster risks and enhancing early warning systems
b. Using indigenous knowledge, innovation, practices, and education to build a culture of safety and resilience at all levels
c. Strengthening disaster preparedness for effective response at all levels
d. Creation of disaster prevention volunteer corps at local and national levels to be fully trained and equipped to identify, assess, and monitor disaster events.

Operational Mechanism

This policy will be implemented through the following strategic actions:
a. Sensitization programs and advocacy on disaster prevention
b. Mainstreaming disaster prevention and management in school curricula and development programs
c. Factor disaster scenarios into economic planning and programs
d. Capacity building and information sharing
e. Monitoring and evaluation.

Agencies Involved During Disaster Management

- **The Adventist Community Services (ACS)** receives, processes, and distributes clothing, bedding, and food products. In major disasters, the agency brings in mobile distribution units filled with bedding and packaged clothing that is presorted according to size, age, and gender. ACS also provides emergency food and counseling and participates in the cooperative disaster child care program.
- **The Red Cross** is required by congressional charter to undertake disaster relief activities to ease the suffering caused by a disaster. Emergency assistance includes fixed mobile feeding stations, shelter, cleaning supplies, comfort kits, first aid, blood and blood products, food, clothing, emergency transportation, rent, home repairs, household items, and medical supplies.
- Additional assistance for long-term recovery may be provided when other relief assistance and personal resources are not adequate to meet disaster-caused needs.
- **The Ananda Marga Universal Relief Team (AMURT)** renders immediate medical care, food and clothing distribution, stress management, and community and social services. AMURT also provides long-term development assistance and sustainable economic programs to help disaster-affected people. AMURT depends primarily on full- and part-

time volunteer help and has a large volunteer base to draw on worldwide. AMURT provides and encourages disaster services training in conjunction with other relief agencies, such as the Red Cross.

- **Children's Disaster Services (CDS)** provides childcare in shelters and disaster assistance centers by training and certifying volunteers to respond to traumatized children with a calm, safe, and reassuring presence. CDS provides respite for caregivers as well as individualized consultation and education about their child's unique needs after a disaster. CDS creates a more favorable work environment for the staff and volunteers of their partner agencies. CDS works with parents, community agencies, schools, or others to help them understand and meet the special needs of children during or after a disaster.
- **The Friends Disaster Service** provides clean-up and rebuilding assistance to the elderly, disabled, low income, or uninsured survivors of disasters.
- **The International Relief Friendship Foundation (IRFF)** has the fundamental goal of assisting agencies involved in responding to the needs of a community after disaster strikes. When a disaster hits, IRFF mobilizes a volunteer group from universities, businesses, youth groups, women's organizations, and religious groups. IRFF also provides direct support and emergency services immediately following a disaster, such as blankets, food, clothing, and relief kits.
- **The National Emergency Response Team (NERT)** meets the basic human needs of shelter, food, and clothing during times of crisis and disaster. NERT provides emergency mobile trailer units (EMTUs) which are self-contained, modest living units for up to 8–10 people, to places where disaster occurs. When EMTUs are not in use, they serve as mobile teaching units used in emergency preparedness programs in communities.
- **The National Organization for Victim Assistance** provides social and mental health services for individuals and families who experience major trauma after disaster including critical incident stress debriefing.

Impact on Health and aftereffects of Disaster

- Mental health problems have proven to be some of the most common side effects of natural disasters. The great loss and devastation disasters make mental health problems, such as post-traumatic stress disorder and depression, rampant among survivors of these horrific acts of nature.
- Communicable diseases: Communities reeling from natural disasters also tend to become breeding grounds for outbreaks of communicable diseases, which are defined as diseases that easily transfer from person to person or animal to person. "Continuing problems with hygiene and diseases related to hygiene are common in refugee camps."
- Health service system: The real damage in the long run is done to the health service infrastructure. The physical damage done to the hospitals and health buildings, the loss of medical equipment and medicines, "there's the issue of the dysfunction of health facilities."

Aftereffects of Disaster

Common reactions experienced following a major traumatic event include:
- Feelings of fear, sadness, or anger
- Feeling overwhelmed
- Feeling numb, detached, or withdrawn
- Difficulty with focusing attention and concentration
- Difficulty in planning ahead
- Tearfulness

- Unwanted and recurring memories or bad dreams related to the event
- Sleep problems
- Constant questioning: "What if I had done x, y, or z, instead?" and "What will happen now?"
- "Replaying" the event and inventing different outcomes in order to be prepared should it happen again?

Grief

Grief after the death of a loved one, a pet, or loss of property, can be felt. Intensely for a long time after the event. Everyone copes differently, but the intensity of the feelings usually diminishes with time. A person may feel one or all of the following:

- A short-lived sense of unreality or feelings of detachment from the world
- Numbness, shock, and confusion
- Anger and self-blame or blaming others for the outcome
- An inability to find anything meaningful and be able to make sense of the experience— "Why has this happened to me?" and spiritual questions—"Where is God in this?"
- Feelings of despair and loneliness
- Sleep disturbances and changes in appetite
- Emotional distress so severe it feels like physical pain
- Fatigue
- Flooding of memories or preoccupation with thinking about the person who has died
- Loneliness or longing for the person who has died
- Stress about financial problems, parenting, and practical concerns.

Dealing with Emotional Impact of Disaster

Following a disaster, it is important to find ways to regain a sense of safety and control. People often need to have access to a safe and secure environment, to find out what happened to family members and friends and to have access to relevant services. There are steps victims can take to make the situation more manageable.

Helping yourself:
- Spending time with family and friends
- Trying to get back to a routine
- Trying to be healthy
- Take time out
- Limiting the amount of media coverage you watch, listen to, or read. While getting information is important, watching or listening to news bulletins too frequently can cause people who have experienced a disaster to feel distressed.
- Write down your worries: You may find it helpful to write down your worries and concerns and use the problem-solving worksheet at the back of this booklet to identify some practical steps you can take to address those issues. Identifying the specific feelings you are experiencing and the concern/worry that may be underlying each of these feelings.
- Expressing your feelings
- Accepting help when it is offered
- Not expecting to have the answers
- Realizing you are not alone: Grief, loss and shock, sadness, and stress can make you feel like isolating yourself from others. It may be helpful to remember that many people are feeling the same as you and will share your journey of recovery. Shutting yourself off from others is unlikely to make the situation any better.

Infectious Diseases after Disaster

- Cryptosporidiosis
- Enteroviruses
- *Escherichia coli*
- Giardiasis
- Hepatitis B, hepatitis C, HIV/AIDS
- Leptospirosis
- Legionnaires' disease
- Methicillin-resistant *Staphylococcus aureus* infection
- Norovirus
- Rotavirus
- Shigellosis
- Skin infections
- Tetanus
- Toxoplasmosis
- Trench foot or immersion foot
- Tuberculosis
- Varicella disease (chickenpox)
- *Vibrio cholerae*
- *Vibrio parahaemolyticus*
- *Vibrio vulnificus*
- West Nile virus

EMERGENCY CONDITIONS

SHOCK

Clinical syndrome characterized by decreased tissue perfusion and impaired cellular metabolism resulting in an imbalance between the supply and demand for oxygen and nutrients.

Etiology and Pathophysiology

Cardiogenic Shock

Occurs when either systolic or diastolic dysfunction of the pumping action of the heart results in compromised cardiac output (CO). Precipitating causes of cardiogenic shock include myocardial infarction, cardiomyopathy, blunt cardiac injury, severe systemic or pulmonary hypertension, cardiac tamponade, and myocardial depression from metabolic problems. Hemodynamic profile will demonstrate an increase in the pulmonary artery wedge pressure (PAWP) and pulmonary vascular resistance.

Signs and Symptoms

Tachycardia, hypotension, a narrowed pulse pressure, tachypnea, pulmonary congestion, cyanosis, pallor, cool and clammy skin, decreased capillary refill time, anxiety, confusion, and agitation.

Hypovolemic Shock

Occurs when there is a loss of intravascular fluid volume.

a. **Absolute hypovolemia** results when fluid is lost through hemorrhage, gastrointestinal (GI) loss (e.g., vomiting, diarrhea), fistula drainage, diabetes insipidus, hyperglycemia, or diuresis.

b. **Relative hypovolemia** results when fluid volume moves out of the vascular space into extravascular space (e.g., interstitial or intracavitary space) and this is called *third spacing*. The physiologic consequences of hypovolemia include a decrease in venous return, preload, stroke volume, and cardiac output (CO) resulting in decreased tissue perfusion and impaired cellular metabolism. Clinical manifestations depend on the extent of injury or insult, age, and general state of health and may include anxiety, an increase in heart rate, CO, and respiratory rate and depth, and a decrease in stroke volume, PAWP, and urine output.

Neurogenic Shock

It is a hemodynamic phenomenon that can occur within 30 minutes of a spinal cord injury at the fifth thoracic (T5) vertebra or above and last up to 6 weeks, or in response to spinal anesthesia. Clinical manifestations include hypotension, bradycardia, temperature dysregulation (resulting in heat loss), dry skin, and *poikilothermia* (taking on the temperature of the environment).

Anaphylactic Shock

It is an acute and life-threatening hypersensitivity (allergic) reaction to a sensitizing substance (e.g., drug, chemical, vaccine, food, insect venom). Immediate reaction causes massive vasodilation, release of vasoactive mediators, and an increase in capillary permeability resulting in fluid leaks from the vascular space into the interstitial space. Clinical manifestations can include anxiety, confusion, dizziness, chest pain, incontinence, swelling of the lips and tongue, wheezing, stridor, flushing, pruritus, urticaria, and angioedema.

Septic Shock

It is the presence of sepsis with hypotension despite fluid resuscitation along with the presence of tissue perfusion abnormalities. In severe sepsis and septic shock, the initiated body response to an antigen is exaggerated resulting in an increase in inflammation and coagulation, and a decrease in fibrinolysis. Endotoxins from the microorganism cell wall stimulate the release of cytokines and other proinflammatory mediators that act through secondary mediators, such as platelet-activating factor.

Clinical presentation for sepsis is complex. Patients will usually experience a hyperdynamic state characterized by increased CO. Persistence of a high CO beyond 24 hours is ominous and often associated with hypotension and multiple organ dysfunction syndrome. Initially, patients will hyperventilate as a compensatory mechanism, resulting in respiratory alkalosis followed by respiratory acidosis and respiratory failure. Other clinical signs include alteration in neurologic status, decreased urine output, and GI dysfunction.

Stages of Shock

Compensatory stage:
a. Decrease in circulating blood volume.
b. Sympathetic nervous system stimulated, release catecholamines (epinephrine and norepinephrine), bronchodilation and increased CO occurs. To maintain blood pressure: Increase heart rate and contractility increases in peripheral vasoconstriction due to stimulation of beta-adrenergic fibers (cause vasoconstriction of blood vessels of skin and abdominal viscera) and increase in heart rate and contractility.
c. Renin–angiotensin release of aldosterone—reabsorb H_2O and sodium, get fluid shift from interstitial to capillaries due to decrease in hydrostatic pressure in capillaries.
d. Shunting blood from the lungs—ventilation–perfusion mismatch.
e. Circulation maintained, but only sustained short time without harm to tissues.

Progressive stage:

a. Altered capillary permeability (third spacing)

b. In the lungs—alveolar or pulmonary edema, ARDS, increased pulmonary artery pressure

c. CO decreases and coronary perfusion is decreased. Decreased myocardial perfusion—arrhythmias and myocardial ischemia

d. Kidneys—elevated BUN and creatinine

e. Metabolic acidosis, anaerobic metabolism, and kidneys cannot excrete acids and reabsorb bicarbonate

f. GI—ischemia causes ulcers and GI bleed

g. Liver—cannot eliminate waste products, elevated ammonia and lactate, bilirubin (jaundice) bacteria released in bloodstream

h. Hematologic—disseminated intravascular coagulopathy (DIC).

Refractory stage:

a. Anaerobic metabolism starts lactic acid build-up.

b. Increased capillary blood leak, worsens hypotension and tachycardia, also get cerebral ischemia.

c. Get profound hypotension and hypoxemia.

d. Cellular death leads, tissue death, vital organs fail and death occurs (lungs, liver, and kidneys result in accumulation of waste products). One organ failure leads to another.

e. Recovery unlikely.

Diagnostic Evaluation

- Blood: RBC, hemoglobin, and hematocrit
- Arterial blood gases (ABGs)—respiratory alkalosis and metabolic acidosis
- Electrolytes (Na level increased early, decreased later if hypotonic fluid given) K decrease later increase K with cellular breakdown and renal failure
- Blood urea nitrogen (BUN) and creatinine increased, specific gravity increased then fixed at 1.010
- Blood cultures—identify causative organism in septic shock
- Cardiac enzymes—diagnosis of cardiogenic shock
- Glucose—increased early then decreased
- DIC screen—fibrinogen level, platelet count, partial thromboplastin time (PTT) and prothrombin time (PT), thrombin time
- Lactic acid—increased
- Liver enzymes, alanine aminotransferase (ALT), aspartate aminotransferase (AST), and g-glutamyltransferase gamma symbol (GGT) increased.

Management

- General management strategies for a patient in shock begin with ensuring that the patient has a patent airway and oxygen delivery is optimized. The cornerstone of therapy for septic, hypovolemic, and anaphylactic shock is volume expansion with the administration of the appropriate fluid.
- It is generally accepted that isotonic crystalloids, such as normal saline are used in the initial resuscitation of shock. If the patient does not respond to 2-3 L of crystalloids, blood administration, and central venous monitoring may be instituted.
- The primary goal of drug therapy for shock is the correction of decreased tissue perfusion.
  - Sympathomimetic drugs cause peripheral vasoconstriction and are referred to as vasopressor drugs (e.g., epinephrine, norepinephrine).

- The goals of vasopressor therapy are to achieve and maintain a mean arterial pressure (MAP) of 60–65 mm Hg and the use of these drugs is reserved for patients unresponsive to other therapies.
- The goal of vasodilator therapy, as in vasopressor therapy, is to maintain MAP at 60–65 mm Hg or greater.
- Vasodilator agents most often used are nitroglycerin (in cardiogenic shock) and nitroprusside.

Collaborative Care

Cardiogenic Shock

- Overall, goal is to restore blood flow to the myocardium by restoring the balance between oxygen supply and demand.
- Definitive measures include thrombolytic therapy, angioplasty with stenting, emergency revascularization, and valve replacement.
- Care involves hemodynamic monitoring, drug therapy (e.g., diuretics to reduce preload), and use of circulatory assist devices (e.g., intra-aortic balloon pump, ventricular assist device).

Hypovolemic Shock

- The underlying principles of managing patients with hypovolemic shock focus on stopping the loss of fluid and restoring the circulating volume.
- Fluid replacement is calculated using a 3:1 rule (3 mL of isotonic crystalloid for every 1 mL of estimated blood loss).

Septic Shock

- Patients in septic shock require large amounts of fluid replacement, sometimes as much as 6–10 L of isotonic crystalloids and 2–4 L of colloids, to restore perfusion.
- Vasopressor drug therapy may be added and vasopressin may be given to patient's refractory to vasopressor therapy.
- Intravenous (IV) corticosteroids are recommended for patients who require vasopressor therapy, despite fluid resuscitation, to maintain adequate blood pressure (BP).
- Antibiotics are early component of therapy and are started after obtaining cultures.
- Drotrecogin alpha, a recombinant form of activated protein C has demonstrated promise in treating patients with severe sepsis.
- Glucose levels should be maintained at <150 mg/dL.
- Stress ulcer prophylaxis with histamine (H_2)-receptor blockers and deep vein thrombosis prophylaxis with low-dose unfractionated heparin or low molecular weight heparin are recommended.

Neurogenic Shock

- Treatment of neurogenic shock is dependent on the cause.
  - In spinal cord injury, general measures to promote spinal stability are initially used.
  - Definitive treatment of the hypotension and bradycardia involves the use of vasopressor and atropine, respectively.
  - Fluids are administered cautiously as the cause of the hypotension is generally not related to fluid loss.
  - The patient is monitored for hypothermia.

Anaphylactic Shock

- Epinephrine is the drug of choice to treat anaphylactic shock.
- Diphenhydramine is administered to block the massive release of histamine.
- Maintaining a patent airway is critical and the use of nebulization with bronchodilators is highly effective.
- Endotracheal intubation or cricothyroidotomy may be necessary.
- Aggressive fluid replacement, predominantly with colloids is necessary.
- IV corticosteroids may be helpful in anaphylactic shock if significant hypotension persists after 1–2 hours of aggressive therapy.

Nursing Management

Acute Intervention

The role of the nurse in shock involves:

1. Monitoring the patient's ongoing physical and emotional status to detect subtle changes in the patient's condition.
2. Planning and implementing nursing interventions and therapy.
3. Evaluating the patient's response to therapy.
4. Providing emotional support to the patient and family and.
5. Collaborating with other members of the health team when warranted by the patient's condition.

Nursing Care

- Neurologic status including orientation and level of consciousness should be assessed every hour or more often.
- Heart rate, rhythm, BP, central venous pressure, and PA pressures including continuous CO should be assessed at least every 15 minutes.
- The patient's ECG should be continuously monitored to detect dysrhythmias that may result from the cardiovascular and metabolic derangements associated with shock. Heart sounds should be assessed for the presence of an S_3 or S_4 sound or new murmurs. The presence of an S_3 sound in an adult usually indicates heart failure.
- The respiratory status of the patient in shock must be frequently assessed to ensure adequate oxygenation, detect complications early, and provide data regarding the patient's acid–base status.
- Pulse oximetry is used to continuously monitor oxygen saturation.
- ABGs provide definitive information on ventilation and oxygenation status, and acid–base balance.
- Most patients in shock will be intubated and on mechanical ventilation.
- Hourly urine output measurements assess the adequacy of renal perfusion and a urine output of <0.5 mL/kg/h may indicate inadequate kidney perfusion.
- BUN and serum creatinine values are also used to assess renal function.
- Tympanic or pulmonary arterial temperatures should be obtained hourly if temperature is elevated or subnormal, otherwise every 4 hours.
- Capillary refill should be assessed and skin monitored for temperature, pallor, flushing, cyanosis, and diaphoresis.
- Bowel sounds should be auscultated at least every 4 hours, and abdominal distention should be assessed.
- If a nasogastric tube is inserted, drainage should be checked for occult blood as should stools.

- Oral care for the patient in shock is essential and passive range of motion should be performed three or four times per day.
- Anxiety, fear, and pain may aggravate respiratory distress and increase the release of catecholamine's.
- The nurse should talk to the patient, even if the patient is intubated, sedated, and paralyzed or appears comatose. If the intubated patient is capable of writing, a pencil and paper should be provided.

SEIZURE OR EPILEPSY

A seizure is a sudden disruption of the brain's normal electrical activity accompanied by altered consciousness and other neurological and behavioral manifestations. Epilepsy is a condition characterized by recurrent seizures with symptoms that vary from a momentary lapse of attention to severe convulsions.

Types of Seizures

- **Grand-mal seizures:** This type of seizure presents as a generalized tonic–clonic seizure that often begins with a loud cry before the person having the seizure loses consciousness and falls to the ground. The muscles become rigid for about 30 seconds during the tonic phase of the seizure and alternately contract and relax during the clonic phase which lasts 30–60 seconds. The skin sometimes acquires a bluish tint and the person may bite his tongue, lose bowel or bladder control, or have trouble breathing. A grand-mal seizure lasts between 2 and 5 minutes, and the person may be confused or have trouble talking when he regains consciousness. The period of time immediately following a seizure is known as the "postictal" state.
- **Primary generalized seizures:** This is a primary generalized seizure that occurs when electrical discharges begin in both halves (hemispheres) of the brain at the same time. Primary generalized seizures are more likely to be major motor attacks than to be absence seizures.
- **Absence (petit mal) seizures:** This type of seizure generally begins at about the age of four, and usually stops by the time the child becomes an adolescent. Petit mal seizures usually begin with a brief loss of consciousness and last between 1 and 10 seconds. A person having a petit mal seizure becomes very quiet and may blink, stare blankly, roll his eyes, or move his lips. A petit mal seizure lasts 15–20 seconds. When it ends, the person who had the seizure resumes whatever he was doing before the seizure began. He will not remember the seizure and may not realize that anything unusual has happened.
- **Myoclonic seizures:** This type of seizure is characterized by brief, involuntary spasms of the tongue or muscles of the face, arms, or legs. Myoclonic seizures are most likely to occur first thing in the morning.
- **Simple partial seizures:** This type of seizure does not spread from the focal area where they arise. Symptoms are determined by what part of the brain is affected. The patient usually remains conscious during the seizure.
- **Complex partial seizures:** This type of seizures presents with a distinctive smell, taste, or other unusual sensation (aura) may signal the start of a complex partial seizure. Complex partial seizures start as simple partial seizures, but move beyond the focal area and cause loss of consciousness. Complex partial seizures can become major motor seizures. Although a person having a complex partial seizure may not seem to be unconscious, he does not know what is happening and may behave inappropriately. He will not remember the seizure but may seem confused or intoxicated for a few minutes after it ends.

Pathophysiology

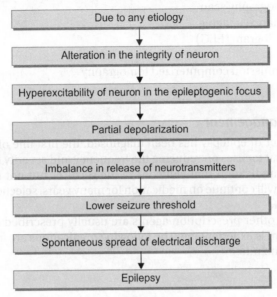

Due to any etiology

↓

Alteration in the integrity of neuron

↓

Hyperexcitability of neuron in the epileptogenic focus

↓

Partial depolarization

↓

Imbalance in release of neurotransmitters

↓

Lower seizure threshold

↓

Spontaneous spread of electrical discharge

↓

Epilepsy

Etiology

Most cases of epilepsy are of unknown origin. Sometimes, however, a genetic basis is indicated, and other cases may be traceable to birth trauma, lead poisoning, congenital brain infection, head injury, alcohol or drug addiction, or the effects of organ disease. Known causes of epilepsy and other seizure disorders can include:

- Brain tumor
- Cerebral hypoxia
- Cerebrovascular accident
- Convulsive or toxic agents
- Alcohol and drug use withdrawal
- Eclampsia
- Hormone changes during pregnancy and menstruation
- Exogenous factors (sound, light, cutaneous stimulation)
- Fever (especially in children)
- Head injury
- Heatstroke
- Infection (acute or chronic)
- Metabolic disturbances (diabetes mellitus, electrolyte imbalances)
- Withdrawal from, or hereditary intolerance of alcohol
- Kidney failure
- Degenerative disorders (**senile dementia**)

Diagnostic Evaluation

- The first step in diagnosing a seizure disorder is to determine whether or not the patient "did" or "did not" actually have seizures. To do this, the following is required:
    - Medial history
    - Careful history of clinical presentation and events related to alleged seizure
- General physical and neurological examination

- Diagnostic testing that includes:
  - Computed tomography scan
  - Magnetic resonance imaging
  - Electroencephalogram (EEG)
  - Video EEG
  - Single proton emission computerized tomography

Management

Pharmacological Management

Once a seizure disorder of epilepsy has been diagnosed, the first line of treatment is usually medication therapy that focuses on reducing the frequency and severity of the seizures.

The goal is to find a medication that will control the seizures but not produce side effects. Because many people will continue on medication for many years, selection of a good first drug is extremely important.

Anticonvulsants and other prescription agents are usually prescribed based on the type of seizures that the patient is experiencing. The following medications are frequently prescribed:

- Benzodiazepines include:
  - Clonazepam
  - Clorazepate
  - Diazepam
- Phenytoin (Dilantin): A synthetic drug that is classified as a hydantoin. It is used for the treatment of simple partial, complex partial and generalized tonic–clonic seizures.
- Carbamazepine: Used as a first-line agent for the treatment of simple partial, complex partial and generalized tonic–clonic seizures.
- Lamotrigine: Used when seizures are focal in onset, tonic–clonic, atypical absence or myoclonic in nature.
- Valproate: Used for the management of myoclonic, tonic, atonic, absence and generalized tonic–clonic seizures especially with patients with one or more types of generalized seizure.
- Phenobarbital: Once a mainstay in the treatment of seizures (especially status epilepticus), phenobarbital is now being replaced by other anticonvulsants but can still be used for the treatment of generalized seizures except for absence and partial seizures.

Surgical Intervention

The most common surgical areas include:

- Temporal lobectomy
- Frontal lobectomy
- Hemispherectomy
- Corpus callosotomy (splitting of the two hemispheres of the brain).

Placement of a vagus nerve stimulator (VNS): A VNS is an implantable device that is used to decrease seizure frequency. In some cases, it eliminates seizure activity altogether. It is a surgically implanted device that is placed in the chest wall (similar to a pacemaker), with a wire that is threaded to the vagus nerve in the neck. Once in place the VNS is programed (using a magnet), to stimulate the vagus nerve at preset intervals. Patients are sent home with a magnet as well to trigger the device at the onset of a seizure.

Nursing Care and Management of Seizures in the Acute Setting

Before (and during) seizure care:

- If the patient is seated when a major seizure occurs, ease them to the floor
- Providing privacy if possible

- If patient experiences an aura, have them lie down to prevent injury
- Removing eyeglasses and loosening restrictive clothing
- Not trying to force anything into the mouth
- Guiding the movements to prevent injuries (do not restrain patient)
- Staying with the patient throughout the seizure to ensure safety
- Note down the time duration of seizure
- Verbalizing events as they happen to assist with more accurate recall later
- If not already available, have someone retrieve O_2 and suction.

Postseizure care:
- Position patient on their side to facilitate drainage of secretions
- Providing adequate ventilation by maintaining a patent airway
- Suction secretions if necessary to prevent aspiration
- Allowing the patient to sleep postseizure.

Status Epilepticus

Seizures lasting at least 5 minutes or two or more seizures in a row without complete recovery in between are termed as status epilepticus

Initial Nursing Management
- ABCs of life support
- Position patient to avoid aspiration or inadequate oxygenation
- If possible as soft oral airway can be placed (again do not force teeth apart)
- Suction and O_2 must be available
- Monitor respiratory function with ongoing pulse oximetry
- IV access should be secured
- Frequent monitoring of neurological examination and vital signs
- Monitoring ABGs
- Monitoring glucose
- Treating hyperthermia

Anticonvulsant Therapy for Management of Status Epilepticus
The following drug therapy regimen is used to treat status epilepticus:
- Time 0–3 minutes: Lorazepam 4–8 mg IVP (2 mg/min)
- Time 4–23 minutes: Phenytoin (Dilantin) 20 mg/kg (about 1 g) in NS at (50 mg/min)
- Time 22–33 minutes: Phenytoin (Dilantin) 5–10 mg/kg
- Time 37–58 minutes: Phenobarbital 20 mg/kg IV
- Time 58–68 minutes: Phenobarbital 5–10 mg/kg

Patient and Family Education for Seizures or Epilepsy

General Health
- Trigger signs (patient specific if possible)
- Regular exercise
- Regular sleep patterns
- Showers or bath
- Good oral hygiene (some anticonvulsant can cause gingival hyperplasia)
- Eat well-rounded meals at routine times
- Avoiding excess sugar, caffeine or other trigger foods
- Noisy environments should be avoided
- Avoiding bright flashing or fluorescent lights
- Using a screen filter on the computer screen to avoid glare
- Not using recreational or street drugs
- Avoiding work/recreation that could cause injury if a seizure was to occur
- Swimming with friends only and avoiding be alone in pool

- Avoiding contact sports
- Avoiding emotional stress
- Counseling for stress reduction or depression may be warranted.

HEATSTROKE

Heatstroke is a condition caused by body overheating, usually as a result of prolonged exposure to or physical exertion in high temperatures. This is the most serious form of heat injury, heatstroke can occur if body temperature rises to 104°F (40°C) or higher.

Heatstroke requires emergency treatment. Untreated heatstroke can quickly damage brain, heart, kidneys, and muscles. The damage worsens the longer treatment is delayed, increasing risk of serious complications or death.

Etiology

Heatstroke can occur as a result of:

- **Exposure to a hot environment:** In a type of heatstroke, called nonexertional or classic heatstroke, being in a hot environment leads to a rise in body temperature. This type of heatstroke typically occurs after exposure to hot, humid weather especially for prolonged periods, such as 2 or 3 days. It occurs most often in older adults and in people with chronic illness.
- **Strenuous activity:** Exertional heatstroke is caused by an increase in body temperature brought on by intense physical activity in hot weather. Anyone exercising or working in hot weather can get exertional heatstroke.
- **Wearing excess clothing** that prevents sweat from evaporating easily and cooling of body.
- **Drinking alcohol** which can affect body's ability to regulate the temperature.
- **Becoming dehydrated**, by not drinking enough water to replenish fluids lost through sweating.

Signs and Symptoms

Heatstroke symptoms include:

- **High body temperature:** A body temperature of 104°F (40°C) or higher is the main sign of heatstroke.
- **Altered mental state or behavior:** Confusion, agitation, slurred speech, irritability, delirium, seizures, and coma can all result from heatstroke.
- **Alteration in sweating:** In heatstroke brought on by hot weather, skin will feel hot and dry to the touch. However, in heatstroke brought on by strenuous exercise, skin may feel moist.
- Nausea and vomiting
- Flushed skin
- Rapid breathing
- Tachycardia
- Headache

Risk Factors

- **Age:** Ability to cope with extreme heat depends on the strength of central nervous system. In the very young, the central nervous system is not fully developed, and in adults over 65, the central nervous system begins to deteriorate, which makes the body less able to cope with changes in body temperature. Both age groups usually have difficulty remaining hydrated, which also increases risk.

- **Exertion in hot weather:** Military training and participating in sports, such as football, in hot weather are among the situations that can lead to heatstroke.
- **Sudden exposure to hot weather,** such as during an early summer heat wave or travel to a hotter climate.
- **A lack of air conditioning:** Fans may make feel better, but during sustained hot weather, air conditioning is the most effective way to cool down and lower humidity.
- **Certain medications:** Beta-blockers, diuretics, or reduce psychiatric symptoms (antidepressants or antipsychotics).
- **Certain health conditions:** Certain chronic illnesses, such as heart or lung disease might increase risk of heatstroke.

Diagnostic Evaluation

- **A blood test** to check blood sodium or potassium and the content of gases in blood to see if there is been damage to central nervous system.
- **A urine test** to check the color of urine, because it is usually darker if have a heat-related condition, and to check kidney function which can be affected by heatstroke.
- **Muscle function tests** to check for serious damage to muscle tissue.
- **X-rays and other imaging tests** to check for damage to internal organs.

Management (Fig. 22.2)

- **Immerse in cold water:** A bath of cold or ice water can quickly lower temperature.
- **Using evaporation cooling techniques:** In this technique, cool water is misted on skin while warm air fanned over body causes the water to evaporate, cooling the skin.
- **Pack with ice and cooling blankets:** Another method is to wrap in a special cooling blanket and apply ice packs to groin, neck, back, and armpits to lower temperature.

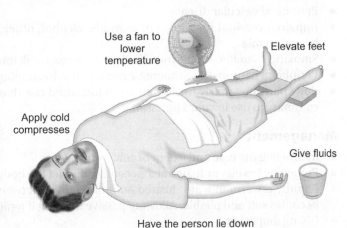

Use a fan to lower temperature

Elevate feet

Apply cold compresses

Give fluids

Have the person lie down

Fig. 22.2: Management of heatstroke.

- **Give medications to stop shivering:** If treatments to lower body temperature make shiver, muscle relaxant, such as a benzodiazepine can be administered. Shivering increases body temperature, making treatment less effective.

Prevention

- **Wear loose fitting, lightweight clothing:** Wearing excess clothing or clothing that fits tightly would not allow body to cool properly.
- **Protect against sunburn:** Sunburn affects body's ability to cool itself, so protect outdoors with a wide-brimmed hat and sunglasses and use a broad-spectrum sunscreen with an SPF of at least 15.
- **Drink plenty of fluid:** Staying hydrated will help the body sweat and maintain a normal body temperature.
- **Take extra precautions with certain medications, such as caffeine.**

- **Never leave anyone in a parked car:** This is a common cause of heat-related deaths in children. When parked in the sun, the temperature in car can rise 20°F (more than 6.7°C) in 10 minutes.

FROSTBITES

It is an emergency condition in with the body fluids freeze because of extreme low temperature. The severity of cold injury depends on the temperature, duration of exposure, environmental conditions, amount of protective clothing, and the patient's general state of health. Exposure to cold can cause localized injury or generalized cooling of the entire body.

Risk Factor

- Lower temperatures—especially windy conditions
- Dehydration
- Infancy, elderly age, malnutrition, exhaustion
- Immobilization
- Open wounds
- Prolonged exposure
- Moisture
- Peripheral vascular disease
- Impaired cerebral function: For example, alcohol, other sedatives, psychiatric illnesses, hypoglycemia
- Smoking, diabetes and Reynaud's disease increase risk due to vasoconstriction
- Peripheral neuropathy, autonomic neuropathy, head injury, spinal cord damage
- Body parts previously frostbitten are at increased risk due to damaged microcirculation a summary to use in your appraisal.

Management

- Identifying the type and extent of cold injury.
- Removing jewelry or material that could constrict the body part.
- Rapidly rewarm in water heated and maintained between 37°C and 39°C until the area becomes soft and pliable. Allowing passive thawing if rapid rewarming is not possible.
- Giving ibuprofen
- Air dry the area
- Applying topical aloe vera cream or gel if available.
- Protect from refreezing and any direct trauma. Using large, dry, bulky dressings and elevate the body part if possible.
- Ensuring the patient is rehydrated.
- Avoiding walking on a thawed lower limb
- Tetanus prophylaxis
- Debridement—this may involve selective drainage of clear blisters. Hemorrhagic blisters should be left intact.
- Systemic hydration with IV fluid
- Systemic antibiotics
- Thrombolytic therapy can be considered.

Complications

- Secondary wound infection
- Tetanus

- Diuresis may cause volume depletion
- Hyperglycemia, acidosis
- Dysrhythmias
- Gangrene
- Paresthesias and sensory deficits, tremor
- Cracking of skin and loss of nails
- Permanent discoloration
- Vasospasm, cold sensitivity
- Joint stiffness
- Premature closure of epiphyses in children
- Muscle atrophy

CARDIOPULMONARY RESUSCITATION

Cardiopulmonary resuscitation (CPR) provides artificial ventilation and circulation until advanced life support can be provided and spontaneous circulation and ventilation can be restored. CPR can keep oxygenated blood flowing to the brain and other vital organs until more definitive medical treatment can restore a normal heart rhythm.

Introduction

In 1954, James Elam was the first to demonstrate experimentally that CPR was a sound technique and, with Dr Peter Safar, he demonstrated its superiority to previous methods. Peter Safar wrote the book *ABC of resuscitation* in 1957.

Definitions

- CPR is a technique of basic life support (BLS) for the purpose of oxygenating the brain and heart until appropriate, definitive medical treatment can restore normal heart and ventilator action. Management of airway obstruction or cricothyroidotomy may be necessary to open the airway before CPR can be performed.
- CPR combines rescue breathing (one person breathing into another person) and chest compression in a lifesaving procedure performed when a person has stopped breathing or a person's heart has stopped beating.

What is Cardiopulmonary Resuscitation?

CPR is:
- Emergency life-saving measure
- Combination of rescue breathing and chest compressions
- Done on unconscious/nonbreathing patient
- Done on persons suffering cardiac arrest
- Also for near-drowning/asphyxiation/trauma cases
- CPR conducts defibrillation
- Supports heart pumping for short duration
- Allows oxygen to reach brain
- Buys time till help arrives
- More effective when done as early as possible

Purpose

- CPR can save lives in such emergencies as loss of consciousness, heart attacks or heart "arrests," electric shock, drowning, excessive bleeding, drug overdose.

- The purpose of CPR is to bring oxygen to the victim's lungs and to keep blood circulating so oxygen gets to every part of the body.

Indications

- **Cardiac arrest:**
  - Ventricular fibrillation
  - Ventricular tachycardia
  - Asystole
  - Pulseless electrical activity (PEA)
- **Respiratory arrest:**
  - Drowning
  - Stroke
  - Foreign-body airway obstruction
  - Smoke inhalation
  - Drug overdose
  - Electrocution/injury by lightning
  - Suffocation
  - Accident/injury
  - Coma
  - Epiglottitis

Complications

- Postresuscitation distress syndrome (secondary derangements in multiple organs)
- Neurological impairment and/or brain damage.

Changes in Basic Life Support Guidelines

New American Heart Association Adult Chain of Survival

New fifth link—postcardiac arrest care

- Immediate recognition and activation of emergency response system
- Early CPR, emphasis on chest compressions
- Rapid defibrillation
- Effective advanced life support
- Integrated postcardiac arrest care **(Fig. 22.3)**.

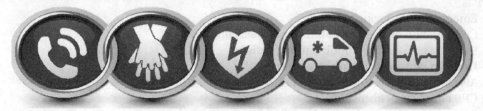

Fig. 22.3: Adult chain of survival.

Key Changes in Revised AHA Guidelines for CPR and ECC

Following are the key changes:

I. The change from "A–B–C" to "C–A–B"

2010 (new): It is necessary to initiate chest compressions before ventilations.

2005 (old): The sequence of adult CPR began with opening of the airway, checking for normal breathing, and then delivery of 2 rescue breaths followed by cycles of 30 chest compressions and 2 breaths.

Why: To reduce delay to CPR, sequence begins with skill that everyone can perform. Emphasize primary importance of chest compressions for professional rescuers. Starting CPR with 30 compressions rather than 2 ventilations leads to improved outcome, chest compressions provide vital blood flow to the heart and brain, and studies of out-of-hospital adult cardiac arrest showed that survival was higher when bystanders made some attempt rather than no attempt to provide CPR. Chest compressions can be started almost immediately, whereas positioning the head and achieving a seal for mouth-to-mouth or bag-mask rescue breathing all take time.

II. Elimination of "look–listen–feel" in breathing

2010 (new): "Look, listen, and feel" was removed from the CPR sequence. After delivery of 30 compressions, the lone rescuer opens the victim's airway and delivers two breaths.

2005 (old): "Look, listen, and feel" was used to assess breathing after the airway was opened.
Why: With the new "chest compressions first" sequence, CPR is performed if the adult is unresponsive and not breathing or not breathing normally (as noted above, lay rescuers will be taught to provide CPR if the unresponsive victim is "not breathing or only gasping"). The CPR sequence begins with compressions (C–A–B sequence). Therefore breathing is briefly checked as part of a check for cardiac arrest; after the first set of chest compressions, the airway is opened, and the rescuer delivers two breaths.

III. Chest Compressions Rate: 100/minute

2010 (new): It is reasonable for lay rescuers and healthcare providers to perform chest compressions at a rate of at least 100/minute.

2005 (old): Compress at a rate of about 100/minute.

Why: The number of chest compressions delivered per minute during CPR is an important determinant of return of spontaneous circulation (ROSC) and survival with good neurologic function. The actual number of chest compressions delivered per minute is determined by the rate of chest compressions and the number and duration of interruptions in compressions [e.g., to open the airway, deliver rescue breaths, or allow automated external defibrillator (AED) analysis].

IV. Chest Compression Depth

2010 (new): The adult sternum should be depressed at least 2 in. (5 cm).
2005 (old): The adult sternum should be depressed approximately 1–2 inch (approximately 4–5 cm).

Why: Compressions create blood flow primarily by increasing intrathoracic pressure and directly compressing the heart. Compressions generate critical blood flow and oxygen and energy delivery to the heart and brain. Confusion may result when a range of depth is recommended, so 1 compression depth is now recommended. Rescuers often do not compress the chest enough despite recommendations to "push hard." In addition, the available science suggests that compressions of at least 2 inch are more effective than compressions of 1.5 inch. For this reason, the 2010 AHA Guidelines for CPR and external chest compression (ECC) recommend a single minimum depth for compression of the adult chest.

V. Cricoid Pressure

2010 (new): Routine use of cricoid pressure during CPR is generally NOT recommended.

Why: Cricoid pressure can interfere with ventilation and advanced airway placement. Not proven to prevent aspiration or gastric insufflation during cardiac arrest.

VI. Team Resuscitation

2005 (old): The steps of BLS consist of a series of sequential assessments and actions. The intent of the algorithm is to present the steps in a logical and concise manner that will be easy for each rescuer to learn, remember, and perform.

2010 (new): The steps in the BLS algorithm have traditionally been presented as a sequence to help a single rescuer prioritize actions. There is increased focus on providing CPR as a team because resuscitations in most EMS and health-care systems involve teams of rescuers, with rescuers performing several actions simultaneously. For example, one rescuer activates the emergency response system while a second begins chest compressions, a third is either providing ventilations or retrieving the bag mask for rescue breathing, and a fourth is retrieving and setting up a defibrillator.

Why: Some resuscitations start with a lone rescuer who calls for help, whereas other resuscitations begin with several willing rescuers. Training should focus on building a team as each rescuer arrives, or on designating a team leader if multiple rescuers are present. As additional personnel arrive, responsibilities for tasks that would ordinarily be performed sequentially by fewer rescuers may now be delegated to a team of providers who perform them simultaneously. For this reason, BLS healthcare provider training should not only teach individual skills but should also teach rescuers to work in effective teams.

VII. Precordial thump

The precordial thump should not be used for unwitnessed out-of-hospital cardiac arrest. The precordial thump may be considered for patients with witnessed, monitored, unstable VT (including pulseless VT) if a defibrillator is not immediately ready for use, but it should not delay CPR and shock delivery.

VIII. Simplified ACLS Algorithm and New Algorithm

2005 (old): ACLS courses focused mainly on added interventions, such as manual defibrillation, drug therapy, and advanced airway management, as well as alternative and management options for special situations.

2010 (new): The conventional ACLS Cardiac Arrest Algorithm has been simplified and streamlined to emphasize the importance of high-quality CPR (including compressions of adequate rate and depth, allowing complete chest recoil after each compression, minimizing interruptions in chest compressions, and avoiding excessive ventilation) and the fact that ACLS actions should be organized around uninterrupted periods of CPR **(Figs. 22.4A and B)**.

Why: For the treatment of cardiac arrest, ACLS interventions build on the BLS foundation of high-quality CPR to increase CPR quality

- Push hard [≥2 inch (5 cm)] and fast (≥100/minute) and allow complete chest recoil
- Minimize interruptions in compressions
- Avoiding excessive ventilation
- Rotate compressor every 2 minutes
- If no advanced airway, 30:2 compression–ventilation ratio

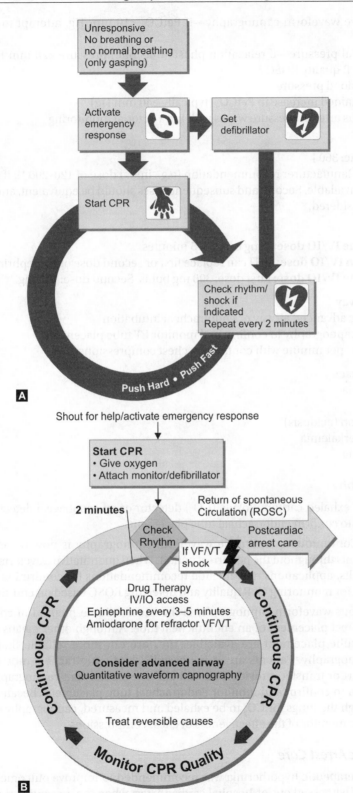

Figs. 22.4A and B: Adult cardiac arrest.

- Quantitative waveform capnography—if PetCO$_2$ <10 mm Hg, attempt to improve CPR quality
- Intra-arterial pressure—if relaxation phase (diastolic) pressure <20 mm Hg, attempt to improve CPR quality ROSC
- Pulse and blood pressure
- Abrupt sustained increase in PetCO$_2$ (typically ≥40 mm Hg)
- Spontaneous arterial pressure waves with intra-arterial monitoring

Shock energy
- **Monophasic:** 360 J
- **Biphasic:** Manufacturer recommendation (e.g., initial dose of 120–200 J); if unknown, use maximum available. Second and subsequent doses should be equivalent, and higher doses may be considered.

Drug therapy
- **Epinephrine IV/IO dose:** 1 mg every 3–5 minutes
- **Vasopressin IV/IO dose:** 40 U can replace first or second dose of epinephrine
- **Amiodarone IV/IO dose:** First dose: 300 mg bolus. Second dose: 150 mg.

Advanced airway
- Supraglottic advanced airway or endotracheal intubation
- Waveform capnography to confirm and monitor ET tube placement
- 8–10 breaths per minute with continuous chest compressions

Reversible causes
- Hypovolemia
- Hypoxia
- Hydrogen ion (acidosis)
- Hypo-/hyperkalemia
- Hypothermia

IX. Capnography

2005 (old): An exhaled carbon dioxide (CO$_2$) detector or an esophageal detector device was recommended to confirm endotracheal tube placement.

2010 (new): Continuous quantitative waveform capnography is now recommended for intubated patients throughout the periarrest period. When quantitative waveform capnography is used for adults, applications now include recommendations for confirming tracheal tube placement and for monitoring CPR quality and detecting ROSC based on end-tidal CO$_2$ value.

Why: Continuous waveform capnography is the most reliable method of confirming and monitoring correct placement of an endotracheal tube. Although other means of confirming endotracheal tube placement are available, they are not more reliable than continuous waveform capnography. Patients are at increased risk of endotracheal tube displacement during transport or transfer; providers should observe a persistent capnographic waveform with ventilation to confirm and monitor endotracheal tube placement. Because blood must circulate through the lungs for CO$_2$ to be exhaled and measured, capnography can also serve as a physiologic monitor of the effectiveness of chest compressions.

X. Postcardiac Arrest Care

2005 (old): Therapeutic hypothermia was recommended to improve outcome for comatose adult victims of witnessed out-of-hospital cardiac arrest when the presenting rhythm was VF.

2010 (new): To improve survival for victims of cardiac arrest who are admitted to a hospital after ROSC, a comprehensive, structured, integrated, multidisciplinary system of postcardiac arrest care should be implemented in a consistent manner. Treatment should include cardiopulmonary and neurologic support. Therapeutic hypothermia and percutaneous coronary interventions should be provided when indicated. Because seizures are common after cardiac arrest, an EEG for the diagnosis of seizures should be performed with prompt interpretation as soon as possible and should be monitored frequently or continuously in comatose patients after ROSC.

Why: Postcardiac arrest care with an emphasis on multidisciplinary programs that focus on optimizing hemodynamic, neurologic, and metabolic function (including therapeutic hypothermia) may improve survival to hospital discharge among victims who achieve ROSC after cardiac arrest either in or out of hospital.

XI. Atropine is "out"; adenosine is "in"

2005 (old): Atropine was included in the BLS Pulseless Arrest Algorithm: for a patient in asystole, atropine could be considered.

2010 (new): Atropine is not recommended for routine use. Adenosine is recommended in the initial diagnosis and treatment of stable, undifferentiated regular, monomorphic wide-complex tachycardia. It is important to note that adenosine should *not* be used for *irregular* wide-complex tachycardias because it may cause degeneration of the rhythm to VF. For the treatment of the adult with symptomatic and unstable bradycardia, chronotropic drug infusions are recommended as an alternative to pacing.

Why: There are several important changes regarding management of symptomatic arrhythmias in adults. Available evidence suggests that the routine use of atropine during PEA or asystole is unlikely to have a therapeutic benefit. Adenosine is recommended in the initial diagnosis and treatment of stable, undifferentiated regular, monomorphic wide-complex tachycardia. This is on the basis of new available evidence of its safety and potential efficacy.

XII. AEDs use in Children now includes Infants

2005 (old): For children 1–8 years of age, the rescuer should use a pediatrics dose–attenuator system if one is available. If the rescuer provides CPR to a child in cardiac arrest and does not have an AED with a pediatric attenuator system, the rescuer should use a standard AED. There are insufficient data to make a recommendation for or against the use of AEDs for infants <1 year of age.

2010 (new): For attempted defibrillation of children 1–8 years of age with an AED, the rescuer should use a pediatrics dose–attenuator system if one is available. If the rescuer provides CPR to a child in cardiac arrest and does not have an AED with a pediatrics dose–attenuator system, the rescuer should use a standard AED. For infants (<1 year of age), a manual defibrillator is preferred.

Why: The lowest energy dose for effective defibrillation in infants and children is not known. The upper limit for safe defibrillation is also not known, but doses >4 J/kg (as high as 9 J/kg) have effectively defibrillated children and animal models of pediatric arrest with no significant adverse effects. AEDs with relatively high-energy doses have been used successfully in infants in cardiac arrest with no clear adverse effects.

XIII. Pediatrics Resuscitation

Revised pediatrics chain of survival. New postarrest care link **(Fig. 22.5)**.

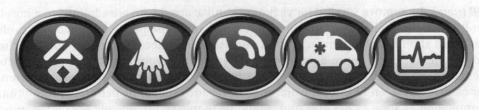

Fig. 22.5: Chain of pediatrics resuscitation.

Pediatrics BLS

- Similarities in pediatrics BLS and adult BLSC–A–B rather than A–B–C sequence
- Continued emphasis on high-quality CPR
- Removal of "look, listen, and feel"
- Deemphasis of pulse check for HCPs
- Using AEDs as soon as available
- AEDs may be used in infants, although manual defibrillation preferred.
- Some differences between pediatrics BLS and adult BLS
- Chest compression depth—at least one third of the anterior–posterior diameter of chest Infants: about 1.5 inch
- Children: about 2 inch
- Lone rescuer provides 2 minutes of CPR before activating emergency response
- Two rescuers use 15:2 compression to ventilation ratio
- Traditional CPR (compressions and ventilations) by bystanders associated with higher survival than chest compressions alone.

Pediatrics advanced life support

- Optimal energy dose for defibrillation of children unknown
    - Initial dose 2–4 J/kg
    - Subsequent dose ≥4 J/kg
- **Post-ROSC:** Titrate oxygen to limit hyperoxemia.
- Therapeutic hypothermia (from 32°C to 34°C) may be beneficial (studies in progress).
- Young victims of sudden, unexpected cardiac arrest should have a complete autopsy with genetic analysis of tissue to look for inherited channelopathy.

Neonatal resuscitation

- For babies born at term, begin resuscitation with room air rather than 100% oxygen.
- Any oxygen administered should be blended with room air, titrated based on oxygen saturation measured from right upper extremity.
- Suctioning after birth reserved for infants with obvious airway obstruction, those requiring ventilation or nonvigorous babies with meconium.
- Therapeutic hypothermia recommended for babies near term with evolving moderate to severe hypoxic–ischemic encephalopathy.

XIV. Ethical Issues

Until recent guidelines, no prognostic indicators had been established for patients undergoing therapeutic hypothermia. According to 2005 guidelines, there were three factors associated with poor outcomes:

1. Absence of pupillary response on day 3
2. Absence of motor response on day 3
3. Bilateral absence of somatosensory evoked potentials

STEPS OF BASIC LIFE SUPPORT

Following are the steps of BLS:

Step 1

- **It is necessary to check responsiveness:** "Are you all right?"
- **At the same time, it is necessary to check for absent/abnormal breathing:** It is necessary to scan the chest for movement for 5–10 seconds.

Step 2

- **Get help!!:** "Code blue team."
- It is necessary to send for AED/defibrillator.

Step 3

- Checking the carotid pulse for 5–10 seconds
- If no pulse (or unsure of pulse), chest compressions should be started.
  - Compressing the lower half of the sternum at a rate of 100/minute at a depth of at least 5 cm
  - Allowing complete chest recoil after each compression
  - Minimizing interruptions in compressions (10 seconds or less)
  - Switching compression providers every 2 minutes
  - Giving breaths at a rate of two breaths for every 30 compressions if no advanced airway is in place or at a rate of one breath every 5–6 seconds (8–10 breaths per minute) if advanced airway is in place
  - Avoiding excessive ventilation!
- If pulse present, giving rescue breaths at one breath every 5–6 seconds and checking pulse every 2 minutes.

Step 4

- No pulse, checking for shockable rhythm with an AED or defibrillation as soon as it arrives
- Shocking as indicated
- Following each shock immediately with CPR, beginning with compressions
- Checking pulse and rhythm after 2 minutes **(Figs. 22.6 and 22.7)**.

Responder/Rescuer

Everyone can be a lifesaving rescuer for a cardiac arrest victim. CPR skills and their application depend on the rescuer's training, experience, and confidence.

All rescuers, regardless of training, should provide chest compressions to all cardiac arrest victims. Rescuers who are able should add ventilations to chest compressions. Highly trained rescuers working together should coordinate their care and perform chest compressions as well as ventilations in a team-based approach.

Precautions

- Not leaving the victim alone.
- Not giving chest compressions if the victim has a pulse. Chest compression when there is normal circulation could cause the heart to stop beating.
- Not giving the victim anything to eat or drink

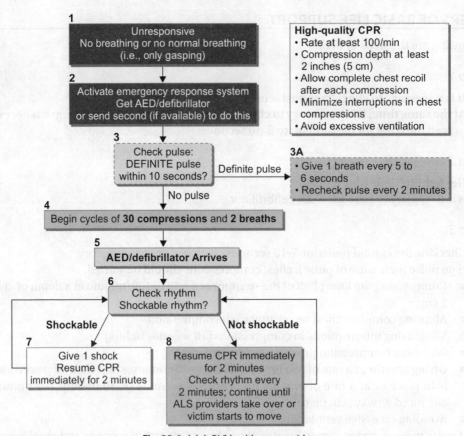

Fig. 22.6: Adult BLS healthcare providers.

- Avoiding moving the victim's head or neck if spinal injury is a possibility. The person should be left as found if breathing freely. To check for breathing when spinal injury is suspected, the rescuer should only listen for breath by the victim's mouth and watch the chest for movement.
- Not slapping the victim's face, or throwing water on the face, to try and revive the person.
- Not placing a pillow under the victim's head
- The description above is not a substitute for CPR training and is not intended to be followed as a procedure.

Drugs Used During Cardiopulmonary Resuscitation

Drug	Dose	Indications	Timing of administration	Other
Adrenaline	1 mg IV (0.01 mg/kg)	➤ Given immediately in nonshockable rhythm ➤ Given after the third shock in shockable rhythm (VT/VF)	➤ Repeated every 4 minutes (every other cycle) ➤ Once adrenaline ALWAYS adrenaline	Given as a vasopressor for its α-adrenergic effect. Not as an inotrope
Amiodarone	300 mg IV bolus (5 mg/kg)	Given after the third shock in shockable rhythm	A further dose of 150 mg if VT/VF persists	If amiodarone is not available, lidocaine can be used instead

Contd...

Contd...

Drug	Dose	Indications	Timing of administration	Other
Lidocaine	100 mg IV (1–1.5 mg/kg)	Given after the third shock in shockable rhythm (IF amiodarone is unavailable)	A further dose of 50 mg can be given if necessary	Total dose must not exceed 3 mg/kg during the first hour
Magnesium	2 g IV	➤ VT ➤ Torsade de pointes ➤ Digoxin toxicity with hypomagnesemia	May be repeated after 10–15 minutes	
Sodium bicarbonate	50 mmol IV	➤ Routine use is not recommended ➤ Hyperkalemia ➤ Overdose of TCA	May be repeated according to ABG	Do NOT give calcium solutions and $NaHCO_3$ simultaneously by the same route

(ABG: Arterial blood gas; IV: Intravenous; TCA: tricyclic antidepressant)

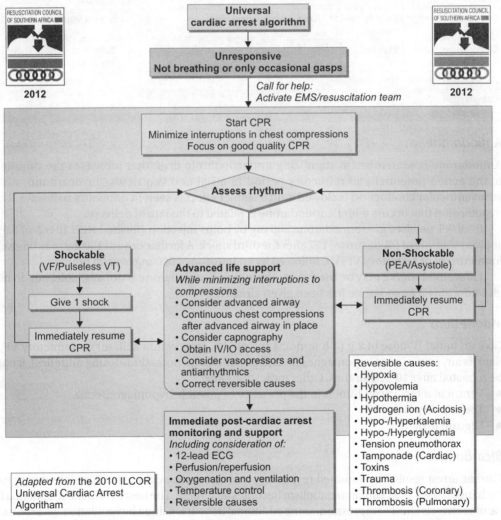

Fig. 22.7: Steps of BLS.

Summary of CPR Steps for Adults, Children and Infants CPR Levels A, B and C

CPR	Adult (8 years of age and older)	Child (1–8 years of age)	Infant (Less than one year)
Check the scene Establish unresponsiveness	Is the scene safe to help? Wake and shout-gently squeeze or tap shoulders—are you OK?		
Activate EMS and get an AED	Yell for help. If you are alone phone EMS right away	Yell for help. If you are alone phone EMS after giving 5 cycles of CPR	
Check for breathing	Open airway using head-tilt/chin-lift, take no more than 5 seconds to look for normal breathing using visual cues, such as chest rise. Gasping is not normal breathing Spinal victims: NLS lifeguards attemt jaw thrust to open the airway		
Start CPR	If victim is unresponsive and not breathing normally, immediately start CPR beginning with chest compressions (30 compressions: 2 breaths)		
Compression location	Center of chest		Just below nipple line on breastbone
Compression method	2 hands: Heel of 1 hand, other hand on top (or 1 hand for children)		2 fingers: Middle and ring
Compression depth	5 cm or 2 inch		1/3 depth of chest or about (5 cm child or 4 cm infant)
Compression rate	100 per minute		
Compression ventilation ratio	30:2 (1 or 2 rescuer CPR)		

Amiodarone

Amiodarone is a membrane-stabilizing antiarrhythmic drug that increases the duration of the action potential and refractory period in atrial and ventricular myocardium. Also, atrioventricular conduction is slowed, and a similar effect is seen in accessory pathways. The hypotension that occurs with IV amiodarone is related to the rate of delivery.

If VF/VT persists, give amiodarone 300 mg by bolus injection (flushed with 20 mL of 0.9% sodium chloride or 5% dextrose) 177 after the third shock. A further dose of 150 mg may be given for recurrent or refractory VF/VT, followed by an infusion of 900 mg over 24 hours.

Lidocaine 1 mg/kg may be used as an alternative if amiodarone is not available, but do not give lidocaine if amiodarone has been given already.

Magnesium

Give an initial IV dose of 2 g (= 8 mmol, 4 mL of 50% magnesium sulfate) for refractory VF if there is any suspicion of hypomagnesemia (e.g., patients on potassium-losing diuretics); it may be repeated after 10–15 minutes. Other indications are:
- Ventricular tachyarrhythmias in the presence of possible hypomagnesemia
- Torsade de pointes VT
- Digoxin toxicity

Bicarbonate

Cardiac arrest results in combined respiratory and metabolic acidosis because pulmonary gas exchange ceases and cellular metabolism becomes anaerobic. The best treatment of acidemia in cardiac arrest is chest compression; some additional benefit is gained by ventilation. Bicarbonate causes generation of CO_2, which diffuses rapidly into cells. It has the following effects:

- It exacerbates intracellular acidosis.
- It produces a negative inotropic effect on ischemic myocardium.
- It presents a large, osmotically active, sodium load to an already compromised circulation and brain.
- It produces a shift to the left in the oxygen dissociation curve, further inhibiting release of oxygen to the tissues.

Giving sodium bicarbonate routinely during cardiac arrest and CPR (especially in out-of-hospital cardiac arrest), or after ROSC, is not recommended. Giving sodium bicarbonate (50 mmol) if cardiac arrest is associated with hyperkalemia or tricyclic antidepressant overdose. Repeating the dose according to the clinical condition of the patient and the results of repeated blood gas analysis.

Calcium

Calcium plays a vital role in the cellular mechanisms underlying myocardial contraction. Give calcium during resuscitation only when indicated specifically, that is, in cardiac arrest caused by hyperkalemia, hypocalcemia, or overdose of calcium channel-blocking drugs.

The initial dose of 10 mL 10% calcium chloride (6.8 mmol Ca^{2+}) may be repeated, if necessary. Calcium can slow the heart rate and precipitate arrhythmias. In cardiac arrest, calcium may be given by rapid IV injection. In the presence of a spontaneous circulation give it slowly. Not giving calcium solutions and sodium bicarbonate simultaneously by the same route.

Equipment

- Oral airway
- Bag and mask device
- Oxygen
- IV setup
- Defibrillator
- Emergency cardiac drugs
- Cardiac monitor
- Electrocardiograph machine
- Intubation equipment
- Suction

Procedure

Nursing action	Rationale
Responsiveness/airway	
Determine unresponsiveness: tap or gently shake patient while shouting, "Are you okay?"	This will prevent injury from attempted resuscitation on a person who is not unconscious
Activate emergency medical service	
Place the patient supine on a firm, flat surface. Kneel at the level of the patient's shoulders. If head or neck trauma is suspected, he should not be moved unless it is absolutely necessary (e.g., at the site of an accident, fire, or other unsafe environment)	This enables the rescuer to perform rescue breathing and chest compression without changing position
Circulation	
Determining the presence or absence of pulse	
While maintaining head-tilt with one hand on the patient's forehead, palpate the carotid or femoral pulse for no more than 10 seconds. If pulse is not palpable, start external chest compressions	Cardiac arrest is recognized by pulselessness in the large arteries of the unconscious, breathless patient. If the patient has a palpable pulse, but is not breathing, initiate rescue breathing at rate of 12 times per minute (once every 5 seconds) after two initial breaths

Contd...

Contd...

Nursing action	Rationale
This procedure consists of serial, rhythmic applications of pressure over the middle third of the sternum	
Kneel as close to side of patient's chest as possible. Placing the heel of one hand on the middle third of the sternum, The fingers may either be extended or interlaced but must be kept off the chest	The long axis of the heel of the rescuer's hand should be placed on the long axis of the sternum so that the main force of the compression is on the sternum, thereby decreasing the chance of rib fracture
While keeping your arms straight, elbows locked, and shoulders positioned directly over your hands, quickly and forcefully depress the middle third of the patient's sternum straight down one-third the depth of the chest	
Releasing the external chest compression completely and allow the chest to return to its normal position after each compression. The time allowed for release should equal the time required for compression. Not lifting your hands from the patient's chest or change position	Releasing the external chest compression allows blood flow into the heart
For CPR performed by one rescuer, do 30 compressions at a rate of 100 per minute and then perform two ventilations; reevaluate the patient. After four cycles of 30 compressions and two breaths each, checking the pulse; checking again every few minutes thereafter. Minimizing interruptions of chest compressions	Rescuing breathing and external chest compressions must be combined. Checking for return of carotid pulse. If absent, resuming CPR with two ventilations followed by compressions. For CPR performed by health professionals, mouth-to-mask ventilation is an acceptable alternative to rescue breathing
For CPR performed by two rescuers, the compression rate is 100/minute. The compression–ventilation ratio is 30:2. Once an advanced airway is in place, the compressing rescuer should give continuous chest compressions at a rate of 100 without pauses for ventilation. The rescuer delivering ventilation provides 8–10 breaths per minute	
Open the airway	
Head-tilt/chin-lift maneuver: Place one hand on the patient's forehead and apply firm backward pressure with the palm to tilt the head back. Then, place the fingers of the other hand under the bony part of the lower jaw near the chin and lift up to bring the jaw forward and the teeth almost to occlusion	In the absence of sufficient muscle tone, the tongue or epiglottis will obstruct the pharynx and larynx. This supports the jaw and helps tilt the head back
Jaw-thrust maneuver: Grasp the angles of the patient's lower jaw, lifting with both hands, one on each side; displacing the mandible forward, while tilting the head backward	The jaw-thrust technique without head tilt is the safest method for opening the airway in the presence of suspected neck injury
Breathing	
Place ear over patient's mouth and nose while ➢ Observing the chest ➢ Looking for the chest to rise and fall ➢ Listening for air escaping during exhalation ➢ Feeling for the flow of air	To determine presence or absence of spontaneous breathing
Perform rescue breathing by mouth-to-mouth, using: Ventilation barrier device. While keeping the patient's airway open, pinch the nostrils closed using the thumb and index finger of the hand you have placed on his forehead. Taking a deep breath, open your mouth wide, and place it around the outside edge of the patient's mouth to create an airtight seal Ventilate the patient with two full breaths (each lasting 1 second), taking a breath after each ventilation. If the initial ventilation attempt is unsuccessful, reposition the patient's head and repeat rescue breathing	This prevents air from escaping from the patient's nose. Adequate ventilation is indicated by seeing the chest rise and fall, feeling the air escape during ventilation, and hearing the air escape during exhalation

Contd...

Contd...

Nursing action	Rationale
Usage of special resuscitation equipment	
While resuscitation proceeds, simultaneous efforts are made to obtain and use special resuscitation equipment to manage breathing and circulation and provide definitive care	Definitive care includes defibrillation, pharmacotherapy for dysrhythmias and acid–base disturbances, and ongoing monitoring and skilled care in an intensive care unit
Utilize the AED as soon as possible. Special circumstances affecting use of AEDs include ➤ AEDs should not be used on children younger than age 8 ➤ The victim should not be lying in water when using an AED. Making sure the patient's chest is dry before attaching the AED ➤ Do not place the AED electrode directly over an implanted pacemaker ➤ Removing any transdermal medication patches from the patient before using the AED	The American Heart Association supports the use of AEDs in public places as well as medical centers ➤ The default energy level of AEDs is too high for children younger than age 8 ➤ Using an AED when patients are wet or lying in water may result in burns and shocks to the rescuer ➤ Placing an AED pad directly over an implanted pacemaker may reduce the effectiveness of the defibrillation ➤ Placing an AED pad over a transdermal medication patch may make the defibrillation less effective and cause a burn
The four basic steps used in AED operation are: 1. Turn the power on 2. Attach the AED pads to the patient's chest, using the diagrams on the pads to show you exactly where to place them 3. Analyze the patient's rhythm by pushing the button on the AED labeled ANALYZES 4. Deliver the shock. During this time, no one should touch the patient	The directions provided for operation of the AED were provided by the device manufacturer ➤ Touching the patient could create artifact and interfere with analysis. Telling you what to do ➤ Charging the AED and deliver the shock if indicated by the AED. Making sure that no one is touching the patient. Pushing the shock button

(AED: automated external defibrillator; CPR: cardiopulmonary resuscitation)

Complications

- Postresuscitation distress syndrome (secondary derangements in multiple organs)
- Neurological impairment and/or brain damage

STRESS

It is an unpleasant psychological and physiological state caused due to some internal and external demands that go beyond our capacity.

Stress may be considered as any physical, chemical, or emotional factor that causes bodily or mental unrest and that may be a factor in causing disease.

Stress is the response of the nervous system to stressors that are too large to handle. It is the internalized result of external overloads. It consists of stored abnormalities that serve to protect us from repeated exposure to the same overloads by limiting our functioning. Meaning of STRESS: Meaning of stress means:

S—Situation

T—That

R—Release

E—Emergency

S—Signal (or)

S—Stimuli

Stress management: Stress management is a process of learning how to live with the inevitable life stressor of people encounter by learning how to counteract or cope efficiency with counterproductive response to stress through enhanced self-activities.

A. Body coping mechanism with stress:

General adaptive syndrome model

Hans Selye (1907–1982) explained his stress model based on physiology and psychobiology as general adaptation syndrome (GAS). Physiologists define stress as how the body reacts to a stressor, real or imagined, a stimulus that causes stress. Acute stressors affect an organism in the short term; chronic stressors over the longer term.

I. **Alarm stage:** It is the first stage, which is divided into two phases—the *shock* phase and the *antishock* phase.

- *Shock phase*: During this phase, the body can endure changes, such as hypovolemia, hypoosmolarity, hyponatremia, hypochloremia, hypoglycemia—the stressor effect. The organism's resistance to the stressor drops temporarily below the normal range and some level of shock (e.g., circulatory shock) may be experienced.

- *Antishock phase*: When the threat or stressor is identified or realized, the body starts to respond and is in a state of alarm. During this stage, the locus coeruleus/sympathetic nervous system is activated and catecholamines such as adrenaline are being produced, hence the fight-or-flight response. The result is—increased muscular tonus, increased blood pressure due to peripheral vasoconstriction and tachycardia, and increased glucose in blood.

Stage 1: Alarm

- Upon encountering a stressor, body reacts with "fight-or-flight" response and sympathetic nervous system is activated.
- Hormones such as cortisol and adrenalin released into the bloodstream to meet the threat or danger.
- The body's resources now mobilized.

Example

- Increased heart rate
- Increased RBC production
- Increased breathing

II. **Resistance stage:** It is the second stage and increased secretion of glucocorticoids play a major role, intensifying the systemic response—they have lipolytic, catabolic, and antianabolic effects: increased glucose, fat, and amino-acid/protein concentration in blood. Moreover, they cause lymphocytopenia, eosinopenia, neutrophilia, and polycythemia. In high doses, cortisol begins to act as a mineralocorticoid (aldosterone) and brings the body to a state similar to hyperaldosteronism. If the stressor persists, it becomes necessary to attempt some means of coping with the stress. Although the body begins to try to adapt to the strains or demands of the environment, the body cannot keep this up indefinitely, so its resources are gradually depleted.

Stage 2: Resistance

- Parasympathetic nervous system returns many physiological functions to normal levels while body focuses resources against the stressor.
- Blood glucose levels remain high, cortisol, and adrenalin continue to circulate at elevated levels, but outward appearance of organism seems normal.
- Increase HR, BP, breathing
- Body remains on red alert

Resistance reaction

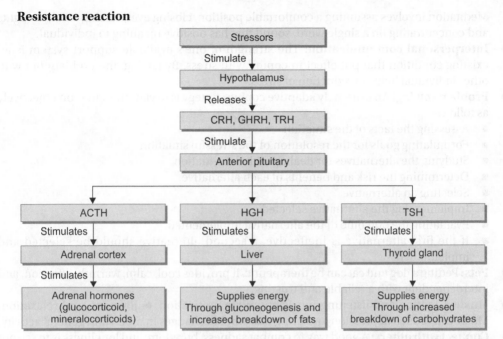

(CRH: corticotropin-releasing hormone; GHRH: growth hormone-releasing hormone; TRH: thyrotropin-releasing hormone; ACTH: adrenocorticotropic hormone; HGH: human growth hormone; TSH: thyroid stimulating hormone)

III. Exhaustion or recovery stage:

- **Recovery** stage follows when the system's compensation mechanisms have successfully overcome the stressor effect (or have completely eliminated the factor which caused the stress). The high glucose, fat and amino acid levels in blood prove useful for anabolic reactions, restoration of homeostasis and regeneration of cells.
- **Exhaustion** is the alternative third stage in the GAS model. At this point, all of the body's resources are eventually depleted and the body is unable to maintain normal function. The initial autonomic nervous system symptoms may reappear (sweating, raised heart rate, etc.). If stage three is extended, long-term damage may result (prolonged vasoconstriction results in ischemia which in turn leads to cell necrosis), as the body's immune system becomes exhausted, and bodily functions become impaired, resulting in decompensation.

Stage 3: Exhaustion

- If stressor continues beyond body's capacity, organism exhausts resources and becomes susceptible to disease and death.

B. Adaptive coping strategies.

- **Awareness:** The initial step in managing stress is awareness:
  - To become aware of the factors that creates stress
  - The feeling associative with a successful response.

  Stress can be controlled only when one recognize that is being experienced. As they aware about stressors, they can omitted, avoided, or accepted.
- **Relaxation:** Individual relaxes by engaging in large motor activities, such as sports, jogging and physical exercise. Still other techniques, such as breathing exercises and progressive relaxation to relieve stress.
- **Meditation:** Practiced 20 minutes once or twice daily, meditation has been shown to produce a lasting reduction in blood pressure and other stress-related symptoms.

Meditation involves assuming a comfortable position, closing eyes, casting off all thoughts and concentrating on a single word, sound that has positive meaning to individual.

- **Interpersonal communication:** The strength of one's available support system is an existing condition that put effect in coping with stress. By talking, the problem out with other individual helps in reduction of stress.
- **Problem solving:** An extremely adaptive coping strategy is to view the situation objectively as follow:
    - Assessing the facts of the situation
    - Formulating goals for the resolution of the stressful situation
    - Studying the alternatives for dealing with the situation
    - Determining the risk and benefits of each alternative
    - Selecting an alternative
    - Implementing the alternative selected
    - Evaluating the outcome of the alternative implemented
    - If the first alternative is ineffective, a second alternative should be selected and implemented.
- **Pets:** Petting a dog and cat can be therapeutic. It provides cool, calm, warmth, affection, and interdependent with a reliable and trusting.
- **Music:** Creating and listening music stimulate motivation, enjoyment, and relaxation. Music can reduce depression and bring measurable changes in mood and general activity.
- **Connect with others:** A good way to combat sadness, boredom, and loneliness is to see out activities involving others.
- **Take a minute vacation:** Imaging a quiet country scene can take you out of the stressful situation. Take a moment to close your eyes and imagine a place where feel you relaxed and comfortable.
- **Laugh:** Maintaining your sense of humor including the ability to laugh at yourself.
- **Think positively:** Refocus the negative to be positive. Making an effort to stop negative thoughts.
- **Compromise:** By cooperation and compromise helps in reduction of strain and help you more comfortable.
- **Have a good cry:** A good cry during periods of stress can be a healthy way to bring relief to your anxiety and prevent headache or others physical consequences.
- **Avoiding self-medications:** Alcohol and other medications do not remove stress. They may provide temporary relief. But it increases more complications.
- **Take care of your body:** Healthy eating and adequate sleep fuels your mind as well as your body. Avoiding consuming too much caffeine and sugar.

Role of Nurse in Stress Management Assessment

Nursing Assessment

Assessment of the person:
- Too much dependence on others for love and affection
- Inability to change or learn new ways of dealing with frustration
- High expectations

Assessment of family: Assessing the family perception of the problem and it is supportive of the client's efforts at coping.

Assessment of environment:
- Occupation with high stress
- Environmental factors, such as lighting and temperature

Nursing Interventions

- Increasing the client's awareness regarding as an actual health problem
- Helping him realize the health problem
- To support the client through the process of changes and cooperation with treatment
- The client encourages talking about the losses that have result in behavior changes
- Family members also need accurate information about health problem.

INTENSIVE CARE UNIT PSYCHOSIS

ICU psychosis is a disorder in which patients in an ICU or a similar setting experience a cluster of serious psychiatric symptoms. Another term that may be used interchangeably for ICU psychosis is ICU syndrome. ICU psychosis is also a form of delirium, or acute brain failure. Delirium is often used to refer to drowsiness, disorientation, and hallucination.

Etiology

Environmental Causes

- **Sensory deprivation:** A patient being put in a room that often has no windows and is away from family, friends, and all that is familiar and comforting.
- **Sleep disturbance and deprivation:** The constant disturbance and noise with the hospital staff coming at all hours to check vital signs, give medications, etc.
- **Continuous light levels:** Continuous disruption with lights (no reference to day or night)
- **Stress:** Patients in an ICU frequently feel the almost total loss of control over their life.
- **Lack of orientation:** A patient's loss of time and date.
- **Medical monitoring:** The continuous monitoring of the patient's vital signs, and the noise monitoring devices produce can be disturbing and create sensory overload.

Medical Causes

- **Pain** that may not be adequately controlled in an ICU.
- **Critical illness:** The pathophysiology of the disease, illness or traumatic event—the stress on the body during an illness can cause a variety of symptoms.
- **Infection** creating fever and toxins in the body.
- **Metabolic disturbances:** electrolyte imbalance, hypoxia (low blood oxygen levels), and elevated liver enzymes.
- Heart failure (inadequate CO)

Signs and Symptoms

The cluster of psychiatric symptoms of ICU psychosis includes:

- Extreme excitement
- Anxiety
- Restlessness
- Hearing voices
- Clouding of consciousness
- Hallucinations
- Nightmares
- Paranoia
- Disorientation
- Agitation
- Delusions
- Abnormal behavior

Diagnostic Evaluation

It is mainly diagnosed with the help of confusion assessment method.

The diagnosis of ICU psychosis can be made only in the absence of a known underlying medical condition that can mimic the symptoms of ICU psychosis. A medical assessment of the patient is important to search for other causes of mental status abnormality such as:

- Stroke
- Low blood sugar
- Drug or alcohol withdrawal
- Any other medical condition that may require treatment.

Treatment

- The treatment of ICU psychosis clearly depends on the cause. Many times the actual cause of the psychosis involves many factors, and many issues will need to be addressed to relieve the symptoms.
- A first step is a review of the patient's medications. The physician in charge of the patient along with the pharmacist can review each of the patient's medications to determine if they may be influencing the delirium.
- Family members, familiar objects, and calm words may help
- Sleep deprivation may be a major contributing factor. Therefore providing a quiet restful environment to allow the patient optimal sleep is important.
- Controlling the amount of time visitors are allowed to stimulate the patient can also help. Dehydration is remedied by administering fluids.
- Heart failure requires treatment with digitalis.
- Infections must be diagnosed and treated.
- Sedation with antipsychotic agents may help. A common medication used in the hospital setting to treat ICU psychosis is haloperidol or other medications for psychosis (antipsychotics).

MULTIPLE CHOICE QUESTIONS

1. **Which of the following is not a phase of disaster?**
   A. Preimpact
   B. Postimpact
   C. Recovery
   D. Mitigation

2. **Which of the following is a part of disaster preparedness?**
   A. Mitigation
   B. Rehabilitation
   C. Recovery
   D. Follow-up

Answers

1. D   2. A

Geriatric Nursing

23

AT THE END OF THIS CHAPTER, THE STUDENT WILL BE ABLE TO UNDERSTAND:

➤ Aging
➤ Demography: myths and realities
➤ Concepts and theories of aging
➤ Cognitive aspects of aging
➤ Normal biological aging
➤ Age-related body system changes
➤ Psychosocial aspects of aging
➤ Medications and elderly
➤ Stress and coping in older adults
➤ Common health problems and nursing management
➤ Cardiovascular, respiratory, and musculoskeletal, endocrine, genitourinary, gastrointestinal (GI) systems
➤ Neurological, skin, and other sensory organs
➤ Psychosocial and sexual
➤ Abuse of elderly person
➤ Role of nurse for care of elderly: ambulation, nutritional, communicational, psychosocial, and spiritual
➤ Role of nurse for caregivers of elderly
➤ Role of family and formal and nonformal caregivers
➤ Use of aids and prosthesis
➤ Legal and ethical issues

TERMINOLOGY

- **Geriatrics:** The study of old age includes the physiology, pathology, diagnosis, and treatment of the diseases affecting older adults.
- **Gerontology:** It is study of the aging process and includes the biological, psychological, and social sciences.
- **Gerontology nursing:** It is the field of nursing that specializes in the care of the elderly.
- **Old age:** The group of people whose age is above 65 years.
- **Aging:** Aging usually refers to the adverse effects of the passage of time but are also referred to the positive process of malnutrition or acquiring a desired quality.

INTRODUCTION AND ASSESSMENT

Aging is a maturational process that creates the need for individual adaptation because of physical and psychological declines that occur during a lifetime.

Normal Biological Changes of Aging

The types of changes in aging, category, and intensity vary from person to person. Heredity, nutritional, health, or tension-related factors might be responsible for this.

The changes in aging may be classified into:

1. Physical
2. Psychological
3. Psychosocial
4. Psychosexual changes
5. Cognitive and intellectual

Physical Changes

Changes, which may occur in different systems, are as follows:

Nervous System Changes

- Enlargement of the ventricular system as people get older the volume of ventricle gets increased (the cells surroundings the ventricles are lost)
- Reduced brain weight and volume probably caused by the loss of neurons
- Delirium, dementia, depression, and agitation
- Irritability
- Expression of feeling of worthlessness, hopelessness, and helplessness
- Diminished memory, orientation, and judgment
- Paranoid delusions (suspicious, false, impression)
- Demanding behavior and anxiety disorder
- Alcohol abuse, impaired concentration, short attention span
- Stress incontinence
- Elder abuse

Integumentary Changes

- Decrease in skin's elasticity and dryness appears
- Thinning in the skin's layer
- Increased pigmentation
- Decreased subcutaneous fat layer of skin
- Decreased perspiration and temperature regulation due to decreased sebaceous and sweat glands
- Wrinkles appear
- Hardness and dryness of nails and decreased nail growth and strength
- Toenails may discolor
- Hair of head, axial, or pubic region become scanty gray or white (decrease in melanin)
- Increased growth of nose, ear, and facial hair
- Slight growth of hair on upper lip and chin in postmenopause women.

Cardiovascular Changes

- Less blood circulation in heart and therefore slowed heart rate
- Blood vessels of head, neck, hands, and legs become prominent
- Decreased stroke volume and carbon monoxide (CO), diastolic murmur is common
- Deceased elasticity of blood vessels
- Increased rigidity and thickening of valves

- Increased blood pressure (BP) and peripheral vascular resistance
- Weaken pedal pulses and colder lower extremities

Respiratory Changes

- Increased potential for respiratory infections
- Increased breathing difficulties
- Decreased gas exchange
- Aspiration
- Decreased elasticity and numbers of alveolar sacs
- Decreased cough strength
- Common diseases are asthma, bronchitis, and emphysema.

Genitourinary Changes

- Decreased kidney size, function, and output
- Decreased glomerular filtration and number of nephrons
- Reduced renal blood flow from decreased CO
- Decreased bladder size and tone
- Incomplete bladder emptying leading to urine retention from weakness of tone
- Increased ease of backflow of urine
- Bladder capacity decreases
- Increased residual urine, incontinence, and nocturia
- Increased incidence of urinary tract infections
- Increased plasma urea and uric acid
- Enlargement of prostate and atrophy of reproductive organs in female.

Gastrointestinal Changes

- The main changes are decrease in contraction of the muscles and more time for the cardiac sphincter to open, thus taking more time for the food to be transmitted to the stomach.
- This will produce loss of appetite and cause deficiency in nutrients. This is the reason why older people eat small quantities of food.
- Changes in taste and smell and falling of teeth
- Less secretion of saliva and gastric juice (hydrochloric acid, HCl) and pepsin
- Decreased abdominal muscle strength
- Alteration in bowl habit—constipation
- Decline in liver enzymes and decreased liver weight and blood flow.

Musculoskeletal Changes

- Older people suffer from arthritis, paralytic stroke in addition to osteoporosis problems. This produces stiffness of joint, making them difficult for easy movement, such as getting up from a chair, turning their neck, and maintaining an erect posture.
- Their shoulder width also reduces due to bone loss and also weakening of muscles and loss of tone and elasticity causes stooping.
- Similarly collapsing of vertebrae causes a hunched back or kyphosis in addition to spondylitis. This occurs as the spongy cartilages decrease and breaks down, causing no or less lubrication between the vertebra.
- Range of motion decreases—stiffness, if no proper exercises are done
- Decreased mobility in joints affecting gait, posture, balance, and flexibility
- Injury due to joint instability and joint pain
- Reduced ability for activities of daily living due to stiff thoracic spine.

Reproductive Changes (Female)

- Ovarian cysts
- Lower esteem in women
- Atrophied ovaries and uterus
- Atrophy of external genitalia
- Scanty vaginal discharge
- Pendulous breasts
- Small flat nipples
- Decreased pubic hair

Reproductive Changes (Male)

- Difficulty in urinating
- Incontinence
- Lower self-esteem
- Enlarge prostate glands
- Pendulous scrotum
- Decreased size of penis and testis
- Decreased pubic hair

Endocrine System Changes

In males, the problems are due to decreased testosterone production and also include fatigue, weight loss, decreased libido, lower esteem, and depression.

In females, problems are due to decreased estrogen and progesterone levels. The problems also include osteoporosis, menopause and associated problems, diabetes (lifelong illness due to faulty carbohydrate rate), etc.

Immune System Changes

- In older people, cells continually wear out and the existing cells cannot repair damaged part within themselves, especially in skeletal and heart muscles and throughout the nervous system
- Aging affects the immune system of the body making it defective, thereby attracting foreign proteins, bacteria, and viruses and also produces antibodies against itself, e.g., cancer, diabetes, and rheumatoid arthritis.

Changes in Sensory Functions

Sensation is the process of taking information through the sense organs. The efficiency of sensory perception reduces as a result of degeneration changes. The ability to respond to the information provided by the sense organs may also be reduced.

Sense of Touch

- Sense of touch deteriorates with age especially in fingertips and palms and in the lower extremities.
- This also causes fewer levels of painful stimuli. But they may complain of pain, and it is due to depression.

Changes in vision

- The loss of vision in older people prevents them from their daily activities.
- The important problem is the changes in the visual pathways of the brain and in the visual cortex that block the transmission of stimuli from the sensory organs.

- The surface of the cornea thickens causing the rounded surface of the cornea to become less smooth and flatter and irregular in shape and also the blood vessels become prominent.

Changes in Hearing
- An older person, who is having some hearing loss, learns to adapt and make changes in behavior and social interactions, so as to reduce the bad social impact of hearing loss.
- High-pitched sounds stimulate hair cells at the base of the cochlea, and low-pitched sounds stimulate the apex.
- The nerve impulses that are sent through the internal auditory nerve and the cochlear nerve to the brain where they are translated into meaningful sounds.

Changes in Taste and Smell
- As they age, their taste also changes, and like children they also prefer more sweet food. Otherwise, they may complain of taste difference. This is due to the weakness of taste buds as they age or their ability to appreciate taste.
- Hence, they may require more salty and spicy food. To avoid giving them more salty and spicy food, their food can be enhanced with good food odors to increase their appetite.

Psychological Changes

- Loss of self-esteem
- Acceptance and nonacceptance of physical changes
- Coping with personal loss
- Slower process of information and possible depression
- Gradual decline in intelligence
- Inaccurate communication
- Disruption of sleep

Psychosocial Changes

The older adults must adapt to psychosocial changes that occur with aging, such as the following:

Retirement
- Retirement often has associations of passivity and seclusion and often leads to psychological stresses.
- Retirement brings about role changes with the spouse or family and therefore the problems of social isolation.
- Retirement is also viewed as the beginning of old age.

Role Changes
- Aging is associated with many role changes and transitions.
- Some roles—such as spouse, friends, or employee—may be lost, while new roles—such as widow or volunteer—may arise.

Loneliness
- Any lose that creates a deficit in intimacy and interpersonal relationships can lead to loneliness.
- Even sensory deprivation increases the risk
- It can provoke or aggravate physical symptoms, sleep disturbances.
- Retirement, poor health, and inactivity also may contribute to loneliness

Depression and Suicide

- More likely in the older individuals, i.e., depression increases in frequency and intensity with age.
- Changes in neurotransmitters, multiple losses, and decreased internal and external resources contribute to its incidence.
- Risk factors for depression include a recent major loss, isolation from family and friends, feeling of hopelessness, absence of an identifiable role in life, and loss of partner or sexual function.

Psychosexual Changes

- Physical incapacity
- Less secretion of hormones
- Degeneration of reproductive organs
- Lack of privacy
- Hesitation or death of life partner
- Ignorance relating to sexuality in old age, etc.

Cognitive and Intellectual Changes

In addition to those physiological changes that occur with advancing age, older patients are also experiencing changes that have an effect on cognition. Cognition includes abilities related to memory, intelligence, orientation, judgment, calculation abilities, learning, attention, language, higher cognitive function, and constructional ability.

Many factors can affect cognition:
- Sensory changes and disease associated with age can cause misinterpretation of information being collected.
- Pain from chronic diseases, such as arthritis, can limit cognition as pain takes over the body and mind.
- Sleep deprivation caused by worry or fear can make it more difficult to perform routine tasks.
- Medications that cause drowsiness as side effects can also impair cognition.

Changes in Mental Functioning

- Decreased adaptation, coping with new situations, perception, comprehension, range of interests, and understanding
- Increased repetitive thoughts and vulnerability to stress

Changes in Memory

- Decreased number of neurons, blood supplies to brain; short-term memory, which is associated with decreased judgment, insight, and orientation.
- Gradual memory loss during sixth decade of life with greater memory decline after mid-seventh decade.
- Long-term memory retrieval is easier to accomplish in old age than short-term memory retrieval.

Learning and Intelligence

- Aging process may affect learning
- Registration of information or reception of new stimuli may be affected through age-associated changes.

- Intelligence does not decline as one ages if it is measured using an appropriate instrument that focus on accuracy, not on response.

THEORIES OF AGING (TABLE 23.1)

The complex process of aging can be described as follows:

- **Chronological age:** Refers to the number of years a person has lived and most commonly uses objective method.
- **Physiological age:** Refers to the determinants of age by function, though age-related changes affect everyone. It is impossible to pinpoint exactly when these changes occur, so it is useful in determining a person's age.
- **Functional age:** Refers to a person's ability to contribute to society and benefit others and himself. It is a fact that not all individuals of the same chronological age function at the same level.

TABLE 23.1: Theories of Aging (A comparison of theories).

Stochastic	Non-stochastic	Psychological
Aging is caused by external forces acting on the body cells and there are ways to slow down the process	Aging is internally regulated by a biological time clock and nothing can change it	Attempt to explain behavior, roles and relationship in the aging process
Free radical theory: Cells are damaged by free radicals which leads to aging	**Programmed aging theory:** A biological clock controls cell behavior and life span	**Disengagement theory:** Older adults and society mutually withdraw from each other. The aging person becomes more introspective and self-focused
Somatic mutation theory: Chromosomes are damaged by exposure to toxins or radiation	**Pacemaker theory:** Neurochromosones (brain) regulated development and aging throughout the life span	**Activity theory:** Continuing the social activities of middle age or those activities must be replaced with others for successful aging
Wear and tear theory: Damage from everyday wear eventually exceeds the body's ability to repair itself	**Immunological theory:** Changes in the immune system are responsible for the effects of aging	**Continuity theory:** Personality and behavior develop over a lifetime and are key to how a person adjusts to aging

Biological Theory

It addresses the anatomic and physiologic changes occurring with age. Biologic theories of aging address questions about the basic aging process that affect all living organisms. These theories answer how cells age and what triggers the process of aging. Leynard Hayflick one of the first gerontologists to propose a theory of aging explains age-related changes are the following:

- **Deleterious:** Reduces function
- **Progressive:** Occurs gradually
- **Intrinsic:** Does not attribute to modifiable environmental changes
- **Universe:** Affects all members of a species.
    - **Genetic theory:** It emphasizes the role of genes in causing age changes. Hayflick estimates that human cell divides 50 times in these many number of years. Moreover cells are genetically programmed to stop all divisions after achieving 50, after which the cells start deteriorating. A genetic theory called mutation theory suggests that aging is the result of mutation of somatic cells or alteration in DNA repair mechanism.
- **Wear and tear theory:** The wear and tear theory suggests that organism have fixed amount of energy, which will wear out on a schedule basis. When enough cells wear out, the body does not function well. The process is aggravated by harmful stress factors, such as smoking, poor diet, muscular strain, or large intake of alcohol. This theory of aging is supported by

microscopic signs of wear and tear in the cells of striated skeletal tissue, heart muscle, and all nerve cells.

- **Immunity theory:** This theory is based on the knowledge that immune system particularly the thymus and immunocompetent cells in the bone marrow is affected by aging process and diminished functioning of the immune system.
- **Free radical theory:** The free radical theory was proposed in the mid-1950 and still provides basic for research on aging. With the aging process, the body's immune system, free radical components that are not being used by the body, will act opposite to antioxidants.

Psychosocial Theory

The four psychosocial theories are as follows:

1. **Activity theory:** The activity theory proposed that older people would remain psychologically and socially fit if they remain active. According to this perspective, the maintenance of optimal physical, mental, and social activity is necessary for successful aging. This theory also assumes that older adults have the same needs as a middle-age person.
2. **Human needs theory:** Maslow's hierarchy is one of the theories used by the gerontologist, i.e., people continually move between the levels, but they always strive toward higher levels.
3. **Continuity theory:** The continuity or developmental theory states that personality remains the same and behavior becomes more predictable as people age. This theory focuses more on the personality and individual behavior over time.
4. **Adjustment theory:** It defines aging as a series of adjustment to retirement to grandparenthood, to changes in income, to changes in social life and marital status, and to potential deterioration of health and well-being.

Role of Nurse in Elderly Care

- Consider individuality
- Consult his/her preferences
- Do not attempt to alter lifelong character and behavior.
- Give time to listen, to learn, and to adapt
- Help him/her to cope with thought of life
- Be patient, kind, and sympathetic; communicate effectively; and demonstrate respect
- Encourage independence and encourage him/her to make choices and decisions; assist elderly individuals to achieve emotional stability
- Praise even their minimal achievements
- Support them even during their period of anxiety
- Give person time to express his/her feelings
- Encourage them to have contact with others
- Stimulate mental acuity and sensory input and physical activity to uplift their self-esteem, self-concept, and confidence
- Make elderly individual's stay at home interesting and lively
- Arrange small library, indoor games, religious place for worship, and festival celebrations.
- Provide diversional or occupational therapy
- Maintain privacy
- Handle them gently
- Make them comfortable by providing comfortable bed, bed linen, etc.
- Protect them from injuries, falls, etc., make arrangements for night lights or under bed lights to avoid confusion and accidents
- Keep their bed dry, smooth, and unwrinkled

- Encourage them to maintain body hygiene, thus regulating the body temperature
- Assist them in changing weather
- Assist them to take care of visual, auditory, and dental

Nursing Care Plan

Impairment of Vision Related to Aging

Nursing intervention
- Provide bright light for reading
- Use dim lights in their bed rooms all through the night
- Provide safety rails at the sides of the bed
- Place the furniture in a convenient place away from the bed
- Regular eye checkup and correction of eyeglasses
- Treatment of eye infections in their early stages.

Impairment of Hearing Related to Aging Process

Nursing intervention
- Face the patient while speaking, so as to enable the patient for lip reading
- Talk slowly and distinctly
- Use simple language and short sentences
- Lower the pitch of the voice
- Use nonverbal communication (facial expressions, use of hands, writing), etc.
- When giving instruction, get feedback from the patient
- Get the cleaning of the auditory canal

Alterations in Smell and Taste

Nursing intervention
- Create a pleasant meal time
- Create pleasant atmosphere by maintaining the patient's unit as clean as possible
- Serve the food attractively
- Maintain good oral hygiene before and after food intake
- Check the gas leaks from gas cylinder as their sensation of smell is impaired

Impaired Skin Integrity Related to Aging and Malnutrition

Nursing intervention
- Special attention should be given to pressure points
- Frequent position change should be done
- Soft, smooth, and wrinkle-free bed should be provided
- Avoid prolonged exposure of the skin to hot and cold application
- Keeping the skin dry and clean
- Adequate nutrition should be given
- Active and passive exercises should be done
- Adequate fluid intake should be given
- Cut long nails to prevent skin injuries by scratching

Impaired Mobility of Bones and Joints Related to Fractures

Nursing intervention
- Active and passive exercise should be given to promote mobility.
- Encourage ambulation

- Prevent fatigue by maintaining balance between exercise and rest period.
- Provide side rails in bed to prevent accidents.
- Provide adequate lighting in the passage to bathrooms to prevent fall
- Physiotherapy should be done.
- Avoid slippery floors
- Never leave the patient alone

Impaired Memory, Impaired Sleep, and Reduced Sensory Perception Related to Aging

Nursing intervention
- Assessment of the vital signs frequently
- Use an effective communication process
- Always face the patient while talking
- Provide with hearing aids, eyeglasses for patient to improve his/her sensory perception
- Arrange for comfortable bed without wrinkles
- Administration of medicine in time
- Never leave the patient alone
- Help the patient to perform his/her activities of daily living (ADLs)
- Daily observation of vital signs, mental status, and body movements.

Dyspnea on Exertion, Edema, Hypertension, and Palpitation Related to Aging Condition of Heart

Nursing intervention
- Complete bed rest should be provided to the patient.
- Cardiac position should be given to the patient.
- Salt-free diet should be provided.
- Frequent observation of temperature, pulse, respiration, and BP
- Allow ambulation with the advice of doctor
- Educate the client not to lift any weight and climb steps
- Administer oxygen inhalation
- Provide assistance to carry out ADLs

Dyspnea Even at Rest, Cough Expectoration, Cyanosis Related to Aging Process

Nursing intervention
- Provide Fowler's position to the patient
- Apply suction in case of pooling of secretions in the respiratory passage
- Administer oxygen if the patient is cyanosed
- Ask the patient to cough out the sputum
- Provide steam inhalation or nebulization to bring out sputum
- Provide frequent mouth care to the patient
- Provide postural drainage to bring out secretions
- Serve small and frequent feeds
- Assist the client in his/her ADLs

Unnoticed Injury to Feet due to Altered Sensory Perception Related to Diabetes Mellitus (DM)

Nursing intervention
- Daily examination of limbs for cuts, blisters, redness areas, scratches should be done.
- Do not allow the patient to walk bare foot

- Use well-fitting shoes and socks
- Keep the feet clean and dry always
- Cut short nails to prevent scratches causing injury
- Check the temperature of the water given to patient for bath to prevent scald
- Check the urine or blood for sugar to evaluate and control DM
- Exercise will help to reduce the blood glucose level and promote circulation to limbs.

Altered GI Function due to Anorexia, Dyspepsia, Dysphagia, Constipation, Diarrhea Related to Aging Process

Nursing intervention

- Always assess the ability of the patient to swallow the food before the next round of feed is given.
- Always start with plain water (sips of water)
- Position the client in an upright position
- Always keep a suction apparatus ready
- Create pleasing surrounding for meals
- Give mouth care before and after every meal.
- Encourage taking a small bite of food at a time to prevent choking
- Check body weight to evaluate adequacy of food intake and encourage large amount of fluid intake

Retention of Urine Related to Old Age

Nursing Intervention

- Always provide enough privacy
- Unless contraindicated, allow the patient to resume normal position for urination
- Always use clean, dry, and warm bedpan
- Cleanliness of the bathroom helps the patient to void
- Offer bed pan at regular intervals
- Apply cold therapy to help in micturating
- Give fluid in large amounts
- Catheterize the bladder, if required

Incontinence Related to Neurological Disorders or Aging Process

Nursing Intervention

- Back care should be given 2 hourly
- Bed linen should be changed as necessary
- Maintain the hygiene of the patient
- Catheterize the bladder, if required
- Encourage the client to empty his/her bladder frequently.

COGNITIVE ASPECT OF AGING

Cognitive abilities are the mental skills that we need to carry out any task from the most simple to the most complex. These mental skills include awareness, information handling, memory, and reasoning. As we get older, our cognitive abilities gradually deteriorate. A certain amount of cognitive decline is a normal part of aging. Some people, however, will experience a severe deterioration in cognitive skills, leading to dementia.

All of these mental functions are critical for carrying out everyday activities, living independently, and for general health and well-being.

Cognition

In addition to physiological changes that occur with advancing age, older patients also experience changes that have an effect on cognition. Cognition includes abilities related to intelligence, memory, orientation, judgment, calculation, and learning.

Cognition focuses on intake, storage, processing, and retrieval of information. For the most part, older patients store information without much conscious efforts. If dealing with information becomes difficult, the older person may begin to worry. Unless this worry is addressed, the patient's concern may result in psychological problems and fear.

I. **Attention:** Attention is a basic but complex cognitive process that has multiple subprocesses specialized for different aspects of attention processing. Some form of attention is involved in virtually all other cognitive domains, except when task performance has become habitual or automatic. Declines in attention can therefore have broad-reaching effects on one's ability to function adequately and efficiently in everyday life.

- Selective attention: Selective attention refers to the ability to attend to some stimuli while disregarding others that are irrelevant to the task at hand.
- Divided attention and attention switching: Divided attention has usually been associated with significant age-related declines in performance, particularly when tasks are complex. Divided attention tasks require the processing of two or more sources of information or the performance of two or more tasks at the same time.
- Sustained attention: Sustained attention refers to the ability to maintain concentration on a task over an extended period of time. Typically, vigilance tasks are used to measure sustained attention, in which people must monitor the environment for a relatively infrequent signal, such as a blip on a radar screen. In general, older adults are not impaired on vigilance tasks.

II. **Intelligence:** Older adults show progressive decline in intelligence. Higher educational level, occupational status, and income have a positive effect on intelligence score in later life. Intellectual process, such as reasoning and abstract thinking is disturbed.

III. **Personality:** Changes may occur in the personality due to the death of life partner, decreased or end of self-dependence, loss of source of income, incapacity, etc. Personality breakdown in old may lead to criminal behavior or suicidal tendencies.

IV. **Memory:** Memory power may decrease with increasing age. Recalling of less frequently used information is difficult. Confused memory may be found.

- **Working memory:** Short-term or primary memory, on the other hand, involves the simple maintenance of information over a short period of time.
- **Long-term memory:** The cognitive domain that has probably received the most attention in normal aging is memory.
- **Episodic memory:** The episodic memory problems experienced by older adults may involve deficient encoding, storage, or retrieval processes. At the input stage, older adults may encode new information less meaningfully or with less elaboration, so that memory traces are less distinctive, more similar to others in the memory system and thereby more difficult to retrieve.
- **Semantic memory:** Semantic memory refers to one's store of general knowledge about the world, including factual information, such as "George Washington was the first president of the United States" and knowledge of words and concepts.
- **Autobiographical memory:** Autobiographical memory involves memory for one's personal past and includes memories that are both episodic and semantic in nature.
- **Recent memories** are easiest to retrieve, those from early childhood are most difficult to retrieve, and there is a monotonic decrease in retention from the present to the most remote past, with one exception.

- **Procedural memory:** Procedural memory refers to knowledge of skills and procedures, such as riding a bicycle, playing the piano, or reading a book. These highly skilled activities are acquired more slowly than episodic memories through extensive practice. Once acquired, procedural memories are expressed rather automatically in performance and are not amenable to description.

For example, although the finger movements of a skilled typist slow down with age, the overall typing speed is maintained because other aspects of the skill adjust. Procedural memory depends on several brain regions, including the basal ganglia and the cerebellum.

- **Implicit memory:** Implicit memory refers to a change in behavior that occurs as a result of prior experience, though one has no conscious or explicit recollection of that prior experience. For example, laboratory experiments have shown that it is easier to identify a degraded stimulus (from a brief exposure or partial information) if the stimulus was seen previously, even if one does not remember the prior occurrence.

Conceptual priming, which requires semantic processing and is observed in response to a conceptual cue, is also preserved in many older adults and has been associated with left frontal and left temporal cortical regions.

- **Prospective memory:** Much of what we have to remember in everyday life involves prospective memory, remembering to do things in the future, such as keep appointments, return a book to the library, or pay bills on time. Older adults do quite well on these daily tasks, using a variety of external aids, such as calendars and appointment books to remind themselves of these activities. Certain habitual tasks, such as taking medications at the appropriate times each day, however, may create difficulties for older people.

V. **Perception:** Most people view perception as a set of processes that occurs prior to cognition. However, the boundaries between perception and cognition are unclear, and much evidence suggests that these domains are interactive with top-down cognitive processes affecting perception, and perceptual processing has a clear impact on cognition.

Declining sensory and perceptual abilities have important implications for the everyday lives of older adults. Hearing loss can isolate older people, preventing them from engaging in conversation and other social interactions. Visual impairments can limit mobility and interact with attention deficits to make driving a particularly hazardous activity. As older people develop strategies to compensate for declining sensory abilities, the ways in which they perform other cognitive tasks may also be altered and may be less efficient. Retraining and practice on these tasks may help the adjustment and improve performance.

VI. **Speech and language:** Older people often tell well-structured elaborate narratives that are judged by others to be more interesting than those told by young. They usually have more extensive vocabularies and although they exhibit the occasional word-finding difficulty, older adults are easily able to provide circumlocutions to mask the problem. They are skilled conversationalists and appear to have few difficulties in processing ongoing speech. Some older adults have hearing loss and so, in conversational settings, may be required to interpret a weak or distorted acoustic signal. Older adults also experience problems with comprehension when individual words are presented at a very rapid rate, but they show sharply reduced impairments when such words form meaningful sentences.

VII. **Decision-making:** Older adults, again possibly because of working memory limitations, tend to rely on expert opinion to a greater degree than young adults. Although this strategy may work reasonably well when the expert is well qualified (e.g., a physician for medical decisions), it may leave older people susceptible to things, such as investment scams. Poor decision-making may also be a result of episodic memory decline, particularly the loss of memory for details or source. For example, remembering that "Stock ABC is a good investment," without remembering where one heard such information, could lead to a bad decision.

VIII. Learning: Ability to learn and acquire new skills decreases in older adults. Physical skills, motivation, etc., have positive influence on the learning. Memory is the integral part of learning, and age-related loss occurs more in short-term memory.

Factors Affecting Cognition of Older People

The following factors have an impact on the cognition of older people:

- Sensory changes and disease associated with age can cause misinterpretation of information being collected.
- Pain from chronic diseases, such as arthritis can limit cognition as pain takes over the body and mind.
- Sleep deprivation caused by worry or fear can make it more difficult to perform routine tasks.
- Medications that cause drowsiness as an effect can also impair cognition.
- Long-term memory retrieval is easier to accomplish in old age compared to short-term retrieval.
- Assist the patient having short-term memory problems by using written lists, visual clues, and other memory-enhancing systems to aid in strengthening the short-term memory skills.

PSYCHOLOGICAL ASPECTS OF AGING

With increasing age, many psychological changes occur in the elderly people, which are described as follows:

Coping Abilities

In addition to the normal aging changes, many patients are coping with compounding changes that occur because of chronic disease. Changes in employment status and societal and family roles and shift from independence to dependence may leave a strong psychological impact on both older patients and significant others. With such combination of losses, an older patient's confidence level may be affected, requiring encouragement of self-care behaviors. Personality, attitude, past life experiences, and the desire to adapt to changes are all intrinsic influencing factors that help the older patient to cope with changes brought on by advancing age.

Depression

There are times when the psychological impact of change is too difficult to cope with, resulting in loneliness and depression with the potential to disable the older person's mind and body. Depression is the most common psychiatric problem among the older adults. This psychological condition, which includes disturbances in mood, increases the risk for suicide, physical health complaints, and sleep disturbances. The changes that often come in later life, such as retirement, the death of loved ones, increased isolation, medical problems, can lead to depression. Depression prevents older people from enjoying life. It also impacts energy, sleep, appetite, and physical health. Depression can result from the physical changes in the brain due to a medication or a condition affecting neurotransmitters or psychological changes at an emotional level, such as maladaptive coping from a perceived loss. It is important, therefore, to know what older person is and is not saying during communications.

Causes

- **Health problems:** Illness and disability, chronic or severe pain, cognitive decline, damage to body image due to surgery or disease.

- **Loneliness and isolation:** Living alone, a dwindling social circle due to deaths or relocation, decreased mobility due to illness or loss of driving privileges.
- **Reduced sense of purpose:** Feelings of purposelessness or loss of identity due to retirement or physical limitations on activities.
- **Fears:** Fear of death or dying, anxiety over financial problems or health issues.
- **Recent bereavements:** The death of friends, family members, and pets; the loss of a spouse or partner.

Some Other Causes

- A move from home, such as to a retirement facility
- Chronic illness or pain
- Children moving away
- Spouse or close friends passing away
- Loss of independence

Risk Factors for Depression

- Lack of a supportive social network or stressful life events
- Damage to body image due to amputation, cancer surgery, or heart attack
- Family history of major depressive disorder
- Fear of death, living alone, or social isolation
- Other illnesses or past suicide attempt
- Presence of chronic or severe pain
- Previous history of depression
- Recent loss of a loved one, or substance abuse

Signs and Symptoms of Depression

- Sadness and fatigue
- Abandoning or losing interest in hobbies or other pleasurable pastimes
- Social withdrawal and isolation: reluctance to be with friends, engage in activities, or leave home
- Weight loss or loss of appetite
- Sleep disturbances: difficulty falling asleep or staying asleep or oversleeping or daytime sleepiness
- Loss of self-worth: worries about being a burden, feelings of worthlessness, self-loathing
- Increased use of alcohol or other drugs
- Fixation on death, suicidal thoughts, or attempts

Management

- Treat any illness that may be causing the symptoms
- Stop taking any medications that may be making symptoms worse
- Avoid alcohol and sleep aids
- If these steps do not help, medicines to treat depression and talk therapy often help.
- Doctors often prescribe lower doses of antidepressants to older people and increase the dose more slowly when compared to younger adults.
- Exercise regularly
- Surround yourself with caring, positive people and do fun activities
- Learn good sleep habits
- Learn to watch for the early signs of depression and know how to react if these occur

- Drink less alcohol and do not use illegal drugs
- Talk about feelings with someone you trust
- Take medications correctly and discuss any side effects with doctor

Dementia

Dementia involves a permanent progressive deterioration of mental function. Dementia is often characterized by confusion, forgetfulness impaired judgment, memory, and personality changes but without impairment of consciousness.

These include the following:

- **Emotional liability:** Marked variation in emotional expressions; thought abnormalities, e.g., delusion, perseveration
- Urinary and fecal incontinence may develop in late stages
- Disorientation in time, place, and person may also develop in late stages
- Neurological signs may/may not be present depending on the underlying cause.

Causes

- Parenchymatous brain disease (Alzheimer's disease)
- Parkinson's disease
- Vascular dementia
- **Metabolic problems and endocrine abnormalities**
- Nutritional deficiency
- Dementias due to infections
- Neoplastic dementias

Risk Factors

- **Age:** As you age, especially after age 65, the risk of Alzheimer's disease, vascular dementia, and several other dementias greatly increases.
- **Family history:** If you have a family history of dementia, you are at greater risk of developing the condition.
- **Down syndrome:** By middle age, many people with Down syndrome develop plaques and tangles in the brain that are associated with Alzheimer's disease. Some may develop dementia.

Clinical Manifestation

- Personality changes, lack of interest in day-to-day activities, early mental fatigability, self-centered
- Memory loss
- Difficulty communicating or finding words
- Difficulty with complex tasks
- Difficulty with planning and organizing
- Difficulty with coordination and motor functions
- Problems with disorientation, such as getting lost
- Inability to reason, inappropriate behavior, paranoia, agitation, hallucinations

Diagnostic Evaluation

- **History taking:** Family history of dementia or any previous history of depression
- **Lab tests:** Simple blood tests can rule out physical problems that can affect brain functions, such as vitamin B_{12} deficiency or an under active thyroid gland, complete blood count (CBC), urinalysis, liver function tests, cerebrospinal fluid (CSF) examination.

- **Radiological examination:** Chest X-ray
- **Computed tomography (CT) scan and magnetic resonance imaging (MRI):** To check for evidence of stroke or bleeding and to rule out the possibility of a tumor.

Management

Treatment depends on the condition causing the dementia. Some people may need to stay in the hospital for a short time. Stopping or changing medicines that make confusion worse may improve brain function.

- **Memantine:** Memantine works by regulating the activity of glutamate. Glutamate is another chemical messenger involved in brain functions, such as learning and memory. A common side effect of memantine is dizziness.
- **Occupational therapy:** Therapists may teach you coping behaviors and ways to adapt to movements and daily living activities as your condition changes.
- **Modifying the environment:** Reducing clutter and distracting noise can make it easier for someone with dementia to focus and function. It also may reduce confusion and frustration.
- **Modifying your responses:** A caregiver's response to a behavior can make the behavior, such as agitation, worse. It is best to avoid correcting and quizzing a person with dementia. Reassuring the person and validating his/her concerns can defuse most situations.
- **Modifying tasks:** Break tasks into easier steps and focus on success, not failure. Structure and routine during the day also help reduce confusion in people with dementia.

Delirium

Delirium is a sudden onset of mental confusion causing changes in behavior.

Clinical Manifestation

- Restless and upset
- Slurred speech, not making sense
- Mix-up days and nights
- Sleepy, then alert
- Forgetful, cannot concentrate
- More alert than normal

Etiology

- Infection
- Medication, not taking medication
- Surgery with anesthesia
- Dehydration
- High/low blood sugar
- Pain
- Constipation, diarrhea

Diagnostic Evaluation

- **Mental status assessment:** A doctor starts by assessing awareness, attention, and thinking. This can be done informally through conversation or more formally with tests or screening checklists that assess mental state, confusion, perception, and memory.
- **Physical and neurological examination:** The doctor will perform a physical examination, checking for signs of dehydration, infection, alcohol withdrawal, and other problems.

The physical examination can also help detect underlying disease. Delirium may be the first or only sign of a serious condition, such as respiratory failure or heart failure. A neurological examination, checking vision, balance, coordination, and reflexes can help determine whether a stroke or another neurological disease is causing the delirium.

Management

Supportive therapies are as follows:

- Clocks and calendars to help a person stay oriented
- A calm, comfortable environment that includes familiar objects from home
- Regular verbal reminders of current location and what is happening
- Involvement of family members
- Avoidance of change in surroundings and caregivers
- Uninterrupted periods of sleep at night, with low levels of noise and minimal light
- Open blinds during the day to promote daytime alertness and a regular sleep–wake cycle
- Avoidance of physical restraints and bladder tubes
- Adequate nutrition and fluid
- Use of adequate light, music, massage, and relaxation techniques to ease agitation
- Opportunities to get out of bed, walk, and perform self-care activities
- Provision of eyeglasses, hearing aids, and other adaptive equipment as needed.

ELDER ABUSE

Elder abuse is any form of mistreatment that results in harm or loss to an older person. Elder abuse tends to take place where the senior lives, most often at home (family members), institutional settings (long-term care facilities), when they face personal losses (loss of independence, homes, lifesaving, health, dignity, and security).

Types of Elder Abuse

- **Physical abuse:** Physical elder abuse is nonaccidental use of force against an elderly person, which results in physical pain, injury, or impairment. Such abuse includes not only physical assaults, such as hitting or shoving but the inappropriate use of drugs, restraints, or confinement.
- **Emotional abuse:** In emotional or psychological abuse, people speak to or treat elderly persons in ways that cause emotional pain or distress.
- Verbal forms of emotional elder abuse include intimidation through yelling or threats, humiliation and ridicule, and habitual blaming.
- Nonverbal psychological elder abuse can take the form of ignoring the elderly person, isolating an elder from friends or activities, or terrorizing or menacing the elderly person.
- **Sexual abuse:** Sexual elder abuse is contact with an elderly person without the elder's consent. Such contact can involve physical sex acts, but activities, such as showing an elderly person pornographic material, forcing the person to watch sex acts, or forcing the elder to undress are also considered sexual elder abuse.
- **Neglect or abandonment by caregivers:** Elder neglect and failure to fulfill a caretaking obligation constitute more than half of all reported cases of elder abuse. It can be intentional or unintentional, based on factors, such as ignorance or denial that an elderly charge needs as much care as he/she does.
- **Financial exploitation:** This involves unauthorized use of an elderly person's funds or property, either by a caregiver or by an outside scam artist.

An Unscrupulous Caregiver Might

- Misuse an elder's personal checks, credit cards, or accounts
- Steal cash, income checks, or household goods
- Forge the elder's signature
- Engage in identity theft

Typical Rackets that Target Elders include

- Announcements of a "prize" that the elderly person has won but must pay money to claim
- Phony charities
- Investment fraud

Healthcare fraud and abuse: Carried out by unethical doctors, nurses, hospital personnel, and other professional care providers; examples of healthcare fraud and abuse regarding elders include the following:

- Not providing health care but charging for it
- Overcharging or double billing for medical care or services
- Getting kickbacks for referrals to other providers or for prescribing certain drugs
- Overmedicating or undermedicating
- Recommending fraudulent remedies for illnesses or other medical conditions
- Medicaid fraud

Risk Factors

- Poor health and functional impairment in older persons
- Cognitive impairment, impairment in memory, personality changes, etc.
- Substance abuse or mental illness
- Shared living arrangements
- External factors causing stress, such as relationship difficulties or a divorce, serious illness in the family, caring for dependents, such as children or elderly persons, bereavement, moving house, debt problems.
- Social isolation
- History of violence
- Dependence of abuse on the victims

Risk Factors Among Caregivers

The stress of caring older individuals can lead to mental and physical health problems among the caregivers, making them feel burned out and impatient; and therefore, the caregivers cannot stop themselves from lashing out against elders in their care.

- Inability to cope with stress (lack of resilience)
- Depression, which is common among caregivers
- Lack of support from other potential caregivers
- Caregiver's perception is burdened without psychological reward
- Substance abuse
- **Institutional settings:** Lack of training, too many responsibilities, unsuited to caregiving, work under poor conditions.

Signs and Symptoms

- General signs of abuse
- Frequent arguments or tension between the caregiver and the elderly person
- Changes in personality or behavior in the elder

- If elder abuse is suspected, but not sure, look for clusters of the following physical and behavioral signs.

Physical Abuse

- Unexplained signs of injury, such as bruises, welts, or scars, especially if they appear symmetrically on two side of the body
- Broken bones, sprains, or dislocations
- Report of drug overdose or apparent failure to take medication regularly
- Broken eyeglasses or frames
- Signs of being restrained, such as rope marks on wrists
- Caregiver's refusal to allow someone meeting the elder alone

Emotional Abuse

- Threatening, belittling, or controlling caregiver behavior that you witness
- Behavior from the elder that mimics dementia, such as rocking, sucking, or mumbling to oneself.

Sexual Abuse

- Bruises around breasts or genitals
- Unexplained venereal disease or genital infections
- Unexplained vaginal or anal bleeding
- Torn, stained, or bloody underclothing
- Neglect by caregivers or self-neglect
- Unusual weight loss, malnutrition, dehydration
- Untreated physical problems, such as bed sores
- Unsanitary living conditions, such as dirt, bugs, soiled bedding and clothes
- Being left dirty or unbathed
- Unsuitable clothing or covering for the weather
- Unsafe living conditions (no heated or running water, faulty electrical wiring, other fire hazards)
- Desertion of the elder at a public place

Financial Exploitation

- Significant withdrawals from the elder's accounts
- Sudden changes in the elder's financial condition
- Items or cash missing from the senior's household
- Suspicious changes in wills, power of attorney, titles, and policies
- Addition of names to the senior's signature card
- Unpaid bills or lack of medical care, though the elder has enough money to pay for them
- Financial activity the senior could not have done, such as an ATM withdrawal when the account holder is bedridden.
- Unnecessary services, goods, or subscriptions

Health-care fraud and abuse

- Duplicate billings for the same medical service or device
- Evidence of overmedication or undermedication
- Evidence of inadequate care when bills are paid in full
- Problems with the care facility, namely, poorly trained, poorly paid, or insufficient staff, crowding, inadequate responses to questions about care
- The caregiver's perception that taking care of the elder is burdensome and without psychological reward
- Substance abuse

Preventing Elder Abuse and Neglect

Elder abuse can be prevented by practicing the following:
- Listening to seniors and their caregivers
- Intervening when you suspect elder abuse
- Educating others about how to recognize and report elder abuse.

Role of Caregivers in Preventing Elder Abuse

- Request help, from friends, relatives, or local agencies, so you can take a break, if only for a couple of hours
- Find an program and stay healthy and get medical care for yourself when necessary
- Adopt stress reduction practices
- Seek counseling for depression, which can lead to elder abuse
- Find a support group for caregivers of the elderly
- If you are having problems with drug or alcohol abuse, get help

Role of a Concerned Friend or Family Member

- Watch for warning signs that might indicate elder abuse
- Take a look at the elder's medications
- Watch for possible financial abuse and ask the elder if you may scan bank accounts and credit card statements for unauthorized transactions
- Call and visit the elders as often as you can and help the elder consider you a trusted person
- Offer to stay with the elders, so the caregiver can have a break—on a regular basis, if possible

Protecting Yourself, as an Elder, Against Elder Abuse

- Make sure your financial and legal affairs are in order. If they are not, enlist professional help to get them in order, with the assistance of a trusted friend or relative, if necessary.
- Keep in touch with family and friends and avoid becoming isolated
- If you are unhappy with the care you are receiving, whether it is in your own home or in a care facility, speak up to someone you trust and ask that person to report the abuse, neglect, or substandard care to an elder abuse helpline or long-term care ombudsman, or make the call yourself.

MYTHS AND REALITIES OF AGING

Myths, more than many forms of word play, create images that inaccurately characterize everyday experiences of the majority of older people. Myths of aging are found in our jokes and conversations, are expressed in the popular literature, and subtly shape social, health, and work experiences in the presence of extraordinary knowledge to the contrary.

Negative stereotypes about older adults abound—they are sickly, frail, forgetful, unattractive, dependent, or otherwise incompetent. Such stereotypes can lead to agism, or prejudice against elderly people. Most elderly adults have internalized these negative views but believe they apply to other older adults and not to themselves.

1. Myth: Older People are all the Same

There is a perception that older people are all the same and that they are boring.
The reality: Far from being boring, many older people find the years between the mid-50s to mid-70s are a time of liberation where a sense of personal freedom allows them to speak their minds and make plans for new and different experiences. To highlight aging as a problem,

there is a tendency to immediately define older people as a separate, single category; when in reality, as they age, they become more diverse. The aging experience of all people is affected by their gender, culture, education, and geographical location, tending to make individual biological variations greater between people the older they become. Older people represent a broad spectrum of economic, political, and social backgrounds, with a composite of lifestyle, beliefs, educational achievement, and personal resources. Adjustment to older age also differs greatly between individuals, consistent with a person's self-image, goals, attitudes, and strategies developed throughout life. Men and women experience aging differently as a result of the different roles they have undertaken throughout their lives. Women tend to live longer than men and are most likely to be the majority of oldest people in most parts of the world. However, longevity results in different outcomes for men and women. Chronic diseases, such as osteoporosis, arthritis, incontinence, diabetes, and hypertension are more likely to afflict women, while men are more likely to suffer from heart disease and stroke. As women age and live longer, they, too, suffer from these major causes of death and disability. Notably, as people grow old, they tend to have less anxiety about aging. This is thought to be because they have gained experience about how to overcome negative stereotypes and learned how to handle social, psychological, and situational changes. In fact, the group most worried about aging is the "young old" group who are approaching retirement. Older people cope very well with the day-to-day problems of life, while those aged 64–74 years have the least worry of all age-groups. Many older people regard aging as being a state of mind that can be seen in people of any age.

2. Myth: All Old People are Unwell

There is a perception that older people must be in poor health, ill, or disabled.

The reality: Recent improvements in health care and prevention now mean that older people will remain in relatively good health and that the years spent being disabled are likely to be compressed into the final years of life.

Aging is a continuous process, rather than a distinct phase with a particular starting time. It includes our genetics, natural developmental stages, and environmental factors. Aging is not an affliction but a natural part of the life cycle. Older people reject the myth that they are in poor health, sick and say that this idea is slowly changing in the media. Growing old does not mean becoming sick. Most are active and living in the community, not in nursing homes. In 2003, only 5% of the population aged 60 and older was in cared accommodation (nursing home or hospital), with the median age being 85 years, those in the oldest age-group.

3. Myth: Disabilities come with age

There is a perception that growing old inevitably means becoming frail and disabled.

The reality: Far from being frail, the majority of older people remain physically fit well into later life, carrying out the tasks of daily living and playing an active part in community life. Advances in medical knowledge and disease prevention mean that people are living longer, and therefore we are seeing an increase in chronic diseases that cannot be cured, but which may be managed over time (e.g., arthritis, heart disease, diabetes). However, it is mostly the very old who reach the point that they need care and assistance with the ADLs. It is important to remember that although the rate of disability is higher for those aged over 60, age in itself does not signify dependence. Older people remain alert and aware, involved, and interested. Some may appear frail, but most are active. Around 40% of the adult population in Australia had either a disability or long-term health condition: 46% of people aged 45–64 years, increasing to around 56% of those 65 years and over. In 2003, less than half who reported having a disability said that they needed help to manage their health conditions or to cope with everyday activities. As people grow older, their need for assistance does increase.

4. Myth: Memory loss and senility come with age

Older people are often stereotyped as having memory loss, lacking in mental sharpness, and being senile.

The reality: Losses are not synonymous with growing old, the later decades of life are not necessarily impoverished, and there are viable alternatives to the inevitability of decline.

Studies have shown that intellect and creativity can be maintained into old age, although being old differs for individuals. Old age can involve losses and gains of varying degrees. Biological changes, individual differences, and lifestyle factors can affect memory, and not surprisingly, the oldest-old, those approaching 90 years, seem to be the most affected by health and memory decline. Unfortunately, the tendency is to include all older people under the umbrella term of decline when there may be other explanations for certain behaviors. Beliefs about the inevitable decline in memory with aging are very strongly entrenched, and some studies are investigating how such stereotypes influence older people into accepting these age-biased beliefs. Dementia is not a normal or inevitable part of aging. It is true that there is a greater risk of Alzheimer's disease or other forms of dementia as age increases, but it affects only about 5% of older people. Most people keep their knowledge and skills. However, as there will be older people in the future, there may be more people with dementia in the oldest age-group, though pharmaceutical developments and improved lifestyle factors may lessen the predicted numbers. Many people assume that memory loss indicates cognitive decline. However, memory loss may occur at any age through factors, such as disease or substance abuse. Studies have found great variability in the effects of normal aging on memory, such as the differences between short- and long-term memory, with long-term memory being most resilient. Aging can slow reaction time and the retrieval of information from memory, requiring a few more seconds. However, in some ways there are indications that older people, with their broader knowledge and perspective, make better learners. While depression and stressful life events can have a negative impact on older people's mental health, remaining in the work force can be a positive influence. Various preventative measures can prolong competencies as people grow older and give them good quality of life. These include minimizing the demands of the home and social environment, following appropriate health behaviors, and even undertaking cognitive training to improve skills. Older adults undertaking challenging mental exercises have shown lower rates of memory loss, proving that the "use it or lose it" hypothesis has merit and that training and practice can offset some mental losses.

5. Myth: The increase in the number of older people is the main reason for the rising health-care costs

A perception is that because of the aging population, a catastrophic impact can be seen on the healthcare system.

The reality: The aging population should be seen as one of the greatest success stories of the 20th century.

As the number of older people increases as a proportion of the population, there are myths emerging about the high costs of medical care for the last years of life, about technology used to needlessly prolong life, and a view that there will be an economic burden on the health budget. Living longer healthier lives should not be seen as a problem, particularly while there is considerable potential for higher incomes as a result of continuing growth in productivity.

Aging is not the principal determinant of rising healthcare costs, and limiting acute care for those at the end of their life would save only a small fraction of healthcare costs. Studies show that the older the age people reach, the less likely they are to receive aggressive and costly treatment. But those who need these treatments survive and do well for extended periods.

6. Myth: Older people are an economic burden on society

There is a myth that older people are a burden on society and that an increase in numbers of older people will be detrimental to the economy.

The reality: Older people are actively involved in Indian society in a number of ways, making important contributions to the family, community, and economy.

Most people aged 45 years and older who have already retired have a government pension or allowance as their main source of income. By contrast, only 25% of those intending to retire in the future expect the government pension or allowance to be their main source of income at retirement; many expect to have superannuation or annuity. Changes to taxation and superannuation are also in place to encourage older people to remain in the workforce longer.

7. Myth: Older people do not contribute

Retirement often signals the onset of poor attitudes toward older people when it is assumed that they are no longer productive.

The reality: Older people make considerable contributions to families and communities as carers and volunteers and continue to be interested in learning new things. Retirees are a diverse group just like the rest of the Indian population. The retirement phase of life can last for 20 or 30 years, perhaps even a third of a person's life. Yet younger retired people can be wrongly thought to have the same limitations that are expected after 85 years of age, such as financial or physical dependency. Volunteering is an important face of social and community life in India that allows people to help others and the community and provides personal satisfaction. It appears that formal volunteering has a direct impact on well-being, functional health, and longevity, apart from other factors, such as health levels and socioeconomic status.

8. Myth: Older people are lonely and will gradually withdraw from society

There is a perception that older people lack vitality and vigor, are sad, depressed, are withdrawn from society, and are lonely.

The reality: It was once thought that older people naturally declined in health and wanted to disengage from social roles and interests. Nothing could be further from the truth. There is a difference between living alone and being lonely. Depression and loneliness can affect people of all ages for various reasons. The milestone of retirement for older people may be felt as an initial depression because of factors, such as role loss, financial concerns, and poor health. Older people reject this myth as generalizing and believe it depends on the individual. Some may be grouchy or lonely, but many older people resent the assumption that they are always at home with nothing to do. Many are busy with family and no other group of people in society has such organized outings and community activities.

9. Myth: Mature age workers are slower and less productive than younger workers

The retirement age once was set at 65 for men and 60 for women in order to make way for the younger generation of workers who were perceived to be more productive than older workers.

The reality: Government policy encourages older workers to stay in employment, reinforcing the usefulness of older people. Unfortunately, mature aged workers are the ones most likely to be retrenched or encouraged to take redundancies due to organizational restructuring and they are likely to face age discrimination when seeking work.

10. Myth: Older people are unable to learn or change

There is a common belief that "You cannot teach an old dog new tricks."

The reality: There are many examples of older people learning new things in later life.

Contrary to what Sigmund Freud believed, early experiences rarely make or break us. Instead, there are opportunities throughout the lifespan—within limits—to undo the damage done by early traumas, to teach new skills, and to redirect lives along more fruitful paths.

Many older people continue to learn new things, often because they did not have the opportunity to receive a formal education when younger. They attend informal classes provided by the university and there are increasing numbers of older people pursuing university studies. Learning is undertaken by older people for reasons other than paid employment, for instance, to gain knowledge and skills, and for interest.

11. Myth: Older people do not want or need close physical relationships

There is a belief that older people have no capacity for or interest in sexual activity.

The reality: Many older people want and are able to lead an active, satisfying sex life. Historically, sexual decline was assumed to be an inevitable and universal consequence of growing older; thus, aging individuals were expected to adjust to it gracefully and to appreciate the special moral benefits of postsexual maturity.

The idea that older people have no interest in sexuality is based on beliefs about their inability to perform, their lack of interest in sex, or thinking that those who are interested are perverted.

Older people reject it, saying that media images are changing. Acknowledging that health problems and lack of a partner hinder some people, they point out that sex is more than a physical act and can be expressed in other loving ways. It can also be more fun without hang ups and there are medications that can help.

12. Myth: Older people are more likely to be victims of crime than other age-groups

There is a belief that older people are more likely to be the victims of criminal assault and robbery.

The reality: People aged 65 and over have lower rates of victimization for all types of offenses than those between 20 and 64 years. They are also less likely to be victims of crime than other adults. Compared to the whole population, people over 65 have the lowest rate of personal offense victimization. Older people or married people with family responsibilities were less likely to be at risk of personal victimization because the time they spend in public places differs from that of the young, single people, students, or the unemployed. However, older people who are victims of assault (usually associated with a robbery) are more likely than younger victims to sustain fatal injuries because of physical vulnerability.

ALZHEIMER'S DISEASE

It was first described by German psychiatrist and pathologist Alois Alzheimer's in 1906. Alzheimer's disease is the most common type of dementia; the term dementia describes a loss of mental activity associated with the gradual death of the brain cells. Alzheimer's disease is a degenerative disease that slowly and progressively destroys brain cells.

It is a progressive, irreversible, degenerative neurologic disease that begins insidiously and is characterized by gradual losses of cognitive function and disturbances in behavior and affect.

Etiology and Risk Factors

- Down syndrome
- Head injury
- DM
- Hypertension
- Hypercholesterolemia
- Hyperglycemia
- Family history
- Genetic factor

- Sedentary lifestyle
- Diets high in saturated fat

Genetic factors: Genetics plays a role in early onset Alzheimer's, a rare form of the disease. At this time, only one gene, apolipoprotein E (*ApoE*) has been definitively linked to late onset Alzheimer's disease. However, only a small percentage of people carry the form of *ApoE* that increases the risk of late onset Alzheimer's.

Environmental factors: It may play a role in Alzheimer's disease or that triggers the disease process in people who have a genetic susceptibility.

Age: Although Alzheimer's is not a normal part of growing older, the greatest risk factor for the disease is increasing age. After age 65, the risk of Alzheimer's doubles every 5 years. After age 85, the risk reaches nearly 50%.

Family history: Another risk factor for Alzheimer's is the family history. The risk increases if more than one family member has this illness. When diseases tend to run in families, either heredity or environmental factors or both may play a role.

Down syndrome: People with Down syndrome are at higher risk of developing Alzheimer's disease. This is because the genetic fault that causes Down syndrome can also cause amyloid plaques to build up in the brain, leading to Alzheimer's disease.

Head injury: People who had a severe head injury or a neck injury caused by a sudden movement of the head have been found at higher risk. Head injury results into the disruption of normal brain function and affects person cognitive abilities, thinking, and learning skills.

Diabetes mellitus: Diabetes can damage our blood vessels, and Alzheimer disease is caused by reduced or blocked blood flow to the brain. Type 2 DM affects the ability of the brain and other body tissues to use sugar and respond to insulin. So it results in the impairment of the brain functions.

Hypertension: High BP can damage the small blood vessels in the brain affecting the parts of the brain responsible for thinking and memory.

High saturated fat diet: People who have high saturated fat or sugar diet results in the change in their *ApoE* such that *ApoE* is less able to clear amyloid. So they are left in brain and are more likely to form plaques that interferes with the neuron function, and high level of amyloid plaques leads to reduced levels of neurotransmitter acetylcholine, which is a neurotransmitter messenger in brain. So amyloid plaque leads to this condition.

Sedentary lifestyles: It leads to obesity, and lack of physical activities is important risk factors for diabetes and high BP.

Ten Warning Signs of Alzheimer's Disease

1. Memory loss
2. Difficulty performing familiar tasks
3. Problems with language
4. Disorientation to time and place
5. Poor or decreased judgment
6. Problems with abstract thinking
7. Misplacing things
8. Changes in mood or behavior
9. Changes in personality
10. Loss of initiative

Stages of Alzheimer's Disease

The various stages in Alzheimer's disease are as follows:

- The first symptoms are often mistakenly attributed to aging or stress.
- Detailed neuropsychological testing can reveal mild cognitive difficulties.
- These early symptoms can affect the most complex daily living activities.
- The most noticeable deficit is memory loss, which shows up as difficulty in remembering recently learned facts and inability to acquire new information.
- Many problems with the executive functions of attentiveness, planning, flexibility, and abstract thinking, or impairments in semantic memory (memory of meanings, and concept relationships) can also be symptomatic of the early stages of AD.
- Apathy remains the most persistent neuropsychiatric symptom throughout the course of the disease. The preclinical stage of the disease has also been termed mild cognitive impairment.

Early Stage of Alzheimer's Disease

The signs and symptoms of the early stage of Alzheimer's disease are as follows:

- Alzheimer's disease is the increasing impairment of learning and memory.
- Difficulties with language, executive functions, perception (agnosia), or execution of movements (apraxia) are more prominent than memory problems.
- Alzheimer's disease does not affect all memory capacities equally. Older memories of the person's life (episodic memory), facts learned (semantic memory), and implicit memory (the memory of the body on how to do things, such as using a fork to eat) are affected to a lesser degree than new facts or memories.
- Language problems are mainly characterized by a shrinking vocabulary and decreased word fluency, which lead to a general impoverishment of oral and written language.
- While performing fine motor tasks, such as writing, drawing, or dressing, certain movement coordination and planning difficulties (apraxia) may be present but they are commonly unnoticed.
- As the disease progresses, person may need assistance or supervision with the most cognitively demanding activities.

Moderate Stage

The signs and symptoms of the moderate stage of Alzheimer's disease are as follows:

- Progressive deterioration eventually hinders independence with subjects being unable to perform most common ADLs.
- Speech difficulties become evident due to an inability to recall vocabulary, which leads to frequent incorrect word substitutions (paraphasias).
- Reading and writing skills are also progressively lost, as time passes and Alzheimer's disease progresses.
- Complex motor sequences become less coordinated, so the risk of falling increases.
- During this phase, memory problems worsen, and the person may fail to recognize close relatives.
- Long-term memory, which was previously intact, becomes impaired.
- Behavioral and neuropsychiatric changes are there. Common manifestations are wandering, irritability, and labile affect, leading to crying, outbursts of unpremeditated aggression, or resistance to caregiving.
- Approximately 30% of people with AD develop illusionary misidentifications and other delusional symptoms.
- Urinary incontinence can develop.

Advanced Stage

The signs and symptoms of the advanced stage of Alzheimer's disease are as follows:
● The person is completely dependent upon caregivers.
● Language is reduced to simple phrases or even single words, eventually leading to complete loss of speech.
● Aggressiveness
● Extreme apathy and exhaustion are common
● Muscle mass and mobility deteriorate to the point where they are bedridden, and they lose the ability to feed themselves.
● The cause of death typically being an external factor, such as infection of pressure ulcers or pneumonia, not the disease itself.

Clinical Manifestation

● Patient has noticeable memory loss
● Frequently uses words inappropriately
● Begins to lose the ability to perform normal tasks of daily living, involving muscle coordination, such as cooking, dressing, bathing, shopping, or signing a checkbook (apraxia)
● May wander off, become agitated, start confusing day from night, and fail to recognize friends and relatives
● Loses the ability to recognize and use familiar objects, such as clothing (agnosia)
● Becomes uncomprehending and mute
● Loses all self-care ability
● Unable to feed, dress, and bath by himself or herself

Diagnostic Evaluation

● **Get the complete history:** Ask the client for present and past illnesses and about the use of medications.
● Ask the client family history related to the Alzheimer's disease
● A complete physical and neurological examination is the first step
● Ask the client about the diet, nutrition, and use of alcohol
● Check the vital signs of client
● Check the symptoms of dementia
● Assess their memory problems
● In neurological examinations, check the client reflexes, their coordination, muscle tone, and strength.
● Check client eye movement
● Assess the client speech
● Evaluate cognitive functioning using Mini-Mental State Examination (MMSE), wherein a health professional asks a patient a series of questions designed to test a range of everyday mental skills. Its total score is 30 points. If the patient scores 20–24, it indicates mild dementia and less than 12 indicates severe dementia.
● Psychiatric assessment involves interviewing someone close to the patient to learn about the patient's daily activity and to understand their emotional state. Memory tests are undertaken for recall of events.
● **Mood assessment:** In addition to assessing the mental status, the doctor will evaluate a person's sense of well-being to detect depression or other mood disorders that can cause memory problems, loss of interest in life, and other symptoms that can overlap with dementia.

- The brain imaging is done using CT scan or MRI or the newer positron emission tomography (PET) scan to understand any apparent changes in the overall size of the brain and the memory-associated areas of the brain and also helps to see any damage from severe head trauma and also a buildup of fluid in the brain.
- Electroencephalograph (EEG) of the brain where the signals are picked up by recorder and analyzed.

Management

There is no cure for the Alzheimer's disease, but the main goals for the management are to maintain the quality of life.
- Maximize the daily activity functions
- Foster a safe environment
- Enhance cognition, mood, and behavior

Pharmacological Management

- In medication, cholinesterase inhibitors are used; 5 mg of donepezil, a acetylcholinesterase inhibitor, is given at bed time, starting dose of 1.5 mg rivastigmine twice daily with food at 2 weeks intervals and increase each dose by 1.5 mg up to a dosage of 6 mg twice daily.
- Galantamine, starting dose of 4 mg twice daily with food at 4 weeks' interval and increase each dose by 4 mg up to a dosage of 12 mg twice daily.
- Antipsychotic drugs, loxapine and haloperidol
- Antidepressants
- Selective serotonin reuptake inhibitors, fluvoxamine, fluoxetine, and citalopram.

Nutritional Management

- A well-balanced diet rich in protein, high in fiber, with adequate amount of calories depending on height and body weight
- The total quantity of food can be calculated by a dietitian
- The diet should take into account other medical illnesses that require diet modification, such as diabetes or high BP
- The safest diet is a semisolid one in the consistency of a puree
- Liquids are the most dangerous type of food, as these can easily get aspirated into the lungs
- Food rich in vitamin C, vitamin E, and vegetables help in reducing the incidence of dementia.

Health Education

It is necessary that family members of patients should be educated about the Alzheimer's disease.
- Advise the family members and caregivers that the client requires as much fluid as normal, sufficient fluid should be given during the day, and only the minimum essential amount of fluid should be given at night.
- Advise to do not give beverages, including tea, coffee, cocoa, or any other caffeine-containing drinks, as all these promote urination.
- Proper fluid management will reduce bed-wetting and also reduce the number of times the patient will need to get up during the night.
- Patients of Alzheimer's disease often lose their geographic orientation and can get lost even in familiar surroundings.
- They may be found wandering aimlessly either in the neighborhood or far away.
- It is advisable to have some identification bracelet or card always in their possession.

- The doors of the house should be securely locked, so that the patient cannot leave unnoticed.
- Great care should be taken to avoid accidents caused by tripping over furniture, falling down the stairs, or slipping in the bathroom.
- The reasons for falling include loose and poorly fitting footwear and wrinkled carpets.
- Advise the patient to wear soft slip-on shoes with straps that fit securely.
- Any floor covering must be firmly secured.
- Once early signs of the disease appear, patients should be gently advised to stop driving as this can cause harm to them and others.
- Particular care should be taken about the patient's personal hygiene, including brushing of teeth, bathing, keeping the skin clean and dry, particularly in areas prone to perspiration, such as the armpits and groin.
- Advise the family members and client to maintain a proper personal hygiene.
- Toilet habits should be established as soon as possible and maintained as a rigid routine.
- The patient should be taken to urinate at fixed intervals, depending on the season and amount of fluid intake.

Nursing Care plan

Nursing management plays a very crucial role in the managing Alzheimer's patients. Listed below are some of the management aspects:

Nursing Assessment

- It includes nurse have to provide emotional support to the patient and family.
- It establishes an effective communication system with the patient and the patient's family to help them adjust to the patient's altered cognitive abilities.
- It administers ordered medications and notes their effects.
- It protects client from injury by providing a safe, structured environment.
- It assists the patient with hygiene and dressing as necessary.

Nursing Diagnosis

- Impaired thought processes related to decline in cognitive function
- Risk for injury related to decline in cognitive function
- Anxiety related to confused thought processes
- Imbalanced nutritional pattern, which is less than body requirements related to cognitive decline
- Activity intolerance related to imbalance in activity or rest pattern.

1. Impaired thought processes related to decline in cognitive function
Interventions
- Assess the condition of patient
- Provide a calm, comfortable environment to the patient to minimize the confusion and disorientation
- Advise the family members to be with the client
- Help the patient to feel a sense of security in a quiet, pleasant manner
- Provide simple explanations to the client
- Make use of memory aides and cues

2. Risk for injury related to decline in cognitive function

Interventions
- Provide a safe environment to client and allow moving as freely as possible
- Prevent falls and other accidents by providing adequate lighting, remove hazards, and install handrails in the home
- Prohibit driving
- Supervise all the activities outside the home to protect the client
- Ensure that patient wears an identification bracelet and neck chain
- Avoid restraints to the client

3. Anxiety related to confused thought processes

Interventions
- Assess the level of anxiety
- Provide emotional support to the client to foster a positive self-image
- Keep the environment simple, familiar, and noise free and limit the changes
- Remain calm and unhurried, even if the client is experiencing agitated state, overreaction to excessive stimulation
- Always be with the client

Prevention

The following are the ways to prevent serious issues in old age:
- Stay active mentally and physically
- Keeping oneself physically fit helps the circulation of the body and helps the brain from delaying the progression or onset of the disease even if a person is genetically prone to get the disease.
- Mental activity is equally important and occupying oneself by doing crossword, sudoku, playing chess, a game of bridge, or a board game, or playing a musical instrument can help in delaying the onset of the disease or keeping the symptoms of the disease mild.

Occupational Health Disorders

AT THE END OF THIS CHAPTER, THE STUDENT WILL BE ABLE TO LEARN ABOUT THE VARIOUS OCCUPATIONAL HEALTH HAZARDS AND THEIR NURSING MANAGEMENT:

➤ Pneumoconioses (*refer* respiratory system)
➤ Silicosis (*refer* respiratory system)
➤ Coal workers' pneumoconiosis (*refer* respiratory system)
➤ Pneumoconiosis associated with tuberculosis
➤ Welders' pneumoconiosis
➤ Asbestosis and other pneumoconioses due to silicates (*refer* respiratory system)
➤ Pneumoconiosis due to talc
➤ Graphite fibrosis
➤ Pneumoconioses due to metal dusts
➤ Allergic contact dermatitis (*refer* skin disorders)
➤ Irritant contact dermatitis (*refer* skin disorders)
➤ Oil acne, chloracne, coal tar acne of diffuse nature

INTRODUCTION

Occupational disease is any illness associated with a particular occupation or industry. Such diseases result from a variety of biological, chemical, physical, and psychological factors that are present in the work environment or are otherwise encountered in the course of employment. Occupational nursing is concerned with the effect of all kinds of work on health and the effect of health on a worker's ability and efficiency and its treatment.

EFFECTS OF OCCUPATIONAL HEALTH DISORDERS

Occupational diseases are essentially preventable and can be ascribed to faulty working conditions. The control of occupational health hazards decreases the incidence of work-related diseases and accidents and improves the health and morale of the workforce, leading to decreased absenteeism and increased worker efficiency. In most cases, the moral and economic benefits far outweigh the costs of eliminating occupational hazards.

Types of Occupational and Industrial Disorders

1. Disorders due to Chemical Agents

Hazardous chemicals can act directly on the skin, resulting in local irritation or an allergic reaction, or they may be absorbed through the skin, ingested, or inhaled. In the workplace, ingestion of toxic chemicals is usually accidental and most commonly results from handling contaminated food, drink, or cigarettes. Substances that occur as gases, vapors, aerosols, and dusts are the most difficult to control, and most hazardous chemicals are therefore absorbed through the respiratory tract. If inhaled, airborne contaminants act as irritants to the respiratory tract or as systemic poisons. Toxicity in such cases depends on the contaminant's concentration, particle size, and physicochemical properties, particularly its solubility in body fluids. An individual's reaction to any hazard depends primarily on the length, pattern, and concentration of exposure but is also affected by such factors as age, sex, ethnic group, genetic background, nutritional status, and coexistent disease, concomitant exposure to other toxic agents, lifestyle, and history of previous exposure to the agent in question. The wide range of both naturally occurring and synthetic chemical compounds that can give rise to adverse health effects can be roughly organized into four major categories: gases, metals, organic compounds, and dusts.

a. Gases

Gases may act as local irritants to inflame mucous surfaces. Common examples include sulfur dioxide, chlorine, and fluorine, which have pungent odors and can severely irritate the eyes and the respiratory tract. Some gases, such as nitrogen oxide and phosgene, are much more insidious. Victims may be unaware of the dangers of exposure because the immediate effects of these gases may be mild and overlooked. Several hours after exposure, however, breathlessness and fatal cardiorespiratory failure may develop due to pulmonary edema.

Gases that interfere with oxygen supply to the tissues are known as asphyxiates. Simple asphyxiants are physiologically inert gases that act by diluting atmospheric oxygen. If the concentration of such gases is high enough, hypoxia may develop. Victims of mild hypoxia may appear to be intoxicated and may even resist rescue attempts. Common examples of simple asphyxiants are methane and carbon dioxide.

In contrast to simple asphyxiants, chemical asphyxiants, such as carbon monoxide and hydrogen sulfide, are highly reactive. They cause a chemical action that either prevents the blood from transporting oxygen to the tissues or interferes with oxygenation in the tissues. For example, carbon monoxide, a frequently encountered gas produced by incomplete combustion, combines with hemoglobin in the blood and reduces its oxygen-carrying capacity. In low concentration, carbon monoxide poisoning can cause symptoms of fatigue, headache, nausea, and vomiting, but heavy exposure leads to coma and death. It is especially dangerous because it is both colorless and odorless. Hydrogen sulfide acts by inhibiting the respiratory enzyme cytochrome oxidase, thus giving rise to severe tissue hypoxia. In addition to its asphyxiant properties, hydrogen sulfide also acts as an irritant to the eyes and mucous membranes.

Prevention

Preventing gas poisoning involves preventing exposure. Workers should never enter enclosed spaces that have suspect atmospheres alone, workplaces should provide adequate ventilation, and air should be regularly tested for contamination. If exposure does occur, treatment involves the removal of the victim from the contaminated atmosphere, artificial respiration, and administration of oxygen or recommended antidotes. Victims exposed to gases with insidious delayed effects should be kept under medical observation for an appropriate period.

b. Metals

Metals and their compounds are among the poisons most commonly encountered in the home and workplace. Even metals essential for life can be toxic if they are present in excessive amounts. Iron, for example, is an essential element and is sometimes given therapeutically; however, if taken in overdose, it can be lethal.

Mercury poisoning, one of the classic occupational diseases, is a representative example of metal poisoning. Exposure to mercury can occur in many situations, including the manufacture of thermometers, explosives, fungicides, drugs, paints, batteries, and various electrical products. The disorders it can cause vary depending on the type of mercury compound and the method of exposure.

Ingestion of mercury salts, such as mercuric chloride leads to nausea, vomiting, and bloody diarrhea. In extreme cases, it can cause kidney damage resulting in death. Inhalation or absorption of mercury vapor through the skin causes salivation, loosening of the teeth, and tremor. It also affects the higher centers of the brain, resulting in irritability, loss of memory, depression, anxiety, and other personality changes. Poisoning with organic mercury compounds (used in fungicides and pesticides) results in permanent neurological damage and can be fatal.

Other hazardous metals commonly encountered in industry include arsenic, beryllium, cadmium, chromium, lead, manganese, nickel, and thallium. Some have been shown to be carcinogenic, including certain compounds of nickel (linked to lung and nasal cancer), chromium (lung cancer), and arsenic (lung and skin cancer).

c. Organic compounds

The organic compounds that pose the greatest occupational hazards are various aromatic, aliphatic, and halogenated hydrocarbons and the organophosphates, carbamates, organochlorine compounds, and bipyridylium compounds used as pesticides.

Pesticides are used world over, and in spite of the precautionary measures (such as using protective clothing and respirators, monitoring contamination of equipment and clothing, keeping workers out of recently sprayed areas, and requiring workers to wash thoroughly after exposure), poisoning not infrequently occurs in agricultural communities. The organophosphates and the generally less toxic carbamates exert their effects by inhibiting cholinesterase, an enzyme that prevents stimulation from becoming too intense or prolonged by destroying the acetylcholine involved in the transmission of impulses in the autonomic nervous system. Cholinesterase inhibitors allow the accumulation of acetylcholine, causing symptoms related to parasympathetic over activity, such as chest tightness, wheezing, blurring of vision, vomiting, diarrhea, abdominal pain, and in severe cases respiratory paralysis. Atropine and certain oxides counteract their effects.

d. Dusts

Inhalation of a variety of dusts is responsible for a number of lung and respiratory disorders, whose symptoms and severity depend on the composition and size of the dust particle, the amount of dust inhaled, and the duration of exposure. The lung diseases known as the pneumoconioses result when certain inhaled mineral dusts are deposited in the lungs, where they cause a chronic fibrotic reaction that leads to decreasing capacity for exercise and increasing breathlessness, cough, and respiratory difficulty. No specific treatment is known, but as with all respiratory disorders, patients are urged to quit smoking, which aggravates the condition. Suggested measures for limiting exposure include using water and exhaust ventilation to lower dust levels and requiring workers to wear respirators or protective clothing, but such procedures are not always feasible. Coal worker's pneumoconiosis, silicosis, and asbestosis are the most common pneumoconioses.

2. Disorders Due to Physical Agents

a. Temperature

When working in a hot environment, humans' maintain normal body temperature by perspiring and increasing the blood flow to the surface of the body. The large amounts of water and salt lost in perspiration then need to be replaced. In the past, miners who perspired profusely and drank water to relieve their thirst experienced intense muscular pain, a condition known as miner's cramps, as a result of restoring their water but not their salt balance. When salt in the requisite amount was added to their drinks, workers no longer developed miner's cramps. Heat exhaustion is characterized by thirst, fatigue, giddiness, and often muscle cramps, and fainting can also occur. Heatstroke, a more serious and sometimes lethal condition, results when prolonged exposure to heat and high humidity prevents efficient perspiration, causing the body temperature to rise above 106°F (41°C) and the skin becomes hot and dry. If victims are not quickly cooled down, coma, convulsions, and death can follow. To prevent heat exhaustion or heatstroke, workers unaccustomed to high temperatures should allow adequate time (ranging from days to weeks) for their bodies to become acclimatized before performing strenuous physical tasks.

Work in cold environments may also have serious adverse effects. Tissue damage that does not involve freezing can cause inflammatory swelling known as chilblains. Frostbite, or the freezing of tissue, can lead to gangrene and the loss of fingers or toes. If exposure is prolonged and conditions (such as wet or tight clothing) encourage heat loss, hypothermia, a critical fall in body temperature, may result. When body temperature falls below 95°F (35°C), physiological processes are slowed; consciousness is impaired; and coma, cardiorespiratory failure, and death may ensue. Workers exposed to extreme cold require carefully designed protective clothing to minimize heat loss, even though a degree of acclimatization occurs with time.

b. Atmospheric pressure
Decompression sickness can result from exposure to high or low atmospheric pressure. Under increased atmospheric pressure (such as that experienced by deep-sea divers or tunnel workers), fat-soluble nitrogen gas dissolves in the body fluids and tissues. During decompression, the gas comes out of solution and, if decompression is rapid, forms bubble in the tissues. These bubbles cause pain in the limbs (known as the bends), breathlessness, angina, headache, dizziness, collapse, coma, and in some cases death. Similarly, the gases in solution in the body tissues under normal atmospheric pressure form bubbles when the pressure rapidly decreases, similar to a situation when aviators in unpressurized aircraft too quickly ascend to high altitudes. Emergency treatment of decompression sickness consists of rapid recompression in a compression chamber with gradual subsequent decompression. The condition can be prevented by allowing sufficient decompression time for the excess nitrogen gas to be expelled naturally.

c. Noise
Exposure to excessive noise can be unpleasant and can impair working efficiency. Temporary or permanent hearing loss may also occur, depending on the loudness or intensity of the noise, its pitch or frequency, the length and pattern of exposure, and the vulnerability of the individual. Prolonged exposure to sound energy of intensity above 80–90 decibels is likely to result in noise-induced hearing loss, developing first for high frequencies and then progressing downward. The condition can be prevented by enclosing noisy machinery and providing effective ear protection. Routine audiometry gives an indication of the effectiveness of preventive measures.

d. Vibration
Whole-body vibration is experienced in surface and air transport, with motion sickness being its most familiar effect. A more serious disorder, known as Raynaud syndrome or vibration white finger (VWF), can result from the extensive use of vibratory hand tools, especially in cold weather. The condition is seen most frequently among workers who handle chain saws, grinders, pneumatic drills, hammers, and chisels. Forestry workers are particularly at risk in cold climates. Initial signs of VWF are tingling and numbness of the fingers, followed by intermittent blanching and redness and pain occur in the recovery stage. In a minority of cases, the tissues, bones, and joints are affected by the vibration, which may cause abnormalities and may even develop gangrene. The VWF can be prevented by using properly designed tools, avoiding prolonged use of vibrating tools, and keeping the hands warm in cold weather.

e. Other mechanical stresses

Muscle cramps often afflict workers engaged in heavy manual labor as well as typists, pianists, and others who frequently use rapid, repetitive movements of the hand or forearm. Tenosynovitis, a condition in which the sheath enclosing a tendon to the wrist or to one of the fingers becomes inflamed, causing pain and temporary disability, which can also be due to prolonged repetitive movement. When the movement involves the rotation of the forearm, the extensor tendon attached to the point of the elbow becomes inflamed, a condition commonly known as tennis elbow.

f. Ionizing radiation

Ionizing radiation damages or destroys body tissues by breaking down the molecules in the tissues into positively or negatively charged particles called ions. Radiation that is capable of causing ionization may be electromagnetic (X-rays and gamma rays) or particulate (radiation of electrons, protons, neutrons, a particles, and other subatomic particles) and has many uses in industry, medicine, and scientific research.

Ionizing radiation injury is in general dose dependent. Whole-body exposure to doses in excess of 1,000 rads results in acute radiation syndrome and is usually fatal. Doses in excess of 3,000 rads produce cerebral edema (brain swelling) within a matter of minutes and death within days. Lesser doses cause acute gastrointestinal symptoms, such as severe vomiting and diarrhea, followed by a week or so of apparent well-being before the development of the third toxic phase, which is characterized by fever, further gastrointestinal symptoms, ulceration of the mouth and throat, hemorrhages, and hair loss. There is an immediate drop in the white-cell elements of the blood, affecting the lymphocytes first and then the granulocytes and platelets, with a slower decline in the red cells. If death does not occur, these symptoms may last for many months before slow recovery begins.

Delayed effects of exposure to radiation include the development of leukemia and other cancers. Examples include the skin cancers that killed many of the pioneering scientists who worked with X-rays and radioactive elements, the lung cancer common among miners of radioactive ores, and bone cancer and aplastic anemia developed among women who painted clock dials with a luminous mixture containing radium and mesothorium, as a result of ingesting small amounts of paint when they licked their paintbrushes to form a point.

g. Nonionizing radiation

Nonionizing forms of radiation include electromagnetic radiation in the radiofrequency, infrared, visible light, and ultraviolet ranges. Exposure to radiation in the radiofrequency range occurs in the telecommunications industry and in the use of microwaves. Microwaves produce localized heating of tissues that may be intense and dangerous. Various other disorders, mainly of a subjective nature, have been reported in workers exposed to this frequency range. Infrared radiation can be felt as heat and is commonly used in industry for drying or baking processes. Prolonged exposure to the radiation can result in severe damage to the skin and especially to the lens of the eye, causing cataract. Working under poor lighting conditions can adversely affect worker efficiency and well-being and may even cause temporary physical disorders, such as headache or dizziness. Proper lighting should provide adequate, uniform illumination and appropriate contrast and color, without any flickering or glare. Exposure to ultraviolet radiation from the sun or such industrial operations as welding or glassblowing causes erythema of the skin, skin cancer, and inflammation of the conjunctiva and cornea. Pigmentation offers natural protection against sunburn, and clothing and glass can also be used as effective shields against ultraviolet radiation. Lasers emit intense infrared, visible, or ultraviolet radiation of a single frequency that is used in surgery; for scientific research; and for cutting, welding, and drilling in industry. Exposure to these beams can burn the skin and cause severe damage to the eye.

h. Disorders due to infectious agents

A large number of infectious diseases are transmitted to humans by animals. Many such diseases have been largely eliminated, but some still pose hazards. Anthrax, for example, can be acquired by workers handling the unsterilized hair, hide, and bone of infected animals; and slaughterhouse workers, farmers, veterinarians, and others in contact with infected animals, milk, and milk products still frequently contract brucellosis.

i. Disorders due to psychological factors

Psychological factors are important determinants of workers' health, well-being, and productivity. Studies have shown the benefits to workers who feel satisfied and stimulated by their jobs, who maintain good relationships with their employers or supervisors and with other employees, and who do not feel overworked. Such workers have lower rates of absenteeism and job turnover and higher rates of output than average.

The two psychological hazards commonly encountered at work are boredom and mental stress. Workers who perform simple, repetitive tasks for prolonged periods are subject to boredom, similar to those who work in bland, colorless environments. Boredom can cause frustration, unhappiness, inattentiveness, and other detriments to mental well-being. More practically, boredom decreases worker output and increases the chances of error and accident. Providing refreshment and relaxation breaks or other outside stimulus can help relieve boredom.

Mental stress often results from overwork, though nonoccupational factors, such as personal relationships, lifestyle, and state of physical health, can play a major role. Job dissatisfaction, increased responsibility, disinterest, competition, feelings of inadequacy, and bad working relationships can also contribute to mental stress. Stress affects both mental and physical health, causing anger, irritation, fatigue, aches, nausea, ulcers, migraine, asthma, colitis, and even breakdown and coronary heart disease. Moderate exercise, meditation, relaxation, and therapy can help workers to cope with stress.

Common Occupational and Industrial Health Hazards

Listed below are the common occupational and industrial health hazards:
- Acute and chronic intoxications with chemical substances and their sequels
- Metallic fever
- Pneumoconioses (*refer* **respiratory system**)
- Silicosis (*refer* **respiratory system**)
- Coal workers' pneumoconiosis (*refer* **respiratory system**)
- Pneumoconiosis associated with tuberculosis
- Welders' pneumoconiosis
- Asbestosis and other pneumoconioses due to silicates (*refer* **respiratory system**)
- Pneumoconiosis due to talc
- Graphite fibrosis
- Pneumoconioses due to metal dusts
- Allergic contact dermatitis (*refer* **skin disorders**)
- Irritant contact dermatitis (*refer* **skin disorders**)
- Oil acne, chloracne, coal tar acne of diffuse nature (*refer* **skin disorders**)
- **Candida infections:** Hand intertrigo, nail dystrophy with paronychia due to working conditions
- Dermatophyte infections due to contact with biological material from animals
- Contact urticaria
- Occupational photodermatoses

MULTIPLE CHOICE QUESTIONS

1. **What is the main purpose of hazard identification?**
   A. To minimize the effect of a consequence
   B. For better risk management
   C. To characterize adverse effect of toxins
   D. To reduce probability of occurrence

2. **The _____ process determines whether exposure to a chemical can increase the incidence of adverse health effect.**
   A. Hazard identification
   B. Exposure assessment
   C. Toxicity assessment
   D. Risk characterization

3. **Which of the following data is not required for hazard identification?**
   A. Land use
   B. Contaminant levels
   C. Affected population
   D. Estimation of risk

4. **Why site history has to be considered for hazard identification?**
   A. To estimate the risk
   B. To calculate carcinogenic exposure
   C. To know the probable source and causes of contamination on site
   D. For determination of remedial actions

5. **Hazard identification mainly focuses on**
   A. Chemical source and concentration
   B. Chemical exposure
   C. Chemical analysis
   D. Chemical pathway

Answers

1. C   2. A   3. D   4. C   5. A

Female Reproductive Disorders

AT THE END OF THIS CHAPTER, THE STUDENTS WILL BE LEARN ABOUT NURSING MANAGEMENT OF:
- ➢ Dysmenorrhea
- ➢ Amenorrhea
- ➢ Pelvic inflammatory disease
- ➢ Ovarian and fallopian tube disorder
- ➢ Cystocele/urethrocele and rectocele
- ➢ Infertility
- ➢ Contraception; types, methods, risks, and effectiveness
- ➢ Emergency contraception methods
- ➢ Sexual dysfunction

TERMINOLOGY

- Premenstrual syndrome (PMS) is the emotional and physical manifestations that occur cyclically in the female before menstruation.
- Dysmenorrhea is characterized by severe and frequent menstrual cramps and pain associated with menstruation.
- Amenorrhea is the medical term used for the absence of menstrual periods.
- Fistula is an abnormal opening between two internal organs and exterior of the body.
- Vaginitis is an inflammation of vagina.
- Cryptorchidism is also called undescended testis.
- Epispadias is congenital anomaly in males, wherein the urethra is on the upper surface of the penis.

REVIEW OF ANATOMY AND PHYSIOLOGY

Vagina

The vagina is an elastic, muscular tube connecting the cervix of the uterus to the vulva and exterior of the body, i.e., located between the bladder and the rectum. Measuring around 3 inches in length and less than an inch in diameter, the vagina stretches to become several inches longer and many inches wider during sexual intercourse and childbirth.

Size

In its normal state, there is anatomical variation in the length of the vagina of a woman of child-bearing age. The length is approximately 7.5 cm (2.5–3 in) across the anterior wall (front) and 9 cm (3.5 in) long across the posterior wall (rear), making the posterior fornix deeper than the anterior. During sexual arousal, the vagina expands in both length and width.

Layers

The three layers of a vagina are as follows:
1. **Epithelial layer:** The epithelial layer is made of connective tissues with many elastin fibers that allow the vagina to stretch. This layer is deep to the lamina propria.
2. **Lamina propria:** A layer of smooth muscle tissues located deep to the lamina propria, allowing the vagina to expand and contract during sexual intercourse and childbirth.
3. **Tunica externa:** Surrounding the smooth muscle is the outermost layer of the vagina known as the tunica externa. The tunica externa is a layer of dense irregular connective tissues that form the outer protective shell of the vagina.

Functions

The vagina provides the passageway for childbirth and menstrual flow and also receives the penis and semen during sexual intercourse. The inner surface of the vagina is folded to provide greater elasticity and to increase friction during sexual intercourse. Watery secretions produced by the vaginal epithelium lubricate the vagina and have an acidic pH to prevent the growth of bacteria and yeast. The acidic pH also makes the vagina an inhospitable environment for sperm, which has resulted in males producing alkaline seminal fluid to neutralize the acid and improve the survival of sperm.

Uterus

Uterus is a hollow muscular pear-shaped organ flattened anteroposteriorly. It lies in the pelvic cavity between the urinary bladder and the rectum. It is about 7.5 cm long and 5 cm wide and its walls are about 2.5 cm thick. It weighs are about 30–40 g.

The parts of the uterus are the fundus, body, and cervix.
1. **Fundus:** This is the dome-shaped part of the uterus found above the openings of the uterine tubes.
2. **Body:** This is the main part. It is narrowest inferiorly at the internal orifice (OS) where it is continuous with the cervix.
3. **Cervix (neck of uterus):** This protrudes through the anterior wall of the vagina, opening into the external OS.

Structure

The walls of the uterus are composed of three layers of tissue: perimetrium, myometrium, and endometrium.
1. **Perimetrium:** This is the peritoneum and is distributed differently on the various surfaces of the uterus. Anteriorly, it lies over the fundus and the body where it is folded on the upper surface of the urinary bladder. This fold of peritoneum forms the vesicouterine pouch. Posteriorly, the peritoneum covers the fundus, the body, and the cervix, then it folds back on the rectum to form the rectouterine pouch.
2. **Myometrium:** It is the thickest layer of the tissue in the uterine wall. It is a mass of smooth muscle fibers interlaced with areolar tissue, blood vessels, and nerves.
3. **Endometrium:** It consists of columnar epithelium containing a large number of mucus secreting tubular glands. It is functionally divided into two layers:
   i. The functional layer is the upper layer and it thickens and becomes rich in blood vessels in the first half of the menstrual cycle. If the ovum is not fertilized and not implanted, this layer is shed during menstruation.
   ii. The basal layer lies next to the myometrium and is not lost during menstruation. It is the layer from which the fresh functional layer is regenerated during each cycle.

Functions of Uterus

The uterus is a dynamic female reproductive organ that is responsible for several reproductive functions, including menstruation, implantation, gestation, labor, and delivery. It is responsive to the hormonal milieu within the body, which allows adaptation to the different stages of a women's reproductive life. The uterus adjusts to reflect changes in the ovarian steroid production during the menstrual cycle and displays rapid growth and specialized contractile activity during pregnancy. It serves two important functions: It is the organ of menstruation and during pregnancy, it receives the fertilized ovum and retains and nourishes it until it expels the fetus during labor.

DISORDERS OF THE FEMALE REPRODUCTIVE SYSTEM

INFERTILITY

According to the World Health Organization (WHO), infertility is a disease of the reproductive system defined by the failure to achieve a clinical pregnancy after 12 months or more of regular unprotected sexual intercourse.

Infertility is the inability of a sexually active, noncontraception couple to achieve pregnancy in 1 year. The male partner can be evaluated for infertility using a variety of clinical interventions and also from a laboratory evaluation of semen.

Types of Infertility

1. **Primary infertility:** Primary infertility is a condition where someone who has never conceived a child in the past and has difficulty in conceiving.
2. **Secondary infertility:** When a person has had one or more pregnancies in the past but is having difficulty in conceiving again.

Etiological Factors

Infertility may be caused by many factors. In women, infertility is most commonly due to ovulation disorders. Some problems stop women releasing eggs at all and some cause an egg to be released during some cycles but not others. Ovulation problems can occur as a result of many problems as listed below:

- **Polycystic ovary syndrome (PCOS):** A condition that makes it more difficult for ovaries to produce an egg.
- **Thyroid problems:** Both an overactive thyroid gland, hyperthyroidism and hypothyroidism can prevent ovulation.
- **Premature ovarian failure:** A condition when a woman's ovaries stop working before she is 40.
- **Womb and fallopian tubes:** The fallopian tubes are the tubes along which an egg travels from the ovary to the womb. The egg is fertilized as it travels down the fallopian tubes, where it reaches the womb; it is implanted into womb lining, where it continues to grow. If the womb or the fallopian tubes are damaged or stop working, it may be difficult to conceive.
- **Scarring from surgery:** Pelvic surgery can sometimes cause damage and scarring to the fallopian tubes. Cervical surgery can also cause scarring or shorten the cervix.
- **Cervical mucus defect:** At the time of ovulation, mucus in the cervix becomes thinner, so that sperm can swim through it more easily; if there is a problem with mucus, conceiving becomes harder.
- **Endometriosis:** It is a condition where small pieces of the womb lining, known as the endometrium, start growing in other places, such as ovaries. This can cause infertility because the new growths form adhesions or cysts that block the pelvis.

- **Pelvic inflammatory disease:** It is an infection of the upper female genital tract and is often the result of a sexually transmitted infection and can damage fallopian tubes.
- **Medicines and drugs:** Long-term use of nonsteroidal inflammatory drugs, such as aspirin, ibuprofen, causes difficulty in conceiving.
- **Chemotherapy:** They make ovaries weak and unable to function properly.
- **Other drugs:** Drugs, such as marijuana and cocaine can affect fertility.
- **Age:** Fertility is also linked to age, the biggest decrease in fertility begins during the mid-30s.

In men, infertility is mainly due to the following:
- Abnormal semen
- Decreased number of sperm
- Decreased sperm mobility
- Abnormal sperm and abnormal shape
- If testicles are damaged it affects semen
- An infection in testicles (orchitis)
- Testicular cancer
- Testicular surgery
- Congenital defect in testicles (cryptorchidism)
- Trauma to testicles
- **Sterilization:** Vasectomy involves cutting and sealing of vas deferens, so that semen will no longer contain sperm
- An abnormally low level of testosterone is referred to as hypogonadism, which is involved in making sperm
- Alcohol which damages the quality of sperm
- Smoking can adversely affect fertility
- If either one of the partners is in stress, it affects the relationship by decreasing the sex drive.

Clinical Manifestation

The main symptom of infertility is not getting pregnant.

In women

- Changes in the menstrual cycle and ovulation may be a symptom of infertility
- Abnormal periods, or bleeding may be heavy or low
- Acne
- Changes in sex drive and desire
- Weight gain
- Milky discharge from nipples but unrelated to breastfeeding
- Pain during sex

In men

- Problems are with the sexual functions, i.e., difficulty in ejaculation, reduced desire, and erectile dysfunction.
- Pain and swelling in testicles
- Having a lower normal sperm count

Diagnostic Evaluation

- **History:**
  - Collect the history related to irregular menstruation.
  - Collect the history related to the known problems with uterus, tubes, or other problems, such as endometriosis.

- Collect history related to male infertility problems.
- Ask about the history of drugs uses and about alcohol and smoking habits.
- Ask the couple about their relationship.
- **Physical examination:** In physical examination, assess the patient for any abnormalities in penis, vas deferens, testicles.
  - Assess the client for skin changes
  - Check the weight of the patient
  - Ask the client for her menstrual history
- **Male partner semen analysis:** It provides information related to the number, movement, and shape of the sperm. It is an essential part of infertility evaluation.
- **Hysterosalpingogram:** This is an X-ray procedure to see whether the fallopian tubes are open and to see the shape of uterine cavity. A catheter is inserted into the opening of the cervix through the vagina. A liquid containing iodine contrast is injected through the catheter.
- **Transvaginal ultrasonography:** An ultrasound probe placed in vagina allows checking uterus and ovaries for abnormalities.
- **Other blood tests**: Thyroid-stimulating hormone and prolactin levels are useful to identify thyroid disorders, because thyroid disorders may cause infertility, menstrual irregularities, and repeated miscarriages. A blood progesterone level drawn in the second half of the menstrual cycle can help to document the occurrence of ovulation.
- **Sonohysterography:** This procedure uses transvaginal ultrasound after filling the uterus with saline. This improves the detection of intrauterine problems, such as endometrial polyps, fibroids.
- **Hysteroscopy:** This is a surgical procedure in which hysteroscope is passed through the cervix to view the inside of the uterus. It helps to diagnose or treat problems inside the uterine cavity, such as fibroids, polyps and adhesions.
- **Laparoscopy:** This is a surgical procedure in which laparoscope is inserted through the wall of the abdomen into the pelvic cavity. It evaluates pelvic cavity for endometriosis and pelvic adhesions.

Management

Only limited numbers of medical treatments are available at improving the chances of conception for patients with known cause of infertility.

- **Endocrinopathies:** A number of patients with hypogonadotropic hypogonadism respond to gonadotropin replacement.
- **Artificial insemination:** Depositing semen into the female genital tract by artificial insemination. If the sperm cannot penetrate the cervical canal normally, artificial insemination using the partner's semen may be considered.
- **Indications for using artificial insemination:** The inability to deposit semen in the vagina, which may be due to premature ejaculation or due to hypospadias or dyspareunia.
- Inability of semen to be transported from the vagina to uterine cavity, which is usually due to faulty chemical conditions and may occur with an abnormal cervical discharge.
- During insemination, women may have received clomiphene and menotropins to stimulate ovulation.
- The success rate for artificial insemination varies, three to six inseminations may be required over 2–4 months, because artificial insemination is likely to be a stressful and difficult situation for couples, and nursing support should be provided.

- **Insemination with donor semen:** When the sperm of the women's partner is defective or absent or when there is a risk of transmitting a genetic disease, donor sperm may be used but written consent is obtained from the patient/couple.
- **In vitro fertilization:** It involves ovarian stimulation, egg retrieval, fertilization, and embryo transfer. This procedure is accomplished by first stimulating the ovary to produce multiple eggs, or ova, usually with medications.
- Most common indications are irreparable tubal damage, endometriosis, immunologic problems, unexplained infertility, and inadequate sperm.

Pharmacological Therapy

- Pharmacologically induced ovulation is performed only when the woman does not ovulate. Various medications are used depending upon the primary cause of infertility. These medications induce ovulation.
- Clomiphene is used when the hypothalamus is not the stimulating pituitary gland to release follicle-stimulating hormone (FSH) and luteinizing hormone (LH).
- Menotropin is a combination of FSH and LH and is used in women deficient in these hormones.
- Urofollitropin containing FSH with a small amount of LH is used to stimulate follicle growth in polycystic ovarian syndrome.
- Chorionic gonadotropin is used to stimulate the release of egg from ovary.

Lifestyle Modifications

- Healthy lifestyle and daily exercise may restore fertility.
- Overweight or underweight can affect the chances of ovulating normally in women. In women with less or more body fat hinders the menstrual cycle, making conception difficult; hence, it is required to maintain a healthy body weight before conception.
- Avoid smoking and alcohol as they also affect conception and in male, it decreases the sperm count.
- Caffeine and drugs should be avoided because they affect the sperm count and also interfere with the menstrual cycle.
- Take healthy diet, including the diet rich in antioxidants, vitamin C, and certain minerals, thereby maintaining ideal body weight.
- A high intake of vitamins C and E increases sperm count and motility of sperm, and in women, it can reduce the stress on eggs or reproductive organs.

Nursing Management

Nursing Assessment

Nursing interventions appropriate when working with couples during fertility evaluations include the following:

- Assist the client in reducing stress in the relationship
- Encourage cooperation, protect privacy, foster understanding, and refer the couple to appropriate resources when necessary.
- Infertility workups are expensive, time-consuming, stressful, so couples need to support in working together to deal with these problems.

Nursing Diagnosis

- Anticipatory grieving related to the loss of pregnancy
- Anxiety related to the diagnosis of infertility

- Disturbed body image related to altered fertility, fears about sexuality, and relationships with partner and family.
- Deficient knowledge related to the disease process
- Community coping impairment related to the diagnosis of infertility.

1. Anticipatory grieving related to the loss of pregnancy.
Interventions
- Assess the client condition
- Client distress may not be expressed verbally, not by the partner.
- So nurse should be present to listen and provide support.
- The client partner should also participate in this process.
- If the client is having severe distress, then refer the client for counseling.

2. Anxiety related to the diagnosis of fertility.
Interventions
- Assess the level of anxiety in the client
- The patient must be allowed to talk and ask questions.
- Assist the patient in expressing their feelings
- Provide support
- Educate them about the disease condition and also about the treatment
- Tell the client partner to be with the patient

3. Disturbed body image related to the altered fertility, fears about sexuality, and relationship between partner and family.
Interventions
- Assess the condition of patient
- The patient may have strong emotional reactions related to the diagnosis of infertility and views of the others who may be involved (family, partner, religious beliefs, and fears about prognosis).
- Provide reassurance to the client
- Provide psychological support
- If the fear or stress level is high, then refer patient for counseling.

PREMENSTRUAL SYNDROME

It is defined as a combination of emotional and physical manifestations that occur cyclically in the female before menstruation and regress or disappear during menstruation.

Etiology

The cause of PMS is unclear. However, neuroendocrine mechanisms appear to be involved. It is not clear whether PMS is a single syndrome or a group of separate disorders. Some suggested causes of PMS are as follow:
- Estrogen–progesterone imbalance, especially in cases with estrogen excess and a progesterone deficiency or estrogen deficiency
- Interaction among estrogen, progesterone, and aldosterone
- Excess of prolactin, hypothyroidism, or hypoglycemia
- Dietary factors, such as deficiency of vitamin B_6, magnesium
- Lifestyle factors, such as increased stress and poor diet.

Pathophysiology

The pathophysiology involved in PMS is as follows:

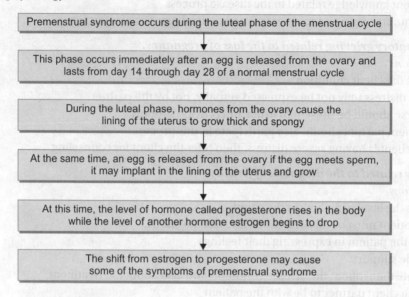

Premenstrual syndrome occurs during the luteal phase of the menstrual cycle

This phase occurs immediately after an egg is released from the ovary and lasts from day 14 through day 28 of a normal menstrual cycle

During the luteal phase, hormones from the ovary cause the lining of the uterus to grow thick and spongy

At the same time, an egg is released from the ovary if the egg meets sperm, it may implant in the lining of the uterus and grow

At this time, the level of hormone called progesterone rises in the body while the level of another hormone estrogen begins to drop

The shift from estrogen to progesterone may cause some of the symptoms of premenstrual syndrome

Clinical Manifestations

The clinical manifestations of PMS are of two types, namely—physical and affective symptoms.

Physical Symptoms

The following are the physical symptoms of PMS:
- Fluid retention
- Sensation of weight gain
- Episodes of binge eating
- Breast discomfort
- Headache
- Peripheral edema
- Abdominal cramp
- Sleep disturbance
- Joint or muscle pain

Affective Symptoms

The following are the affective symptoms of PMS:
- Depression
- Anger
- Anxiety
- Irritability
- Confusion
- Insomnia
- Tendency to cry easily
- Poor concentration

Diagnostic Evaluation

There is no objective of diagnosing PMS. Diagnosis usually made by documenting the cyclic nature of the symptoms on a menstrual calendar. A diagnosis of PMS requires a reoccurrence of symptoms for a minimum of three menstrual cycles. Diagnosis is made on the time of symptoms, rather than on the presence of particular symptoms.

Management

Daily intake of vitamin B_6 and minerals and the elimination of caffeine have improved some premenstrual manifestations.

Medications Management

- Spironolactone is a synthetic steroid aldosterone antagonist that inhibits the physiologic effect of aldosterone on the distal tubules. It is commonly used to treat the edema associated with excessive aldosterone secretions.
- Progesterone may relieve physiologic and psychological manifestations.
- Bromocriptine reduces serum prolactin concentrations by inhibiting prolactin release from the anterior pituitary gland. It has been successfully used to reduce breast pain in some PMS cases.
- **Antidepressants:** Selective serotonin reuptake inhibitors, which include fluoxetine, paroxetine, sertraline, and others, have been successful in reducing symptoms and are also considered the first-line agents for PMS treatment.
- **Analgesic:** These are commonly given for menstrual cramps, headache, and pelvic discomfort. The most effective group of analgesic appears to be the nonsteroidal anti-inflammatory medications, e.g., ibuprofen.

Heath Education

- Avoid salt before menstrual period
- Reduce caffeine intake
- Quit smoking
- Reduce alcohol intake
- Increase fiber intake
- Adequate rest and sleep
- Eat smaller more frequent diet to reduce fluid retention

DYSMENORRHEA

It is a menstrual condition characterized by severe and frequent menstrual cramps and pain associated with menstruation. The degree of pain and discomfort varies with the individual.

Types

Dysmenorrhea are of the following two types:
1. Primary dysmenorrhea
2. Secondary dysmenorrhea

Primary dysmenorrhea: It is believed to be caused by either an excess prostaglandin or an increased sensitivity to prostaglandins, with no underlying pathologic pelvic disorders.

Secondary dysmenorrhea: It is caused by other medical condition other than menstruation and also involves natural production of prostaglandins. The cramps caused by other medical problems, such as endometriosis, uterine fibroid, pelvic inflammatory disease, etc.

Etiology

- Early age of menarche (<12 years)
- Nulliparity
- Heavy and prolonged menstrual flow
- Smoking
- Alcohol
- Family history

The characteristics of secondary dysmenorrhea are as follows:

- Pelvic inflammatory disease
- Endometriosis
- Uterine prolapsed
- Uterine myomas
- Polyps

Pathophysiology

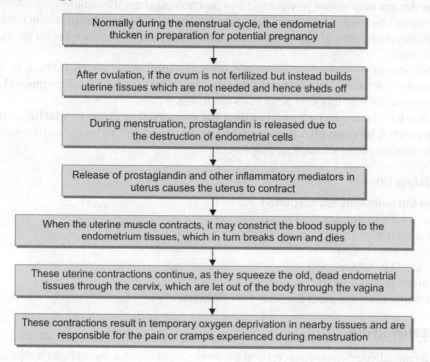

Normally during the menstrual cycle, the endometrial thicken in preparation for potential pregnancy

↓

After ovulation, if the ovum is not fertilized but instead builds uterine tissues which are not needed and hence sheds off

↓

During menstruation, prostaglandin is released due to the destruction of endometrial cells

↓

Release of prostaglandin and other inflammatory mediators in uterus causes the uterus to contract

↓

When the uterine muscle contracts, it may constrict the blood supply to the endometrium tissues, which in turn breaks down and dies

↓

These uterine contractions continue, as they squeeze the old, dead endometrial tissues through the cervix, which are let out of the body through the vagina

↓

These contractions result in temporary oxygen deprivation in nearby tissues and are responsible for the pain or cramps experienced during menstruation

Clinical Manifestations

- Pain concentrated in the lower abdomen, i.e., in the umbilical region or in the suprapubic region of the abdomen; may radiate to thighs and lower back
- Nausea and vomiting
- Headache
- Dizziness
- Fainting
- Fatigue
- Diarrhea
- Back pain

Diagnostic Evaluation

- Understanding the past history
- **Physical examination:** Manual vaginal examination to examine for masses, tenderness, or enlarged uterus. Examine for discharge coming from the cervix, which suggests pelvic inflammatory disease.
- **Pelvic ultrasound:** To reveal the function of internal organs, i.e., examine for an enlarged uterus or fallopian tube or ovarian mass found on physical examination.
- **Blood test:** Full blood count and erythrocyte sedimentation rate (ESR)
- Thyroid function test
- Pregnancy test in case of a suspicion of ectopic pregnancy
- **Hysteroscopy:** A visual examination of the canal of the cervix and the interior of the uterus using an instrument (hysteroscope) inserted through the vagina.

Management

- **Administer prostaglandin synthesis inhibitors:** Prostaglandin synthesis inhibitors may provide relief by decreasing prostaglandin activity, even in the presence of ovulatory cycle. Some commonly prescribed medications for this are ibuprofen and indomethacin.
- **Analgesics:** Aspirin and paracetamol may be useful in the starting point especially when NSAIDs are contraindicated.
- **Administer oral contraceptives:** If contraception as well as relief of dysmenorrhea is desired, a combination oral contraceptives may be of help. The combination inhibits ovulation, resulting in decreased endometrial prostaglandin production and a concurrent reduction in uterine activity.

Nonpharmacological Treatment

- Women should be advised that during acute pain, relief may be obtained by lying down for a short period
- Drinking hot beverages, such as herbal teas
- Applying heat on the abdomen or back
- Taking bath using warm water
- Regular exercise is thought to be beneficial because it may reduce endometrial hyperplasia and subsequently reduce prostaglandin production
- Acupuncture and transcutaneous nerve stimulation also provide varying degrees of relief.

Nursing Care Plan

Nursing Assessment

- Assess the general condition of the patient and also assess the level of discomfort and vital signs of the patient.
- Obtain full history of the illness

Nursing Diagnosis

- Acute pain related to increased uterine contractility, hypersensitivity
- Imbalanced nutrition, which is less than that required by the body and this is related to the nausea and vomiting
- Ineffective individual coping related to emotional excess
- Activity intolerance related to pain
- Disturbed sleeping pattern related to discomfort

1. Acute Pain Related to Increased Uterine Contractility

Interventions

- Assess the level and severity of pain
- Provide warm application to the patient like hot water bottle
- Massage the abdominal area as it reduces the pain due to the stimulus of therapeutic touch
- Provide diversion therapy to the patients, such as music, meditation, etc.
- Provide comfort devices to the patients
- Administer analgesic to the patient

2. Imbalanced Nutrition, which is less than that Required by the Body Requirement and this is Related to Nausea and Vomiting

Interventions

- Assess the condition of the patient
- Provide small and frequent meals to the patient
- Monitor the intake and output of the patient
- Provide liquid diet to the patient

3. Ineffective Individual Coping Related to Emotional Excess

Interventions

- Assess the patient's understanding of her illness
- Determine additional pain that accompanies it
- Provide an opportunity to the patient to discuss about the severity of the pain
- Provide relaxation therapy and deep breathing exercise to the patient
- Advise the patient to sleep and rest
- Provide psychological support to the patient
- Counsel the patient

AMENORRHEA

Amenorrhea is the medical term used for the absence of menstrual periods, either permanently or temporarily in women of reproductive age. The physiological state of amenorrhea is seen during pregnancy and lactation. Other than reproductive years, menses is absent during childhood and after menopause.

Classification of Amenorrhea

Amenorrhea are of two types:
1. Primary amenorrhea
2. Secondary amenorrhea

Primary Amenorrhea

It is the absence of menstrual bleeding and secondary sexual characteristics (e.g., breast development, pubic hair) in girls aged 14 years and also the absence of menstrual bleeding with normal development of secondary sexual characteristics in girls aged 16 years. It may be because of the following:

- Congenital absence of uterus
- Failure of ovary to receive or maintain egg cells
- Delay in pubertal development

Secondary Amenorrhea

It is the absence of menstrual bleeding in a woman who had been menstruating but later stops menstruating for 3 or more months even in the absence of pregnancy, lactation, and menopause. It may be because of the following:

- Hormonal disturbance
- Premature menopause
- Intrauterine scar formation

Etiology

a. Lifestyle factors

Sometimes lifestyle factors contribute to amenorrhea, for instance:

- **Low body weight:** Excessively low body weight, i.e., about 10% under normal weight interrupts many hormonal functions in our body, potentially halting ovulation. Women who have an eating disorder, such as anorexia or bulimia, often stop having periods because of these abnormal hormonal changes.
- **Excessive exercise:** Women who participate in activities that require rigorous training, such as ballet, may find their menstrual cycles interrupted. Several factors together contribute to the loss of periods in athletes, including low body fat, stress, and high energy expenditure.
- **Stress:** Mental stress can temporarily alter the functioning of the hypothalamus, an area of brain that controls the hormones that regulate the menstrual cycle. As a result, ovulation and menstruation may stop. Regular menstrual periods usually resume after stress decreases.

b. Hormonal Imbalance

Hormonal imbalances occur when there is too much or too little of a hormone in the bloodstream. Because of their essential role in the body, even small hormonal imbalances can cause side effects throughout the body.

c. Many types of medical problems can cause hormonal imbalance, including:

- **Polycystic ovary syndrome (PCOS):** PCOS causes relatively high and sustained levels of hormones, rather than the fluctuating levels seen in the normal menstrual cycle.
- **Thyroid malfunction:** An overactive thyroid gland (hyperthyroidism) or underactive thyroid gland (hypothyroidism) can cause menstrual irregularities, including amenorrhea.
- **Pituitary tumor:** A noncancerous (benign) tumor in pituitary gland can interfere with the hormonal regulation of menstruation.
- **Premature menopause:** Menopause usually begins around the age of 50. But, for some women, the ovarian supply of eggs diminishes before the age of 40 and menstruation stops.

d. Structural Problems

- Problems with the sexual organs themselves also can cause amenorrhea. Examples include:
- **Uterine scarring:** Asherman's syndrome, a condition in which the scar tissue builds up in the lining of the uterus, which sometimes occur after a dilation and curettage (D&C), cesarean section, or treatment of uterine fibroids. Uterine scarring prevents the normal buildup and shedding of the uterine lining.
- **Lack of reproductive organs:** Sometimes problems arise during fetal development that leads to the birth of a girl without some major parts of her reproductive system, such as uterus, cervix, or vagina. Because her reproductive system did not develop normally, she cannot have menstrual cycle.

- **Structural abnormality of the vagina:** An obstruction of the vagina may prevent visible menstrual bleeding. A membrane or wall may be present in the vagina that blocks the outflow of blood from the uterus and cervix.

Clinical Manifestations

Symptoms of primary amenorrhea may include:

- Headache
- Galactorrhea
- Acne
- Excessive hair growth (hirsutism)
- Excessive anxiety

Symptoms of secondary amenorrhea may include:

- Nausea
- Breast tenderness
- Headache
- Being very thirsty
- Weight gain or weight loss
- Goiter (an enlarged thyroid gland)
- Darkening skin
- Vaginal dryness
- Hot flashes
- Night sweats
- Mood changes

Diagnostic Evaluations

- History and physical examination
- Lab tests
  - **Pregnancy test:** This will probably be the first test doctor suggests to rule out or confirm a possible pregnancy.
  - **Thyroid function test:** Measuring the amount of thyroid-stimulating hormone (TSH) in blood can determine whether thyroid is working properly.
  - **Ovary function test:** Measuring the amount of FSH in blood to determine whether ovaries are working properly.
  - **Prolactin test:** Low levels of the hormone prolactin may be a sign of a pituitary gland tumor.
  - **Male hormone test:** If someone is experiencing increased facial hair and a lowered voice, doctor may assess the level of male hormones in blood.
- **Ultrasound:** This test uses sound waves to produce images of internal organs. Ultrasound test is used to check for any abnormalities in reproductive organs.
- **Computerized tomography (CT):** CT scans combine many X-ray images taken from different directions to create cross-sectional views of internal structures. A CT scan can indicate whether uterus, ovaries, and kidneys look normal.
- **Magnetic resonance imaging (MRI):** MRI uses radio waves with a strong magnetic field to produce exceptionally detailed images of soft tissues within the body.
- **Hysteroscopy:** A test in which a thin, lighted camera is passed through vagina and cervix to view the inside of uterus.

Management

Treatment of both primary and secondary amenorrhea is determined by the precise cause of the amenorrhea.

Goals

- Relive symptoms of hormonal imbalance
- Establish menstruation
- Prevent complications associated with amenorrhea
- Achieve fertility

Drug Therapy

- **Dopamine agonists**, such as bromocriptine or pergolide, are effective in treating hyperprolactinemia. In most women, treatment with dopamine agonists restores normal ovarian endocrine function and ovulation.
- **Hormonal replacement therapy**, consisting of an estrogen or a progestin, is needed for women with estrogen deficiency.
- **Metformin** is a drug that has been successfully used in women with PCOS to induce ovulation.

Surgical Management

- Some pituitary and hypothalamic tumors may require surgery and in some cases, only radiation therapy will suffice.
- Women with intrauterine adhesions require dissolution of the adhesions.
- Surgical procedures required for other genital tract abnormalities depend on the specific clinical situation.

VAGINAL FISTULA

A fistula is an abnormal opening between two internal organs and exterior of the body. Fistula indicates the two areas that are connected abnormally. It may be congenital or due to tissue damage in the particular areas.

A fistula is an abnormal connection between the two different organs. Vaginal fistula is of five types:

1. **Rectovaginal fistula:** It is an opening between the rectum and vagina.
2. **Vesicovaginal fistula:** It is an opening between the bladder and vagina.
3. **Uterovaginal fistula:** Uterovaginal fistula is an opening between the uterus and vagina.
4. **Urethrovaginal fistula:** It is an opening between the urethra and vagina.
5. **Vaginoperineal fistula:** Vaginoperineal fistula is an opening between the vagina and the perineum.

Etiology

- A vaginal fistula starts with some kind of tissue damage. After days to years of tissue breakdown, a fistula opens up. Vaginal fistulas are not a common problem in the developed countries.
- A vaginal fistula may result from an injury during childbirth.
- Crohn's disease or other inflammatory bowel disease can cause vaginal fistula.
- Radiation treatment for pelvic cancer.
- Surgery of the back wall of the vagina, perineum, anus, or rectum.
- A deep tear in the perineum or an infected episiotomy after childbirth.

Pathophysiology

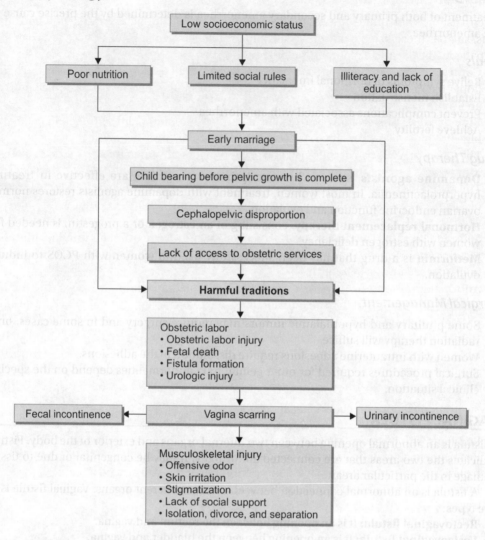

Low socioeconomic status

Poor nutrition | Limited social rules | Illiteracy and lack of education

Early marriage

Child bearing before pelvic growth is complete

Cephalopelvic disproportion

Lack of access to obstetric services

Harmful traditions

Obstetric labor
- Obstetric labor injury
- Fetal death
- Fistula formation
- Urologic injury

Fecal incontinence ← Vagina scarring → Urinary incontinence

Musculoskeletal injury
- Offensive odor
- Skin irritation
- Stigmatization
- Lack of social support
- Isolation, divorce, and separation

Signs and Symptoms

Depending on the size and location of the fistula, the patient may have minor symptoms or significant problems with continence and hygiene. Signs and symptoms of a rectovaginal fistula may include the following:

- A vaginal fistula is painless. But a fistula lets urine or feces pass into the vagina. This is called incontinence
- Passing stool via the vagina
- Inability to control bowel movements
- Foul-smelling vaginal discharge
- Pain during sexual intercourse
- Persistent pain in the pelvic area
- The symptoms of a rectovaginal fistula often cause emotional distress as well as physical discomfort, which can impact self-esteem and intimate relationships.

Diagnostic Evaluation

Often a fistula is not found during the physical examination. The doctor may recommend other tests, such as those listed below, to locate and evaluate a vaginal fistula. These tests can also help the medical team in planning for surgery.

- **Contrast tests:** A vaginogram or a barium enema can help identify a fistula located in the upper rectum. These tests use a contrast material to show either the vagina or the bowel on an X-ray image.
- **Blue dye test:** This test involves placing a tampon into the vagina and then injecting the blue dye into the rectum. Blue staining on the tampon shows the presence of a fistula.
- **The CT scan:** A CT scan of abdomen and pelvis provides more detail compared to a standard X-ray. The CT scan can help locate a fistula and determine its cause.
- **The MRI:** This test produces images of soft tissues in the body, which can show the location of a fistula as well as involvement of pelvic organs or the presence of a tumor.
- **Anorectal ultrasound:** This procedure uses sound waves to produce a video image of the anus and rectum. The doctor inserts a narrow, wand-like instrument into the anus and rectum. Anorectal ultrasound can evaluate the structure of anal sphincter and may show injury caused during childbirth.
- **Anorectal manometry:** This test measures the sensitivity and functions of the rectum and can provide useful information about rectal sphincter and the ability to control stool passage. This test does not locate fistulas, but it can help in planning to repair the fistula.
- **Urinalysis:** This test is used to check for infection, and blood test (complete blood count) is also used to check for signs of infection in the body.

Complication

Physical complications of rectovaginal fistula may include the following:
- Incontinence
- Problems with hygiene
- Recurrent vaginal or urinary tract infections
- Irritation or inflammation of the vagina, perineum, or the skin around anus
- Infected fistula that forms an abscess, a problem that can become life threatening, if not treated
- Fistula recurrence

Management

- **Education:** The majority of patients with fistula are from rural areas, where people have low literacy levels and lack of physical and economic access to good medical care. Since many expectant mothers do not attend antenatal clinics, they are exposed to high-risk conditions and medical and obstetric complications that endanger the life or harm the health of the mother and her baby. These high-risk conditions and complications are not be detected early enough for precautionary measures to be taken. To avoid such situations, pregnant women should be educated about such risks and complications.
- **Healthcare facilities:** In the short-term, better use of the existing obstetric services and increased provision of effective health services in rural areas will lower the incidence of fistula. Such improvements would lead women to seek safer obstetric practices, including the use of family planning, delayed childbearing, and prenatal and antenatal care during pregnancy. Good hygiene can help ease discomfort and reduce the chance of vaginal or urinary tract infections while waiting for repair.

Personal Hygiene

- **Wash with water:** Gently wash the outer genital area with warm water each time when the patient experiences vaginal discharge or passage of stool.
- **Avoid irritants:** Soap can dry and irritate skin, but a gentle unscented soap may be of help. Avoid harsh or scented soap and scented tampons. Vaginal douches can increase the chance of infection.
- **Dry thoroughly:** Allow the area to air-dry after washing or gently pat dry the area with toilet paper or a clean washcloth.
- **Avoid rubbing with dry toilet paper:** Premoistened, alcohol-free wipes or moistened cotton balls may be a good alternative for cleaning the area.
- **Use a cold compress:** Apply a cold compress, such as a washcloth, at the folds of the vaginal opening.
- **Apply a cream or powder:** Moisture-barrier creams help keep irritated skin from having direct contact with liquid or stool. Nonmedicated talcum powder or cornstarch also may help relieve discomfort. Be sure the area is clean and dry before applying any cream or powder.
- **Wear loose clothing:** Tight clothing can restrict airflow, making skin problems worse. Products, such as absorbent pads, disposable underwear, or adult diapers can help if patient passes liquids or stool.

Pharmacological Management

Depending on the circumstances, the doctor may recommend the following medications:

- **Antibiotics:** Antibiotics may also be recommended for women with Crohn's disease who develop fistula.
- **Nonsteroidal anti-inflammatory drugs (NSAIDs):** The NSAIDs are the mostly commonly used drugs for arthritis-related pain, swelling, and stiffness. They interfere with the body's production of hormone-like chemicals called prostaglandins. Prostaglandins are one of the biggest contributors to inflammation in the body. The NSAIDs are available over-the-counter or with a prescription. They include aspirin, ibuprofen, naproxen, etc.

Surgical Management

The main treatment for fistulas is surgical repair. The success and recovery rate from an operation to correcting simple fistula is very high, i.e., almost 90%. However, the success of the repair is dependent not only on good surgery but also on excellent nursing care and the prevention of complications. Sometimes fistulas heal on their own, but most people need surgery to close or repair the abnormal connection. Before an operation can be done, the skin and other tissue around the fistula must be healthy, with no signs of infection or inflammation.

Urinary or colorectal bypass surgery: This essentially involves repairing a hole in the bladder or rectum and can usually take place through the vagina without the need for major incision. The operation is delicate and can be performed by especially trained surgeons and support staff.

- Sewing an anal fistula plug or patch of biologic tissue into the fistula to allow the tissue to grow into the patch and heal the fistula.
- Using a tissue graft taken from a nearby part of the body or folding a flap of healthy tissue over the fistula opening.
- Doing more complicated surgical repair if the anal sphincter muscles also are damaged or if there is scarring or tissue damage from radiation or Crohn's disease.
- Performing a colostomy before repairing a fistula in more complex or recurrent cases to divert stool through an opening into the abdomen instead of passing through the rectum.

This may be needed if the patient had tissue damage or scarring from previous surgery or radiation treatment, an ongoing infection, significant fecal contamination, a cancerous tumor, or an abscess. If a colostomy is needed, the surgeon may wait 8–12 weeks before repairing the fistula. Usually, after about 3–6 months and confirmation that the fistula has healed, the colostomy can be reversed and normal bowel function is restored.

Nursing Care plan

- **History taking:** The nurse will first consider history of vaginal infections or sexually-transmitted infections and perform a physical or pelvic examination. If the discharge is from the vagina, a sample will be sent for analysis to the lab to determine the possibility of an infection.
- **Psychological assessment:** Psychosocial assessment should include evaluation of the patient's home situation and a sexual history. Ask the patient about the type of contraception that she and her partner use. Provide a private environment to allow the patient to answer questions without making the patient feel embarrassed.

Nursing Diagnoses

1. Risk for infection related to contamination of urinary tract by flora or contamination of the vagina by rectal organisms
2. Impaired urinary elimination related to fistula
3. Anxiety related to the diagnosis of fistula, surgery, and possible loss of femininity
4. Sexual dysfunction related to change in vaginal structure
5. Self-care deficit related to the lack of understanding of perinea care and general health status

1. Risk for infection related to contamination of urinary tract by flora or contamination of the vagina by rectal organisms.
Interventions
- Encourage frequent sitz baths
- Perform vaginal irrigation as ordered, and teach patients the procedure
- Before repair surgery, administer prescribed antibiotics to reduce pathogenic flora in the intestinal tract
- Maintain patient on clear liquids as prescribed to limit bowel activity for several days
- Encourage rest because of debilitation
- Administer warm perinea irrigations to decrease healing time and increase comfort.

2. Impaired urinary elimination related to fistula.
Interventions
- Suggest the use of perinea pads or incontinence products preoperatively.
- Maintain proper drainage from indwelling catheter to prevent pressure on the newly sutured tissue.
- Administer vaginal or bladder irrigations gently because of tenderness at the operation site.
- Maintain strict intake and output records.
- Encourage the patient to express feelings about her altered route of elimination and share them with significant other.

Prevention
Prevention of fistulas requires skilled attendants at birth and a swift surgical intervention especially if obstructed labor occurs. The pressure of the fetal head during obstructed labor causes ischemia to the pelvic organs, and a spectrum of injuries follows as a consequence.

Education and Health Maintenance

- Teach patients to report early the signs of infection
- Teach patients to clean perineum gently and to follow surgeon's instructions on when to resume sexual intercourse and strenuous activity.
- Advise patient to go for regular follow-up appointments.

OVARIAN CYST OR POLYCYSTIC OVARIAN SYNDROME

Ovaries are two small organs located on both side of the uterus. They are responsible for production of estrogens and maintaining the menstruation cycle. The ovaries release egg every month. This cycle of egg release is called ovulation. In PCOS, the follicles fail to open and become cysts.

Etiology and Risk Factors

- Endometriosis
- Cystadenomas
- Dermoid cysts
- Age
- Smoking
- Obesity
- Nulliparity or not breastfeeding
- Intake of fertility drugs
- Hormone replacement therapy
- Family or personal history of ovarian, breast cancer.

Clinical Manifestations

- Pain or bloating in the abdomen
- Difficulty urinating
- Dull ache in the lower back
- Painful sexual intercourse
- Painful menstruation
- Weight gain
- Nausea or vomiting
- Loss of appetite

Histopathology

Gross description: Ovarian cysts are rarely greater than 8 cm and have glistening membrane with thin and toned wall. Cyst can be unilocular or multilocular filled with clear or serous fluid contents.

Micro description: The outer layer of theca interna cells become luteinized and surrounded by reticulum. Cyst lining is convoluted and composed of luteinized granulosa cells and an outer layer of theca cells. Cysts usually have prominent inner layer of fibrous tissues.

VAGINITIS

Vaginitis is an inflammation of vagina.

Etiology and Types

There are many different causes and types of vaginitis. These are as listed as follows:

Noninfectious Vaginitis

It refers to vaginal inflammation caused due to chemical irritants or allergies. Spermicides, douches, detergents, fabric softeners, and latex condoms can all irritate the vaginal lining. Also, some sanitary napkins can cause irritation at the entrance to the vagina.

Atrophic Vaginitis

It may occur after a woman reaches menopause. It results from lower hormone (estrogen) levels and the thinning of the vaginal lining caused by hormonal changes. This makes the vagina more prone to irritation.

Infectious Vaginitis

It is caused by an bacterial or yeast infection. Trichomoniasis is caused by a parasite called *Trichomonas vaginalis* and spreads through unprotected sex with an infected partner. Other types of vaginal infections can occur when a woman has a fistula, i.e., an abnormal passage connecting the intestine to the vagina. This allows stool to enter the vaginal area, greatly increasing the risk of infections.

Bacterial Vaginitis

It may be due to an imbalance between normally occurring bacteria that protect the vagina and potentially infectious ones. Cigarette smoking, using intrauterine devices, douching, and having multiple sexual partners all will increase the risk of infection. Bacterial vaginitis is not considered a sexually-transmitted infection, as it can occur even in women who have never had vaginal intercourse.

Yeast Infection

Also known as vaginal candidiasis. It occurs when there is an overgrowth of the yeast called *Candida* that normally lives in the vagina. Anything that changes the type and amount of bacteria normally present in the vagina, such as douching or irritation from inadequate vaginal lubrication, can increase the risk. A yeast infection can be sexually transmitted, especially through oral–genital sexual contact. However, yeast infection is not considered a sexually-transmitted infection because it happens in women who are not sexually active, and *Candida* is naturally present in the vagina. Newborns can also have vaginal inflammation and discharge for the first couple weeks of their life, which is caused by exposure to the mother's estrogen just prior to birth.

Pathophysiology

The vagina is protected against infection by its normal pH 3.5–4.5 which is maintained by the actions of *Lactobacillus acidophilus*, which maintains normal vaginal ecosystem. These bacteria suppress the growth of anaerobes and produce lactic acid that maintains a normal pH.

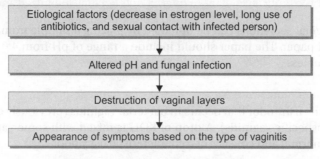

Signs and Symptoms

Bacterial Infection

In some cases, women have no symptoms even if they have a bacterial infection. Generally, bacterial vaginitis causes itching and burning during urination or after sexual intercourse. There may also be whitish discharge with an unpleasant (fishy) odor. The discharge may be more noticeable after sex.

Trichomoniasis Infection

This can be quite severe in some women, whereas others may have no symptoms at all. Trichomoniasis causes vaginal soreness and sometimes abdominal discomfort. It can lead to heavy yellow-green or gray discharge accompanied by an unpleasant odor. Urination and sexual intercourse can be painful. If left untreated during pregnancy, trichomoniasis can lead to premature labor.

Yeast Infections

They include vaginal itching and painful urination. The labia often swell and can be quite sore. There may be a thick and whitish discharge that may look, such as cottage cheese.

Irritant or Allergic Vaginitis

This can cause mild to severe itching or burning of the vagina, which often becomes swollen and red. This type of vaginitis does not cause a vaginal discharge.

Atrophic Vaginitis

This often causes no symptoms. However, some women have dry, sore vaginas, which may be red and irritated. Sexual intercourse is painful and is often followed by a burning feeling. Occasional spotting and watery discharge are common with rectovaginal fistula.

Diagnostic Evaluation

Wet Mount

A vaginitis test called a **wet mount** is used to help diagnose vaginal infections that do not affect the urinary tract. It is also called a "wet prep." The doctor will make patient lie down on the examination table, with her feet in stirrups, such as a regular gynecologic examination. He/she will insert a speculum into the vagina to help him/her see the area. A sterile, moist cotton swab is inserted into the vagina to obtain a sample of vaginal discharge. The swab is then used to transfer the sample onto a slide. The slide is then examined under a microscope to check for infection.

pH Test

The pH of the vaginal secretions can be obtained by placing a sample from the lateral wall of the vagina on pH paper. The paper should include a range of pH from 4.0 to above 5.0. The normal pH is 4.5 or less.

Whiff Test

This is to test for the fishy odor that occurs in bacterial vaginitis (previously called *Gardnerella vaginitis* and nonspecific vaginitis). A drop of KOH is mixed with some vaginal discharge. A positive test is abnormal and consists of a characteristic fishy odor.

Gram Staining

Gram stain of the endocervical mucous may be helpful in the evaluation of cervicitis. An excess of leukocytes (more than 10/hpf) in the endocervical mucous suggests chlamydial cervicitis, and appropriate studies should be obtained.

Pap Smear

In addition to information about cervical cytology, the Pap smear will often add information regarding possible vaginal and cervical pathogens.

Culture Test

Depending on the results of a vaginal culture and without microscopic examination of the secretions, it will result in frequent treatment errors. Nevertheless, cervical cultures may be especially helpful in some cases.

Management

Nonpharmacological Management

The nurse will first consider the history of vaginal infections or sexually transmitted infections and perform a physical or pelvic examination. In case of vaginal discharge, a sample will be sent to the lab for analysis to determine the presence of infection. If infection is ruled out, ask questions about what the chemicals or irritants (e.g., douches or latex condoms) vagina has been exposed to. In some cases, vaginitis can be diagnosed simply by considering a woman's age, as postmenopausal women are prone to irritation of the vaginal lining.

Treatment of Vaginitis

- **Tablets, gels, or creams are used to treat bacterial vaginitis:** Some treatments might not be safe to use with alcohol or during pregnancy. Talk to doctor or pharmacist about how to safely use the medication prescribed. Trichomoniasis requires a single dose of prescription antibiotics, and sexual partners should also be treated at the same time to prevent them from reinfecting each other.
- **Antifungal pills or cream are available for vaginal yeast infections:** It is a good idea to seek doctor's opinion before purchasing nonprescription products. It is especially important to detect whether:
  - It is the first yeast infection.
  - Woman is pregnant or breastfeeding.
  - The treatments tried earlier but did not work.
  - The recurrence of infection.
  - Other signs pelvic pain, fever, or a colored or unpleasant-smelling vaginal discharge.
- **Steroid ointments:** The doctor can also recommend a steroid ointment or cream to reduce the redness, swelling, and itching that can be caused by irritative or allergic vaginitis. Baking soda 4–5 tablespoons should be added to a lukewarm water and have bath in that water. This can provide some relief. It is important to identify the cause of the vaginitis, so that irritants can be avoided in the future.

Tips to keep vaginal skin healthy and prevent noninfectious vaginitis include the following:
- Avoid prolonged moisture and friction, for instance, rubbing vigorously with a towel.
- Do not wear bathing suits or exercise clothes for long periods of time.
- Wear cotton underwear that provides some air flow
- Wear loose-fitting slacks

- Find alternative contraceptives if skin is irritated by lubricated condoms, jellies, creams, or sponges.
- Keep the area around the genitals clean and dry
- Avoid irritants, such as douches, feminine hygiene sprays, deodorized sanitary pads or tampons, and colored or perfumed toilet paper.

Pharmacological Management

The goals of pharmacotherapy in vaginitis are to reduce morbidity, prevent complications, and eradicate the infection. Drugs used for infectious causes of vaginitis may be applied topically or may require oral or parenteral administration.

- **Antibiotics:** It may inhibit bacterial protein synthesis. The antibiotics metronidazole, clindamycin, and tinidazole are used to treat bacterial vaginosis. Depending on the antibiotic that is prescribed, patient may take it by mouth or use it vaginally.
- **Antifungals:** Believed to bind to sterol of the fungal cell membrane, thereby altering cell permeability. Some of the antifungal are fluconazole, clotrimazole, miconazole, etc.
- **Antiprotozoal:** They act by entering into the cells of microorganisms, containing nitroreductase, which interferes and finally causes cell death, e.g., metronidazole. Avoid drinking alcohol during treatment with metronidazole or tinidazole. These medicines can cause severe nausea and vomiting if patients consume alcohol when taking one of them.

Surgical Management

- **Radial hysterectomy:** Radical hysterectomy includes removal of the uterus with parametrial and paracervical tissues, proximal vagina, and proximal uterosacral ligaments. The uterine artery is transected at its origin, lateral to the ureter. In order to complete this dissection, the ureter is unroofed from the paracervical tunnel until the point of entry into the bladder. In order to resect the parametrial and paracervical tissues and unroof the ureter, the paravesical and pararectal spaces must be developed.
- **Vaginectomy:** Partial and total vaginectomy refer to procedures in which the vaginal epithelium is removed without disruption of the adjacent tissues of the paracolpium. Partial vaginectomy may also be utilized to do biopsy of large vaginal lesions of unknown etiology. Radical vaginectomy is performed for pelvic malignancy involving or encroaching upon the vagina. It is rarely indicated. More commonly, at the time of radical hysterectomy for early cervix cancer or endometrial cancer involving the cervix, the upper third (2–3 cm) of the vagina is removed.

Nursing Care Plan

Nursing Assessment

History taking

- Elicit the history of onset and description of symptoms, with particular attention to the nature and amount of vaginal discharge, which may be frothy, thick, or malodorous.
- Question the patient to determine whether the patient is experiencing discomfort, such as external inflammation and pain, and pruritus.
- Patients may describe exertional dysuria, dyspareunia, and vulvular inflammation. Determine the medications that the patient is taking, with particular attention to antibiotics, hormone replacement therapy, and contraceptives.
- Ask about the patient's rest, sleep, nutrition, exercise, and hygiene practices. Ask the patient whether she is pregnant or diabetic, both of which place the patient at risk of vaginitis.

Vaginal examination

Vaginal examination should take place under the following conditions—not on menses, no douching, or vaginal sprays for 24 hours prior to examination, no sexual intercourse without a condom for 24 hours prior to the examination. Physical examination generally reveals some type of discharge, such as frothy, malodorous, greenish-yellow, purulent vaginal discharge (trichomoniasis), thick, cottage cheese like discharge (candidiasis) or malodorous, thin, grayish-white, foul, fishy odor discharge.

Psychological assessment

Psychosocial assessment should include evaluation of the patient's home situation and a sexual history. Ask the patient about the type of contraception her and his partner use. Provide a private environment to allow the patient to answer questions without being embarrassed.

Nursing Diagnosis

1. Risk for infection related to invasion or proliferation of microorganisms
2. Acute pain related to inflammation and subsequent wound care
3. Impaired skin integrity related to the inflammation and drainage from vagina
4. Sexual dysfunction related to change in vaginal structure
5. Self-care deficit related to lack of understanding of perineal care and general health status.

1. Risk of infection related to invasion or proliferation of microorganisms.

Interventions

- Encourage the patient to get adequate rest and nutrition
- Encourage the patient to use appropriate hygiene techniques by wiping from front to back after urinating or defecating
- Teach the patient to avoid wearing tight-fitting clothing (pantyhose, tight pants, or jeans) and to wear cotton underwear rather than synthetics
- Explain to patients that the risk of getting vaginal infections increases if one has sex with more than one person.
- Teach the patient to abstain from sexual intercourse until the infection is resolved

2. Acute pain related to inflammation and subsequent wound care.

Interventions

- Assess the level, intensity, and severity of pain by pain scale
- Provide wet compresses and then using a hair dryer on a cool setting several times a day provides some relief of itching
- Suggest the patient for sitz bath as it provides comfort
- For yeast infections, tepid sodium bicarbonate baths and drying the area may increase comfort during treatment
- Be informed about which sexually transmitted diseases need to be reported to the local health department

3. Impaired skin integrity related to the inflammation and drainage from vagina.

Interventions

- Assess the condition of the skin
- A pressure reducing mattress may be used to prevent pressure ulcers
- Change the position of the patient frequently
- Clothes should be changed every day
- The wound is cleaned everyday with normal saline, antiseptic solutions, etc.

Health Education

Home healthcare guidelines involve teaching the patient how to maintain lifestyle changes with regard to rest, nutrition, and medication management. Make sure that the patient understands all aspects of the treatment regimen with particular attention to taking the full course of medication therapy. Make sure the patient understands the necessity of any follow-up visits.

PELVIC ORGAN PROLAPSE

Common prolapse are cystocele, urethrocele, enterocele, and rectocele. These disorders involve protrusion of an organ into the vaginal canal: cystocele (bladder), urethrocele (urethra), enterocele (small intestine and peritoneum), and rectocele (rectum).

Types of Prolapse

1. **Anterior:** Cystocele, urethrocele
2. **Posterior:** Enterocele, rectocele

Cystocele

It is a downward displacement of the bladder toward the vaginal orifice, resulting from the damage of the anterior vaginal support structures. Cystocele and cystourethrocele commonly develop when the pubocervical vesical fascia is weakened.

Etiology

The origin of cystocele is as follows:
- It usually results from injury and strain during childbirth
- Being overweight or obese
- Repeated lifting of heavy things
- Straining with bowel movements
- A chronic cough or bronchitis

Risk Factors
- **Childbirth:** Women who have vaginally delivered one or more children have a higher risk of anterior prolapse.
- **Aging:** Risk of anterior prolapse increases as you age. This is especially true after menopause, when body's production of estrogen, which helps keep the pelvic floor strong, decreases.
- **Hysterectomy**
- **Obesity:** Women who are overweight or obese are at higher risk of anterior prolapse.

Clinical Manifestations
- Feeling of fullness or pressure in pelvis and vagina
- Discomfort when you strain, cough, bend down, or lift
- A feeling that you have not completely emptied your bladder after urinating
- Repeated bladder infection
- Pain or urinary leakage during sexual intercourse

Rectocele

It is an upward pouching of the rectum that pushes the posterior wall of the vagina forward. The thin wall of fibrous tissue that separates the rectum from the vagina weakens, allowing the vaginal wall to bulge.

Etiology
- Weight on pelvic floor
- Constipation
- Chronic cough or bronchitis
- Repeated lifting of heavy objects
- Being overweight or obese
- Pregnancy and childbirth

Risk Factors
- **Genetics:** Some women are born with weaker connective tissues in the pelvic area, making them naturally more likely to develop posterior prolapse.
- **Childbirth:** Women who have vaginally delivered multiple children have a higher risk of developing posterior prolapse.
- **Aging:** Risk of posterior prolapse increases as they age because the muscle mass is lost and elasticity and nerve functions are also lost, causing the muscles to stretch or weaken.
- **Obesity:** A high body mass index is linked to an increased risk of posterior prolapse. This is likely due to the chronic stress that excess body weight places on the pelvic floor tissues.

Clinical Manifestations
The clinical manifestations of rectocele are the following:
- A soft bulge of the tissue in vagina which may/may not protrude through the vaginal opening
- Difficulty having a bowel movement with the need to press
- Sensation of rectal pressure or fullness
- A feeling that the rectum has not completely emptied after a bowel movement.

Enterocele
Occurs when the small intestine descends into the lower pelvic cavity and pushes the top part of the vagina, creating a bulge.

Etiology
- Pregnancy and childbirth
- Aging
- Chronic constipation or straining with bowel movements
- Chronic cough or bronchitis
- Repeated lifting of heavy objects
- Being overweight or obese

Risk Factors
- **Pregnancy and childbirth:** Vaginal delivery of one or more children contributes to the weakening of pelvic floor support structures, increasing the risk of prolapse. The more pregnancies one has, the greater your risk of developing any type of pelvic organ prolapse.
- **Age:** As the person gets older, she tends to lose muscle mass and muscle strength in pelvic muscles as well as other muscles.
- **Pelvic surgery:** Removal of uterus (hysterectomy) or surgical procedures to treat incontinence may increase the risk of developing small bowel prolapse.
- **Increased abdominal pressure:** Being overweight increases the pressure inside the abdomen, which increases the risk of developing small bowel prolapse.
- **Smoking:** Smoking is associated with developing prolapse because smokers frequently cough, increasing abdominal pressure. Also, smokers may have problems with healing of damaged connective tissues, which can contribute to prolapse.
- **Family history**

Clinical Manifestations
- Feeling of pelvic fullness, pressure or pain
- Low back pain that eases when lying down
- A soft bulge of tissue in the vagina
- Vaginal discomfort and painful intercourse

Urethrocele

It is the prolapse of urethra into the vagina.

Etiology
- Multiple pregnancies and deliveries
- Obesity
- Aging related to muscle changes
- Pelvic tumor
- Excessive strain during bowel movement

Risk Factors
- **Multiple pregnancies and vaginal deliveries:** Women most at risk for this condition are those who have had multiple pregnancies and deliveries.
- **Age:** Decreased muscle tone due to aging, excessive strain during bowel movement, and complications of pelvic surgery have also been associated with prolapse of the uterus.
- Chronic coughing
- Lifting of heavy things

Clinical Manifestation
- Backache
- Perinea pain
- Sense of "heaviness" in the vaginal area
- Pain
- Urinary incontinence

Diagnostic Evaluation
- **History:** Pregnancies, any surgical procedure, family history
- **Pelvic examination:** During the examination, look for a tissue bulge into the vagina and check the strength of the pelvic floor muscle
- **Bladder and urine tests:** To see how well and completely the bladder empties. Run a test on a urine sample to look for signs of a bladder infection.
- **Imaging test:** X-ray or MRI is done to determine the size of tissue bulge
- **Defecography:** To know how efficiently the bladder empties.

Management
- **Pessary:** This device is inserted into the vagina and positioned in such a manner to properly align the organ.
- **Colpexin sphere:** It is an intrauterine device similar to pessary, and it supports the pelvic floor muscles.
- **Kegel exercises:** These involve contracting or tightening of the vaginal muscles and are prescribed to help strengthen these weakened muscles.

Surgical Management
- **Anterior colporrhaphy:** Procedure to repair anterior vaginal wall
- **Perineorrhaphy:** The repair of perinea lacerations.

Nursing Management
Nursing Diagnosis
Acute pain related to pelvic pressure
Interventions
- Encourage period of rest with legs elevated to relieve strain on pelvis
- Psychologically support the patient
- Check for proper placement of pessary
- Advise mild analgesics as prescribed by the physician
- Encourage fluid intake and void frequently to prevent bladder infection

Urinary retention related to displaced organ.
Interventions
- Encourage fluid to decrease bacterial flora in the bladder
- Catheterize the patient if retention is suspected
- Obtain urine sample if infection is suspected

Constipation related to displaced rectum or bowel.
Interventions
- Teach patients to increase the intake fluids and fibers.
- Use stool softeners or bulk laxatives to make easy passage of stool.
- Use of enema may be necessary to prevent straining.

Critical Care Unit

> **AT THE END OF THIS CHAPTER, THE STUDENTS WILL BE LEARN ABOUT:**
> ➤ Principles of critical care nursing
> ➤ Concept of critical care nursing
> ➤ Scope of critical care nursing
> ➤ Role of nurse in critical care unit
> ➤ Organization, physical setup, policies, staffing norms
> ➤ Special equipment, ventilators, cardiac monitors, defibrillators, and cardioversion
> ➤ CPR (see Chapter 22 Emergency and Disaster Nursing)
> ➤ Physical setup of ICU

CONCEPT OF CRITICAL CARE NURSING

Critical care nursing is that specialty within nursing that deals specifically with human responses to life-threatening problems. These problems deal dynamically with human responses to actual or potential life-threatening illnesses.

The framework of critical care nursing is a complex, challenging area of nursing practice that utilizes the nursing process by applying assessment, diagnosis, outcome identification, planning, implementation, and evaluation. The critical care nursing practice is based on a scientific body of knowledge and incorporates specific professional competencies and is focused on restorative, curative, rehabilitative, maintainable, or palliative care, based on identified patient need. It upholds multi- and interdisciplinary collaboration in initiating interventions to restore stability, prevent complications, and achieve and maintain optimal patient responses. The critical care nursing profession requires a clear description of the attributes, guidelines, and nursing practice standards in guiding the critical care nursing practice to fulfill this purpose.

Critical care nursing reflects a holistic approach in patient care. It places great emphasis on caring the biopsycho–social–spiritual nature of human beings and their responses to illnesses rather than the disease process. It helps to maintain the individual patient's identity and dignity. The caring focus includes preventive care, risk factor modification, and education to decrease future patient admission to acute care facilities.

Goals of Critical Care Nursing

The major goals of critical care nursing are the following:

- To promote optimal delivery of safe and quality care to the critically ill patients and their families by providing highly individualized care, so that the physiological dysfunction and the psychological stress in the intensive care unit (ICU) are under control.
- To care for the critically ill patients with a holistic approach, it is necessary to consider the patient's biological, psychological, cultural, and spiritual dimensions regardless of diagnosis or clinical setting.

- To use appropriate and up-to-date knowledge, caring attitude, and clinical skills supported by advanced technology for prevention, early detection, and treatment of complications in order to facilitate recovery.
- To provide palliative care to the critically ill patients in situations where their health status is progressing to unavoidable death.

Scope of Critical Care Nursing

The scope of critical care nursing is defined by the dynamic interaction of the critically ill patient, the critical care nurse and the critical care environment in order to bring about optimal patient outcomes through nursing proficiency within an environment conducive to the provision of this highly specialized care.

Constant intensive assessment, timely critical care interventions, and continuous evaluation of management through multidisciplinary efforts are required to restore stability, prevent complications, and achieve optimal health. Palliative care should be instituted to alleviate pain and sufferings of the patient and family in situations where death is imminent.

Critical care nurses are registered nurses who are trained and qualified to practice critical care nursing. They possess the standard critical care nursing competencies in assuming specialized and expanded roles in caring for the critically ill patients and their family. Likewise, the critical care nurse is personally responsible and committed to continue learning and updating of knowledge and skills. The critical care nurses carry out interventions and collaborate patient care activities to address life-threatening situations that will meet patient's biological, psychological, cultural, and spiritual needs.

The critical care environment constantly supports the interaction between the critically ill patients, their family, and the critical care nurses to achieve the desired patient outcomes. It entails readily available and accessible emergency equipment, sufficient supplies, and effective supporting system to ensure quality patient care as well as staff safety and productivity.

ROLES OF THE CRITICAL CARE NURSES

The roles of critical care nurses are the following:

Care Provider

Direct Patient Care

- Detects and interprets indicators that signify the varying conditions of the critically ill with the assistance of advanced technology and knowledge
- Plans and initiates nursing process to its full capacity in a need-driven and proactive manner
- Acts promptly and judiciously to prevent or halt deterioration when conditions warrant
- Coordinates with other health-care providers in the provision of optimal care to achieve the best possible outcomes.

Indirect Patient Care—Care of the Family

- Understands family needs and provides information to allay fears and anxieties
- Assists family to cope with the life-threatening situation and/or patient's impending death.

Critical care nurses have roles beyond their professional boundary. With proper training and established guidelines, algorithms, and protocols that are continuously reviewed and updated, critical care nurses also perform procedures and therapies that are otherwise done by doctors. Such procedures and therapies are:

- Sampling and analyzing arterial blood gases
- Weaning patients off ventilations

- Adjusting intravenous (IV) analgesia/sedations
- Performing and interpreting electrocardiographs (ECGs)
- Titrating IV and central line medicated infusion and nutrition support
- Initiating defibrillation to patient with ventricular fibrillation (VF) or lethal ventricular tachycardia (VT)
- Removal of pacer wire, femoral sheaths, and chest tubes

Educator

- Provides health education to patient and family to promote understanding and acceptance of the disease process and to facilitate recovery
- Participates in the training and coaching of novice health-care team members to achieve cohesiveness in the delivery of patient care.

Patient Advocate

- Acts in the best interest of the patient
- Monitors and safeguards the quality of care which the patient receives.

Management and Leadership Role

The critical care nurse in management and leadership role will be able to render the following responsibilities:
- Perform management and leadership skills in providing safe and quality care
- Accountability for safe critical care nursing practice
- Delivery of effective health programs and services to critically ill patients in the acute setting
- Management of the critical care nursing unit or acute care setting
- Take lead and supervision among nursing support staff
- Utilize appropriate mechanism for collaboration, networking, linkage–building, and referrals.

Researcher Role

The critical care nurse in her researcher role will be able to render the following responsibilities:
- Engage self in nursing or other health-related research with or under supervision of an experienced researcher.
- Utilize guidelines in the evaluation of research study or report.
- Apply the research process in improving patient care infusing concepts of quality improvement and in partnership with other team players.

PRINCIPALS OF CRITICAL CARE NURSING PRACTICE

The principals of critical care nursing practice are as follows:
- The critical care nurse should function in accordance with legislation, common laws, organizational regulations, and bylaws, which affect nursing practice.
- The critical care nurse should provide care to meet individual patient needs on a 24-hour basis.
- The critical care nurse should competently practice the current critical care nursing.
- The critical care nurse should deliver nursing care in a way that can be ethically justified.
- The critical care nurse should demonstrate accountability for his/her professional judgment and actions.
- The critical care nurse should create and maintain an environment which promotes safety and security of patients, visitors, and staff.

- The critical care nurse should master the use of all essential equipment, available services, and supplies for immediate care of patients.
- The critical care nurse must protect patients from developing environmental-induced infection.
- The critical care nurse must utilize the nursing process in an explicit systematic manner to achieve the goals of care.
- The critical care nurse should carry out health education for promotion and maintenance of health.
- The critical care nurse acts to enhance the professional development of self and others.

PHYSICAL SETUP OF CRITICAL CARE UNIT

Introduction

The development of coronary care units (CCUs) in the mid-20th century was a major advance in cardiology practice as it allowed the concentration of patients with ST elevation myocardial infarction (STEMI) in an area with specialist monitoring, nursing, and medical care. This became particularly important as the medical management of STEMI became more aggressive and specialized.

A CCU or cardiac ICU (CICU) is a hospital ward specialized in the care of patients with heart attacks, unstable angina, cardiac dysrhythmia, and (in practice) various other cardiac conditions that require continuous monitoring and treatment.

Definition

- The CCU is a dedicated cardiac ICU designed to treat patients with acute myocardial infarction (AMI) and other acute cardiac conditions.
- After a heart attack or major cardiac surgery, patients typically are treated in a hospital's cardiac care unit, or CCU, which offers highly specialized care until their condition stabilizes.
- An ICU is for critically ill patients with other types of conditions, and a CCU contains extensive heart monitoring and testing equipment as well as a staff trained and certified in heart conditions and procedures and their aftermath.

Concept of Intermediate Cardiac Care Units

The ICCUs form an essential part of the cardiology service and aim to attend to heart patients who require a higher level of monitoring, nursing care, and medical response than that offered by conventional wards of the cardiology service but whose risk does not justify using the technical and human resources of a care unit (CU). This suggests that these units should have the equipment (continuous monitoring system and equipment for emergency cardiac care), staff (nurses training in cardiology with a sufficiently high ratio of nurses per bed), and a setup such that, in emergencies, they can temporarily offer medical and nursing care similar to those of CU through specifically defined care protocols.

History

The CCUs were developed in the 1960s when it became clear that cardiopulmonary resuscitation (CPR) and medical measures performed under close monitoring by specially trained staff could reduce the mortality from complications of cardiovascular disease. The first description of a CCU was given in 1961 to the British Thoracic Society, and the first CCU was located at the Toronto General Hospital in 1965. Early CCUs were also located in Sydney, Kansas city, and Philadelphia. Studies published in 1967 revealed that those observed in a coronary care setting had consistently better outcomes.

Types of Coronary Care Unit

Acute coronary care: Acute CCUs (ACCUs), also called "critical CCUs" (CCCUs) is equivalent to intensive care in the level of service provided. Patients with AMI, cardiogenic shock, or postoperative "open-heart" patients commonly abide here.

Subacute coronary care: Subacute CCUs (SCCUs), also called progressive care units (PCUs), intermediate CCUs (ICCUs), or step-down units, and provide a level of care intermediate to that of the ICU and that of the general medical floor. These units typically serve patients who require cardiac telemetry, such as those with unstable angina.

What Happens in the CCU?

Now we should understand how a CCU is different from the ICU. The following list clearly provides the differences:

- Like normal ICUs, CCUs are designed to limit stress to patients during the initial, critical phase of their treatment. Visitors are typically restricted to immediate family members, and visiting hours are often limited to two or three short periods of time daily. Food and other items brought from outside the hospital, such as plants and flowers, are usually prohibited as well. Patients in CCUs tend to be on supervised diets, and plants can introduce potential infection-causing bacteria into the environment.
- Often patients are hooked up to wires and tubes during their CCU stays, which can prove disconcerting to family members but is necessary for close monitoring. All patients are connected to heart monitors, and some patients also require ventilators to assist their breathing. Additionally, a variety of tests are often done during a stay in the CCU, such as blood work or ECGs, which measures the electrical activity of the heart. Many different cardiac medications may be given, including those to treat heart failure or to reduce the workload of the heart.
- Stress-inducing noise, however, can be a hard-to-control problem in CCUs. Many medical devices, including heart monitors and respirators, emit periodic beeps and buzzes, and the around-the-clock movement of medical personnel through the unit can make the CCU less restful than intended.

Characteristics of Coronary Care Unit

The main feature of coronary care is the availability of telemetry or the continuous monitoring of the cardiac rhythm by ECG. This allows early intervention with medication, cardioversion, or defibrillation, improving the prognosis. As arrhythmias are relatively common in this group, patients with myocardial infarction or unstable angina are routinely admitted to the CCU. For other indications, such as atrial fibrillation (AF), a specific indication is generally necessary, while for others, such as heart block, CCU admission is standard.

Importance of Acute Cardiac Care

Roughly 30% of the acute medical take is comprised of patients with a primary cardiac problem. The majority of these acute cardiac patients are admitted to district general hospitals, under the initial care of acute or general physicians. Advantage of primary percutaneous coronary intervention (PPCI) centers has had little impact on this, as STEMI patients comprise a limited and decreasing proportion of the acute cardiac workload.

- Patients presenting with cardiac conditions managed in specialized cardiac wards have demonstrably better outcomes.
- A significant proportion of these patients are not currently managed within a cardiac service, leading to a greater morbidity and mortality, and cost to the NHS.

- Patients presenting with acute cardiac conditions should be managed by a specialist, multidisciplinary cardiac team and have access to key cardiac investigations and interventions, at all times.
- All hospitals admitting unselected acute medical patients should have an appropriately sized, staffed, and equipped ACCU, where high-risk patients with a primary cardiac diagnosis should be managed.
- All high-risk cardiac patients must have access to ACCUs, and access should not be restricted to patients with acute coronary syndrome (ACS).

UNIT MODELS

Model Integrated into the Intensive Cardiac Care Unit

According to this model, the ICCUs and CUs are located in the same physical space. In this type of unit, care resources are assigned according to the severity and progression of the patients, and the care resources stay in the same place throughout the process until they are moved to the conventional hospital ward. The advantage of this model is that it favors continuity in care and minimizes how often patients are moved. It also allows for the training of nursing staff and maintains a high standard. In contrast, it makes selection of patients with direct admission criteria to intermediate care units more difficult; increases equipment costs, complicates staff management because of the range of types of patient, and is less convenient for the patients. For these reasons, this is the least recommended model for intermediate cardiac care although it may be more appropriate for surgical units.

Model with the Unit Adjacent to the Intensive Cardiac Care Unit

In this model, the intermediate care unit is in close proximity to the CU, so that care resources can be shared. Although such units were originally created with the idea of easing the burden on the CUs, they are currently designed to ensure continuity in the levels of care and to attend to patients who may have to be admitted directly to these units. Unlike the previous model, their physical separation from the CU provides more comfortable and private surroundings for the patients. With the proximity of the CU, transfer of patients who present with a sudden complication is made easier. This model is suitable for cardiology services that have their own CU.

Model Integrated into the Cardiology Ward

In this model, the unit is located within but structurally differentiated from the cardiology ward of the hospital. The unit is sufficiently well equipped and staffed in accordance with its needs as described in the section on infrastructure. Like the previous model, its main advantage is that it is a flexible unit that allows direct admission, thus reducing the number of admissions to the ICUs and ensuring continuity in care. The cases admitted are predictable, controllable, and homogeneous, thereby facilitating resource management and staff training. The advantages of these units disappear if they are very small, as the nursing staff would be similar to that of ICUs, resulting in lost efficiency, and savings in human resources would no longer be made. This model is the most appropriate one in hospitals in which the coronary unit does not belong to the cardiology service.

INFRASTRUCTURE OF INTERMEDIATE CORONARY CARE UNITS

The infrastructure of ICCUs must be appropriate for the target group of patients. The patients with indications for admission to these units basically need:

- More medical and nursing care because their management is more complex (IV medication that affects vital functions, such as vasodilators, antiarrhythmic, inotropic agents).
- Constant monitoring by the nursing staff because of the higher risk of arrhythmias, sudden and profound hemodynamic changes, and clinical instability (angina, heart failure) as a result of disease progression or effects of the medication they are receiving.
- More instrumentation and an appropriate physical space. However, these patients do not need intensive care or other complex techniques or devices (invasive mechanical respiration, dialysis, ultrafiltration, mechanical circulatory assistance, or invasive monitoring) to be properly managed to sustain their clinical state. Likewise their clinical state is such that their life is not at immediate risk.

Physical Structure

The physical structure of coronary units is listed below:

The physical structure of the units should be functional—not rigid or hermetic—and adapted to the architectural characteristics of their hospital to maximize operational efficiency. The following structural considerations apply:

- The physical structure of the ICCU should be integrated into the cardiology service. It should be located next or near to the CU and/or the conventional hospital ward of the cardiology service.
- A traditional requirement of all the units with specialized care has been that the layout allows a direct line of sight between the patients and the normal work stations of the nursing staff. Such arrangements limit the privacy of the patients (large rooms with boxes separated in different ways) and reduce the comfort. At present, the situation has changed substantially. On the one hand, the need for comfort and a relaxed and quiet atmosphere of the patients who need to be admitted to these units is recognized as an inherent part of their treatment. On the other hand, most patients admitted to these units do not require a direct line of sight for sufficient monitoring of their clinical state, given that monitoring of vital signs can provide sufficient information. At present, high-quality and cheap video surveillance systems are available. Therefore, there is no reason not to structure the ICCU into individual rooms; in fact, such an arrangement is preferable.
- The rooms of the ICCU must be readily accessible for the health professionals, and it must be possible to readily move beds and equipment (resuscitation trolley, portable X-ray equipment, etc.) at times of emergency. The doors should be wide (approximately 1.5 m). The rooms should also be sufficiently soundproofed and air-conditioned, preferably with windows with natural light.
- The rooms should be large enough to deal with emergencies and it is recommended that they have 15 m^2 of usable space (and certainly not <12 m^2) in the case of single rooms and approximately 25 m^2 in the case of double rooms. They should have an appropriately designed en-suite bathroom. The doors should be wide and open outward.
- The rooms should have a bedside call button/alarm and one in the bathroom that the patients can use easily, and the tone should preferably be different to the emergency alarm used by the staff.
- There should be at least one connection to the oxygen supply and one vacuum line per patient.
- The ICCU should have a spacious working area for nursing staff (control area) where the center for monitoring vital signs and, if required, closed-circuit television screens for monitoring the patients are located. Likewise, the ICCU should have staff rest areas, offices for medical staff, and a room for attending to family members, either for exclusive use or shared with other units (CU or hospital ward), depending the size of the unit.

- The electrical system of the ICCU should be compliant with the current legislation for specialized hospital units, which requires connection to their own power generators and, if possible, to a continuous power supply system. As for other areas of the hospital, the unit should have its own disaster management plan for a planned evacuation.

Diagnostic Requirements for Acute Cardiac Care/Equipment

Electrocardiography

Electrocardiography is a basic tool in cardiovascular medicine; it should be immediately available on every unit, performed by someone with formal training in ECG lead placement, and read by someone of suitable experience in interpretation. Likewise continuous ECG monitoring is required for patients judged to be at risk of cardiac arrhythmias after an acute cardiac presentation. The facility for central monitoring is an important component of every CCU. The provision of telemetry elsewhere in the hospital allows extended expert remote monitoring for patients whose primary problem may not be cardiac but in whom cardiac complications are possible.

Imaging

X-ray Fluoroscopy

All ACCUs should ideally have access to emergency fluoroscopy for temporary transvenous pacing and positioning of IABPs at all times. The C-arm should be operated by a radiographer experienced in its use and with the requirements for temporary pacing. Where not available at present, a formal network solution must be in place to offer these services.

Coronary Angiography Suite

Not all hospitals offering acute cardiac care services run a coronary angiography suite. The ACS patients managed in such units must be transferred to centers possessing the capability of coronary angiography and percutaneous coronary intervention (PCI).

Some hospitals have access to coronary angiography facilities in either a dedicated cardiac laboratory or a shared vascular cardiac facility, but without the capability of performing PCI. Other hospitals may perform PCI during normal working hours only, covering out of hours for complications. Some centers (or occasionally linked hospitals) provide a full PPCI service.

Transthoracic Echocardiography

The provision of cardiac ultrasound is fundamental to the diagnosis of many heart diseases but in particular acute heart failure, suspected cardiac tamponade, complications postmyocardial infarction, acute valvular heart disease including endocarditis, and acute disease of the ascending aorta.

Transthoracic echocardiography (TTE) of suitable quality should be available to all patients who require it. Where this is not currently achievable and in particular where patients may require urgent or emergent out-of-hours scanning a formal network protocol for emergency echocardiography must be in place.

Out-of-hours TTE should not be undertaken by junior members of the medical team unless they have British Society of Echocardiography (BSE) accreditation, have undergone a documented locally approved competency assessment, or can have the images rapidly reviewed by someone with the appropriate expertise.

Transesophageal Echocardiography

Transesophageal echocardiography (TEE) is a vital tool in the assessment of a variety of cardiac diagnosis. Within the context of acute care the most frequent indications are in the diagnosis of endocarditis and in searching for structural complications, to rule out intracardiac thrombus particularly in the setting of AF and in the assessment of acute aortic disease.

Good quality TEE should be available to all patients who require it. Where this is not achievable and in particular where patients may require out-of-hours TEE, a network solution should be in place.

As with TTE, the appropriate governance and quality assurance arrangements should be in place for both in-hours and out-of-hours TEE.

Functional Cardiac Assessment or Advanced Anatomical Imaging

Despite the increased use of other assessment modalities for ischemic heart disease, exercise ECG remains a vital investigation for acute assessment of patients with a variety of heart diseases and should be available in every unit. However, the advanced assessment of cardiac function either in relation to reversible ischemia or myocardial viability is vital in the assessment and triage of complex coronary patients, particularly in those with complex presentations. Local expertise varies between hospitals, but a modern cardiac assessment unit would be expected to have access to stress echocardiography, nuclear perfusion imaging, or cardiac magnetic resonance imaging (MRI) and preferably more than one of these modalities. Cardiac-gated computer tomography (CT) scanning is an emerging technology. It is main use is currently in the diagnosis of chronic chest pain and particularly in the exclusion of coronary artery disease (CAD) in low-risk individuals.

Cardiac Device Management

With the increasing use and complexity of cardiac devices, it is important that all units are able to manage device complications out of hours and program and interrogate devices in hours. Where an out-of-hours service is not available, a formal network solution should be in place.

1. **Brady pacing:** To check pacing and sensing (thresholds, under- and oversensing) and to detect arrhythmic events from pacemaker recordings
2. **Automatic internal cardiac defibrillator (AICD):** Override the device in the appropriate clinical context (e.g., VT storm), diagnose inappropriate shocks, check pacing and sensing (both thresholds, under- and oversensing), deactivate the device in the case of terminal care or dying patients, and deliver an emergency shock via the device.
3. **Biventricular devices:** To check pacing and sensing (both thresholds under- and oversensing) and deactivate coronary sinus lead in the case of significant diaphragmatic pacing.
4. **Implantable loop recorders:** Device interrogation.

Electrophysiological Studies and Radiofrequency Ablation

Electrophysiological study and ablation are becoming a major component of the management of acute arrhythmias. At present, they remain specialist services and as such fall outside the expectations of a general ACCU. Protocols should be in place for the emergency transfer of patients to a unit providing electrophysiology (EP)/radiofrequency (RF).

Laboratory-based Diagnostics

- The use of biomarkers is now a vital component in the diagnosis of non-ST-segment-elevation acute coronary syndrome and increasing heart failure. All ACCUs should have access to urgent troponin assessment, whether this be troponin I, troponin T, or high-sensitivity troponin T. These biomarkers should be provided by a locally agreed protocol and with an acceptable margin of error.

- Likewise serum natriuretic peptides (BNPs or NTpro-terminal BNP) are increasingly important, and there is good evidence for their use in triage for patients admitted with suspected heart failure.
- Where near patient testing is integrated into care, rather than laboratory tests, it should be with appropriate evidence of accuracy and regular calibration.

Human Resources

Suitably qualified and trained staffs are essential to ensure that the ICCUs run as smoothly as the CUs.

Medical Staff

There should be a person in charge of the unit who is responsible for organization, clinical management, and training programs for the other staff. This person should be a specialist in cardiology with appropriate experience in managing acute heart disease. Like the person in charge, the staff physicians should also be cardiology specialists. It is recommended to regularly rotate the staff physicians of this unit, those of the CU of the cardiology service, and/or other physicians in the cardiology service, particularly those responsible for continued care. This aspect should be adapted to each specific situation according to the characteristics of each cardiology service, but in general, rotation is considered advantageous, not only from the point of view of training those who form part of the service and are on call, but also because these rotations motivate staff and strengthen commitment to the institution. With regard to the number of cardiologists, the recent guidelines published by the Working Group on Acute Cardiac Care of the European Society of Cardiology recommend one physician for every six beds. If the unit has more than 12 beds, then the recommendation is one physician for every 8 beds. This number could well vary according to the functional setup of the cardiology service.

To ensure continuous medical care, a cardiologist should be on call 24 hours in the hospital. However, it is not deemed necessary—given the characteristics of the patients who should be admitted to this type of unit—that this physician is always present in the unit and he or she could be assigned other tasks related to continuous cardiac care. The structure of the duty roster should be adapted to the characteristics of the hospital, the cardiology service, the CU, and the ICCU.

Level I

The level I features are listed as follows:
- It is recommended for small district hospital, small private nursing homes, and rural centers
- Ideally six to eight beds
- Provides resuscitation and short-term cardiorespiratory support including defibrillation and arterial blood gas (ABG) test desirable
- It should be able to ventilate a patient for at least 24 to 48 hours and noninvasive monitoring, such as SPO_2, HR and rhythm (ECG), noninvasive blood pressure (NIBP), temperature, etc.
- Able to have arrangements for safe transport of the patients to secondary or tertiary centers
- The staff should be encouraged to do short training courses, such as fundamental critical care support (FCCS) or ICU course
- In charge should be preferably a knowledgeable, trained doctor in ICU technology

- Blood bank support
- Should have basic clinical laboratory [complete blood count (CBC), blood sugar (BS), electrolyte, liner function test (LFT), and right function test (RFT)] and imaging backup [X-ray and ultrasonography (USG)], ECG.

Level II

- Recommended for larger general hospitals
- Bed strength of 6–12
- Director be a trained/qualified intensivist
- Multisystem life support
- Invasive ventilation and noninvasive ventilation (NIV)
- Invasive monitoring
- Long-term ventilation ability
- Access to ABG, electrolytes, and other routine diagnostic support for 24 hours
- Strong microbiology support with facility for fungal identification desirable
- Nurses and duty doctors should be trained in critical care
- Computed tomography must, and MRI desirable
- Protocols and policies for ICUs are observed
- Research will be highly recommended
- Should be supported ideally by cardiology and other super specialties of medicine and surgery
- High dependency unit (HDU) facility will be desirable
- Blood banking

Level III

- Recommended for tertiary-level hospitals
- Bed strength 10–16 with one or multiple ICUs per the requirement of the institution
- Headed by intensivist
- Preferably closed ICU
- Protocols and policies are observed
- Have all recent methods of monitoring, invasive and noninvasive including continuous cardiac output, central venous sample monitoring, etc.
- Long-term acute care of highest standards; intra- and interhospital transport facilities available
- Multisystem care and referral available for 24 hours
- Should become lead centers for Indian Diploma in Critical Care Course (IDCC) and fellowship courses
- Bedside X-ray, USG, 2D echo should be available
- Own or outsourced CT scan and MRI facilities should be available
- Bedside bronchoscopy
- Bedside dialysis and other forms of renal replacement therapy (RRT) available
- Adequately supported by blood banks and blood component therapy
- Optimum patient/nurse ratio is maintained
- Protocols observed about prevention of infection
- Provision for research and participation in National and International research programs
- Patient area should not be <100 sq. ft per patient
- Doctors, nurses, and other support staff should be continuously updated in newer technologies and have updated knowledge in critical care.

Staffing Pattern of Critical Care Unit

- Intensivist
- Resident doctors
- Nurses
- Respiratory therapists
- Nutritionist
- Physiotherapist
- Technicians, computer programmers
- Biomedical engineer
- Clinical pharmacist
- Other support staff, such as cleaning staff, etc.

ADVANCE PROCEDURES IN INTENSIVE CARE UNIT

Cardioversion and Defibrillator

Introduction

Electrical cardioversion has now become a routine procedure and is used electively or emergently to terminate cardiac arrhythmias. The delivered shock in both defibrillation and cardioversion causes electric current to go from the negative to the positive electrode of the defibrillator, passing the heart on its way. It causes all the heart cells to contract simultaneously, thereby interrupting and terminating the abnormal electrical rhythm without damaging the heart and thus allowing the sinus node to resume normal pacemaker activity.

Definition

- Cardioversion is a procedure that can restore a fast or irregular heartbeat to a normal rhythm. A fast or irregular heartbeat is called arrhythmia.
- Arrhythmias can prevent heart from pumping enough blood to body. They also can raise the risk of stroke, heart attack, and sudden cardiac arrest.

Indications

- Supraventricular tachycardia
- Atrial fibrillation
- Atrial flutter
- Ventricular tachycardia
- Any patient with re-entrant tachycardia with narrow or wide QRS complex (ventricular rate >150) who is unstable (e.g., chest pain, pulmonary edema, hypotension).

Indications for defibrillation include the following:
- Pulseless VT
- Ventricular fibrillation
- Cardiac arrest due to or resulting in VF

Types of Cardioversion

Cardioversion can be "chemical" or "electrical."
a. **Chemical cardioversion:** It refers to the use of antiarrhythmia medications to restore the heart's normal rhythm, such as amiodarone, diltiazem, verapamil, and metoprolol.
b. **Electrical cardioversion** (also known as "direct-current" or DC cardioversion): It is a procedure whereby a synchronized electrical shock is delivered through the chest wall to

the heart through special electrodes or paddles that are applied to the skin of the chest and back.

Contraindications

- Dysrhythmias due to enhanced automaticity, such as in digitalis toxicity and catecholamine-induced arrhythmia
- Multifocal atrial tachycardia.

For dysrhythmias due to enhanced automaticity, such as in digitalis toxicity and catecholamine-induced arrhythmia, a homogeneous depolarization state already exists. Therefore, cardioversion is not only ineffective but also associated with a higher incidence of postshock VT/VF.

Anesthesia

- Cardioversion is almost always performed under induction or sedation (short-acting agent, such as midazolam). The only exceptions are if the patient is hemodynamically unstable or if cardiovascular collapse is imminent.
- Defibrillation is an emergent maneuver and when necessary should be promptly performed in conjunction with or prior to the administration of induction or sedative agents.

Equipment

- Defibrillators [automated external defibrillators (AEDs), semiautomated AED, standard defibrillators with monitors]
- Paddle or adhesive patch
- Conductive gel or paste
- Electrocardiograph monitor with recorder
- Oxygen equipment
- Intubation kit
- Emergency pacing equipment

The use of handheld paddle electrodes may be more effective than self-adhesive patch electrodes. The success rates are slightly higher for patients assigned to paddled electrodes because these handheld electrodes improve electrode-to-skin contact and reduce the transthoracic impedance.

Positioning

Paddle placement on the chest wall has two conventional positions, namely, anterolateral and anteroposterior.

In the anterolateral position, a single paddle is placed on the left fourth or fifth intercostal space on the midaxillary line. The second paddle is placed just to the right of the sternal edge on the second or third intercostal space.

In the anteroposterior position, a single paddle is placed to the right of the sternum, as above, and the other paddle is placed between the tip of the left scapula and the spine. An anteroposterior electrode position is more effective than the anterolateral position for external cardioversion of persistent AF. The anteroposterior approach is also preferred in patients with implantable devices to avoid shunting current to the implantable device and damaging its system.

Technique

Emergent application, which may be lifesaving and elective cardioversion should be used cautiously, with attention to patient selection and proper techniques. Repetitive, futile attempts at direct current cardioversion should be avoided.

Advanced cardiac life support (ACLS) measures should be instituted in preparing the patient, such as obtaining IV access and preparing airway management equipment, sedative drugs, and a monitoring device.

Before Procedure

Before undergoing the technique, patients will have to be prepared in the following manner:

- Patient cannot have any food or drinks for about 12 hours before cardioversion.
- Patient is at higher risk for dangerous blood clots during and after a cardioversion. The procedure can dislodge blood clots that have formed as the result of an arrhythmia.
- Doctor may prescribe anticlotting medicine to prevent dangerous clots. Doctor may recommend that the patient take this medicine for several weeks before and after the cardioversion procedure.
- To find out whether the patient needs anticlotting medicine, the patient might have to undergo TEE before the cardioversion. Transesophageal echocardiography is a special type of ultrasound. An ultrasound is a test that uses sound waves to look at the organs and structures in the body.
- Transesophageal echocardiography involves a flexible tube with a device at its tip that sends sound waves. Doctor will guide the tube down the throat and into the esophagus (the passage leading from the patient's mouth to stomach). Medicines will be given to the patient to make him or her sleep during the procedure.
- Doctor will place the tube close to heart, and the sound waves will create pictures of heart. Doctor will look at these pictures to see whether the patient has any blood clots.
- Transesophageal echocardiography will be done at the same time as the cardioversion or just before the procedure. If the doctor finds blood clots, he or she may delay cardioversion for a few weeks. During this time, patient is advised to take anticlotting medicine.
- Even if no blood clots are found, doctor may prescribe anticlotting medicine during and after the cardioversion to prevent the formation of dangerous blood clots.
- Before the cardioversion procedure, patients must be given medicine to sleep. This medicine can affect the patients' awareness when they wake up. So someone has to accompany the patient to hospital and back home.

During Cardioversion

- A nurse or technician will stick soft pads called electrodes on the patient's chest and possibly on the back also. He or she may need to shave some areas on the patient's skin to get the pads to stick.
- The electrodes will be attached to a cardioversion machine. The machine will record the patient's heart's electrical activity and send low-energy shocks through the pads to restore a normal heart rhythm.
- Nurse will use a needle to insert an IV line into a vein in arm. Through this line, the patient gets medicine to fall asleep.
- While the patient is asleep, a cardiologist (heart specialist) will send one or more low-energy electrical shocks to heart. The patient would not feel any pain from the shock.

After Cardioversion

- Health-care team will closely watch patient after the procedure for any signs of complications. Doctor or nurse will let you know when patient can go home. Patients are likely to be discharged home the same day after the procedure.

- Patients may feel drowsy for several hours after the cardioversion because of the medicine used to make the patients sleep. Patients should not drive or operate heavy machinery on the day of the procedure.
- Patients need to arrange for someone to drive them back home from the hospital. Until the medicine wears off, it may also affect patients' awareness and the ability to make decisions.
- After cardioversion, patients may have some redness or soreness on chest where the electrodes were placed. This may last for a few days after the procedure. Patient may also have slight bruising or soreness at the site where the IV line was inserted.
- Doctors will likely prescribe anticlotting medicine for several weeks after the procedure to prevent blood clots. During this time, patients may also take medicine to prevent repeat arrhythmias.

Synchronized cardioversion is a low-energy shock that uses a sensor to deliver electricity that is synchronized with the peak of the QRS complex (the highest point of the R wave). When the "sync" option is engaged on a defibrillator and the shock button pushed, there will be a delay in the shock. During this delay, the machine reads and synchronizes with the patient's ECG rhythm. This occurs so that the shock can be delivered with the peak of the R-wave in the patient's QRS complex. The most common indications for synchronized cardioversion are unstable AF, atrial flutter, atrial tachycardia, and supraventricular tachycardia. If medications fail in the stable patient with the before mentioned arrhythmias, synchronized cardioversion will most likely be indicated.

Unsynchronized cardioversion is a high-energy shock that is delivered as soon as the shock button is pushed on a defibrillator. This means that the shock may fall randomly anywhere within the cardiac cycle (QRS complex). Unsynchronized cardioversion (defibrillation) is used when there is no coordinated intrinsic electrical activity in the heart (pulseless VT/VF) or the defibrillator fails to synchronize in an unstable patient.

DEFIBRILLATOR

Introduction

Defibrillation is a common treatment of life-threatening cardiac dysrhythmias, VF, and pulse less VT. Defibrillation consists of delivering a therapeutic dose of electrical energy to the heart with a device called defibrillator. This depolarizes a critical mass of the heart muscle, terminates the dysrhythmia, and allows normal sinus rhythm to be re-established by the body's natural pacemaker, in the sinoatrial node of the heart. Defibrillators can be external, transvenous, or implanted, depending on the type of device used or needed. Some external units, known as AEDs, automate the diagnosis of treatable rhythms, meaning that lay responders or bystanders are able to use them successfully with little or no training at all.

Definition

Defibrillation is the treatment of immediately life-threatening arrhythmias with which the patient does not have a pulse, i.e., VF or pulseless VT.

Types of Defibrillators

1. **Manual external defibrillator:** The health-care provider will then decide what charge (in Joules) to use, based on the proven guidelines and experience, and will deliver the shock through paddles or pads on the patient's chest. As they require detailed medical knowledge, these units are generally only found in hospitals and on some ambulances.

2. **Manual internal defibrillator:** These are the direct descendants of the work of Beck and Lown. They are virtually identical to the external version, except that the charge is delivered through internal paddles in direct contact with the heart. These are almost exclusively found in operating theaters (rooms), where the chest is likely to be open or can be opened quickly by a surgeon.

3. **Implantable cardioverter-defibrillator (ICD):** Also known as AICD. These devices are implants similar to pacemakers (and many can also perform the pacemaking function). The device is programmed in such a manner that it constantly monitors the patient's heart rhythm and automatically administer shocks for various life-threatening arrhythmias. Many modern devices can distinguish between VF, VT, and more benign arrhythmias, such as supraventricular tachycardia and AF. Some devices may attempt overdrive pacing prior to synchronized cardioversion. When the life-threatening arrhythmia is VF, the device is programmed to proceed immediately to an unsynchronized shock.

4. **Wearable cardiac defibrillator:** A development of the AICD is a portable external defibrillator that is worn like a vest. The unit monitors the patient 24 hours a day and will automatically deliver a biphasic shock if needed. This device is mainly indicated in patients awaiting an implantable defibrillator.

5. **Modeling defibrillator:** The efficacy of a cardiac defibrillator is highly dependent on the position of its electrodes. Most internal defibrillators are implanted in octogenarians, but a few children need the devices. Implanting defibrillators in children is particularly difficult because children are small, will grow over time, and possess cardiac anatomy that differs from that of adults. Recently, researchers were able to create a software modeling system capable of mapping an individual's thorax and determining the optimal position for an external or internal cardiac defibrillator. With the help of the pre-existing surgical planning applications, the software uses myocardial voltage gradients to predict the likelihood of successful defibrillation. According to the critical mass hypothesis, defibrillation is effective only if it produces a threshold voltage gradient in a large fraction of the myocardial mass. Usually a gradient of 3–5 V/cm is needed in 95% of the heart. Voltage gradients of over 60 V/cm can damage tissue. The modeling software seeks to obtain safe voltage gradients above the defibrillation threshold. Early simulations using the software suggest that small changes in electrode positioning can have large effects on defibrillation; and despite engineering hurdles that remain, the modeling system promises to help guide the placement of implanted defibrillators in children and adults.

Difference between Monophasic and Biphasic Systems

- In monophasic systems, the current travels only in one direction—from one paddle to the other.
- In biphasic systems, the current travels toward the positive paddle and then reverses and goes back; and this occurs several times.
- Biphasic shocks deliver one cycle every 10 milliseconds.
- They are associated with fewer burns and less myocardial damage.
- With monophasic shocks, the rate of first shock success in cardiac arrests due to a shockable rhythm is only 60%; whereas with biphasic shocks, this increases to 90%.
- However, this efficacy of biphasic defibrillators over monophasic defibrillators has not been consistently reported.

Energy Levels for Defibrillation

The energy levels required for the two types of defibrillation are as listed below:
- **Monophasic:** The CPR algorithm recommends single shocks started at and repeated at 360 J.

- **Biphasic:** The CPR algorithm recommends shocks initially of 150–200 J and subsequent shocks of 150–360 J.

Complications

The complications involved in defibrillation are as follows:
- Dysrhythmias pulmonary edema
- Cardiac arrest pulmonary or systemic emboli
- Respiratory arrest due to equipment malfunction
- Neurologic impairment death
- Altered skin integrity

Precautions

- Check all equipment for proper grounding to prevent current leakage
- Disconnect temporary pacemaker and other electrical equipment
- Do not defibrillate directly over an implanted pacemaker. Defibrillation may result in damage to equipment.

Nursing Considerations

- May be mistaken for artifact or leads may be off
- Assess situation. If a second person is getting the defibrillator, establish an airway and begin CPR
- Convert to pediatric size for children or internal if the patient has an open chest
- Enhance electrical conduction through subcutaneous tissue and assist in minimizing burns
- Limit to paddle area. Use 2 J/kg for children
- Will not fire if it is in synchronous mode due to the absence of R wave
- Establish a visual recording and a permanent record of current ECG status and response to intervention
- Defibrillation is achieved by passing an electric current through cardiac muscle mass to restore a single source of impulse generation. Decreases transthoracic resistance and improves flow of current across axis of heart.
- This will charge unit with current
- Maintain safety to caregivers, since electric current can be conducted from the patient to another individual if contact occurs
- The ECG rhythm may change; ensure it is a rhythm that requires defibrillation
- Premature release may result in failure to discharge energy. May also be delivered by depressing discharge button on the defibrillator
- If rhythm is converted, then reassessment is a must
- Immediate action increases the chance for successful depolarization of cardiac muscle. Transthoracic resistance decreases by approximately 8% with the second shock
- Immediate action increases the chance of successful depolarization of cardiac muscle. "Stacked shocks" sequence is more important than adjunctive drug therapy and delays between shocks to deliver medications are detrimental
- It is necessary to maintain the delivery of oxygenated blood to vital organs
- Conductive gel accumulated on defibrillator paddles impedes surface contact and increases transthoracic resistance.

MECHANICAL VENTILATION

Mechanical ventilation is a method to mechanically assist or replace spontaneous breathing. This may involve a machine called a ventilator or the breathing may be assisted by a physician, respiratory therapist, or other suitable person compressing a bag or set of bellows.

Mechanical ventilator device functions as a substitute for the bellow action of the thoracic cage and diaphragm. The mechanical ventilator can maintain ventilation automatically for prolonged periods. It is indicated when the patient is unable to maintain safe levels of oxygen or carbon dioxide by spontaneous breathing even with the assistance of other oxygen delivery devices.

Types of Mechanical Ventilation

The two types of mechanical ventilation are the following:
1. Invasive ventilation
2. Noninvasive ventilation

Modes of Mechanical Ventilation

The two main modes of mechanical ventilation are the following:
1. Positive pressure ventilation, where air (or another gas mix) is pushed into the trachea
2. Negative pressure ventilation, where air is essentially sucked into the lungs

Indications for Use

Mechanical ventilation is indicated when the patient's spontaneous ventilation is inadequate to maintain life. It is also indicated as prophylaxis for imminent collapse of other physiologic functions or ineffective gas exchange in the lungs. Because mechanical ventilation only serves to provide assistance for breathing and does not cure a disease, the patient's underlying condition should be correctable and should resolve over time. In addition, other factors must be taken into consideration because mechanical ventilation is not without its complications.

Common Medical Indications

- Acute lung injury [including acute respiratory distress syndrome (ARDS), trauma]
- Apnea with respiratory arrest, including cases from intoxication
- Chronic obstructive pulmonary disease (COPD)
- Acute respiratory acidosis with partial pressure of carbon dioxide (pCO_2) >50 mm Hg and pH <7.25, which may be due to paralysis of the diaphragm due to Guillain-Barré syndrome, myasthenia gravis, spinal cord injury, or the effect of anesthetic and muscle relaxant drugs.
- Increased work of breathing as evidenced by significant tachypnea, retractions, and other physical signs of respiratory distress
- Hypoxemia with arterial partial pressure of oxygen (PaO_2) <55 mm Hg with supplemental fraction of inspired oxygen (FiO_2) = 1.0
- Hypotension including sepsis, shock, or congestive heart failure
- Neurological diseases, such as muscular dystrophy and amyotrophic lateral sclerosis.

Application and Duration

It can be used as a short-term measure, for example, during an operation or critical illness (often in the setting of an ICU). It may be used at home or in a nursing or rehabilitation institution if patients have chronic illnesses that require long-term ventilator assistance. Owing to the anatomy of the human pharynx, larynx, and esophagus and the circumstances for which ventilation is required then additional measures are often required to secure the airway during positive pressure ventilation to allow unimpeded passage of air into the trachea and avoid air passing into the esophagus and stomach. Commonly this is achieved by insertion of a tube into the trachea which provides a clear route for the air. This can be either an endotracheal tube, inserted through the natural openings of mouth or nose or a tracheostomy inserted through an artificial opening in the neck. In other circumstances simple airway maneuvers, an oropharyngeal airway, or laryngeal mask airway (LMA) may be employed. If the patient is able to protect his or her own airway and NIV or negative-pressure ventilation is used then an airway adjunct may not be needed.

CLASSIFICATION OF VENTILATORS

Negative-Pressure Ventilators

Negative-pressure ventilators exert a negative pressure on the external chest. Decreasing the intrathoracic pressure during inspiration allows air to flow into the lungs, filling its volume. Physiologically this type of assisted ventilation is similar to spontaneous ventilation. It is used mainly in chronic renal failure (CRF) associated with neuromuscular conditions, such as poliomyelitis, muscular dystrophy, amyotrophic lateral sclerosis, and myasthenia gravis. It is inappropriate for the patient whose condition is unstable or complex or who requires frequent ventilator changes. It is simple to use and does not require intubation of airway; consequently they are especially adaptable for home use.

Types of Negative-Pressure Ventilators

The negative-pressure ventilators are of three types, namely, iron lung, body wrap, and chest cuirass.

1. **Iron lung (drinker respirator tank):** The iron lung is also known as the Drinker and Shaw tank. The machine is effectively a large elongated tank, which encases the patient up to the neck. The neck is sealed with a rubber gasket so that the patient's face (and airway) is exposed to the room air. While the exchange of oxygen and carbon dioxide between the bloodstream and the pulmonary airspace works by diffusion and requires no external work, air must be moved into and out of the lungs to make it available to the gas exchange process. In spontaneous breathing, a negative pressure is created in the pleural cavity by the muscles of respiration, and the resulting gradient between the atmospheric pressure and the pressure inside the thorax generates a flow of air.

   In the iron lung, by means of a pump, the air is withdrawn mechanically to produce a vacuum inside the tank, thus creating negative pressure. This negative pressure leads to the expansion of the chest, which causes a decrease in intrapulmonary pressure and increases the flow of ambient air into the lungs. As the vacuum is released, the pressure inside the tank equalizes to that of the ambient pressure, and the elastic coil of the chest and lungs leads to passive exhalation.

2. **Body wrap (pneumo-wrap):** It is a portable device that required rigid cage or shell to create a negative pressure chamber around abdomen. However, when the vacuum is created, the abdomen also expands along with the lungs, cutting off venous flow back to the heart, leading to the pooling of venous blood in the lower extremities. There are large portholes for nurse or home assistant access. The patients can talk and eat normally and can see the world through a well-placed series of mirrors. Some could remain in these iron lungs for years at a time quite successfully.

3. **Chest cuirass:** The prominent device used is a smaller device known as the cuirass. The cuirass is a shell-like unit, creating negative pressure only to the chest using a combination of a fitting shell and a soft bladder. Its main use is in patients with neuromuscular disorders, who have some residual muscular function. However, it was prone to falling off and caused severe chafing and skin damage and was not used as a long-term device. In recent years, this device has resurfaced as a modern polycarbonate shell with multiple seals and a high-pressure oscillation pump to carry out biphasic cuirass ventilation.

Positive-Pressure Ventilators

Positive-pressure ventilators work by increasing the patient's airway pressure through an endotracheal or tracheostomy tube. The positive pressure allows air to flow into the airway until the ventilator breath is terminated. Subsequently, the airway pressure drops to zero, and the elastic recoil of the chest wall and lungs push the tidal volume—the breath—out through passive exhalation.

Types of Positive-Pressure Ventilators

On the basis of method of ending the inspiratory phase of respiration, positive-pressure ventilators are of three types:

1. **Pressure-cycled ventilators:** When the pressure-cycled ventilator is on it delivers a flow of air (inspiration) until it reaches a preset pressure and then cycles off and expiration occurs passively. Its major limitation is that the volume of air or oxygen can vary as the patient's airway resistance or compliance changes. As a result, the tidal volume delivered may be inconsistent, possibly compromising ventilation. Consequently in adults, pressure-cycled ventilators are intended only for short-term use. The most common type is the intermittent positive pressure breathing (IPPB) machine.

2. **Time-cycled ventilators:** Time-cycled ventilators terminate or control inspiration after a preset time. The volume of air the patient receives is regulated by the length of inspiration and the flow rate of the air. Most ventilators have a rate control that determines the respiratory rate but pure time cycling is rarely used for adults. These ventilators are used for newborns and infants.

3. **Volume-cycled ventilators:** Today, the volume-cycled ventilators are by far the most commonly used positive-pressure ventilators. The volume of air delivered with each inspiration is preset. Once this preset volume is delivered to the patient, the ventilator cycles off and exhalation occurs passively. From breath to breath the volume of air delivered by the ventilator is relatively constant, ensuring consistent, adequate breaths despite varying airway pressures.

Associated Risk

- **Barotrauma:** Pulmonary barotrauma is a well-known complication of positive pressure mechanical ventilation. This includes pneumothorax, subcutaneous emphysema, pneumomediastinum, and pneumoperitoneum.
- **Ventilator-associated lung injury:** Ventilator-associated lung injury (VALI) refers to ALI that occurs during mechanical ventilation. It is clinically indistinguishable from ALI or ARDS.
- **Diaphragm:** Controlled mechanical ventilation (CMV) may lead to a rapid type of disuse atrophy involving the diaphragmatic muscle fibers, which can develop within the first day of mechanical ventilation. This cause of atrophy in the diaphragm is also a cause of atrophy in all respiratory-related muscles during CMV.
- **Motility of mucocilia in the airways:** Positive pressure ventilation appears to impair mucociliary motility in the airways. Bronchial mucus transport was frequently impaired and associated with retention of secretions and pneumonia.

Types of Ventilators

Ventilators come in many different styles and method of giving a breath to sustain life. There are manual ventilators, such as bag valve masks and anesthesia bags that require the user to hold the ventilator to the face or to an artificial airway and maintain breaths with their hands. Mechanical ventilators are ventilators not requiring operator effort and are typically computer controlled or pneumatic controlled.

Mechanical Ventilators

Mechanical ventilators typically require power by a battery or a wall outlet (DC or AC), though some ventilators work on a pneumatic system not requiring power.

- **Transport ventilators:** These ventilators are small, more rugged, and can be powered pneumatically or via AC or DC power sources.
- **Intensive-care ventilators:** These ventilators are larger and usually run on AC power (though virtually all contain a battery to facilitate intrafacility transport and as a backup in the event of a power failure). This style of ventilator often provides greater control of a wide variety of ventilation parameters (such as inspiratory rise time). Many ICU ventilators also incorporate graphics to provide visual feedback of each breath.
- **Neonatal ventilators:** Designed with the preterm neonate in mind, these are a specialized subset of ICU ventilators that are designed to deliver the smaller, more precise volumes and pressures required to ventilate these patients.
- **Positive airway pressure (PAP) ventilators:** These ventilators are specifically designed for NIV. This includes ventilators for use at home for treatment of chronic conditions, such as sleep apnea or COPD.

Breath Delivery

- **Trigger:** The trigger is what causes a breath to be delivered by a mechanical ventilator. Breaths may be triggered by a patient taking his or her own breath, a ventilator operator pressing a manual breath button, or by the ventilator based on the set breath rate and mode of ventilation.
- **Cycle:** The cycle is what causes the breath to transition from the inspiratory phase to the exhalation phase. Breath may be cycled by a mechanical ventilator when a set time has been reached, or when a preset flow or percentage of the maximum flow delivered during a breath is reached depending on the breath type and the settings. Breath can also be cycled when an alarm condition, such as a high-pressure limit has been reached, which is a primary strategy in pressure-regulated volume control (PRVC).
- **Limit:** Limit is how the breath is controlled. Breath may be limited to a set maximum circuit pressure or a set maximum flow.
- **Breath exhalation:** Exhalation in mechanical ventilation is almost always completely passive. The ventilator's expiratory valve is opened, and expiratory flow is allowed until the baseline pressure [positive end-expiratory pressure (PEEP)] is reached. Expiratory flow is determined by patient factors, such as compliance and resistance.
- **Dead space:** Mechanical dead space is defined as the volume of gas rebreathed as the result of use in a mechanical device.

MODES OF MECHANICAL VENTILATION

Modes of mechanical ventilation are one of the most important aspects of the usage of mechanical ventilation. The mode refers to the method of inspiratory support. Mode selection is generally based on clinician familiarity and institutional preferences since there is a paucity of evidence indicating that the mode affects clinical outcome. The most frequently used forms of volume-limited mechanical ventilation are intermittent mandatory ventilation (IMV) and continuous mandatory ventilation (CMV). There have been substantial changes in the nomenclature of mechanical ventilation over the years, but more recently it has become standardized by many respirology/pulmonology groups. Writing a mode is most proper in all capital letters with a dash between the cycle and the strategy (i.e., PC-IMV or VC-MMV, etc.)

Cycling is the method for how a ventilator knows to give a breath and stop a breath. Cycling is the governing system for how a breath will ultimately be applied. Parameters vary but rate (f), inspiratory expiratory (I:E) ratio, and other similar parameters are almost always set by the clinician alongside the cycle.

Volume controlled systems of ventilation are based on a measured volume variable that is set by the clinician. When the ventilator detects the set volume having been applied, the ventilator cycles to exhalation. This is measured using various ways based on the brand and model. Some ventilators measure using a flow sensor at the circuit, while some measure where the expiratory circuit plugs into the expiratory port on the ventilator body.

Pressure-controlled cycling is based on an applied positive pressure that is set by the clinician. In pressure-controlled modes, the total volume is variable as the ventilator is using only the pressure as a measurement for cycling. Most ventilators calculate pressure at the expiratory circuit though some measure near the circuit with a proximal pressure line.

Spontaneously controlled cycling is a flow-sensed mode dependent on a spontaneously breathing patient to cycle. Spontaneously controlled ventilation is typically only in reference to continuous spontaneous ventilation also called continuous PAP (CPAP).

Negative-pressure-controlled ventilation cycles by producing a negative pressure around the chest and abdomen. Negative pressure moves across the chest and diaphragm and causes air to move into the lungs in the normal fashion. When the negative pressure stops being applied, the chest returns to atmospheric pressure and the inspired air is then exhaled.

STRATEGY

Airway pressure release ventilation (APRV) is a time-cycled alternant between two levels of PAP, with the main time on the high level, and a brief expiratory release to facilitate ventilation.

The APRV is usually utilized as a type of inverse ratio ventilation. The exhalation time (T_{low}) is shortened to usually <1 second to maintain alveoli inflation. Fundamentally this is a continuous pressure with a brief release. The APRV is currently the most efficient conventional mode for lung protective ventilation.

Continuous mandatory ventilation (formerly known as assist control or AC) is a mode of ventilation where breaths are delivered based on set variables. The patient may initiate breaths by attempting to breathe. Once a breath is initiated, either by the patient or by the ventilator, the set tidal volume is delivered. CMV is also called volume control (VC) or AC, though this is no longer recommended. Since nomenclature of mechanical ventilation is only recently standardized, there are many different names that historically were used to reference CMV but now referred to as AC. Names, such as volume control ventilation and volume-cycled ventilation in the modern usage refer to the AC mode.

The CMV in its original form had no patient sensitivity. A breath set was a breath delivered. Continuous mandatory ventilation was created out of the need for patient initiation in breaths. Fundamentally, CMV is a mode of ventilation with a sensitivity for patient breathing. The use of CMV requires the patient to be completely unconscious, either pharmacokinetically or otherwise in a coma.

Continuous mandatory ventilation is associated with profound diaphragm muscle dysfunction and atrophy. CMV is no longer the preferred mode of mechanical ventilation.

Intermittent mandatory ventilation is similar to CMV in two ways: the minute ventilation (V_E) is determined (by setting the respiratory rate and tidal volume), and the patient is able to increase the minute ventilation. However, IMV differs from CMV in the way that the minute ventilation is increased. Specifically, patients increase the minute ventilation by spontaneous breathing, rather than patient-initiated ventilator breaths. The ventilator breaths are synchronized with patient inspiratory effort. The IMV with pressure support is the most efficient and effective mode of mechanical ventilation.

Intermittent mandatory ventilation has not always had the synchronized feature, so the division of modes was understood to be SIMV (synchronized) versus IMV (not synchronized). Since the American Association for Respiratory Care established a nomenclature of mechanical ventilation the "synchronized" part of the title has been dropped and now there is only IMV. It is indicated for patients who are breathing spontaneously but at a tidal volume and/or rate less than adequate for their needs. Allow patients to do some of the work of breathing.

Mandatory minute ventilation (MMV) allows spontaneous breathing with automatic adjustments of mandatory ventilation to the meet the patient's preset minimum minute volume requirement. If the patient maintains the minute volume settings for V_T x f, no mandatory breaths are delivered.

If the patient's minute volume is insufficient, mandatory delivery of the preset tidal volume will occur until the minute volume is achieved. The method for monitoring whether the patient is meeting the required minute ventilation (V_E) differs by ventilator brand and model, but generally there is a window of monitored time, and a smaller window checked against the larger window (i.e., in the Dräger Evita® line of mechanical ventilators, there is a moving 20-second window, and every 7 seconds the current tidal volume and rate are measured) to decide whether a mechanical breath is needed to maintain the minute ventilation.

The MMV has been considered to be an optimal mode for weaning in neonatal and pediatric populations and has been shown to reduce long-term complications related to mechanical ventilation.

Pressure-regulated Volume Control

The PRVC is an IMV-based mode. The PRVC utilizes pressure-limited, volume-targeted, time-cycled breaths, which can be either ventilator or patient initiated. The peak inspiratory pressure delivered by the ventilator is varied on a breath-to-breath basis to achieve a target tidal volume that is set by the clinician.

For example, if a target tidal volume of 500 mL is set but the ventilator delivers 600 mL, the next breath will be delivered with a lower inspiratory pressure to achieve a lower tidal volume. Although PRVC is regarded as a hybrid mode because of its tidal volume (VC) settings and pressure-limiting (PC) settings. Fundamentally PRVC is a volume-control mode.

Continuous Positive Airway Pressure

The CPAP is a noninvasive positive pressure mode of ventilation (NPPV). The CPAP is simply a pressure applied at the end of exhalation to keep the alveoli open, not fully deflate. This mechanism for maintaining inflated alveoli helps increase the partial pressure of oxygen in arterial blood, and an appropriate increase in CPAP increases the PaO_2.

Continuous positive airway pressure is indicated for patient who are capable of maintaining an adequate tidal volume, but who have pathology preventing maintenance of adequate levels of tissue oxygenation or for sleep apnea.

Bilevel Positive Airway Pressure

The bilevel PAP (BPAP) is a mode used during NPPV. First used in 1988 by Professor Benzer in Austria, it delivers a preset inspiratory PAP (IPAP) and expiratory PAP (EPAP). The BPAP can be described as a CPAP system with a time-cycled change in the applied CPAP level. The CPAP, BPAP, and other NIV modes have been shown to be effective management tools for COPD and acute respiratory failure.

High-frequency Ventilation (Active)

The term **active** refers to the ventilators forced expiratory system. In a high-frequency ventilation (active) (HFV-A) scenario, the ventilator uses pressure to apply an inspiratory breath and then applies an opposite pressure to force an expiratory breath. In high-frequency oscillatory ventilation (sometimes abbreviated HFOV), the oscillation below and piston force positive pressure in and apply negative pressure to force an expiration.

High-frequency Ventilation (Passive)

The term **passive** refers to the ventilator's nonforced expiratory system. In an HFV-P scenario, the ventilator uses pressure to apply an inspiratory breath and then simply returns to atmospheric pressure to allow for a passive expiration. This is seen in high-frequency jet ventilation, sometimes abbreviated as HFJV.

Volume Guarantee

Volume guarantee is a mode or an additional parameter available in many types of ventilators that allows the ventilator to change its inspiratory pressure setting to achieve a minimum tidal volume. This is utilized most often in neonatal patients who need a pressure controlled mode with a consideration for volume control to minimize volutrauma.

SPONTANEOUS BREATHING AND SUPPORT SETTINGS

Positive-end Expiratory Pressure

Positive-end expiratory pressure is pressure applied upon expiration, and PEEP is applied either using a valve that is connected to the expiratory port and set manually or using a valve managed internally by a mechanical ventilator.

Positive-end expiratory pressure is simply a pressure that an exhalation has to bypass, effectively causing alveoli to remain open, not fully deflate. This mechanism for maintaining inflated alveoli helps increase the partial pressure of oxygen in arterial blood, and an increase in PEEP increases the PaO_2.

Purpose

The purpose is to increase functional residual capacity [(FRC) or the amount of air left in the lungs at the end of expiration]. This aids in the following:
- Increasing the surface area of gas exchange
- Preventing collapse of alveolar units and development of atelectasis
- Decreasing intrapulmonary shunt

Benefits

- Because greater surface area for diffusion is available and shunting is reduced, it is often possible to use a lower FiO_2 than otherwise would be required to obtain adequate arterial

oxygen levels. This reduces the risk of oxygen toxicity in conditions, such as acute respiratory distress syndrome.
- Increased lung compliance resulting in decreased work of breathing
- Positive intra-airway pressure may be helpful in reducing the transudation of fluid from the pulmonary capillaries in situations where capillary pressure is increased.

Hazards

- Because the mean airway pressure is increased by PEEP, venous return is impeded. This results in a decrease in cardiac output.
- There is disagreement that the increased airway pressure may possibly result in alveolar rupture. The likelihood of damage is greater due to peak airway pressure during mechanical than due to end-expiratory pressure. This barotraumas may result in pneumothorax, tension pneumothorax, or development of subcutaneous emphysema.
- This decreased venous return may stimulate the formation of antidiuretic hormones, resulting in decreased urine output.

Pressure Support

Pressure support is a spontaneous mode of ventilation also named pressure support ventilation (PSV). The patient initiates every breath and the ventilator delivers support with the preset pressure value. With support from the ventilator, the patient also regulates their own respiratory rate and their tidal volume.

In pressure support, the set inspiratory pressure support level is kept constant and there is a decelerating flow. The patient triggers all breaths. If there is a change in the mechanical properties of the lung/thorax and patient effort, the delivered tidal volume will be affected. The user must then regulate the pressure support level to obtain desired ventilation.

Pressure support improves oxygenation and ventilation and decreases the work of breathing.

OTHER VENTILATION MODES AND STRATEGIES

Adaptive Support Ventilation

Adaptive support ventilation is a brand name of a closed-loop system on the Hamilton ventilators and is the only commercially available mode to date that uses "optimal targeting." This targeting scheme was first described by Tehrani in 1991 and was designed to minimize the work rate of breathing, mimic natural breathing, stimulate spontaneous breathing, and reduce weaning time.

Automatic Tube Compensation

Automatic tube compensation (ATC) is the simplest example of a computer-controlled targeting system on a ventilator. The goal of ATC is to support the resistive work of breathing through the artificial airway.

Neurally Adjusted Ventilatory Assist

Neurally adjusted ventilatory assist (NAVA) is adjusted by a computer (servo) and is similar to ATC but with more complex requirements for implementation.

In terms of patient-ventilator synchrony, NAVA supports both resistive and elastic work of breathing in proportion to the patient's inspiratory effort.

Proportional Assist Ventilation

Proportional assist ventilation (PAV) is a mode in which the ventilator guarantees the percentage of work regardless of changes in pulmonary compliance and resistance. The ventilator varies the tidal volume and pressure based on the patient's work of breathing. The amount it delivers is proportional to the percentage of assistance it is set to give.

Like NAVA, PAV supports both resistive and elastic work of breathing in proportion to the patient's inspiratory effort.

Liquid Ventilation

Liquid ventilation (LV) is a technique of mechanical ventilation in which the lungs are insufflated with an oxygenated perfluorochemical (PFC) liquid rather than an oxygen-containing gas mixture. The use of PFCs, rather than nitrogen, as the inert carrier of oxygen and carbon dioxide, offers a number of theoretical advantages for the treatment of ALI, including the following:

- Reducing surface tension by maintaining a fluid interface with alveoli
- Opening of collapsed alveoli by hydraulic pressure with a lower risk of barotraumas
- Providing a reservoir in which oxygen and carbon dioxide can be exchanged with pulmonary capillary blood
- Functioning as a high-efficiency heat exchanger.

Despite its theoretical advantages, efficacy studies have been disappointing and the optimal clinical use of LV has yet to be defined.

Total Liquid Ventilation

In total liquid ventilation (TLV), the entire lung is filled with an oxygenated PFC liquid, and a liquid tidal volume of PFC is actively pumped into and out of the lungs. A specialized apparatus is required to deliver and remove the relatively dense, viscous PFC tidal volumes and to extracorporeally oxygenate and remove carbon dioxide from the liquid.

Partial Liquid Ventilation

In partial liquid ventilation (PLV), the lungs are slowly filled with a volume of PFC equivalent or close to the FRC during gas ventilation. The PFC within the lungs is oxygenated and carbon dioxide is removed by means of gas breaths cycling in the lungs by a conventional gas ventilator.

INVASIVE MECHANICAL VENTILATION

Invasive mechanical ventilation is defined as mechanical ventilation via an artificial airway, which can be either via endotracheal tube or tracheostomy tube.

Invasive mechanical ventilation is indicated for patients with severe hypoxemia, which cannot be oxygenated by other less invasive means. It is also indicated for patients incapable of maintaining adequate alveolar hypoventilation.

Common Indications for Invasive Mechanical Ventilation

Listed are the common indications for invasive mechanical ventilation:

- Acute pulmonary edema
- Pneumonia
- Acute respiratory distress syndrome
- Severe asthmatic attack
- Severe acute exacerbation of COPD
- Guillain-Barré syndrome

- Myasthenia gravis
- Drug overdose
- Shock
- Severe sepsis

Artificial Airways as a Connection to the Ventilator

There are various procedures and mechanical devices that provide protection against airway collapse, air leakage, and aspiration:

- **Face mask:** In resuscitation and for minor procedures under anesthesia, a face mask is often sufficient to achieve a seal against air leakage. Airway patency of the unconscious patient is maintained either by manipulation of the jaw or by the use of nasopharyngeal or oropharyngeal airway. These are designed to provide a passage of air to the pharynx through the nose or mouth, respectively. Poorly fitted masks often cause nasal bridge ulcers, a problem for some patients. Face masks are also used for NIV in conscious patients. A full face mask does not, however, provide protection against aspiration.
- **Laryngeal mask airway:** The LMA causes less pain and coughing than a tracheal tube. However, unlike tracheal tubes it does not seal against aspiration, making careful individualized evaluation and patient selection mandatory.
- **Tracheal intubation:** Tracheal intubation is often performed for mechanical ventilation of hours to weeks' duration. A tube is inserted through the nose (nasotracheal intubation) or mouth (orotracheal intubation) and advanced into the trachea. In most cases, tubes with inflatable cuffs are used for protection against leakage and aspiration. Intubation with a cuffed tube is thought to provide the best protection against aspiration. Tracheal tubes inevitably cause pain and coughing. Therefore, unless a patient is unconscious or anesthetized for other reasons, sedative drugs are usually given to provide tolerance of the tube. Other disadvantages of tracheal intubation include damage to the mucosal lining of the nasopharynx or oropharynx and subglottic stenosis.
- **Esophageal obturator airway:** Sometimes used by emergency medical technicians and basic emergency medical services (EMS) providers not trained to intubate. It is a tube that is inserted into the esophagus, past the epiglottis. Once it is inserted, a bladder at the tip of the airway is inflated, to block (obturate) the esophagus, and oxygen is delivered through a series of holes in the side of the tube, which is then forced into the lungs.
- **Cricothyrotomy:** Patients who require emergency airway management, in whom tracheal intubation has been unsuccessful, may require an airway inserted through a surgical opening in the cricothyroid membrane. This is similar to a tracheostomy, but a cricothyrotomy is reserved for emergency access.
- **Tracheostomy:** When patients require mechanical ventilation for several weeks, a tracheostomy may provide the most suitable access to the trachea. A tracheostomy is a surgically created passage into the trachea. Tracheostomy tubes are well tolerated and often do not necessitate any use of sedative drugs. Tracheostomy tubes may be inserted early during treatment in patients with pre-existing severe respiratory disease, or in any patient who is expected to have difficulty weaning from mechanical ventilation, i.e., patients who have little muscular reserve.
- **Mouthpiece:** Less common interface and does not provide protection against aspiration. There are lip seal mouthpieces with flanges to help hold them in place if patient is unable.

NONINVASIVE VENTILATION

The NPPV is a ventilator-assist technique used in the management of impending respiratory failure as an alternative to endotracheal intubation. The bi-level PAP (BiPAP) is a low-pressure, electronically driven device intended for use as a ventilatory support system for patients who have an intact respiratory drive. The device provides noninvasive ventilatory assistance through the use of a nasal or face mask. The device may also be used for invasive ventilatory support (refer to the Guideline for Invasive Applications with BiPAP Vision Systems). The device uses an electronic pressure control sensing mechanism to sense patient breathing. It accomplishes this through its ability to monitor pressure differential in the patient circuit. This feedback allows for adjustment of the flow and pressure output to assist in inhalation or exhalation through the administration at two distinct levels of positive pressure. During inspiration, the level is variably positive and is always higher than the expiratory level. During exhalation, pressure is variably positive or near ambient.

In addition, this device has the ability to compensate for leaks through automatic adjustment of the trigger threshold. This capability allows for the application of BiPAP for mask-applied ventilation assistance.

Indications for Noninvasive Ventilation

- Acute respiratory failure
- Hypercapnic acute respiratory failure
- Acute exacerbation of COPD
- Post-extubation difficulty
- Weaning difficulties
- Postsurgical respiratory failure
- Thoracic wall deformities
- Cystic fibrosis
- Status asthmaticus
- Acute respiratory failure in obesity hypoventilation syndrome
- Chronic respiratory failure
- Immunocompromised patients
- Patients "not for intubation".

Selection Criteria

Acute Respiratory Failure

At least two of the following criteria should be present:
- Respiratory distress with dyspnea
- Use of accessory muscles of respiration
- Abdominal paradox respiratory rate >25/min
- Arterial blood gas shows pH <7.35 or $PaCO_2$ >45 mm Hg or PaO_2/FiO_2 <200.

Chronic Respiratory Failure (Obstructive Lung Disease)

The criteria to put patients with chronic respiratory failure on NIV are the following:
- Fatigue, hypersomnolence, dyspnea
- Arterial blood gas shows pH <7.35, $PaCO_2$ >55 mm Hg, $PaCO_2$ 50–54 mm Hg.
- Oxygen saturation <88% for >10% of monitoring time despite O_2 supplementation
- Thoracic restrictive/cerebral hypoventilation diseases
- Fatigue, morning headache, hypersomnolence, nightmares, enuresis, dyspnea
- ABG shows $PaCO_2$ >45 mm Hg
- Nocturnal SaO_2 <90% for more than 5 minutes

Contraindications

- Respiratory arrest/unstable cardiorespiratory status
- Uncooperative patients
- Unable to protect airway-impaired swallowing and cough
- Facial/esophageal or gastric surgery
- Craniofacial trauma/burns
- Anatomic lesions of upper airway

Relative Contraindications

- Extreme anxiety
- Morbid obesity
- Copious secretions
- Need for continuous or nearly continuous ventilatory assistance

Choice of Ventilator

Noninvasive ventilation can be given by conventional critical care ventilators or portable pressure or volume limit ventilators. When a critical care ventilator is used for applying NIV, the presence of variable leaks produces frequent alarming. Therefore, a close monitoring of leaks is mandatory. Noninvasive ventilation may be delivered more successfully using especially designed portable pressure ventilators. These provide a high-flow CPAP or cycle between high inspiratory and low expiratory pressures (BiPAP generators). These devices are sensitive enough for detection of inspiratory efforts even in the presence of leaks in the circuits.

Interfaces are devices that connect the ventilator tubing to the face allowing the entry of pressurized gas to the upper airway. Nasal, oronasal masks, and mouth pieces are currently available. Masks are usually made from a nonirritant material, such as silicon rubber. It should have minimal dead space and a soft inflatable cuff to provide a seal with the skin. Face and nasal masks are the most commonly used interfaces. Nasal masks are used most often in chronic respiratory failure, while face masks are more useful in acute respiratory failure.

Modes of Ventilation

Continuous Positive Airway Pressure

The CPAP by nasal mask provides a pneumatic splint that holds the upper airway open in patients with nocturnal hypoxemia due to episodes of obstructive sleep apnea. It provides PAP throughout all phases of spontaneous ventilation. The CPAP increases the FRC and opens collapsed alveoli. The CPAP reduces left ventricular transmural pressure and therefore increases cardiac output. Hence, it is very effective for treatment of pulmonary edema. Pressures are usually limited to 5–12 cm of H_2O, since higher pressure tends to result in gastric distension requiring continual aspiration through a nasogastric tube.

Biphasic Positive Airway Pressure

The BiPAP provides two levels of positive pressure. During exhalation, pressure is variably positive. Airflow in the circuit is sensed by a transducer and augmented to a preset level of ventilation. Cycling between inspiratory and expiratory modes may be either triggered by the patient's breaths or preset.

Volume-limited Ventilation

In this mode, ventilators are usually set in assist-control mode with high tidal volume (10–15 mL/kg) to compensate for air leaks. This mode is suitable for patients with obesity or chest wall deformity (need high inflation pressure) and in patients with neuromuscular diseases who need high tidal volumes for ventilation.

Proportional Assist Ventilation

This is a newer mode of ventilation. In this mode, the ventilator has the capacity for responding rapidly to the patients' ventilatory efforts. By adjusting the gain on the flow and volume signals, one can select the proportion of breathing work that is to be assisted.

EQUIPMENT AND SUPPLIES

Biphasic Positive Airway Pressure

- The BiPAP ST/D ventilatory support system with detachable control panel (DCP) and airway pressure monitor
- BiPAP ST/D disposable circuit with disposable proximal pressure line and exhalation port
- Main flow bacteria filter
- Nasal or face mask and disposable head strap or airway adapter
- Smooth inner lumen tubing for use in connecting the humidifier system to the BiPAP unit
- Oxygen-enrichment adapter and extension tubing
- Pulse oximetry equipment and supplies
- Continuous ventilation record
- Device-specific humidification system (if necessary)
- BiPAP sizing gauge for nasal masks

BiPAP Vision

- BiPAP vision ventilatory support system
- BiPAP vision disposable circuit with disposable proximal pressure line and exhalation port
- Main flow bacterial filter
- Nasal or face mask and disposable head strap or airway adapter
- Smooth inner lumen tubing for use in connecting the humidifier system to the BiPAP unit
- Pulse oximetry equipment and supplies
- Oxygen analyzer with circuit adapter
- Continuous ventilation record
- Device-specific humidification system (Note: A heated humidification system must be used for all invasive ventilation).

PROCEDURE

Biphasic Positive Airway Pressure

- Determine the appropriate circuit adapter. If a nasal mask is required, use the mask-sizing gauge to select the appropriate size. Assemble the circuit with exhalation port proximal to the patient.
- Connect the mask with head strap or airway adapter to the circuit. Oxygen may be added at two points in the circuit. For use with an airway adapter, an oxygen-enrichment attachment should be placed between the mainstream bacteria filter and the tubing going to the patient. For use with a mask, oxygen tubing should be connected directly from a flow meter to one of the sample ports on the patient's mask.
- Plug electrical cord into A/C outlet. Turn the power switch "ON" to the unit (located on the top right corner).

- Assess appropriateness of physician's orders and set ventilatory parameters accordingly. Initial settings as well as changes in ventilatory parameters must be accompanied by a physician order.
- Adjust the DCP according to the desired mode, IPAP, EPAP, frequency beat per minutte (BPM) and %IPAP (timed mode only). Consult the BiPAP ventilatory support system clinical manual for specific information on the modes of operation. The IPAP and EPAP controls are electrically coupled. The unit will not deliver an EPAP level that is higher than the set IPAP level [If the EPAP control is set higher than IPAP pressure, the unit will be locked to the IPAP setting and the IPAP light-emitting diode (LED) will remain lit]. The maximal achievable peak inspiratory pressure is 20 cm H_2O.
  Note: If the unit fails to read zero when not connected to the patient circuit (i.e., in ambient pressure), mechanically zero the pressure gauge using the zero adjust screw at the rear of the monitor.
- Connect the patient to the circuit. Adjust head strap to minimize leaks at the patient–mask interface. Assess the patient for tolerance and the ventilator system for proper function and adjust accordingly.
- Adjust the oxygen liter flow as needed to achieve an appropriate oxygen saturation.
  Note: The BiPAP system should be turned ON prior to the introduction of oxygen to the circuit; the oxygen should be turned OFF prior to turning the BiPAP unit off.
- Set high and low airway pressure monitor alarms as appropriate.
- Observe the estimated exhaled tidal volume (Est Vte). The number should approximate the desired tidal volume. If the Est Vte flashes beyond 15 respiratory cycles, there is a leak too great for compensation to occur. If this is observed, adjust the patient–unit interface as needed to achieve a steady Est Vte. The Est leak display may be utilized to aid in correcting a persistent leak.
- Perform a thorough assessment of the patient–ventilator system according to the Critical Care Therapy and Respiratory Care System (CCTRCS) Patient Assessment Policy. Monitor the patient continuously via cardiopulmonary monitor and pulse oximetry. Perform blood gas analysis as necessary per physician order.
- Administration of aerosolized medications through the BiPAP system: Small-volume nebulizers or adapters allowing the use of metered dose inhalers (MDIs) may be added to the patient circuit. The liter flow used to drive the nebulizer does not impact on the functioning of the BiPAP system, provided the nebulizer or MDI is added to the circuit on the patient side of the exhalation valve. A main flow bacteria filter must remain in-line during the treatment to prevent the aerosol from entering the BiPAP unit via the patient circuit. The use of a mouthpiece during the treatment may aid in treatment efficacy.

Biphasic Positive Airway Pressure Vision

- Assemble the circuit with exhalation port proximal to the patient. A bacterial filter and oxygen analyzer should be placed between the machine's patient interface port and the patient circuit.
- If using the O_2 module, connect to a 50psi O_2 source. Set parameters. Occlude the end of the circuit to adjust the ventilating pressures.
  Note: Plug electrical cord in A/C outlet. Press START on the back of the machine. The Vision will perform a self-test as indicated by the display screen, "System Self-Test in Progress."
- Perform the "Test Exh Port," second button from top, left of screen.
- Occlude circuit with thumb throughout the test.
- Press START TEST, top button, right of screen. This tests the leak of the circuit.

- Assess appropriateness of physician's orders and set ventilatory parameters accordingly. Initial settings as well as changes to ventilatory parameters must be accompanied by a physician order.
- Select the proper mode by first selecting the mode button at the bottom of screen.
- Choose CPAP or S/T mode, top button, right side of screen, per physician's order.
- Activate view mode by pressing the "activate view mode" button, bottom right of screen.
- Select the "parameters" button below the screen.
- Choose a parameter from the left and right sides of screen. Press the soft button for the parameter of choice. Once it is highlighted, spin the knob clockwise to increase value and counterclockwise to decrease value in the parameter block. Repress the button for that particular parameter to activate the new value.
  Note: Consult the BiPAP Vision Ventilatory Support System Clinical Manual for specific information on the modes of operation and set parameters.
- Connect the patient's properly fitted mask or airway adapter to the BiPAP Vision circuit and then apply the mask to the patient.
- Select "alarms" button below the screen. Set values for Hi Pressure, Lo Pressure, Lo Pressure Delay, Apnea, Lo MinVent, Hi Rate, and Lo Rate as appropriate for the patient.

POSTPROCEDURES

Cleaning and Sterilization for the Biphasic Positive Airway Pressure ST/D

- Disconnect the BiPAP and DCP before cleaning. Do not immerse in water. Unplug the DCP unit.
- Discard the disposable circuit parts.
- Wipe the outside of the DCP enclosure using a standard hospital disinfectant. Do not allow liquids to enter the DCP enclosure. The protective plexiglass cover should always be covering the DCP, except when setting changes are being performed. The DCP should be thoroughly dried before reconnection.
- Using a cloth slightly dampened with water and mild dish detergent, wipe the outside of the BiPAP enclosure. The BiPAP unit should be thoroughly dried before reconnection. **Note: Do not clean any parts of the system with alcohol or cleaning solutions containing alcohol.** Do not clean the system by steam or gas sterilization methods. These cleaning processes may harden or deform the flexible plastic parts of the system and adversely affect the performance of the DCP.

Cleaning and Sterilization for the Biphasic Positive Airway Pressure Vision

After the procedure is done, the BiPAP Vision should be cleaned and sterilized as mentioned below:

- Before cleaning the unit, turn the "Start/Stop" switch to the "Stop" position and unplug the electrical cord from the wall and from the rear of the unit.
- Clean the front panel with water or 70% isopropyl alcohol only. **Do not immerse the Vision unit in water.**
- Clean the exterior of the enclosure with a clinical center-approved disinfectant. **Do not allow any liquid to enter the inside of the ventilator.**

Routine Maintenance: Changing the Intake Filter

In order to protect the patient from breathing dirt and other irritating particles, an air intake filter should be in place at all times when the BiPAP is being used. The white filter (on the front of the BiPAP ST/D and the back of the BiPAP Vision) is disposable and need to be replaced after 30 days of use and in between patients.

Caution: Failure to replace a dirty filter may produce high operating temperature in the BiPAP unit, reduce the flow, and reduce the output pressure.

Biphasic Positive Airway Pressure ST/D

- Turn off the unit and unplug the electrical cord.
- Discard the dirty filter.
  Note: The filter is not washable.
- Center a new filter over the filter holder. Carefully push in on the center button and tuck the filter in on all four sides.
- Release the button. The filter should be intact and fit securely, covering the entire holder. Remove and readjust the filter as necessary.

NURSING CARE OF THE VENTILATED PATIENT

Principles

- The registered nurse is responsible for the assessment, planning, and delivery of care to the patient.
- Care of the ventilated patient can vary from the basic nursing care of activities of daily living to caring for highly technical invasive monitoring equipment and managing and monitoring the effects of interventions.

Care of the Airway

- It is of paramount importance that all cares and procedures are carried out by maintaining a patent airway.
- Always check the patient first. Observe the patient's facial expression, color, respiratory effort, vital signs, and ECG tracing.
- Ensure the endotracheal tube (ETT) or tracheostomy tube is held securely in position but not too tightly to result in pressure area lesions.
- Check the placement of the ETT by listening for equal bilateral breath sounds, checking the chest X-ray (CXR) and noting the distance marks on the tube and the teeth, checking the previously documented level.
- Check and adjust (if necessary) the cuff pressure of the ETT/trachi. In order to minimize tracheal damage, the cuff pressure should be at the lowest pressure necessary to prevent an air leak.

Check the Bedside Emergency Equipment

- An alternative means of ventilation, e.g., Laerdal bag must be available and functional
- Yankauer sucker, suction catheters and functioning suction unit, airways, and masks should be available.

Ventilation

While ventilating a patient, the following must be ensured and checked:
- Ensure the ventilation tubing is not kinked and that it is adequately supported, so as not to drag on the ETT/trachi. Take care of the tube while turning or moving the patient.
- Check the ventilator and document the settings. Look at the alarm parameters and reset if necessary.

- Ensure the ventilator and the cardiac monitor is plugged into emergency power supply in case of power failure.
- Ensure that you have enough room to access the head of the bed in case of emergency.
- Check the type of humidification, and also check when the filters and ventilation tubing were last changed.
- Heat and moisture exchanger (HME) filters and end expiratory filters are changed routinely (and marked with the date and time) every 24 hours or more frequently if condensation is visible.
- Ventilator circuits are changed weekly.

Indications for an Actively Humidified Circuit

- Minute volume greater than 10 L
- Chest trauma with pulmonary contusion
- Airway burns
- Severe asthma
- Hypothermia (<34°C)
- Pulmonary hemorrhage
- Severe sputum plugging/pulmonary edema leading to HME occlusion
- Consultant order

Suction of an Artificial Airway

- Maintain a patent airway
- Promote improved gas exchange
- Obtain tracheal aspirate specimens.
- Prevent effects of retained secretions, e.g., infection, consolidation, atelectasis, increased airway pressures, or blocked tube.
- It is important to oxygenate before and after suctioning. Closed suction catheters should be rinsed postsuctioning to remove mucous and to reduce the likelihood of bacterial growth.
- Tracheal suctioning should be attended 2–3 hourly, more often if necessary (see Suctioning an Artificial Airway Guideline).
- Suction the oropharynx to remove potentially infected secretions.

Monitors

The following aspects have to be checked in the monitor on a regular basis:

- Check the level of any invasive monitoring transducers and zero them (Hemodynamic Monitoring Guideline).
- Check the alarm parameters and reset if necessary.
- Document the patient's vital signs hourly and **when there is a deviation** from the usual.
- Check and document a manual blood pressure to assess the accuracy of the arterial trace once a shift.

NURSING STAFF

The role of the nursing staff in the ICCU, as in the CU, is essential for high-quality care. Thus, there should be a sufficient number of properly trained nurses who should be able to interpret frequent arrhythmias, detect the first indications of deterioration in patients, and take decisions quickly in emergencies (start CPR maneuvers or perform defibrillation). It is desirable that, in addition to appropriate training, the nursing staff assigned to an ICCU have previous experience in attending to patients in ICUs or CUs. An appropriately trained and qualified full-time or part-time (also head of the CU or hospital ward of the cardiology service) supervisor should be present. The degree of preparation necessary has forced the government to consider recognizing specialization in the field of cardiology. The task of the supervisor could also be essential in investigational studies done in the ICCU itself. The rotation of nursing staff from the ICCU with the other units of the cardiology service, and particularly the CU, is a useful way of ensuring commitment, sense of duty, and the degree of training necessary for a suitable level of care.

In order to run smoothly, the ICCUs also need sufficient auxiliary staff (one for every eight beds); hospital porters who work exclusively for the unit or in nearby units, depending on the size of the ICCU; and administrative staff who, depending on the size of the ICCU, may be shared with other units or work exclusively for the ICCU.

INDICATIONS FOR ADMISSION

The criteria for admission to the ICCU should be guided by the basic objective of attending to patients with acute heart disease, particularly ACS, whose clinical condition does not require admission to a CU but who nevertheless are not sufficiently stable to be admitted to a conventional cardiology ward (because of the appearance of arrhythmias or risk of recurrence of ischemia). These patients therefore need closer monitoring and more intensive care, as described at the beginning of this document. In general, we only have data from a few observational studies. Therefore, the recommendations made in this document are based solely on the consensus of an expert committee (level C of evidence). The indications for admission recommended in this document are described below.

Patients with nSTE-ACS who are hemodynamically stable (without hypertension, heart failure, or ventricular arrhythmias) can be considered for admission if they have one or more of the following characteristics: (a) prolonged resting angina with ECG abnormalities (ST-segment depression, T-wave alterations) and/or elevated troponin; (b) impaired ventricular function, kidney failure, or a combination of other comorbidities (infarction or prior revascularization, age, diabetes mellitus, peripheral vascular disease); (c) recurrent angina (two or more episodes of angina in the past 24 hours); and (d) patients with nSTE-ACS initially admitted to the CU because of their high-risk profile, after stabilization with medical treatment (>24 hours without recurrence of ischemia).

Patients with Uncomplicated ST-Elevation Acute Myocardial Infarction

The following patients can be admitted to the ICCU:
- Patients with early reperfusion after percutaneous coronary interventions [(PCIs) primary angioplasty] who are free of severe ventricular dysfunction or other clinical or anatomical risk factors
- Patients treated with thrombolytic agents with evidence of coronary reperfusion and without complications, once 24 hours have elapsed since the onset of AMI.
- Patients with extensive AMI who have not received thrombolytic therapy, without complications, once 48 hours have elapsed.

Immediate Monitoring after Invasive Procedures

Patients who have undergone high-risk PCI are candidates for admission to the ICCU in the following situations:
1. Stable chronic ischemic heart disease during the first 6–24 hours after high-risk PCI (e.g., percutaneous transluminal coronary angioplasty [PTCA] of the left main coronary artery or

the only patent vessel, PTCA patients with severe left ventricular dysfunction or prior kidney failure).
2. Patients with reversible complications during the procedure (excluding major complications, such as AMI, severe heart failure or shock, candidates for admission to the CU), or who need specific treatments (e.g., glycoprotein IIb/IIIa inhibitors, etc.).
3. Recipients of an implantable cardioverter-defibrillator (ICD) or those who have undergone other invasive procedures, such as percutaneous ablation, pacemaker placement, etc., who need temporary monitoring (complicated procedure or high-risk findings).

Other Acute Heart Diseases

Although the main aim of the ICCU is to attend to patients with ischemic heart disease, at the discretion of the cardiologist in charge—and according to the needs for care at the time—certain other patients with acute heart diseases can be considered for admission:
1. **Heart failure:** The ideal treatment for these patients might include administration of inotropic agents or vasodilators, or noninvasive mechanical ventilation (CPAP, BiPAP). Two types of well-defined candidates can be considered: (a) patients with acute heart failure (acute pulmonary edema) with good response to initial treatment that does not require invasive interventions and (b) patients with chronic decompensated heart failure or heart failure refractory to optimum medical treatment (excluding patients with severe hypotension or cardiogenic shock requiring admission to the CU).
2. Patients with advanced atrioventricular block or sick sinus syndrome with good hemodynamic tolerance, or those who are stable after implantation of temporary pacing electrodes, while awaiting definitive pacemaker implantation.
3. Treatment of certain supraventricular arrhythmias (usually fibrillation or atrial flutter) or ventricular arrhythmias according to the available protocols. Patients who are awaiting ICD implantation or who are admitted to the emergency room after an ICD discharge can also be admitted to the ICCU (but not patients with repeated discharges or electrical storm; these patients should be admitted to the CU).
4. At the discretion of the cardiologist in charge of the ICCU, admission can be considered for patients with other cardiovascular diseases, such as hypertensive crises, type B aortic dissection (after initial stabilization in the coronary unit), bacterial endocarditis in patients awaiting emergency surgery, etc.

Other Clinical Situations in which Admission to Intermediate Coronary Care Units could be Considered

In exceptional circumstances, heart surgery patients with cardiac complications (heart failure, arrhythmias, etc.) that would make their admission to a general ward inadvisable can be admitted once 36–48 hours have elapsed since the operation (and the patient has been extubated and the chest drains and so on have been withdrawn), provided no other serious extracardiac problems are present that would indicate admission to the general ICU or the specific resuscitation unit.

INTRODUCTION

The physician determines the blood component that is needed to treat a client's medical condition. Blood products are ordered to restore circulating blood volume, improve hemoglobin levels, or correct serum protein deficiencies. Clinical indicators differ among blood products and the nurse is responsible for understanding the components that are appropriate in various situations.

A blood transfusion is a safe, common procedure in which you receive blood through an intravenous (IV) line inserted into one of your blood vessels. Blood transfusions are used to replace blood lost during surgery or a serious injury. A transfusion also might be done if your body cannot make blood properly because of an illness. During a blood transfusion, a small needle is used to insert an IV line into one of your blood vessels. Through this line, you receive healthy blood. The procedure usually takes 1–4 hours, depending on how much blood you need. Blood transfusions are very common. Each year, almost 5 million Americans need a blood transfusion. Most blood transfusions go well. Mild complications can occur. Very rarely, serious problems develop.

DEFINITION

Blood administration or transfusion therapy is the IV administration of whole blood or blood products.

Purposes

- To restore blood volume after severe hemorrhage
- To restore the oxygen carrying capacity of the blood
- To maintain the hemoglobin levels in severe anemia
- To replace specific blood component
- To assess or focus on clinical signs of reaction (e.g., sudden chills, nausea, itching rash, and dyspnea), status of infusion, site, and any unusual symptoms.

Blood Types

Every person has one of the following blood types: A, B, AB, or O. Also, every person's blood is either Rhesus (Rh) positive or Rh negative. So if you have type A blood, it is either A positive or A negative.

The blood used in a transfusion must match with your blood type. If it does not match, antibodies (proteins) in your blood will attack the new blood and make you sick.

Type O blood is safe for almost everyone. About 40% of the population has type O blood. People who have this blood type are called universal donors. Type O blood is used for emergencies when there is no time to test a person's blood type.

People who have type AB blood are called universal recipients. This means they can get any type of blood.

If you have Rh-positive blood, you can get Rh-positive or Rh-negative blood. But if you have Rh-negative blood, you should only get Rh-negative blood. Rh-negative blood is used for emergencies when there is no time to test a person's Rh type.

Blood types	RBC antigens	Plasma antibodies
A	A	B
B	B	A
AB	—	A and B
O	A and B	—

Rhesus Factor

The Rh factor antigen is present on RBCs of approximately 85% of the people. Blood that contains the Rh factor is known as Rh positive, when it is not present the blood is said to be Rh negative.

Blood Banks

Blood banks collect, test, and store blood. They carefully screen all donated blood for infectious agents (such as viruses) or other factors that could make the receiver sick. Blood banks also screen each blood donation to find whether it is type A, B, AB, or O and whether it is Rh positive or Rh negative. Thus, blood banks carefully test the donated blood.

To prepare blood for a transfusion, some blood banks remove white blood cells. This process is called white cell or leukocyte reduction. Although rare, some people are allergic to white blood cells received as donated blood. Removing these cells makes allergic reactions less likely.

Not all transfusions use blood donated from a stranger. If you are undergoing a surgery, you may need a blood transfusion because of blood loss during the operation. If it is surgery that you are able to schedule months in advance, your doctor may ask your preference of using your own blood, rather than donated blood.

Blood Typing and Crossmatching

To avoid transfusion of incompatible red blood cells, both blood donor and recipient are typed and crossmatched. Blood typing is done to determine the ABO blood group and Rh status. This test is performed on pregnant women and neonates to assess for possible intrauterine exposure of incompatible blood type. Because blood typing only determines the presence of major ABO and Rh antigens, crossmatching also is necessary prior to transfusion.

Selection of Blood Donors

The following points must be remembered while selecting donors:
1. **Age >18:** Our program will not consider donation from individuals under the age of 18.
2. **Smoking:** Candidates will not be considered for donation unless they have been tobacco free (including chewing tobacco) for at least 8 weeks prior to donation and smoking is strongly discouraged after donation to protect long-term health.
3. **Drug use:** Potential donors must not use any illicit drugs. This includes periodic use of any drug, such as marijuana in any form (including orally). Potential donors who use chronic pain medication experience a higher incidence of postoperative pain after donation. These individuals may be requested to see a surgeon and/or psychiatrist prior to being considered for donation. The transplant team may request random drug screening if there is concern

regarding drug use. Failure to comply with requests for drug screening would be considered the cause for declining donation.

4. **Health problems:** Donors must be healthy individuals. If a donor has a past history of suffering from the following problems or if these are discovered during the medical evaluation, a donor may be declined.
   - High blood pressure treated with medication
   - Diabetes
   - Gestational diabetes
   - Systemic lupus erythematosus
   - Polycystic kidney disease
   - Substance abuse
   - Psychiatric illness
   - Heart/heart valve disease or peripheral vascular disease
   - Lung disease with impaired oxygenation or ventilation
   - Low kidney function (usually creatinine clearance of <80 mL/min (a test of kidney function)
   - Protein in the urine >300 mg/24 hours (a test of kidney function)
   - Active hepatitis B or C infection or HIV infection
   - Use of medicines that are known to cause kidney damage
   - History of blood clots or risk factors for the development of blood clots.

5. **Obesity:** Obesity is an independent risk factor for kidney disease. Candidates with a body mass index (BMI) of over 35 will generally not be considered for donation unless an individual is very muscular. Individuals with a BMI of >25 will need to meet a dietitian to discuss strategies to remain at a healthy weight for life.

6. **Psychosocial issues:** The social worker will evaluate many psychosocial aspects of living donation with the potential donor. Donors may be declined if they have inadequate support for recovery, questionable donor–recipient relationship or motivation for donation, a history of poor coping or psychiatric illness, a history of not taking good care of their health, or other similar concerns.

Blood Products for Transfusion

Products	Uses
Whole blood	Use in case of hemorrhage; replace blood volume and all blood products: plasma, fresh platelets, red blood cells, plasma protein, and clotting factors
Packed red blood cells	Used to increase the oxygen-carrying capacity of blood, anemia, surgery, and disorder with slow bleeding
Autologous red blood cells	➤ Use for blood replacement following planned elective surgery ➤ Client denotes blood for autologous transfusion 4–5 weeks prior to surgery
Platelets	Replace in cases of platelet disorder
Fresh frozen plasma	Expand blood volume and provides clotting factors
Albumin and plasma protein fraction	Blood volume expander; provide plasma protein
Clotting factors and cryoprecipitate	Used for patients with clotting factor deficiencies

Patient Instructions and Preparation

Informed Consent

The patients undergoing blood transfusion will have to be informed of the following:
- Informed consent may be obtained by a physician, a nurse, or a physician extender who is knowledgeable about blood transfusion and the patient's condition, so as to be able to explain the elements of informed consent above.

- The **risks of transfusion**, including adverse symptoms and alternatives to homologous (allogeneic) transfusion, must be discussed with the patient well before the transfusion.
- The patient is then given a choice to accept or decline transfusion.
- Consent should be documented in the medical chart using the form.

Refusal of Blood Transfusion

Under the following conditions blood transfusion can be refused to the patients:
The form "patient's release form for refusal of blood or treatment" should be used to document the patient's refusal of transfusion. The form is available on the blood bank website.

Receipt of Blood Components

Steps to follow during receipt of blood:

Step	Action		
1.	Verify ➢ Product is designated for a patient at the receiving location ➢ Name and admission number recorded on the transfusion record form attached to the unit correspond with that of the intended recipient ➢ Unit has a normal appearance		
2.	The person receiving the blood component should: ➢ Record on the blood delivery form the date and time that the blood was received/removed from the pneumatic tube ➢ Sign the blood delivery form		
3.	Return the signed and dated blood delivery form to the blood bank using hospital mail		
4.	Verify that red blood cells and plasma components were received within 30 minutes of the dispensed time stamp on the form		
	If more than 30 minutes have elapsed since the time stamp on the blood delivery form	The red blood cells or plasma may be used for immediate transfusion that will be completed within 4 hours of the time stamp, the transfuse the component	
		Do not store red blood cells and plasma that have been out of refrigeration for more than 30 minutes in patient care unit blood refrigerators	
		If the blood component is not needed for immediate transfusion, return the red blood cells or plasma to the blood bank for proper disposal	

Special Labels

The following are the special labels to look for as soon as the blood bank release blood for transfusion:

- When blood is released for transfusion under unusual circumstances, a special notation will be indicated on the transfusion record form.
- This information will often suggest to physicians and nurses that particular caution must be exercised during transfusion and that the blood transfusion should be terminated at the first sign of an untoward reaction.
- If the personnel initiating the transfusion have questions concerning the significance of this information, then they should contact the blood bank.

Immediately Prior to Blood Transfusion

Pretransfusion Vital Sign Documentation

Before initiating blood transfusion, the following vital documents need to be signed:

- To provide a baseline, record the patient's blood pressure, pulse, respiration, and temperature in the chart or on the transfusion record form.
- If a patient is febrile, consideration should be given to postpone the blood transfusion, since the fever may mask the development of a febrile reaction to the blood component itself.

- Verify physician's orders for transfusion and that any pretransfusion medications have been administered.
- Perform bedside verification of patient and component using the labels on the bag
- Transfusion record form
- Patient's attached positive patient identifier

These steps must never be bypassed.

1.	Ask the patient to state his/her name. Verify patient and component identification information
2.	Verify the blood type, donor number, component name
3.	Verify compatibility
4.	Verify the product is not outdated
5.	Sign the Transfusion Record Form before blood transfusion is initiated
6.	The person who hangs the blood must record the date and time the transfusion was started
7.	Record the date, time, component, and unit number on the appropriate sheet on the patient's chart, and refer to unit policy and procedures

DO NOT START the transfusion if there is any discrepancy. Contact the Blood Bank.

Initiating the Transfusion

To initiate the transfusion, the following steps have to be checked:
- Immediately before transfusion, mix the unit of blood thoroughly by gentle inversion.
- Follow the manufacturer's instruction for the use of special filters and ancillary devices. Additional administration instructions for selected components are printed at the end of this chapter and are available upon request from the blood bank.
- If any part of the unit is transfused, the unit is considered transfused.

Flow Rates

Initial flow rate	Slowly at no more than 1 mL/minute to allow for recognition of an acute adverse reaction; proportionately smaller volume for pediatric patients
Standard flow rate—adults	If no reaction occurs in the first 15 minutes, the rate may be increased to 4 mL/minute
Pediatrics	10–20 mL/kg over 30–60 minutes
Usual infusion time	➢ Red blood cells: 2 hours unless the patient can tolerate only gradual expansion of the intravascular volume ➢ Platelets, plasma, and cryoprecipitate: 10 mL per minute; the transfusion may be administered as rapidly as the patient can tolerate, usually 30 minutes
Maximum infusion time	Infusion time should not exceed 4 hours for any component

If rate slows appreciably	➢ Investigate immediately
	➢ Consider measures that may enhance blood flow
	  – Repositioning the patient's arm
	  – Changing to a larger gauge needle
	  – Changing the filter and tubing
	  – Elevating the IV pole, if gravity rather than a pump is being used

During the Transfusion Document

What	➢ Temperature, blood pressure, respirations, and pulse; and examine the skin for urticaria ➢ Assess flow rate
When	➢ Before initiating the transfusion ➢ After the first 15 minutes ➢ After 30 minutes ➢ Hourly until 1 hour after completion of the transfusion
Outpatient posttransfusion vital signs	For outpatient transfusions, the vital signs may be taken at 30 minutes posttransfusion

If the Patient Has a Preexisting Fever

The need for transfusion must be balanced with the risk of transfusion. Contact the patient's physician to determine whether pretransfusion medications should be administered.

If a Patient is Being Transported with Blood Hanging

Patients should not be transported with blood components infusing unless accompanied by a clinician who can monitor and respond to a potential reaction.

Medications

- Do not add medications directly to a unit of blood during transfusion.
- Medications that can be administered "IV push" may be administered by stopping the transfusion, clearing the line at the medication injection site with 5–10 mL of normal saline, administering the medication, reflushing the line with saline, and restarting the transfusion.

At the Termination of Transfusion

- Document the date and time when transfusion was stopped, volume of blood infused
- Check the box documenting the presence/absence of a transfusion reaction.
- Discontinue the isotonic saline solution used to initiate the transfusion after the completion of the transfusion unless specifically ordered.
- Document the patient's response to the transfusion in the patient's medical record.

If a Transfusion Reaction is Suspected

In case of suspicion of any reaction during transfusion, the below points will have to be followed:
- Stop the transfusion
- Maintain the IV
- Save the bag and attached tubing

Articles

The following articles are required for blood transfusion:
- Blood administration set
- 250 mL NaCl IV solution of 0.9%
- Alcohol swabs
- Disposable clean gloves
- Adhesive tape
- Blood pressure cuff and stethoscope
- Thermometer
- Signed transfusion consent form

Steps	Rationale
1. Complete preprocedure 2. Verify that IV cannula is patent and without complication such as infiltration or phlebitis. In emergency situations that require rapid transfusions, 16 or 18 gauge cannula is preferred; transfusion for therapeutic indications may be infused with cannulas ranging from 20 to 24 gauge 3. Obtain client's transfusion history 4. Review physician's order for blood component transfusion. Check that consent has been properly completed and signed by client	➤ It ensures that transfusion will be infiltrated infused on time. Gauge of IV cannula should be appropriate. Large cannula promotes optimal flow of blood components. Uses of smaller cannula such as 22–24 gauges may require to blood bank to divide unit, so that each half can be infused within allotted time ➤ Identifies client's prior response to transfusion of blood components ➤ For checking physician's order must be present before transfusing blood products and to provide complete information to patient about procedure

Contd...

Contd...

Steps	Rationale
5. Obtain and record vital signs before administration of transfusion	➤ To check the baseline data and to alert the patient about warning signs
6. **Pre-administration:**	➤ To ensure that product is safe to administer
– Obtain blood component from blood bank	➤ Strict adherence to verification procedure before administration of blood or blood components reduces the risk of administering wrong blood to client
– Correctly verify product and identify client with person considered qualified by your agency:	
♦ Check client's first and last names by having client state name, if available	➤ Notify blood bank and appropriate personnel as indicated by agency policy
♦ Verify that component received from blood bank is the component ordered by physician	➤ Ensures that client receive correct therapy
♦ Check that client's blood types and Rh types are compatible with donor blood type and Rh type	➤ Verifies accurate donor blood type; air bubbles, clots, or discoloration may be indicating bacterial contamination or inadequate coagulation of stored component
♦ Check that unit number on unit of blood and on blood bank match	
♦ Check expiration date and time on unit of blood	➤ Expired blood should never be used, because cell components deteriorate and may contain excess citrate ions
♦ Record verification process as directed by agency policy	
7. **During administration:**	➤ Documentation on legal medical record
– Autologous transfusion only:	➤ Allow collection of client's blood for reinfusion, storage no longer than 6 hours or washing and spinning
♦ Connect drainage tubes to collection container or cell processing system	➤ Tubing is used to facilitate maintenance of IV access in case client needs more than 1 unit of blood. Both a unit of blood and container of 0.9% NaCl are connected to system
♦ Minimize air bubbles by establishing secure connections	
– Open Y tubing blood administration set	
– Set roller clamp to "off" position	➤ Moving roller clamps to "off" position prevents accidental spilling and wasting of product
– Spike 0.9% NaCl IV bag with one of Y tubing spikes invert filter, open roller clamps of IV bag, and component side of Y, keeping common tubing clamp below filter closed; set IV bag on table and gently press down to squeeze IV bag to fill both sides of Y tubing; close tubing clamp of component side of Y and open common tubing clamp below filter; continue to press down on IV saline bag to completely fill the filter and half of drip chamber; close both tubing clamps; all three tubing clamps should be closed	➤ Primes tubing with fluid to eliminate air on both sides of Y tubing, inverting filter to fill from top to bottom reduces the formation of air pockets, closing roller clamp prevents spillage and waste of fluid
	➤ This will completely prime tubing with saline and IV line is ready to be connected to client's vascular access device
– Hang on IV pole, open common tubing clamp to finish priming tubing to distal end of tubing connector, close tubing clamp when tubing is filled with saline, maintain protective sterile cap on tubing connector	➤ Protective barrier drape may be used to catch any potential blood spillage, tubing is primed with blood unit and ready for transfusion into client
	➤ This initiates infusion of blood product into client's vein
	➤ Most transfusion reactions occur within first 5–15 minutes of transfusion
Prepare blood component for administration, remove protective covering from access port. Spike blood component unit with other Y connection, hang on IV pole, open clamp of Y connected to blood unit and open common tubing clamp to prime tubing with blood, allow saline in tubing to flow into receptacle, being careful to ensure that any blood spillage is contained in blood precaution container	➤ Frequent monitoring of vital sign will help quickly alert nurse to transfusion reactions
	➤ Maintaining prescribed rate of flow decrease the risk of fluid volume excess while restoring vascular volume
	➤ Infusing IV saline solution infuses remainder of the blood in IV tubing and keep IV line patent for supportive measures in case of transfusion reaction
Nurse alert: Normal saline is compatible with blood products, unlike solutions that contain dextrose, which cause coagulation of donor blood	➤ Standard precautions during transfusions reduce transmission of microorganisms
– Maintaining asepsis, attach primed tubing to client's vascular access device (VAD), and open common tubing clamp	➤ Detects presence of infiltration or phlebitis and verifies continuous and safe infusion of blood products
	➤ These may be early signs of transfusion reaction

Contd...

Contd...

Steps	Rationale
– Remain with client during first 5–15 minutes of transfusion, initial flow rate during this time should be 2 mL/minute **Nurse alert:** If signs of a transfusion reaction occur, stop infusion, start normal saline with new primed tubing directly into VAD at keep vein open (KVO) (5–10 mL/hour), and notify the physician immediately – Monitor client's vital signs 5 minutes after blood product has begun infusing and per agency policy after that – Regulate rate of transfusion according to physician's orders (drop factor for blood tubing is 10 gtt/mL) **Nurse alert:** A unit of whole blood should not hang for more than 4 hours because of the danger of bacterial growth – After blood has infused, clear IV line with normal saline and discard blood bag according to agency policy – Appropriately dispose of all supplies. Remove gloves and perform hand hygiene 8. Monitor IV site and status of infusion each time vital signs are taken 9. Observe for any change in vital signs and for chills, flushing, itching, dyspnea, rashes, or other signs of transfusion reaction 10. Complete postprocedure protocol	

AFTERCARE: RECORDING AND REPORTING

The aftercare following blood transfusion are listed below:
- Record the type of blood component and amount administered.
- Record the starting and finishing time of blood administration.
- Report signs and symptoms of transfusion reaction immediately.

NURSING MANAGEMENT

Unexpected outcomes	Nursing interventions
Hemolytic reaction: Client displays signs and symptoms of transfusion reaction which include: ➤ Fever with/without chills ➤ Tachycardia ➤ Tachypnea ➤ Wheezing ➤ Dyspnea ➤ Headache ➤ Flushing of skin ➤ Hives or itching ➤ Hypotension ➤ Gastrointestinal system	➤ Stop transfusion ➤ Normal saline should be connected at vascular access hub to prevent subsequently blood from infusing from tubing ➤ Disconnect blood tubing at VAD hub and cap the distal end with sterile connector to maintain sterile system ➤ Keep vein open with slow infusion of normal saline at 10–12 gtt/minute to ensure venous patency ➤ It is important to regulate flow rate to minimize administration of excess IV fluid, especially in client who are prone to fluid overload

Client develops infiltration or phlebitis at vein puncture site	➢ Remove IV and insert new VAD in different sites ➢ Product may be restarted if reminder can be transfused within 4 hours of initiation of transfusion ➢ Nursing measures to reduce discomfort at infiltration site
Fluid overload: Client exhibits difficulty in breathing and crackles upon auscultation	➢ Slow and stop transfusion ➢ Elevate head end side of the bed ➢ Inform physician about physical findings ➢ Administer diuretics, morphine, and oxygen as doctors order ➢ Continue frequent assessment ➢ Check vital signs at regular intervals of time
Sepsis: High-grade fever, chills, vomiting, diarrhea, hypotension	➢ Stop transfusion ➢ Keep the vein open with normal saline ➢ Notify the primary care provider ➢ Administer IV fluids, antibiotics ➢ Obtain a blood specimen from the client for culture ➢ Send remaining blood and tubing to the laboratory
Febrile reactions: High-grade fever, chill, headache, flushing of skin, anxiety, muscle pain	➢ Stop transfusion ➢ Keep the vein open with normal saline ➢ Notify the primary care provider ➢ Give antipyretic to the patient
Allergic reactions: Flushing, itching, urticaria, bronchial wheezing, chest pain, cardiac arrest	➢ Stop transfusion ➢ Keep the vein open with normal saline ➢ Notify the primary care provider ➢ Give antihistamine to the patient

Cardiac Catheterization

DEFINITION

Cardiac catheterization is a test that uses a catheter and X-ray machine to check the heart and its blood supply.

PURPOSE

- Chest pain characterized by prolonged heavy pressure or a squeezing pain
- Abnormal treadmill stress test
- Myocardial infarction
- Congenital heart defects
- A diagnosis of valvular heart disease
- A need to measure the heart muscle's ability to pump blood
- Diagnosis of ventricular aneurysms, narrowing of the aortic valve, enlargement of the left ventricle
- Insufficiency of the aortic or mitral valve.

INDICATIONS

- Identify narrowed or clogged arteries of the heart
- Measure blood pressure within the heart
- Evaluate how well the heart valves and chambers are working
- Check heart defects
- Evaluate an enlarged heart
- Decide on an appropriate treatment

COMPLICATIONS

- Bleeding at the point of the catheter insertion
- Damage to arteries
- Heart attack or abnormal heart beats known as arrhythmia
- Allergic reaction to X-ray dye
- Blood clot formation
- Infection

Risk of Complications

- Allergies to medications or X-ray dye
- Obesity
- Smoking

- Bleeding disorder
- Increased age
- Recent pneumonia
- Recent heart attack
- Diabetes
- Kidney disease

PROCEDURE

- A cardiac catheterization is an invasive, **nonsurgical procedure** done to study the arteries that bring blood to the heart muscle and to check the function of the main pumping chamber of heart.
- During cardiac catheterization, the cardiologist inserts a small, hollow tube (catheter) into an artery or vein and then guides it into the heart using X-ray.
- The cardiologist injects contrast through the catheter to outline the arteries and to show any blockages or narrowing that may exist.
- The results of these tests will assist the doctor in making the diagnosis of coronary artery disease (CAD).
- Most patients have little or no discomfort during a cardiac catheterization.
- However, patient may feel a hot, flushing sensation for several seconds when the contrast is injected into the main pumping chamber of the heart.
- The nursing and medical staff will give medication and reassurance throughout the procedure to ensure comfort.
- Percutaneous coronary intervention (PCI) is a treatment procedure that unblocks narrowed coronary arteries without performing surgery. During this procedure, your cardiologist determines the best treatment for your condition. Treatment will vary from patient to patient.
- **Balloon catheter angioplasty:** During this procedure, the cardiologist inserts a cardiac catheter with a small balloon around it into the coronary artery. The cardiologist then places the balloon in the narrowed area of the artery and expands it with liquid. This pushes the plaque (blockage) to the sides of the artery where it remains. This technique reduces the narrowing in the artery and restores the normal size of the artery. The cardiologist removes the balloon catheter at the end of the procedure.
- **Stent:** The cardiologist places a small, hollow metal (mesh) tube called a "stent" in the artery to keep it open following a balloon angioplasty. The stent prevents constriction or closing of the artery during and after the procedure. Drug-eluting stents are now used. These stents are coated with medication that helps prevent narrowing of the artery.
- **Rotational atherectomy:** During this procedure, the cardiologist uses a specialized instrument to break into tiny pieces the rock-hard plaque with calcium build up from the blood vessel walls. Patient may experience some discomfort, such as chest pain, pressure, or tightness in your chest during this procedure. Medications may be given to ease the discomfort. This procedure may last from 30 seconds to 1 minute.

PREPARATION OF THE PATIENT

- Consult with doctor about your medications
- Bring a list of all current medications, including strength (dose) and frequency (time taken). This includes any over-the-counter medications, herbal preparations, or vitamins.
- Ask your doctor about whether routine medications can be taken with a sip of water before coming to the hospital.

- Usually, aspirin should be taken prior to cardiac catheterization and PCI.
- If patient is taking blood-thinning medications, such as Coumadin (warfarin), the patient has to check with the doctor as to when to stop taking these medications prior to the procedure.
- If taking medications for diabetes, e.g., Glucophage (metformin) or Glucovance (glyburide and metformin), the patient may be advised to stop these medications before the procedure and restart these medications after the procedure, as directed by doctor.
- Be sure to tell about any allergic reaction to X-ray dye (contrast), iodine, seafood, or history of bleeding problems.

Prepare the Night Before

For this procedure, the patient will have to be prepared the previous night as follows:

- Drink plenty of fluids the evening before the test, unless otherwise directed by doctor.
- Do not eat or drink anything after midnight, the night before procedure.
- You must arrange for a relative or friend to drive you home. You may not drive for 24 hours following the procedure.
- Take medications that doctor has **specifically** instructed to take on the day of procedure with a **sip** of water
- Arrive at least 2 hours before scheduled procedure. If you are scheduled for a 7 AM procedure, please arrive at 6 AM

While you are in the ambulatory care unit (ACU) and cath lab holding area:

- Take consent form before the procedure.
- Nurse places a small intravenous (IV) catheter (tube) in arm. The IV is needed to give you medications to help you relax and ensure that you are comfortable throughout the procedure.
- Prepare the insertion site either groin and/or arm area to remove hair and prevent infection.
- Urinary catheterization is done if needed.

During the Procedure

- For the procedure, lie on back on an X-ray table. Because the table may be tilted during the procedure, safety straps may be fastened across chest and legs. X-ray cameras may move over and around head and chest to take pictures from many angles.
- An IV line is inserted into a vein in arm.
- Electrodes placed on chest to monitor heart throughout the procedure.
- A blood pressure cuff is placed to monitor blood pressure and a pulse oximeter to measure the amount of oxygen in blood.
- You may receive medication (anticoagulants) to help prevent your blood from clotting in the catheter and in your coronary arteries.
- A small amount of hair may be shaved from groin or arm where the catheter is to be inserted.
- The area is washed and disinfected and then numbed with an injection of local anesthetic.
- Dye (contrast material) is injected through the catheter.
- The dye is easy to see on X-ray images and as it moves through blood vessels.

After the Procedure

- When the angiogram is over, the catheter is removed from arm or groin and the incision is closed with manual pressure, a clamp, or a small plug.
- Keep the recovery area under observation and monitoring

Postoperative Care: At the Care Center

- Electrocardiogram (ECG) and blood studies may be done.
- If the catheter was inserted in the groin area, patients will likely need to lie still in bed and flat on their back for a period of time.
- If the catheter was in arm, patient will likely have to be out of bed sooner.
- A pressure dressing may be placed over the area where the catheter was inserted to help prevent bleeding. It is important to follow the nurse's instructions.

Call Your Doctor

- You notice bleeding, new bruising, or swelling at the catheter site
- You develop increasing pain or discomfort at the catheter site
- You have signs of infection, such as redness, drainage, or fever
- There is a change in temperature or color of the leg or arm that was used for the procedure.
- You feel faint or weak.
- You develop chest pain or shortness of breath.

At Home

When you return home, do the following to help ensure a smooth recovery:
- Do not drive for 72 hours
- Do not lift heavy objects or engage in strenuous exercise or sexual activity for at least 5–7 days.
- Change the dressing around the incision area as instructed
- Your doctor will explain which medications you can take and which ones to avoid. Take medications as instructed.
- You can make lifestyle changes to lower your risk for further complications of heart disease. These include eating a healthier diet, exercising regularly, and managing stress.
- Change the dressing around the incision area as instructed
- Ice may help decrease discomfort at the insertion site. You may apply ice for 15–20 minutes each hour, for the first few days.
- Ask your doctor about when it is safe to shower, bathe, or soak in water.
- Be sure to follow your doctor's instructions.

Chest Physiotherapy

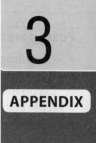

3

APPENDIX

DEFINITION

Chest physiotherapy can be defined as follows:
- Chest physiotherapy (CPT) is a technique used to mobilize or loosen secretions in the lungs and respiratory tract.
- This is especially helpful for patients with large amount of secretions or ineffective cough.
- Chest physiotherapy consists of external mechanical maneuvers, such as chest percussion, postural drainage, vibration, to augment mobilization and clearance of airway secretions, diaphragmatic breathing with pursed lips, coughing, and controlled coughing.
- During forced exhalation, as when blowing out a candle, expiratory muscles including the abdominal muscles and internal intercostal muscles generate abdominal and thoracic pressure, which forces air out of the lungs.
- Chest physical therapy is defined as improving respiratory efficiency, promoting expansion of the lungs, strengthening respiratory muscles, and eliminating secretions from the respiratory system.

PURPOSE

- Help patients breathe more freely.
- Get more oxygen into the body.

INDICATIONS

- Cystic fibrosis
- Bronchiectasis
- Atelectasis
- Lung abscess
- Neuromuscular diseases
- Pneumonia in dependent lung regions.

CONTRAINDICATIONS

- Increased intracranial pressure (ICP)
- Unstable head or neck injury
- Active hemorrhage with hemodynamic instability or hemoptysis
- Recent spinal injury or injury
- Empyema
- Bronchopleural fistula
- Rib fracture
- Fail chest
- Uncontrolled hypertension

- Anticoagulation
- Rib or vertebral fractures or osteoporosis

ASSESSMENT

Nursing care and selection of CPT skills are based on specific assessment findings. The following are the assessment criteria:

- **Know the normal range of patient's vital signs:** Conditions requiring CPT, such atelectasis, and pneumonia, affect vital signs.
- **Know the patient's medications:** Certain medications, particularly diuretics, antihypertensive, cause fluid and hemodynamic changes. These decrease patient's tolerance to positional changes and postural drainage.
- **Know the patient's medical history:** Certain conditions such as increased ICP, spinal cord injuries, and abdominal aneurysm resection contraindicate the positional change to postural drainage. Thoracic trauma and chest surgeries also contraindicate percussion and vibration.
- **Know the patient's cognitive level of functioning:** Participating in controlled cough techniques requires the patient to follow instructions.
- **Beware of patient's exercise tolerance:** The CPT maneuvers are fatiguing. Gradual increase in activity, and through CPT, patient tolerance to the procedure improves.

CLINICAL FINDINGS AND INVESTIGATIONS

- Detailed history
- Physical examination
- Inspection
- Palpation
- Percussion
- Auscultation.

Investigation can be achieved using the following:

- X-ray
- Blood investigations, i.e., bleeding and clotting parameters

CHEST PHYSICAL THERAPY

Chest physiotherapy involves the following techniques:

- Chest percussion
- Chest vibration
- Postural drainage
- Turning
- Deep breathing exercises
- Coughing

TECHNIQUES

- A nurse or respiratory therapist may administer CPT, though the techniques can often be taught to patients' family members.
- The most common procedures used are postural drainage and chest percussion, in which the patient is rotated to facilitate drainage of secretions from a specific lobe or segment while being clapped with cupped hands to loosen and mobilize retained secretions that can then be expectorated or drained.
- The procedure is somewhat uncomfortable and tiring for the patient.

Percussion

The following steps are involved in percussion:

- Usually the patient will be positioned in supine or prone and should not experience any pain.
- Chest percussion involves striking the chest wall over the area being drained.
- Percussing lung areas involves the use of cupped palm to loosen pulmonary secretions, so that they can be expectorated with ease.
- Percussing with the hand held in a rigid dome-shaped position, the area over the lung lobes to be drained in rhythmic pattern.
- Cupping is never done on bare skin or performed over surgical incisions, below the ribs, or over the spine or breasts, because of the danger of tissue damage.
- Typically, each area is percussed for 30–60 seconds several times a day.
- If the patient has tenacious secretions, the area must be percussed for 3–5 minutes several times per day. Patients may learn how to percuss the anterior chest as well.

Hand Position for Chest Percussion (Fig. A-3.1)

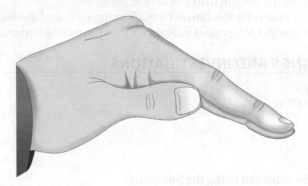

Fig. A-3.1: Correct hand position for chest percussion.

Chest Percussion

- It involves using a cupped hand and alternately clapping with both hands on the patient's chest wall. This should be performed over the lung segment that is to be drained. Hand should be NOT be flat.
- The percussion technique should be vigorous and rhythmical, but it should not involve pain.
- If the patient complains of pain, it means that your hand may not be cupped properly and needs to be softened or readjusted.
- When done properly, you should hear a hollow sound with each percussion.
- Chest percussion should be done over the ribs, with careful attention to avoiding percussing over the spine, breastbone, or lower back to prevent damage to internal organs. Percussion may or may not be accompanied by vibration.
- Mechanical percussive devices are also available as an alternative to manual chest percussion.

VIBRATION

- In vibration, the nurse uses rhythmic contractions and relaxations using his or her arm and shoulder muscles while holding the patient flat on the patient's chest as the patient exhales.

- The purpose is to help loosen respiratory secretions, so that they can be expectorated with ease. Vibration (at a rate of 200 per minute) can be done for several times a day.
- To avoid patient causing discomfort, vibration is never done over the patient's breasts, spine, sternum, and rib cage.
- Vibration can also be taught to family members or accomplished with mechanical device.

Correct Hand Position for Vibration (Fig. A-3.2)

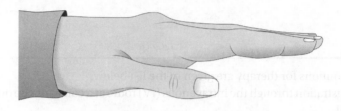

Fig. A-3.2: Correct hand position for vibration.

- Vibration is an airway clearance technique that, coupled with chest percussion, is applied during postural drainage to help chronic obstructive pulmonary disease (COPD) patient's clear mucus from the airways. Vibration helps to gently shake mucus and secretions into the large airways, making it easier to cough up.
- During vibration, place your flat hand firmly against the chest wall, atop the appropriate lung segment to be drained. Stiffen your arm and shoulder, apply light pressure and create a shaking movement, similar to that of a vibrator.
- Tell the patient to breathe in deeply during vibration therapy and exhale slowly and completely. Taking a deep breath and then exhaling slowly and forcefully without straining will hopefully stimulate a productive cough.

PROCEDURE: PERCUSSION AND VIBRATION

- Instruct the patient to breathe diaphragmatically.
- Position the patient in prescribed postural drainage positions. Spine should be straight to promote rib cage expansion.
- Percuss or clap with cupped hands or chest wall for 5 minutes over each segment, i.e., for 5 minutes for cystic fibrosis and 1–2 minutes for other conditions.
- Avoid clapping over spine, liver, spleen, breast, scapula, clavicle, or sternum.
- Instruct the patient to inhale slowly and deeply. Vibrate the chest wall as the patient exhales slowly through the pursed lips.
- Place one hand on top of the other affected area or place one hand on each side of the rib cage.
- Tense the muscles of the hands while applying moderate pressure downward and vibrate arms and hands.
- Relieve pressure on the thorax as the patient inhales.
- Encourage the patient cough, using abdominal muscles, after three or four vibrations.
- Allow the patient to rest several times.
- Listen with stethoscope for changes in breathe sounds.
- Repeat the percussion and vibration cycle according to the patient's tolerance and clinical response: usually 15–30 minutes.

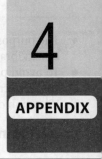

Intravenous Therapy

DEFINITION

The various definitions for therapy are given in the list below:
- Drug administration through the intravenous (IV) route at a constant rate over a determined time interval.
- A solution administered into a vein through an infusion set that includes a plastic or glass vacuum bottle or bag containing the solution and tube connecting the bottle to a catheter or a needle in the patient's vein.
- The process of administering a solution IV or directly into a vein.

PURPOSES

The many purposes of administering therapies are the following:
- Intravenous therapy may be used to correct electrolyte imbalances.
- To deliver medications
- Blood transfusion
- Fluid replacement (dehydration)
- Chemotherapy (the treatment for any kind of cancer)

COMMON INTRAVENOUS SITES

The following are the most common IV sites for administering therapies:
- Cephalic vein
- Basilic vein
- Median cubital vein
- Radial vein
- Superficial dorsal veins
- Dorsal venous arch basilic vein (hand)
- Great saphenous veins
- Dorsal plexus of foot

INFUSED SUBSTANCES

Volume Expanders

The two main types of volume expanders are the following:
1. Crystalloids
2. Colloids

Crystalloids

- **Crystalloids** are aqueous solutions of mineral salts or other water-soluble molecules. Crystalloids generally are much cheaper than colloids.
- The most commonly used crystalloid fluid is normal saline (sodium chloride at 0.9% concentration, isotonic).
- Lactated Ringer (also known as Ringer lactate which is mildly hypotonic solution) is also used as a common crystalloid.

The Table A-4.1 provides a list of intravenous solutions.

TABLE A.4.1: List of intravenous solution.	
Solution	**Concentration**
Dextrose in water solution	
Dextrose 5%	Isotonic
Dextrose 10%	Hypertonic
Saline solution	
0.45% Sodium chloride	Hypotonic
0.9% Sodium chloride	Isotonic
3–5% Sodium chloride	Hypertonic
Dextrose in saline solution	
Dextrose 5% in 0.9% sodium chloride	Hypertonic
Dextrose 5% in 0.45% sodium chloride	Hypertonic
Multiple electrolyte solution	
Lactated Ringer	Isotonic
Dextrose 5% in lactated Ringer	Hypertonic

Colloids

- Colloids contain larger insoluble molecules, such as gelatin. Blood is a colloid.
- Colloids preserve a high colloid osmotic pressure in the blood, while, on the other hand, this parameter is decreased by crystalloids due to hemodilution.

Blood-based Products

A blood product (or blood-based product) is any component of blood that is collected from a donor for use in a blood transfusion.

The following are the indications for blood transfusion:
- Trauma
- Surgery
- Severe anemia
- Thrombocytopenia
- Hemophilia
- Sickle cell disease

Examples:
- Hemophilia usually need a replacement of clotting factor, which is a small part of the whole blood.
- Sickle cell disease may require frequent blood transfusions. Earlier blood transfusions consisted of whole blood.
- Fresh frozen plasma
- Cryoprecipitate

Buffer Solutions

Buffer solutions are used to correct acidosis or alkalosis.
- Lactated Ringer solution also has some buffering effect.
- Intravenous sodium bicarbonate are specifically used for buffering purpose.

Other Medications

The below list provides the method of using other medications:
- Medications may be mixed into the fluids mentioned above. Certain types of medications can only be given IV, such as when there is insufficient uptake by other routes of administration such as enterally. Examples include: IV immunoglobulin and propofol.
- Parenteral nutrition is feeding a person IV and bypassing the usual process of eating and digestion. The person receives nutritional formulas containing salts, glucose, amino acids, lipids, and added vitamins.
- Drug injection used for recreational substances usually enters by the IV route.

INTRAVENOUS DEVICES

The seven most common intravenous devices are the following:

Peripheral Cannula

A peripheral IV line consists of a short catheter inserted through the skin into a peripheral vein. This is usually in the form of a cannula-over-needle device, which consists of a flexible plastic cannula.

Sites

Any accessible vein can be used though arm and hand veins are used most commonly, with leg and foot veins used to a much lesser extent. In infants, the scalp veins are sometimes used.

Sizes of Cannula

- 12–14 gauge (used in resuscitation settings)
- 16 gauge (used for blood donation and transfusion)
- 18–20 gauge (for infusions and blood draws)
- 22 gauge (pediatric line)
- 24–26 the smallest

Colors of Cannula

- Green: 18 G
- Pink: 20 G
- Blue: 22 G
- Yellow: 24 G

Central IV Lines

Central IV lines flow through a catheter with its tip within a large vein, usually the superior vena cava or inferior vena cava, or within the right atrium of the heart. This has several advantages over a peripheral IV:

- It can deliver fluids and medications that would be overly irritating to peripheral veins because of their concentration or chemical composition. These include some chemotherapy drugs and total parenteral nutrition.
- Medications reach the heart immediately and are quickly distributed to the rest of the body.
- There is room for multiple parallel compartments (lumen) within the catheter, so that multiple medications can be delivered at once even if they would not be chemically compatible within a single tube.
- Caregivers can measure central venous pressure and other physiological variables through the line.

Complications

- Bleeding
- Infection
- Gangrene
- Thromboembolism
- Gas embolism

Peripherally Inserted Central Catheter

The PICC lines are used when IV access is required over a prolonged period of time or when the material to be infused would cause quick damage and early failure of a peripheral IV and when a conventional central line may be too dangerous to attempt. Typical uses for a PICC include long chemotherapy regimens, extended antibiotic therapy, or total parenteral nutrition.

Advantage of a PICC: It is safer to insert with a relatively low risk of uncontrollable bleeding and essentially no risks of damage to the lungs or major blood vessels.

Disadvantage: It must be inserted more technically.

Central Venous Lines

Several types of catheters are available that take a more direct route into central veins. These are collectively called central venous lines. A catheter is inserted into a subclavian, internal jugular, or (less commonly) a femoral vein and advanced toward the heart until it reaches the superior vena cava or right atrium.

Implantable Ports

A port is a central venous line that does not have an external connector; instead, it has a small reservoir that is covered with silicone rubber and is implanted under the skin. Medication is administered intermittently by placing a small needle through the skin, piercing the silicone, into the reservoir. When the needle is withdrawn the reservoir cover reseals itself. The cover can accept hundreds of needle sticks during its lifetime.

Syringe Driver

A syringe driver or syringe pump is a small infusion pump (some include infuse and withdraw capability) used to gradually administer small amounts of fluid (with or without medication) to a patient or for use in chemical and biomedical research. A syringe driver is a small portable pump that can be used to give you a continuous dose of painkiller and other medicines. It is often used in instances of vomiting or unable to swallow.

Guidelines for Procedure

- A syringe driver takes 3–4 hours to establish a steady state drug level in plasma. If the patient is in pain, vomiting or very agitated give a stat subcutaneous injection of appropriate medication while setting the syringe driver up.
- Only use drugs that are known to be effective via the subcutaneous route. Diazepam, chlorpromazine, and prochlorperazine are too irritating to be given subcutaneously.
- Check drug compatibility before mixing. If you are unable to discuss or get advice regarding the concerning drug combinations with either the palliative care team or the hospital drug information service, information can also be found at the palliative drug's Web site.
- Always use water for injection to dilute the drugs. Saline may be used if there are problems with site irritation. Saline should not be used with cyclizine as it can cause precipitation.
- Calculate the total dose of drug required in 24 hours and then divide volume of solution by 24, to give a rate per hour.
- Never use solutions that have precipitated or discolored.
- Always consider alternative routes, such as buccal, rectal, sublingual, or transdermal. The patient may not want a syringe driver.

An Infusion Pump

It infuses fluids, medication, or nutrients into a patient's circulatory system. It is generally used IV, though subcutaneous, arterial, and epidural infusions are occasionally used.

TYPES OF INFUSION

The four major types of infusion are the following:

- **Continuous infusion**: It usually consists of small pulses of infusion, usually between 500 nanoliters and 10,000 microliters, depending on the pump's design, with the rate of these pulses depending on the programmed infusion speed.
- **Intermittent infusion**: It has a "high" infusion rate, alternating with a low programmable infusion rate to keep the cannula open. The timings are programmable. This mode is often used to administer antibiotics or other drugs that can irritate a blood vessel.
- **Patient-controlled infusion is on demand**: It usually has a preprogrammed ceiling to avoid intoxication. The rate is controlled by a pressure pad or button that can be activated by the patient. It is the method of choice for patient-controlled analgesia (PCA), in which repeated small doses of opioid analgesics are delivered, with the device coded to stop administration before a dose reaches the limit, which may cause hazardous respiratory depression.
- **Total parenteral nutrition**: It usually requires an infusion curve similar to normal mealtimes.

TYPES OF PUMP

The two basic classes of pumps are the following:

1. **Large-volume pumps** usually use some form of peristaltic pump. Classically, they use computer-controlled rollers compressing a silicone-rubber tube through which the medicine flows. Another common form is a set of fingers that press on the tube in sequence. Large-volume pumps can pump nutrient solutions large enough to feed a patient.
2. **Small-volume pumps** usually use a computer-controlled motor by turning a screw that pushes the plunger on a syringe. Small-volume pumps infuse hormones, such as insulin, or other medicines, such as opiates.

SYRINGES

A **syringe** is a simple pump consisting of a plunger that fits tightly in a tube. The plunger can be pulled and pushed along inside a cylindrical tube (called a barrel), allowing the syringe to take in and expel a liquid or gas through an orifice at the open end of the tube. The open end of the syringe may be fitted with a hypodermic needle, a nozzle, or tubing to help direct the flow into and out of the barrel.

- **Hypodermic syringes:** Hypodermic syringes are used with hypodermic needles to inject liquid or gases into body tissues or to remove from the body.
- **Tip designs:** Syringes come with a number of designs for the area in which the blade locks to the syringe body. Perhaps the most well known of these is the Luer lock, which simply twists the two together.
- **Standard U-100 insulin syringes:** These are designed for insulin users. The dilution of insulin is such that 1 ml of insulin fluid has 100 standard "units" of insulin.
- **Multishot needle syringes:** There are needle syringes designed to reload from a built-in tank after each injection, so they can make several or many injections on a filling. An exception is the personal insulin autoinjector used by diabetic patients.
- **Venom extraction syringes:** Venom extraction syringes are different from standard syringes, because they usually do not puncture the wound. The most common types have a plastic nozzle which is placed over the affected area and then the syringe piston is pulled back, creating a vacuum that allegedly sucks out the venom.
- **Oral:** An oral syringe is a measuring instrument used to accurately measure doses of liquid medicine that are expressed in milliliters (mL). Oral syringes are available in various sizes, from 1 to 10 mL and larger.
- **Dental syringes:** A dental syringe is used by dentists for the injection of an anesthetic. It consists of a breech-loading syringe fitted with a sealed cartridge containing anesthetic solution.

ARTICLES FOR AN INTRAVENOUS INFUSION

During an IV infusion, the following articles should be placed in a tray:
- Intravenous cannula
- Intravenous set
- Tourniquet
- Medication
- Syringes (2 and 5 mL)
- Spirit cotton swab
- Adhesive tape
- Kidney tray

PROCEDURE FOR AN INTRAVENOUS INFUSION

The procedures involved in an IV infusion are as listed below:
- Select a suitable vein for venipuncture.
- Prepare the venipuncture site.
  - Apply a constricting band 2 inches above the venipuncture site. The constricting band should be tight enough to occlude venous flow, but not so tight that distal pulses are lost.
  - Select and palpate a prominent vein.
  - Cleanse the skin with an alcohol swab using a spiral motion starting with the entry site and extending outward about 2 inches. Allow the site to dry.

- Put gloves
- Perform the venipuncture
  - Using your nondominant hand, pull all local skin taut to stabilize the vein.
  - With your dominant hand, position the distal level of the needle up and insert the cannula into the vein at approximately 30° angle.
  - Continue inserting the needle until blood is observed in the flash chamber of the catheter.
  - Decrease the angle to 15° to 20° and carefully advance the cannula approximately 0.5 cm farther.
  - While holding the needle stationary, advance the catheter into the vein with a twisting motion. Insert the catheter all the way to the hub.
  - Place a finger over the vein at the catheter tip and put pressure on the vein to prevent blood from flowing out the catheter.
  - Remove the needle while maintaining firm catheter control.
- Remove the constricting band
- Obtain venous blood samples as required.
- Attach the administration tubing to the cannula hub while maintaining stabilization of the hub with the nondominant hand.
- Open the flow-regulator clamp and observe for drips in the drip chamber. Allow the fluid to run freely for several seconds.
- Adjust to the desired flow rate

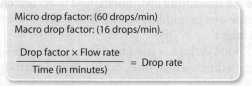

Micro drop factor: (60 drops/min)
Macro drop factor: (16 drops/min).

$$\frac{\text{Drop factor} \times \text{Flow rate}}{\text{Time (in minutes)}} = \text{Drop rate}$$

- Clean the area of blood, if necessary, and secure the hub of catheter with tape, leaving the hub and tubing connection visible. Make a small loop in the IV tube and place a second piece of tape over the first to secure the loop.
- Apply a transparent dressing over the venipuncture site.

INTRAVENOUS MEDICATION ADMINISTRATION

The following is a guideline for commencing IV therapy or loading IV medication into an IV flask or vial:

- Perform routine handwash
- Consult all patient documentation of the patient status [includes patient ID and medical record number (MRN)].
- Check all sections of the medication chart
- Confirm that the fluid order meets legal requirements (i.e., legible, signed, and dated by the doctor and has all essential components including patient's name, drug, dose, route, and frequency).
- Introduce self to patient
- Provide explanation to patient
- Seek permission to perform the procedure
- Identify patient with medical order
- Check for allergies
- Prepare patient and provide privacy as appropriate
- Organize equipment

- Confirm the compatibility of the drug and IV solution.
- Review the literature on the drug if unfamiliar with its action, usual dosages, routes of administration, side effects, and nursing implications.
- Perform first drug check including diluent (if applicable) with second RN. Ensure five rights are adhered to and calculate the dosage correctly.
- Prime the line according to the skill "managing a peripheral IV line."
- Open and attach syringe and drawing up device without causing contamination.

Dose calculations:

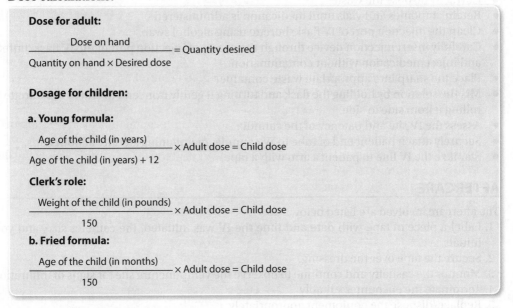

Dose for adult:

$$\frac{\text{Dose on hand}}{\text{Quantity on hand} \times \text{Desired dose}} = \text{Quantity desired}$$

Dosage for children:

a. Young formula:

$$\frac{\text{Age of the child (in years)}}{\text{Age of the child (in years)} + 12} \times \text{Adult dose} = \text{Child dose}$$

Clerk's role:

$$\frac{\text{Weight of the child (in pounds)}}{150} \times \text{Adult dose} = \text{Child dose}$$

b. Fried formula:

$$\frac{\text{Age of the child (in months)}}{150} \times \text{Adult dose} = \text{Child dose}$$

- **For powdered medications:**
  - Draw up diluent.
  - Remove the protective cap (if applicable).
  - Cleanse the rubber stopper with alcohol swab.
  - Inject the compatible type and amount of diluent using aseptic technique and avoiding excessive pressure build up.
  - Ensure the powder is completely dissolved.
  - Draw up the correct dose.
  - Remove device from vial without causing contamination.
  - Change drawing up device without causing contamination.
  - Expel air.
  - Maintain sterility of drawing up device and plunger.
    Ampoule Preparation: The following steps are followed for preparing ampoule:
    - Tap the top of ampoule lightly and quickly until the fluid moves from the neck of the ampoule.
    - Hold the ampoule upside down or set it on a flat surface and insert syringe or drawing up device without causing contamination.
  - Aspirate medication into the syringe by gently pulling back on the plunger without causing contamination of the plunger.
  - Change drawing up device without causing contamination.
  - Expel air.
  - Maintain sterility of the drawing up device and plunger throughout the procedure.

Liquid medication in a vial: The following steps are followed for liquid medication in a vial:

♦ Remove the protective cap.
♦ Cleanse the rubber stopper with alcohol swab.
♦ Inject volume of air equivalent to dosage into vial.
♦ Draw up medication, expel air, and expel excess medication.
♦ Change drawing up device without causing contamination.
♦ Maintain the sterility drawing up device and plunger throughout the procedure.

- Correctly dispose the waste
- Retain ampoules and vials until medication is administered.
- Clean the injection port of IV flask/burette using alcohol swab.
- Carefully insert injection device through the center of injection port of the IV flask/burette and inject medication without contamination.
- Place the sharp into appropriate waste container
- Mix the solution by holding the flask and turning it gently from end to end or the burette by rolling it from side to side.
- Assess the IV site and patency of the cannula
- Securely attach patient end of tube to IV cannula, maintaining sterility at both ends.
- Stabilize the IV line to patient's arm with a tape.

AFTERCARE

The aftercare involved are listed below:

1. Label a piece of tape with date and time the IV was initiated, the catheter size, and your initials.
2. Secure the tape over the dressing.
3. Monitor the casualty and continue to observe the venipuncture site for signs of infiltration.
4. Terminate the encounter suitably.
5. Replace/dispose the equipment appropriately.
6. Perform routine handwash.
7. Discontinue the infusion if signs of infiltration are observed.
8. Remove your gloves and disposes them appropriately.
9. Document the procedure on the appropriate medical form.

COMPLICATIONS

1. *Infection*: Any break in the skin carries a risk of infection. Although IV insertion is an aseptic procedure, skin-dwelling organisms such as *Candida albicans* may enter through the insertion site around the catheter, or bacteria may be accidentally introduced inside the catheter from contaminated equipment.
2. *Phlebitis*: Phlebitis is inflammation of a vein that may be caused by infection, the mere presence of a foreign body (the IV catheter), or the fluids or medication being given. Symptoms: Warmth, swelling, pain, or redness **around the vein**.
3. *Infiltration/extravasation*: Infiltration occurs when an IV fluid or medication accidentally enters the surrounding tissue rather than the vein. It is also known as extravasation (which refers to something escaping the vein). For example, if a cannula is in a vein for some time, the vein may scar and close and the only way for fluid to leave is along the outside of the cannula where it enters the vein.
4. *Fluid overload*: This occurs when fluids are given at a higher rate or in a larger volume than the system can absorb or excrete. The possible consequences include hypertension, heart failure, and pulmonary edema.

5. *Hypothermia:* The human body is at risk of accidentally induced hypothermia when large amounts of cold fluids are infused. Rapid temperature changes in the heart may precipitate ventricular fibrillation.
6. *Electrolyte imbalance:* Administering too dilute or too concentrated solution can disrupt the patient's balance of sodium, potassium, magnesium, and other electrolytes. Hospital patients usually receive blood tests to monitor these levels.
7. *Embolism:* A blood clot or other solid mass, as well as an air bubble, can be delivered into the circulation through an IV and end up blocking a vessel, and this is called embolism.

HEPARIN LOCK/HEPLOCK FLUSH

Introduction

- The device is referred to as an Hep-Lock because a medication called heparin or a similar blood thinner is injected to flush the site and keep the vein open by stopping a clot from forming.
- Heparin lock flush solution is intended for maintenance of patency of IV injection devices only and is not to be used for anticoagulant therapy.

Definition

Hep-Lock (preservative-free heparin lock flush solution) is intended to maintain patency of an indwelling venipuncture device designed for intermittent injection or infusion therapy or blood sampling. Heparin lock flush solution may be used following initial placement of the device in the vein, after each injection of a medication, or after withdrawal of blood for laboratory tests.

An Hep-Lock is a small tube that a medical professional inserts into the arm or other site on a patient's body. The tube has a catheter on one end. The health-care provider administers medication or fluids in an efficient manner through the catheter lock, which works by keeping a vein accessible.

Description

The details of heparin lock flush solution, USP, are given below:
- TUBEX heparin lock flush solution, USP, is a sterile solution. Each milliliter contains either 10 or 100 USP unit heparin sodium derived from porcine intestinal mucosa (standardized for use as an anticoagulant), in normal saline solution, and not more than 10 mg benzyl alcohol as a preservative. The pH range is 5.0–7.5.
- When medication is not being administered, the tube must be flushed with heparin and saline on a regular basis to keep the site viable. With this slight maintenance, the site is kept viable for days longer than a traditional IV. Although saline locks are often used to secure administration sites, many in the medical profession also refer to them as Hep-Locks because they accomplish the same goal.
- In many instances, this tube is a viable and preferred alternative to an IV line. In patients who require multiple but not continuous doses of medication, for example, it allows the administration of medication without the hassle of a cumbersome IV. Medication can be administered through a lock injection directly with a syringe or by hooking up IV to the catheter.

Clinical Pharmacology

The clinical pharmacology of heparin are as follows:
- Heparin inhibits reactions that lead to the clotting of blood and the formation of fibrin clots both in vitro and in vivo.

- Heparin acts at multiple sites in the normal coagulation systems. Small amounts of heparin in combination with antithrombin III (heparin cofactor) can inhibit thrombosis by inactivating activated factor X and inhibiting the conversion of prothrombin to thrombin.
- Once active thrombosis develops, larger amounts of heparin can inhibit further coagulation by inactivating thrombin and preventing the conversion of fibrinogen to fibrin.
- Heparin also prevents the formation of a stable fibrin clot by inhibiting the activation of the fibrin stabilizing factor.
- Bleeding time is usually unaffected by heparin. Clotting time is prolonged by full therapeutic doses of heparin; in most cases, it is not measurably affected by low-dose heparin.
- Patients over 60 years of age, following similar doses of heparin, may have higher plasma levels of heparin and longer activated partial thromboplastin times (APTTs) compared with patients under 60 years of age.
- Heparin does not have fibrinolytic activity; therefore, it will not lyse the existing clots.

Indications and Usage

The usage of heparin are as follows:

- Heparin lock flush solution, USP, is intended to maintain patency of an indwelling venipuncture device designed for intermittent injection or infusion therapy or blood sampling.
- Heparin lock flush solution, USP, may be used following initial placement of the device in the vein, after each injection of a medication, or after withdrawal of blood for laboratory tests.
- Heparin lock flush solution, USP, is not to be used for anticoagulant therapy.

Contraindications

Heparin sodium should not be used in patients with the following conditions:

- *Severe thrombocytopenia*: An uncontrollable active bleeding state, except when this is due to disseminated intravascular coagulation.
- *Hypersensitivity:* Patients with documented hypersensitivity to heparin should be given the drug only in clearly life-threatening situations.

Warnings

- This product contains benzyl alcohol as a preservative. Benzyl alcohol has been reported to be associated with a fatal "gasping syndrome" in premature neonates.
- Neonatologists do not advise the use of 100 units/mL concentration because of the risk of bleeding, especially in low-birth-weight neonates.
- Heparin is not intended for intramuscular use.

Precautions when Taking Preservative-free Heparin Lock Flush Solution

- Before using heparin, tell your doctor or pharmacist if you are allergic to it, to pork products, or if you have any other allergies. This product may contain inactive ingredients that can cause allergic reactions or other problems. Talk to your pharmacist for more details.
- This medication should not be used if you have a certain medical condition. Before using this medicine, consult your doctor or pharmacist if you have uncontrollable bleeding.
- Before using this medication, tell your doctor or pharmacist your medical history, especially of severe high blood pressure (hypertension), infection of the heart, recent surgery/procedure, bleeding/clotting disorders (e.g., hemophilia, antithrombin III deficiency, thrombocytopenia), stomach/intestinal ulcers, or tumor.

Dosage and Administration

- Preservative-free heparin lock flush solution in the 100 unit/mL concentration is available and is not recommended for use in neonates and infants.
- Parenteral drug products should be inspected visually for particulate matter and discoloration prior to administration, whenever solution and container permit. Slight discoloration does not alter potency.

  Description: Heparin lock flush solution, USP, is available in **TUBEX BLUNT POINTE™** Sterile Cartridge Units and in **TUBEX** Sterile Cartridge-Needle Units.
- Each 1 mL size **TUBEX** contains one of the following concentrations of heparin sodium in packages of 50 **TUBEX**:
  - Ten USP units per mL: 25 gauge × 5/8 inches needle
  - One hundred USP units per mL: 25 gauge × 5/8 inches needle
- Each 2.5 mL size **TUBEX** contains one of the following concentrations of heparin sodium in packages of 50 **TUBEX**:
  - Twenty-five USP units per **TUBEX** (10 USP units per mL): 25 gauge × 5/8 inches needle.
  - Two hundred fifty USP units per **TUBEX** (100 USP units per mL): 25 gauge × 5/8 inches needle.

Precautions

General

General precautions to be observed are the following:
- In infants, the cumulative amounts of heparin and benzyl alcohol received from the frequent administration of heparin lock flush solution, USP, during a 24-hour period should be considered.
- Precautions must be exercised when drugs that are incompatible with heparin are administered through an indwelling IV catheter containing heparin lock flush solution, USP.

White Clot Syndrome

It has been reported that patients on heparin may develop new thrombus formation in association with thrombocytopenia, resulting from irreversible aggregation of platelets induced by heparin, the so-called "white-clot syndrome." The process may lead to severe thromboembolic complications like skin necrosis, gangrene of the extremities that may lead to amputation, myocardial infarction, pulmonary embolism, stroke, and possibly death. Therefore, heparin administration should be promptly discontinued if a patient develops new thrombosis in association with thrombocytopenia.

- *Hemorrhage:* Heparin sodium should be used with extreme caution in infants and patients with disease states in which there is increased danger of hemorrhage. Some of the conditions in which increased danger of hemorrhage exists are:
- *Cardiovascular:* Subacute bacterial endocarditis, severe hypertension.
- *Surgical*: During and immediately following (a) spinal tap or spinal anesthesia or (b) major surgery, especially involving the brain, spinal cord, or eye.
- *Hematologic:* Conditions associated with increased bleeding tendencies, such as hemophilia, thrombocytopenia, and some vascular purpuras.
- *Gastrointestinal:* Ulcerative lesions and continuous tube drainage of the stomach or small intestine.
- *Other:* Menstruation, liver disease with impaired hemostasis.
- A higher incidence of bleeding has been reported in patients, particularly women, over 60 years of age.

Laboratory Tests

Periodic platelet counts, hematocrits, and tests for occult blood in stool are recommended during the entire course of heparin use.

Drug Interactions

The most common drug interactions are the following:

Platelet inhibitors: Drugs such as acetylsalicylic acid, dextran, phenylbutazone, ibuprofen, indomethacin, dipyridamole, hydroxychloroquine, and others that interfere with platelet-aggregation reactions (the main hemostatic defense of heparinized patients) may induce bleeding and should be used with caution in patients receiving heparin sodium.

Other interactions: Digitalis, tetracyclines, nicotine, or antihistamines may partially counteract the anticoagulant action of heparin sodium.

Considerations

Heparin administration in various age group of patients should be considered only after appropriate discussion and analysis because of the following reasons:

- **Pregnancy**
  - *Teratogenic effects: Pregnancy category C*: Heparin sodium should be given to a pregnant woman only if clearly needed.
  - *Nonteratogenic effects:* Heparin does not cross the placenta barrier.
- **Nursing mothers:** Heparin is not excreted in human milk.
- **Pediatric use:** Heparin lock flush solution, USP, is not recommended for use in the neonates.
- **Geriatric use:** A higher incidence of bleeding has been reported in patients 60 years of age, especially women.

Adverse Reactions

Hemorrhage

Hemorrhage is the chief complication that may result from heparin use. An overly prolonged clotting time or minor bleeding during therapy can usually be controlled by withdrawing the drug.

Local Irritation

Local irritation and erythema have been reported with the use of heparin lock flush solution, USP.

Hypersensitivity

Generalized hypersensitivity reactions have been reported, with chill, fever, and urticaria as the most usual manifestations, and asthma, rhinitis, lacrimation, headache, nausea and vomiting, and anaphylactoid reactions, including shock, occurring more rarely. Itching and burning, especially on the plantar side of the feet, may occur.

Thrombocytopenia

It has been reported to occur in patients receiving heparin with a reported incidence of 0–30%. While often mild and of no obvious clinical significance, such thrombocytopenia can be accompanied by severe thromboembolic complications such as skin necrosis, gangrene of the extremities that may lead to amputation, myocardial infarction, pulmonary embolism, stroke, and possibly death.

Certain episodes of painful, ischemic and cyanosed limbs have been attributed, in the past, to allergic vasospastic reactions. Whether these are, in fact, identical to the thrombocytopenia-associated complications remains to be determined.

Overdosage

Symptoms: Bleeding is the chief sign of heparin overdosage. Nosebleeds, blood in urine, or tarry stools may be noted as the first sign of bleeding. Easy bruising or petechial formation may precede frank bleeding.

Treatment: Neutralization of heparin effect.

When clinical circumstances (bleeding) require reversal of heparinization, protamine sulfate (1% solution) by slow infusion will neutralize heparin sodium. No more than 50 mg should be administered, very slowly, in any 10-minute period. Each milligram of protamine sulfate neutralizes approximately 100 USP heparin units. The amount of protamine required decreases over time as heparin is metabolized. Although the metabolism of heparin is complex, it may, for the purpose of choosing a protamine dose, be assumed to have a half-life of about 1/2 hour after IV injection.

Administration of protamine sulfate can cause severe hypotensive and anaphylactoid reactions. Because fatal reactions, often resembling anaphylaxis, have been reported, the drug should be given only when resuscitation techniques and treatment of anaphylactoid shock are readily available.

Maintenance of Patency of Intravenous Devices

The patency of IV devices can be maintained as follows:

- To prevent clot formation in a heparin lock set or central venous catheter following its proper insertion, preservative-free heparin lock flush solution, USP, is injected via the injection hub in a quantity sufficient to fill the entire device.
- This solution should be replaced each time the device is used. Aspirate before administering any solution via the device to confirm patency and location of needle or catheter tip.
- If the drug to be administered is incompatible with heparin, the entire device should be flushed with normal saline before and after the medication is administered; following the second saline flush, preservative-free heparin lock flush solution, USP, may be reinstilled into the device.
- The device manufacturer's instructions should be consulted for specifics concerning its use. Usually this dilute heparin solution will maintain anticoagulation within the device for up to 4 hours.

Note: Since repeated injections of small doses of heparin can alter tests for APTT, a baseline value for APTT should be obtained prior to insertion of an IV device.

Withdrawal of Blood Samples

- Preservative-free heparin lock flush solution, USP, may also be used after each withdrawal of blood for laboratory tests.
- When heparin would interfere with or alter the results of blood tests, the heparin solution should be cleared from the device by aspirating and discarding it before withdrawing the blood sample.

Administration Technique/Directions for Use

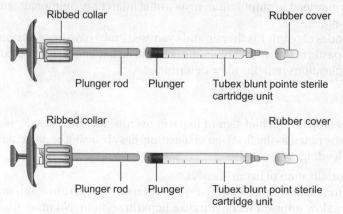

Fig. A-4.1: Blood sample syringe.

Tubex blunt pointe sterile cartridge unit is used with injection sets specifically manufactured as "needle-less" injection systems.

Note: Use aseptic technique for all manipulations of sterile parts.

Loading a Tubex Sterile Cartridge Unit into the Tubex Injector

Loading a Tubex Sterile Cartridge Unit into the Tubex Injector can be achieved as follows:

1. Turn the ribbed collar to the "OPEN" position until it stops.
2. Hold the injector with the open end up and fully insert the **TUBEX** Sterile Cartridge Unit. Firmly tighten the ribbed collar in the direction of the "CLOSE" arrow.
3. Thread the plunger rod into the plunger of the **TUBEX** Sterile Cartridge Unit until slight resistance is felt. The injector is now ready for use in the usual manner.

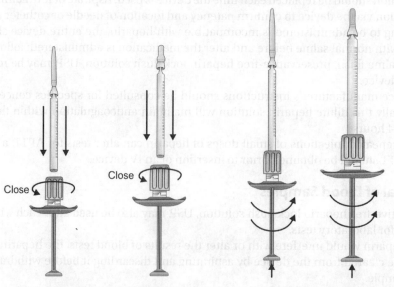

Fig. A-4.2: Opening and closing of syringe.　　　**Fig. A-4.3:** Opening and closing of syringe.

Administering Tubex Sterile Cartridge-Needle Units

Method of administration is the same as with conventional syringe. Remove needle cover by grasping it securely; twist and pull. Introduce needle into patient, aspirate by pulling back slightly on the plunger, and inject.

Administering Tubex Blunt Pointe Sterile Cartridge Units

"Needle-less" opening and closing of syringe IV set administration is similar to administration with conventional syringes. Remove rubber cover by grasping it securely and twist and pull.

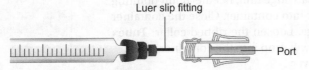

Luer slip fitting

Port

Fig. A-4.4: "Needle-less" IV set.

*For SafSite reflux valves, aseptically swab the luer slip fitting of the **Tubex blunt pointe** sterile cartridge tip assembly with a sterile, individually wrapped, saturated 70% isopropyl alcohol swab. This action will remove the lubricant coating from the tip to facilitate a tight seal. Introduce **Tubex blunt pointe** sterile cartridge unit into the "needle-less" IV set per manufacturer's "Directions for Use."

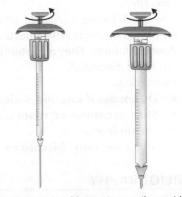

Removing the Empty Tubex Cartridge Unit and Disposing into a Vertical Disposal Container

Fig. A-4.5: Tubex blunt pointe sterile cartridge.

Removal of the empty TUBEX Cartridge Unit can be achieved by the following steps:

1. Do not recap the needle/point. Disengage the plunger rod.
2. Hold the injector, needle/point down, over a vertical disposal container and loosen the ribbed collar. **Tubex** cartridge unit will drop into the container.
3. Discard the cover

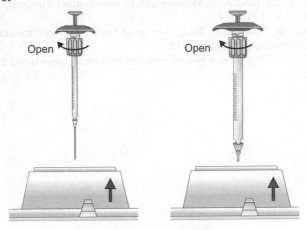

Open

Open

Fig. A-4.6: Empty tubex cartridge.

Removing the Empty Tubex Cartridge Unit and Disposing into a Horizontal (Mailbox) Disposal Container

Removal of the empty Tubex cartridge unit can be achieved by the following steps:

1. Do not recap the needle/point. Disengage the plunger rod.
2. Open the horizontal (mailbox) disposal container. Insert **Tubex** cartridge unit, needle/point pointing down, halfway into container. Close the container lid on cartridge. Loosen the ribbed collar; **Tubex** cartridge unit will drop into the container.
3. Discard the cover.

The **Tubex** injector is reusable and should not be discarded.

The used **Tubex** cartridge units should not be employed for successive injections or as multiple-dose containers. They are intended to be used only once and discarded.

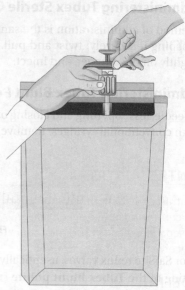

Fig. A-4.7: How to discard Tubex cartridge.

Instructions:

- **Do not use if solution is discolored or contains a precipitate.**
- **Store at controlled room temperature, 20–25°C (68–77°F).**
- **Do not freeze.**
- **Single use only. Discard any unused solution after the initial use.**

BIBLIOGRAPHY

1. Dieck JA, Rizo-Patron C. A new manifestation and treatment alternative for heparin-induced thrombosis. Chest. 1990;98:1524-6.
2. Kappa JR, Fisher CA, Ber kowitz HD. Heparin-induced platelet activation in sixteen surgical patients: diagnosis and Management. J Vasc Surg. 1987;5(1):101-7.
3. King DJ, Kelton JG. Heparin-associated thrombocytopenia. Ann Intern Med. 1984;100:535-40.
4. Rice L, Attisha W, Drexler A, et al. Delayed-onset heparin induced thrombocytopenia. Ann Intern Med. 2002;136:210-5.
5. Smythe MA, Stephens JL, Mattson JC. Delayed-onset heparin induced thrombocytopenia. Ann Emerg Med. 2005;45(4):417-9.
6. Tahata T, Shigehito M, Kusuhara K. Delayed-onset of heparin induced thrombocytopenia—A case report. J Jpn Assn Torca Surg. 1992;40(3):110-1.
7. Warkentin T, Kelton J. Delayed-onset heparin-induced thrombocytopenia and thrombosis. Ann Intern Med. 2001;135:502-6.

Intra-aortic Balloon Pump

INTRODUCTION

Intra-aortic balloon counterpulsation (IABC) is the most widely used therapy for support of a compromised left ventricle (LV). Intra-aortic balloon counterpulsation is the most widely used form of left ventricular mechanical support today; more than 160,000 patients worldwide receive this therapy annually.

DEFINITION

Intra-aortic balloon pump (IABP) therapy is used to improve coronary artery perfusion and to decrease LV afterload. The IABP increases myocardial and systemic blood flow in the incidences of LV failure, unstable refractory angina, septic shock, valvular disease, prophylaxis prior to cardiac surgery, postcardiac surgery cardiogenic shock and provides support for failed angioplasty and valvuloplasty.

PRINCIPLES OF INTRA-AORTIC BALLOON CONTERPULSATION: GENERAL CONCEPTS

Placement

The placement of IAB is as follows:

- A flexible catheter with a balloon mounted on the end is inserted in the femoral artery and passed into the descending thoracic aorta.
- Once the balloon catheter is passed into the descending aorta, placement must be confirmed by fluoroscopy or chest X-ray (CXR).
- The balloon is situated 1–2 cm below the origin of the left subclavian artery and above the renal artery branches.
- On daily CXR, the tip should be visible between the second and third intercostal space.
- This placement is critical for proper operation and avoidance of arterial tributary obstruction.
- If the balloon is placed too low, then the origin of the renal arteries could become obstructed, thereby compromising renal perfusion.
- If the catheter is placed too high, obstruction of the origin of the left subclavian or even the left carotid artery could result.
- The IAB should not totally occlude the aortic lumen during inflation. Ideally, it should be 85–90% occlusive. Total occlusion could result in aortic wall trauma and damage to red blood cells (RBCs) and platelets.

Volume Displacement

The volume displacement changes are as follows:

- The IAB exerts its effect by volume displacement and pressure changes caused by rapidly shuttling helium gas in and out of the balloon chamber. This principle is known as counterpulsation.
- At a precisely timed interval, the gas enters the balloon chamber within the aorta.
- As the gas is shuttled into the balloon, it occupies a space within the aorta equal to its volume.
- The usual adult balloon volume is 40 cc (though it can range from 30 to 50 cc).
- The sudden occupation of space by the gas upon inflation causes blood to be moved from its original position superiorly and inferiorly to the balloon. Since, the volume in the aorta is suddenly increased and the aortic wall is fairly rigid, the intra-aortic pressure increases sharply.
- With deflation of the IAB, the chain of events is in the reverse. A sudden 40 cc fall in aortic volume causes a sudden decrease in aortic pressure within that localized area.
- In response to the local fall in pressure, the blood in adjacent areas moves to normalize the pressure within the aortic cavity as a whole.
- Displacement of blood volume (both away from the balloon on inflation and towards the balloon on deflation) is the mechanism by which the IABP alters the hemodynamic state.
- T obtain beneficial hemodynamic changes, the inflation and deflation of the balloon must occur at optimum times in the cardiac cycle.

Balloon Inflation: Hemodynamics

Inflation of the balloon is set to occur at the onset of diastole. At the beginning of diastole, maximum aortic blood volume is available for displacement. If balloon inflation occurs later in diastole, the pressure generation from volume displacement will be lower. This is because during late diastole, much of the blood has flowed out to the periphery and there is less blood volume in the aorta to displace.

Benefits of Accurately Timed Inflation

The benefits of accurately timed inflation are as follows:
- Coronary artery blood flow and pressure are increased. Increased perfusion may increase the oxygen delivered to the myocardium.
- Increased diastolic pressure also increased the perfusion to distal organs and tissues, i.e., increased urine output, cerebral perfusion.
- Coronary collateral circulation is potentially increased from the increased carebral perfusion pressure (CPP).
- System perfusion pressure is increased.

Balloon Deflation: Hemodynamics

The balloon remains inflated throughout the diastolic phase. Deflation of the balloon should take place at the onset of systole during the inferior vena cava (IVC) phase. At the beginning of systole, the LV has to generate a pressure greater than the accelerated experiential-dynamic psychatherapy (AEDP) to achieve ejection. The sudden evacuation of the 40-cc volume will cause a fall in pressure in the aorta. Properly timed deflation will cause a fall in pressure; therefore, the LV will not have to generate as much pressure to achieve ejection. The IVC phase is shortened, thereby decreasing the oxygen demands of the myocardium. Since, the LV will be ejection against a lower pressure, the peak pressure generated during systole will be less.

Benefits of Accurately Timed Deflation

The benefits of accurately timed deflation are as follows:

- The pressure that the LV must generate is less throughout the systolic phase. Therefore, afterload is reduced, which in turn decreases myocardial the oxygen demands.
- The IVC phase is shortened, which decreases the oxygen demands.
- Reduced afterload allows the LV to empty more effectively, so stroke volume (SV) is increased. In addition, preload is reduced if elevated.
- Enhanced forward cardiac output (CO) also decreases the amount of blood shunted from left to right in case of intraventricle septal defects and incompetent mitral valve.

INDICATIONS

Indications for IABC are as follows:

A. Medical indications

- Cardiogenic shock
- Preshock syndrome
- Threatening extension of myocardial infarction (MI)
- Unstable angina
- Intractable ventricle dysrhythmias
- Septic shock syndrome
- Cardiac contusion
- Prophylactic support for:
  - Coronary angiography
  - Coronary angioplasty
  - Thrombolysis
  - High-risk interventional procedures (i.e., stents).
- Bridging device to other mechanical assist: ventricular—assist device
- Support during transport
- Cardiac support for hemodynamically challenged patients with mechanical defects prior to correction:
  - Valvular stenosis
  - Valvular insufficiency—mitral
  - Ruptured papillary muscle
  - Ventricular septal defect
  - Left ventricular aneurysm.

B. Surgical indications

- Postsurgical myocardial dysfunction
- Support for weaning from cardiopulmonary bypass (CPB).

CONTRAINDICATIONS

Contraindications for IABC are as follows:

A. Absolute

- Severe aortic insufficiency—as the balloon inflates, blood may be forced across the valve, thereby overloading the ventricle and increasing cardiac work.

- Aortic aneurysm—the increased pressure generated by counterpulsation may cause the aneurysm to rupture.
- Severe peripheral vascular disease may limit the ability to advance the catheter through atherosclerotic vessels.
- Severe coagulopathy

B. Relative

- End-stage cardiomyopathies—unless bridging to ventricular assist device (VAD)
- Severe atherosclerosis
- End-stage terminal disease
- Abdominal aortic aneurysm, not resected
- Blood dyscrasias (thrombocytopenia)

EQUIPMENT

The equipment used for IABP are as follows:
- Insertion kit (introducer and sheath) and IAB
- Electrocardiograph (ECG)/pressure cable from external source into the IABP console
- Pressure monitoring setup (transducer, pressure cable, heparinized saline (10–20 cc), pressure bag)
- Major procedure tray, gowns, gloves, masks, and drape sheets
- Ten-milliliter syringe, 21 gauge needle, lignocaine 1% or 2% **(without adrenaline)**
- Sutures and sterile transparent dressing
- Balloon sizing—balloon size should be chosen with respect to patient size (patient's height and possible aortic diameter), so that balloon is positioned above renal vasculature.

Patient height	IAB volume (cc)	Body surface area (m²)
4'10"–5'4" (147–162 cm)	30	Less than 1.8
5'4"–6'0" (162–182 cm)	40	Greater than 1.8
>6'0" (182 cm) or aortic diameter >20 mm	50	Greater than 1.8

Balloon size can be evaluated by monitoring the balloon, pressure waveform, and the arterial pressure during inflation of the balloon.

PROCEDURE

The Balloon Catheter

The percutaneous technique requires only 5–10 minutes for insertion in an uncomplicated case. Insertion of the catheter can be performed by any physician skilled in catheterization techniques.

Preinsertion Nursing Assessment

It includes the following:
- Skin color of both legs
- Skin temperature of both legs
- Capillary refill ability of both legs
- Quality of pulses in both legs
- Baseline sensation and movement of both legs
- Ankle–brachial index of both legs

- Preinsertion hemodynamics including CO, cardiac index (CI), pulmonary capillary wedge pressure (PCWP), and central venous pressure (CVP)
- Complete neuro check
- Patient's family understanding of the procedure.

Intra-Aortic Balloon Insertion

The IAB insertion can be achieved as follows:
Percutaneous insertion:
- Sheathed
- Sheathless

Preparation of Intra-Aortic Balloon for Insertion

The following list provides the preparation of TAB required for insertion:
- Attach the one-way valve to the IAB connector
- Connect the 60 cc syringe to the one-way valve
- Apply full vacuum
- Do not remove one-way valve until IAB is fully inserted into the patient
- Flush through central lumen with heparinized saline just prior to insertion
- Do not remove IAB from tray until time to insert into the patient
- If IAB is to be inserted through a sheath, remove the premounted hemostasis device if present.

After the IAB is positioned in the patient, the following are to be performed:
- Aspirate blood from central lumen and gently flush with approximately 3 cc heparinized saline
- Immediately hookup pressurized heparinized saline flush system to central lumen
- Remove one-way valve and connect IAB to pump
- Suture at both the sheath hub and catheter site
- Setup pressure monitoring system to be connected to the central lumen of the catheter and the pump console. The arterial pressure waveform should appear on the monitor
- Set initial timing for inflation and deflation.

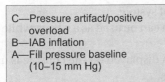
C—Pressure artifact/positive overload
B—IAB inflation
A—Fill pressure baseline (10–15 mm Hg)

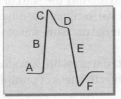

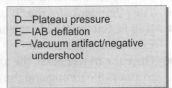
D—Plateau pressure
E—IAB deflation
F—Vacuum artifact/negative undershoot

Fig. A-5.1: Normal balloon pressure waveform.

High balloon pressure plateau may be caused by hypertension, a balloon too large for the aorta, or a restriction to gas flow within the system. The top of the plateau may be squared or rounded.

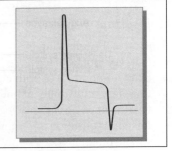

Low balloon pressure plateau could be caused by hypotension, hypovolemia, low systemic vascular resistance, low balloon inflation volume, a balloon sized too small for the patient or positioned too low in the aorta.	*High balloon pressure plateau*
Balloon pressure baseline elevation may be caused by a restriction of gas flow or gas system overpressurization.	*Balloon pressure baseline elevation*
Balloon pressure baseline depression usually indicates a helium leak. Other possible causes not related to helium leak include inappropriate timing settings (early inflation or late deflation) that do not permit enough time for gas to return to the console or a mechanical defect that causes failure to autofill.	*Balloon pressure baseline depression*

SETTING TRIGGERING AND TIMING

Timing and trigger are set as follows:

- For the IABP to "pump" effectively, two waveforms need to be set. The ECG signal to "trigger" the balloon and the arterial pressure signal to "time" the counterpulsation. The arterial waveform, a less reliable trigger, uses the systolic upstroke.
    - The trigger allows the pump to identify the start of the cardiac cycle.
    - The pump looks for the "R" wave to signal the onset of systole.
    - If an ECG is unreliable, the arterial pressure waveform can be used as a trigger while the ECG trace is optimized.
    - Once the trigger is set, the arterial pressure waveform displayed on the console is used to assess the timing and the effectiveness of pumping.
- Timing: Set the mode to 1:2.
- Compare the unassisted cardiac cycle with the assisted (augmented) cycle.

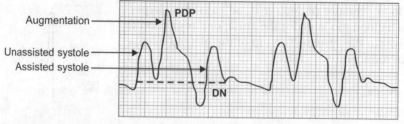

Fig. A-5.2: ECG pattern during IABP.

There is a sharp "V" on the waveform at the dicrotic notch (DN). The DN is when the aortic valve closes—this is the point at which the IAB starts to inflate.

Inflation of the balloon is timed to occur at the DN (aortic valve closure) on the arterial pressure tracing.

- As the balloon inflates and the pressure rises, there will be an upward deflection following the DN, which is referred to as diastolic augmentation and represents the pressure produced early in diastole by the inflated balloon.
- Because inflation increases pressure in the aorta, the peak of diastolic augmentation is higher than the peak of systole.
- As the balloon deflates, the assisted aortic end-diastolic pressure (pressure in the aorta) at the end of diastole dips down to create a "U-" or "V-"shaped waveform.

In early deflation, note the U shape rather than V shape of the waveform and indication of a brief shelf (arrow) before the next systole

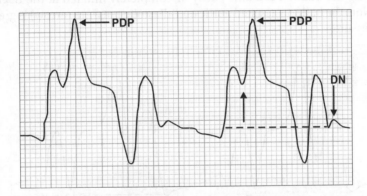

Fig. A-5.3: Peak diastolic pressure (PDP).

In late balloon inflation a significant portion of the dicrotic notch (arrows) is visible

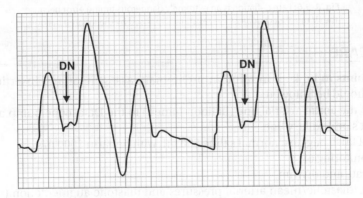

Fig. A-5.4: Dicrotic notch (DN).

In early deflation, note the U shape rather than V shape of the waveform and indication of a brief shelf (arrow) before the next systole.

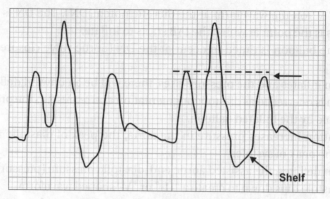

Fig. A-5.5: Early deflation, during IABP.

In late deflation, the balloon remains partly or completely inflated at the beginning of the next systole. Note the balloon assisted aortic end-diastolic pressure (arrow) is greater than the unassisted pressure.

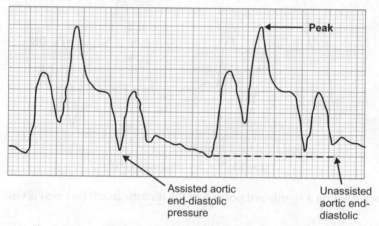

Fig. A-5.6: Late deflation is an extremely dangerous timing error because the LV must eject against the resistance imposed by the inflated balloon.

NURSING CARE

Along with points to be kept in mind in preliminary assessment and insertion, the given instructions should be followed:
- Transduce the aortic arterial line (balloon lumen) to the Datascope pump and level with the patient's midaxillary line.
- For arterial flush bag, use normal saline 500 mL with heparin 1000 u/s.
- Hourly monitoring of:
  - Heart rate and rhythm.
  - Systolic/diastolic/mean arterial pressures and diastolic augmentation (use the blood pressure (BP) obtained from the Datascope pump when titrating drugs).
  - Pedal pulses distal to the catheter site (Doppler may be necessary to assess pulse).
  - L) radial pulse (If the catheter migrates forward it could compromise blood flow to the L) subclavian artery).

- Color, temperature, and capillary refill
- Sensation and movement of both lower extremities
- Patient to be log rolled or Jordan lifted and the end of the bed elevated no more than 30° to prevent catheter migration and arterial puncture.
- Careful monitoring of renal function. (The catheter sits above the bifurcation of the renal arteries—backward migration may compromise blood flow to the kidneys.)
- The balloon should not remain immobile for >20 minutes while in situ due to the risk of thrombus formation.
- Assess insertion site during each shift for redness, ooze, etc.
- Change dressing as recommended
- Carefully monitor the insertion site for signs of bleeding, infection, hematoma, or compartment syndrome of the affected limb.
- Heparinization according to protocol may be initiated at 24 hours.

WEANING

Weaning can be accomplished as follows:
- Counterpulsation may be reduced from 1:1 to 1:2 and finally 1:3 depending on the patient's hemodynamics.
- Do not set the pump at 1:3 unless for weaning and prior to removal. There is an increased risk of thrombus formation at counterpulsation of 1:3.

REMOVAL

Balloon catheters are removed as follows:
- Balloon catheters are removed by medical officers experienced in this procedure.
- When the catheter is removed, allow a very small volume of arterial bleed to occur to expel any small clots. Apply a pressure device, e.g., Fem-stop to provide continuous pressure to the site for at least 30 minutes. Then cover site with a sandbag for 2–4 hours (with frequent checks for signs of bleeding). Contact cardiology cardioneuromuscular center (CNC) in hours or A5a/b after hours for assistance if required.

CARDIAC ARREST

During cardiac arrest, the following have to be performed:
- Switch to pressure triggering once the pump alarms due to loss of ECG rhythm (remember to select "assist" after changing trigger modes). Reduce the pressure threshold if balloon fails to pump from pressure trigger (decrease arrows in auxiliary box under trigger options).
- The balloon pump does not need to be disconnected during defibrillation.
- If the cardiopulmonary resuscitation (CPR) cannot generate a consistent and reliable trigger, then switch to "INTERNAL" mode which will maintain movement of the IAB and therefore reduce the risk of thrombus formation.

> **WARNING:**
> The use of "INTERNAL" trigger will produce asynchronous counterpulsation and should never be used in the event that the patient has an ECG or arterial pressure source available. Once the ECG or arterial signal has been reestablished, the trigger mode must be changed from "INTERNAL" to an acceptable patient trigger.

COMPLICATIONS

The following complications are to be kept in mind:

- Limb ischemia due to occlusion of the femoral artery either by the catheter or by emboli from thrombus formation on the balloon.
- Aortic dissection during insertion or rupture during pumping
- Hemorrhage from insertion site
- Helium emboli from the balloon
- Infection at the site of insertion or catheter related
- Leaks of the membrane or catheter
- Balloon entrapment
- Insertion difficulty/inability to insert the IAB
- Failure of the balloon to unwrap
- Malposition of the balloon in the patient
- Vessel occlusion resulting in infarction to an organ (including paraplegia)
- Thrombocytopenia

Intravenous Drug Administration and Intravenous Infusion

DEFINITION

Intravenous (IV) drug administration and infusion can be defined as follows:
- Drug administration through the IV route at a constant rate over a determined time interval
- A solution administered into a vein through an infusion set that includes a plastic or glass vacuum bottle or bag containing the solution and tube connecting the bottle to a catheter or a needle in the patient's vein
- The process of administering a solution IV or directly into a vein.

PURPOSES

The main purposes of IV administration or infusion are the following:
- To correct electrolyte imbalances
- To deliver medications
- For blood transfusion
- For fluid replacement (dehydration)
- For chemotherapy (the treatment for any kind of cancer).

COMMON INTRAVENOUS SITES

The common IV sites are the following:
- Cephalic vein
- Basilic vein
- Median cubital vein
- Radial vein
- Superficial dorsal veins
- Dorsal venous arch basilic vein (hand)
- Great saphenous veins
- Dorsal plexus of foot

INFUSED SUBSTANCES

Volume Expanders

The two main types of volume expanders are the following:
1. Crystalloids
2. Colloids

Crystalloids

- Crystalloids are aqueous solutions of mineral salts or other water-soluble molecules. Crystalloids generally are much cheaper than colloids.

- The most commonly used crystalloid fluid is normal saline (sodium chloride at 0.9% concentration, isotonic).
- Lactated Ringer' (also known as Ringer' lactate which is mildly hypotonic solution) is also used as a common crystalloid.

The Table A-6.1 provides a list of intravenous solutions.

TABLE A-6.1: List of intravenous solution.

Solution	Concentration
Dextrose in water solution	
Dextrose 5%	Isotonic
Dextrose 10%	Hypertonic
Saline solution	
0.45% sodium chloride	Hypotonic
0.9% sodium chloride	Isotonic
3–5% sodium chloride	Hypertonic
Dextrose in saline solution	
Dextrose 5% in 0.9% sodium chloride	Hypertonic
Dextrose 5% in 0.45% sodium chloride	Hypertonic
Multiple electrolyte solution	
Lactated Ringer	Isotonic
Dextrose 5% in lactated Ringer	Hypertonic

Colloids

- Colloids contain larger insoluble molecules, such as gelatin. Blood is a colloid.
- Colloids preserve a high colloid osmotic pressure in the blood, while on the other hand, this parameter is decreased by crystalloids due to hemodilution.

Blood-based Products

A blood product (or blood-based product) is any component of blood that is collected from a donor for use in a blood transfusion.

The following are the indications for blood transfusion:

- Trauma
- Surgery
- Severe anemia
- Thrombocytopenia
- Hemophilia
- Sickle cell disease

Examples:

- Hemophilia usually need a replacement of clotting factor which is a small part of the whole blood.
- Sickle cell disease may require frequent blood transfusions. Earlier blood transfusions consisted of whole blood.
- Fresh frozen plasma
- Cryoprecipitate

Buffer Solutions

Buffer solutions are used to correct acidosis or alkalosis.

- Lactated Ringer solution also has some buffering effect.
- Intravenous sodium bicarbonate are specifically used for buffering purpose.

Other Medications

The below list provides the method of using other medications:

- Medications may be mixed into the fluids mentioned above. Certain types of medications can only be given IV, such as when there is insufficient uptake by other routes of administration, such as enterally. Examples include IV immunoglobulin and propofol.
- Parenteral nutrition is feeding a person IV and bypassing the usual process of eating and digestion. The person receives nutritional formulas containing salts, glucose, amino acids, lipids, and added vitamins.
- Drug injection used for recreational substances usually enters by the IV route.

INTRAVENOUS DEVICES

The seven most common intravenous devices are the following:

Peripheral Cannula

A peripheral IV line consists of a short catheter inserted through the skin into a peripheral vein. This is usually in the form of a cannula-over-needle device, which consists of a flexible plastic cannula.

Sites:

Any accessible vein can be used though arm and hand veins are used most commonly with leg and foot veins used to a much lesser extent. In infants, the scalp veins are sometimes used.

Sizes of Cannula

- 12–14 gauge (used in resuscitation settings).
- 16 gauge (used for blood donation and transfusion).
- 18–20 gauge (for infusions and blood draws).
- 22 gauge (pediatric line).
- 24–26 the smallest.

Colors of Cannula

- Green-18 G
- Pink-20 G
- Blue-22 G
- Yellow-24 G

Central IV Lines

Central IV lines flow through a catheter with its tip within a large vein, usually the superior vena cava or inferior vena cava, or within the right atrium of the heart. This has several advantages over a peripheral IV:

- It can deliver fluids and medications that would be overly irritating to peripheral veins because of their concentration or chemical composition. These include some chemotherapy drugs and total parenteral nutrition.
- Medications reach the heart immediately and are quickly distributed to the rest of the body.
- There is room for multiple parallel compartments (lumen) within the catheter, so that multiple medications can be delivered at once even if they would not be chemically compatible within a single tube.
- Caregivers can measure central venous pressure and other physiological variables through the line.

Complications

- Bleeding
- Infection
- Gangrene
- Thromboembolism
- Gas embolism.

Peripherally Inserted Central Catheter

The peripherally inserted central catheter (PICC) lines are used when IV access is required over a prolonged period of time or when the material to be infused would cause quick damage and early failure of a peripheral IV and when a conventional central line may be too dangerous to attempt. Typical uses for a PICC include long chemotherapy regimens, extended antibiotic therapy, or total parenteral nutrition.

Advantage of PICC

It is safer to insert with a relatively low risk of uncontrollable bleeding and essentially no risks of damage to the lungs or major blood vessels.

Disadvantage

It must be inserted more technically.

Central Venous Lines

Several types of catheters are available that take a more direct route into central veins. These are collectively called central venous lines. A catheter is inserted into a subclavian, internal jugular, or (less commonly) a femoral vein and advanced toward the heart until it reaches the superior vena cava or right atrium.

Implantable Ports

A port is a central venous line that does not have an external connector; instead, it has a small reservoir that is covered with silicone rubber and is implanted under the skin. Medication is administered intermittently by placing a small needle through the skin, piercing the silicone, into the reservoir. When the needle is withdrawn the reservoir cover reseals itself. The cover can accept hundreds of needle sticks during its lifetime.

Syringe Driver

A *syringe* driver or syringe pump is a small infusion pump (some include infuse and withdraw capability) used to gradually administer small amounts of fluid (with or without medication) to a patient or for use in chemical and biomedical research. A syringe driver is a small portable pump that can be used to give you a continuous dose of painkiller and other medicines. It is often used in instances of vomiting or unable to swallow (**Fig. A-6.1**).

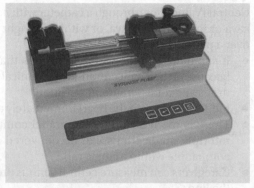

Fig. A-6.1: Syringe driver.

Guidelines for Procedure

- A syringe driver takes 3–4 hours to establish a steady state drug level in plasma. If the patient is in pain, vomiting or very agitated give a stat subcutaneous (SC) injection of appropriate medication while setting up the syringe driver.
- Only use drugs that are known to be effective via the subcutaneous route. Diazepam, chlorpromazine, and prochlorperazine are too irritating to be given subcutaneously.
- Check drug compatibility before mixing. If you are unable to discuss or get advice regarding the concerning drug combinations with either the palliative care team or the hospital drug information service, information can also be found at the palliative drugs website.
- Always use water for injection to dilute the drugs. Saline may be used if there are problems with site irritation. Saline should not be used with cyclizine as it can cause precipitation.
- Calculate the total dose of drug required in 24 hours and then divide volume of solution by 24, to give a rate per hour.
- Never use solutions that have precipitated or discolored.
- Always consider alternative routes, such as buccal, rectal, sublingual, or transdermal. The patient may not want a syringe driver.

An Infusion Pump

It infuses fluids, medication, or nutrients into a patient's circulatory system. It is generally used IV, though subcutaneous, arterial, and epidural infusions are occasionally used.

TYPES OF INFUSION

The four major types of infusion are the following:

Continuous Infusion

It usually consists of small pulses of infusion, usually between 500 nanoliters and 10,000 microliters depending on the pump's design, with the rate of these pulses depending on the programmed infusion speed.

Intermittent Infusion

It has a "high" infusion rate, alternating with a low programmable infusion rate to keep the cannula open. The timings are programmable. This mode is often used to administer antibiotics or other drugs that can irritate a blood vessel.

Patient-controlled Infusion is on Demand

It usually has a preprogrammed ceiling to avoid intoxication. The rate is controlled by a pressure pad or button that can be activated by the patient. It is the method of choice for patient-controlled analgesia (PCA), in which repeated small doses of opioid analgesics are delivered, with the device coded to stop administration before a dose reaches the limit, which may cause hazardous respiratory depression.

Total Parenteral Nutrition

It usually requires an infusion curve similar to normal mealtimes.

TYPES OF PUMP

The two basic classes of pumps are the following **(Fig. A-6.2):**

Large-volume Pumps

Large-volume pumps usually use some form of peristaltic pump. Classically, they use computer-controlled rollers compressing a silicone-rubber tube through which the medicine flows. Another common form is a set of fingers that press on the tube in sequence. Large-volume pumps can pump nutrient solutions large enough to feed a patient.

Small-volume Pumps

Small-volume pumps usually use a computer-controlled motor by turning a screw that pushes the plunger on a syringe. Small-volume pumps infuse hormones, such as insulin, or other medicines, such as opiates.

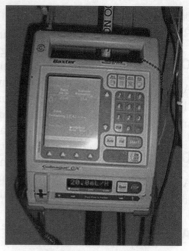

Fig. A-6.2: Infusion pump.

SYRINGES

A **syringe** is a simple pump consisting of a plunger that fits tightly in a tube. The plunger can be pulled and pushed along inside a cylindrical tube (called a barrel), allowing the syringe to take in and expel a liquid or gas through an orifice at the open end of the tube. The open end of the syringe may be fitted with a hypodermic needle, a nozzle, or tubing to help direct the flow into and out of the barrel **(Fig. A-6.3)**.

Fig. A-6.3: Syringe.

Hypodermic Syringes

Hypodermic syringes are used with hypodermic needles to inject liquid or gases into body tissues or to remove from the body.

Tip Designs

Syringes come with a number of designs for the area in which the blade locks to the syringe body. Perhaps the most well-known of these is the Luer lock, which simply twists the two together.

Standard U-100 Insulin Syringes

These are designed for insulin users. The dilution of insulin is such that 1 mL of insulin fluid has 100 standard "units" of insulin **(Fig. A-6.4)**.

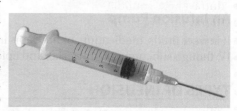

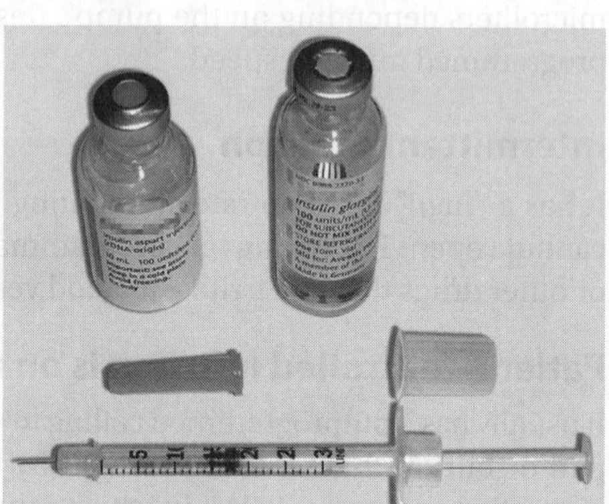

Fig. A-6.4: Standard U-100 insulin syringe.

Multishot Needle Syringes

There are needle syringes designed to reload from a built-in tank after each injection, so they can make several or many injections on a filling. An exception is the personal insulin autoinjector used by diabetic patients.

Venom Extraction Syringes

Venom extraction syringes are different from standard syringes, because they usually do not puncture the wound. The most common types have a plastic nozzle which is placed over the affected area and then the syringe piston is pulled back, creating a vacuum that allegedly sucks out the venom.

Oral

An oral syringe is a measuring instrument used to accurately measure doses of liquid medicine that are expressed in milliliters (mL). Oral syringes are available in various sizes from 1 to 10 mL and larger.

Dental Syringes

A dental syringe is used by dentists for the injection of an anesthetic. It consists of a breech-loading syringe fitted with a sealed cartridge containing anesthetic solution.

ARTICLES FOR AN INTRAVENOUS INFUSION

During an IV infusion, the following articles should be placed in a tray:

- Intravenous cannula
- Intravenous set
- Tourniquet
- Medication
- Syringes (2 and 5 mL)
- Spirit cotton swab
- Adhesive tape
- Kidney tray

Intravenous Tubing Parts, Parts of Intravenous Infusion Set

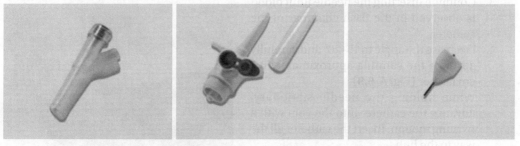

Fig. A-6.5: Assembled Y injection site assembled vented spike microdrip adapter.

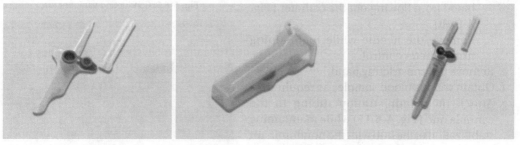

Fig. A-6.6: Vented spike assembled roller clamp IV drip chamber W/Vented spike.

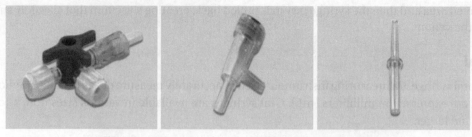

Fig. A-6.7: 3-Way stopcocks assembled T-connector connector.

PROCEDURE FOR AN INTRAVENOUS INFUSION

The procedures involved in an IV infusion are as listed below:

a. Select a suitable vein for venipuncture
b. Prepare the venipuncture site:
1. Apply a constricting band 2 inches above the venipuncture site. The constricting band should be tight enough to occlude venous flow, but not so tight that distal pulses are lost.
2. Select and palpate a prominent vein.
3. Cleanse the skin with an alcohol swab using a spiral motion starting with the entry site and extending outward about 2 inches. Allow the site to dry.
c. Put gloves.
d. Perform the venipuncture (**Fig. A-6.8**):
1. Using your nondominant hand, pull all local skin taut to stabilize the vein.
2. With your dominant hand, position the distal level of the needle up and insert the cannula into the vein at approximately 30° angle.
3. Continue inserting the needle until blood is observed in the flash chamber of the catheter.

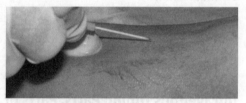

Fig. A-6.8: Performing venipuncture.

4. Decrease the angle to 15–20° and carefully advance the cannula approximately 0.5 cm farther (**Fig. A-6.9**).
5. While holding the needle stationary, advance the catheter into the vein with a twisting motion. Insert the catheter all the way to the hub.
6. Place a finger over the vein at the catheter tip and put pressure on the vein to prevent blood from flowing out the catheter (**Fig. A-6.10**).

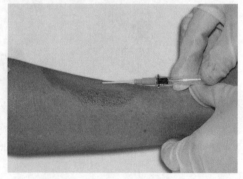

Fig. A-6.9: Conducting venipuncture.

7. Remove the needle while maintaining firm catheter control.
e. Remove the constricting band.
f. Obtain venous blood samples as required.
g. Attach the administration tubing to the cannula hub (**Fig. A-6.11**) while maintaining stabilization of the hub with the nondominant hand.

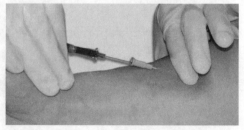

Fig. A-6.10: Using pressure to limit bleeding.

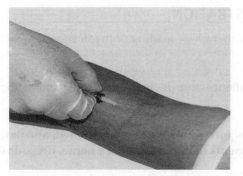

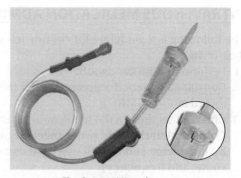

Fig. A-6.11: Connecting the IV tubing.   **Fig. A-6.12:** Micro drop set.

h. Open the flow-regulator clamp and observe for drips in the drip chamber. Allow the fluid to run freely for several seconds **(Fig. A-6.12)**.

i. Adjust to the desired flow rate.

> Micro drop factor: (60 drops/min).
> Macro drop factor: (16 drops/min).
>
> $$\frac{\text{Drop factor} \times \text{flow rate}}{\text{Time (in minutes)}} = \text{Drop rate}$$

j. Clean the area of blood, if necessary, and secure the hub of catheter with tape, leaving the hub and tubing connection visible. Make a small loop in the IV tube and place a second piece of tape over the first to secure the loop **(Fig. A-6.13)**.

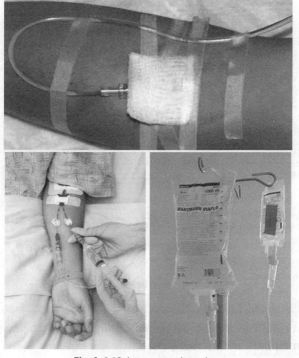

Fig. A-6.13: Intravenous insertion.

k. Apply a transparent dressing over the venipuncture site.

INTRAVENOUS MEDICATION ADMINISTRATION

The following is a guideline for commencing IV therapy or loading IV medication into an IV flask or vial:

1. Perform routine handwash.
2. Consult all patient documentation of the patient status [includes patient ID and medical record number (MRN)].
3. Check all sections of the medication chart.
4. **Confirm that the fluid order meets legal requirements (i.e., legible, signed, and dated by the doctor and has all essential components including patient's name, drug, dose, route, and frequency).**
5. Introduce self to patient.
6. Provide explanation to patient.
7. Seek permission to perform the procedure.
8. **Identify patient with medical order.**
9. Check for allergies.
10. Prepare patient and provide privacy as appropriate.
11. Organize equipment.
12. Confirm the compatibility of the drug and IV solution.
13. Review the literature on the drug if unfamiliar with its action, usual dosages, routes of administration, side effects, and nursing implications.
14. **Perform first drug check including diluent (if applicable) with second registered nurse (RN). Ensure five rights are adhered to and calculate the dosage correctly.**
15. **Prime the line according to the skill "managing a peripheral IV line."**
16. Open and attach syringe and drawing up device without causing contamination.

Dose calculations:

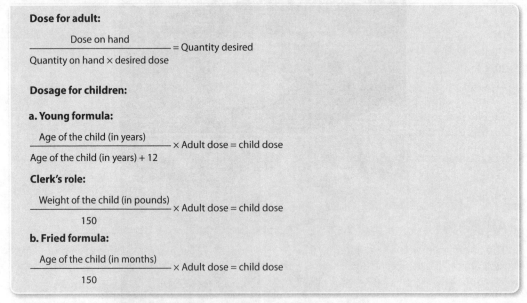

Dose for adult:

$$\frac{\text{Dose on hand}}{\text{Quantity on hand} \times \text{desired dose}} = \text{Quantity desired}$$

Dosage for children:

a. Young formula:

$$\frac{\text{Age of the child (in years)}}{\text{Age of the child (in years)} + 12} \times \text{Adult dose} = \text{child dose}$$

Clerk's role:

$$\frac{\text{Weight of the child (in pounds)}}{150} \times \text{Adult dose} = \text{child dose}$$

b. Fried formula:

$$\frac{\text{Age of the child (in months)}}{150} \times \text{Adult dose} = \text{child dose}$$

17. Prepare the medication according to the medication described below:
    For powdered medications:
    - Draw up diluent.
    - Remove the protective cap (if applicable)

- Cleanse the rubber stopper with alcohol swab.
- Inject the compatible type and amount of diluent using aseptic technique and avoiding excessive pressure build up.
- Ensure the powder is completely dissolved.
- Draw up the correct dose.
- Remove device from vial without causing contamination.
- Change drawing up device without causing contamination.
- Expel air
- Maintain sterility of drawing up device and plunger.

Ampoule Preparation

The following steps are followed for preparing ampoule:
- Tap the top of ampoule lightly and quickly until the fluid moves from the neck of the ampoule.
- Hold the ampoule upside down or set it on a flat surface and insert syringe or drawing up device without causing contamination.
- Aspirate medication into the syringe by gently pulling back on the plunger without causing contamination of the plunger.
- Change drawing up device without causing contamination.
- Expel air
- Maintain sterility of the drawing up device and plunger throughout the procedure.

Liquid Medication in a Vial

The following steps are followed for liquid medication in a vial:
- Remove the protective cap.
- Cleanse the rubber stopper with alcohol swab.
- Inject volume of air equivalent to dosage into vial.
- Draw up medication, expel air, and expel excess medication.
- Change drawing up device without causing contamination.
- Maintain the sterility drawing up device and plunger throughout the procedure.

18. Correctly dispose the waste.
19. Retain ampoules and vials until medication is administered.
20. Clean the injection port of IV flask/burette using alcohol swab.
21. Carefully insert injection device through the center of injection port of the IV flask/burette and inject medication without contamination.
22. Place the sharp into appropriate waste container.
23. Mix the solution by holding the flask and turning it gently from end to end or the burette by rolling it from side to side.
24. Assess the IV site and patency of the cannula.
25. Securely attach patient end of tube to IV cannula, maintaining sterility at both ends.
26. Stabilize the IV line to patient's arm with a tape.

AFTERCARE

The aftercare involved are listed below:
1. Label a piece of tape with date and time the IV was initiated, the catheter size, and your initials.
2. Secure the tape over the dressing.
3. Monitor the casualty and continue to observe the venipuncture site for signs of infiltration.
4. Terminate the encounter suitably.
5. Replace/dispose the equipment appropriately.
6. Perform routine handwash

7. Discontinue the infusion if signs of infiltration are observed.
8. Remove your gloves and disposes them appropriately.
9. Document the procedure on the appropriate medical form.

COMPLICATIONS

Listed below are the various complications involved:

1. **Infection:** Any break in the skin carries a risk of infection. Although IV insertion is an aseptic procedure, skin-dwelling organisms, such as *Candida albicans* may enter through the insertion site around the catheter, or bacteria may be accidentally introduced inside the catheter from contaminated equipment.

2. **Phlebitis:** Phlebitis is inflammation of a vein that may be caused by infection, the mere presence of a foreign body (the IV catheter), or the fluids or medication being given. **Symptoms: Warmth, swelling, pain, or redness around the vein.**

3. **Infiltration/extravasation:** Infiltration occurs when an IV fluid or medication accidentally enters the surrounding tissue rather than the vein. It is also known as extravasation (which refers to something escaping the vein). For example, if a cannula is in a vein for some time, the vein may scar and close and the only way for fluid to leave is along the outside of the cannula where it enters the vein.

4. **Fluid overload:** This occurs when fluids are given at a higher rate or in a larger volume than the system can absorb or excrete. The possible consequences include hypertension, heart failure, and pulmonary edema.

5. **Hypothermia:** The human body is at risk of accidentally induced hypothermia when large amounts of cold fluids are infused. Rapid temperature changes in the heart may precipitate ventricular fibrillation.

6. **Electrolyte imbalance:** Administering too dilute or too concentrated solution can disrupt the patient's balance of sodium, potassium, magnesium, and other electrolytes. Hospital patients usually receive blood tests to monitor these levels.

7. **Embolism:** A blood clot or other solid mass, as well as an air bubble, can be delivered into the circulation through an IV and end up blocking a vessel, and this is called embolism.

Nursing Assessment of a Patient with Obstructive Airway and Use of Artificial Airways

AIRWAY OBSTRUCTION

Introduction

In unanesthetized person, vomitus or laryngeal spasm is due to the presence of foreign material in the larynx. In the nonintubated anesthetized animal, it is caused by caudal displacement of the tongue and epiglottis, accumulation of mucus, saliva and blood in the pharynx, or laryngeal spasm resulting from that accumulation. In the intubated person, faulty placement or functioning of the endotracheal (ET) tube or kinking of it can cause airway obstruction. The signs of obstruction are deep, asphyxial respirations and struggling and great agitation in the conscious animal. Deeply anesthetized animals simply show a decline in respiratory efficiency.

Definition

The various definitions of airway obstruction are the following:
- Airway obstruction is a blockage of respiration in the airway.
- Partial or complete blockage of the breathing passages to the lungs.

Classification

It can be broadly classified as follows:
1. **Upper airway obstructions** occur in the area from your nose and lips to your larynx.
2. **Lower airway obstructions** occur between your larynx and the narrow passageways of your lungs.
3. **Partial airway obstructions** allow some air to pass. You can still breathe with a partial airway obstruction, but it will be difficult.
4. **Complete airway obstructions** do not allow any air to pass. You cannot breathe if you have a complete airway obstruction.
5. **Acute airway obstructions** are blockages that occur quickly. An example of an acute airway obstruction is choking on a foreign object.
6. **Chronic airway obstructions** can occur in one of the two ways. These can be blockages that take a long time to develop. They may also be blockages that last for a long time. For example, emphysema can cause a chronic airway obstruction.

Causes

Upper Airway Obstruction: Choking

Causes of upper airway obstruction, foreign body aspiration, blunt laryngotracheal trauma, penetrating laryngotracheal trauma, tonsillar hypertrophy, paralysis of the vocal cord or vocal fold, acute laryngotracheitis, such as viral croup, bacterial tracheitis, epiglottitis, peritonsillar abscess, pertussis, retropharyngeal abscess, spasmodic croup.

Lower Airway Obstruction: Obstructive Lung Disease

Lower airway obstruction is mainly caused by increased resistance in the bronchioles that reduces the amount of air inhaled in each breath and the oxygen that reaches the pulmonary arteries. It is different from airway restriction that prevents air from diffusing into the pulmonary arteries because of some kind of blockage in the lungs. Diseases that cause lower airway obstruction are termed obstructive lung diseases.

Signs and Symptoms of Airway Obstruction

The following are the signs and symptoms of airway obstruction:
- Agitation
- Cyanosis (bluish-colored skin)
- Confusion
- Difficulty breathing
- Gasping for air
- Panic
- Breathing noises, such as wheezing
- Unconsciousness

AIRWAY ASSESSMENT

Mechanisms of Airway Obstruction

The mechanisms involved in airway obstruction are the following:
- Supine posture in an unconscious child
- Displaced teeth
- Foreign body, such as food/vomit/blood/saliva
- Hemorrhage in the mouth, tongue, neck
- Burn-associated edema of mouth, pharynx, and larynx

Patient Assessment

Before the initiation of sedation, patients should be evaluated for anatomical characteristics and relevant medical history that could increase the risk of airway management problems. Nurse assessments of oxygenation status include a history, physical examination, and review of relevant diagnostic data.

Medical and Nursing History

The following factors may contribute to a potentially higher risk of airway difficulties. If any of these conditions are present, the clinician will determine the patient's level of risk on an individual basis.
- Previous problems with anesthesia, sedation, or airway management
- Stridor, snoring, or sleep apnea
- Advanced rheumatoid arthritis
- Abnormal anatomy in head/neck, such as tumors
- Obese patients
- Congenital syndromes that involve the airway
- Radiation therapy or previous surgery to head/neck may distort airway and complicate airway manipulations
- Large beard such that mask ventilation is more difficult
- A short, thick, muscular neck

Physical Examination

The preprocedure physical examination should include the following assessments to evaluate the patient's airway and uncover physical traits that could contribute to respiratory complications.

- **Oral cavity inspection:** The patient's oral cavity should be carefully inspected for the following abnormalities prior to sedation. Findings should be documented in the patient's record.
  - Small mouth opening (<3 cm in an adult)
  - Protruding incisors
  - Loose or capped teeth
  - Missing teeth
  - Dental appliances, such as crowns, bridges, and dentures
  - Enlarged tonsils
  - Nonvisible faucial pillars, which are vertical folds of tissue created by muscles that surround the palatine tonsils
  - Nonvisible uvula
  - Tumor that could obstruct air flow
- **Temporomandibular joint examination:** Pain or limited range of motion in the temporomandibular joint can be assessed by palpating the joint while the patient's mouth is open to the widest point. In an adult, the normal mouth opening is 4–6 cm. Patients with temporomandibular joint disease who have an opening of less than 4 cm (approximately 2 finger breadths) may have limited airway mobility if mechanical devices are needed to treat respiratory distress.
- **Thyromental distance evaluation:** The thyromental distance should be at least 5–7 cm as measured from the thyroid cartilage to the point of the chin when the neck is extended fully and the mouth closed. A distance of less than 7 cm can indicate difficulty with intubation should the need develop.
- **Neck mobility:** Assessment of the movement of the atlanto-occipital joint through flexion, extension, and side to side is necessary before sedation is initiated. Ability to align the oral, pharyngeal, and laryngeal axes is required for successful ET intubation.
- **Physical characteristics:** Patients should be examined for physical traits that can indicate a potential for airway complications.
  - Significant obesity especially in the region of the neck and face
  - High, arched palate
  - Enlarged tongue
  - Short, immobile neck
  - Protruding teeth
  - Recessed or protruding jaw

Diagnostic Studies

It includes different tests of evaluation of obstructive airway:

- Sputum examination
- Throat culture
- Visualization procedure
- Arterial blood gas analysis
- Pulmonary function tests

Sputum examination

Description

Sputum is the mucous secretion from the lungs, bronchi, and trachea. It is obtained for evaluation of gross appearance, microscopic examination, Gram's stain, culture, and cytology.

- For culture and sensitivity to identify a specific microorganism and its drug sensitivity

- For cytology to identify origin, structure, function, and pathology of cells. Specimen for cytology often require serial collection of three early morning specimens and are tested to identify cancer in the lung and its specific cell type
- For acid-fast bacillus (AFB), which also requires, serial collection, often for 3 consecutive days, to identify the presence of tuberculosis (TB)
- To assess the effectiveness of therapy

Sputum specimen is often collected in the morning. Upon awakening, the client can cough up the secretions that have accumulated during the night. Sometimes specimens are collected during postural drainage, when the client can usually produce sputum. When a client cannot cough, the nurse must sometimes use pharyngeal suctioning to obtain a specimen.

To collect a sputum specimen, the nurse should follow these steps:

- Offer mouth care, so that the specimen will not be contaminated with microorganisms from the mouth.
- Ask the client to breathe deeply and then cough up 15–30 mL of sputum.
- Wear gloves and personal protective equipment to avoid direct contact with the sputum. Follow special precautions if TB is suspected, wear a mask capable of filtering droplet nuclei.
- Ask the client to expectorate the sputum into the specimen container. Make sure the sputum does not contact the outside of the container. If the outside of the container does become contaminated, wash it with a disinfectant.
- Following sputum collection, offer mouthwash to remove any unpleasant taste.
- Label and transport the specimen to the laboratory. Arrange for the specimen to be sent to the laboratory immediately or refrigerated. Bacterial cultures must be started immediately before any contaminating organism can grow, multiply, and produce false results.
- Document the collection of the sputum specimen's on the client's chart. Include the amount, color, consistency (thick, tenacious, watery), presence of hemoptysis, odor of the sputum, any measures needed to obtain the specimen (e.g., postural drainage) and any discomfort experienced by the client.

Throat Culture
Definition
A throat culture sample is collected from the mucosa of the oropharynx and tonsillar regions using a culture swab. The sample is then cultured and examined for the presence of disease producing microorganisms.

To obtain a throat culture specimen, they should follow the steps listed below:

1. Wear clean gloves.
2. Insert the swab into the oropharynx and run the swab along the tonsils and areas on the pharynx that are reddened or contain exudates.
3. The gag reflex, active in some clients, may be decreased by having the client sit upright if health permits, open the mouth, extend the tongue, and say "ah" and by taking the specimen quickly.
4. If the posterior pharynx cannot be seen, use a light and depress the tongue with a tongue blade.

Visualization Procedures
Bronchoscopy: It is the direct inspection and examination of the larynx, trachea, and bronchi through either a flexible fiberoptic bronchoscope or a rigid bronchoscope.

The **purposes** of diagnostic bronchoscopy:

- To examine tissues or collect secretions.
- To determine whether a tumor can be surgically resected.
- To diagnose bleeding sites (source of hemoptysis).

The **purposes** of therapeutic bronchoscopy:
- To remove foreign bodies from the tracheobronchial tree.
- To remove secretions obstructing the tracheobronchial tree when the patient cannot clear them.
- To destroy and excise lesions.

Arterial Blood Gases (ABG) Analysis
Description
- A measurement of oxygen, carbon dioxide, as well as the pH of the blood that provides a means of assessing the adequacy of ventilation and oxygenation.
- Also helps to assess the acid-base status of the body—whether acidosis or alkalosis is present and to what degree (compensated or uncompensated).
- Blood can be obtained from any artery but is most often drawn from radial, brachial, or femoral site. It can be drawn directly by arterial puncture or assessed by way of indwelling arterial catheter.

Nursing/Patient Care Considerations
- After blood sample is withdrawn, apply firm pressure over the puncture site with a dry sponge for 5 minutes.
- Remove air bubbles from syringe and needle after taking sample.
- If the patient is on anticoagulant medication, apply direct pressure over puncture site for 10–15 minutes and then apply a firm pressure dressing.

Interpret ABGs by looking at the following:
- **PaO$_2$:** Partial pressure of oxygen in arterial blood (greater than 95–100 mm Hg).
- **PaCO$_2$:** Partial pressure of carbon dioxide in arterial blood (35–45 mm Hg).
- **SpO$_2$:** Saturation of oxygen in arterial blood (greater than 95%)
- **pH:** Hydrogen ion concentration or degree of acid–base balance (7.35–7.45).

Management of Obstructive Airway
Manual Maneuver

- **Jaw trust method:** This maneuver moves the tongue forward with the mandible, which reduces tongue's ability to obstruct the airway. Standing at the head of the bed, middle finger of the right hand is placed at the angle of the patient's jaw on the right. The middle finger of the left hand is similarly placed at the angle of the patient's jaw on the left side. An upward pressure is applied to elevate the mandible which will lift the tongue from the posterior pharynx.
- **Head tilt and chin lift method (Fig. A-7.1):** The fingers of one hand

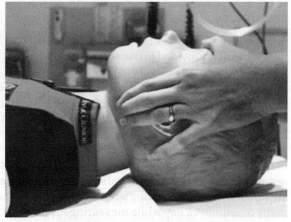

Fig. A-7.1: Head tilt and chin lift method.

are placed under the mandible, which is gently lifted upward to bring the chin anterior. The thumb of the same hand depresses the lower lip to open the mouth.

Pharmacologic Antagonists

Specific antagonists are available to reverse the effects of opioids and benzodiazepines. Naloxone or flumazenil (for benzodiazepines) may be administered to improve patient's spontaneous ventilatory efforts.

Bag Mask Ventilation

Bag mask ventilation is a basic but critical airway management. It is provided to maintain adequate ventilation for patient requiring airway support and allow enough time to establish a more controlled approach to airway management, such as ET intubation.

Successful Bag Mask Ventilation Depends on the Following Three Things

Patent Airway

Airway patency can be established by using manual maneuver.

Adequate Mask Seal

Mask must be placed and held adequately and correctly. The nasal portion of mask must be placed on the bridge of patient's nose. The body of the mask is then placed on to the patient's face covering the nose and mouth.

Proper Ventilation

Bag should not be squeezed explosively. It should be squeezed steadily over appropriately for one full second. Ventilation rate should not exceed 10–12 breaths/minute.

Deep Breathing Exercises

Deep breathing helps expand the lungs and forces an improved distribution of the air into all sections of the lungs. The patient either sits in a chair or sits upright in bed and inhales and then pushes the abdomen out to force the maximum amount of air into the lung. The abdomen is then contracted and the patient exhales. Deep breathing exercises are done several times each day for short periods. Because of the mind–body awareness required to perform coughing and deep breathing exercises, they are unsuitable for most children under the age of 8 years.

Incentive Spirometry

An incentive spirometer is a medical device used to help patients improve the functioning of their lungs. It is provided to patients who have had any surgery that might jeopardize respiratory function, particularly surgery to the lungs themselves, but also commonly to patients recovering from cardiac or other surgery involving extended time under anesthesia and prolonged in-bed recovery. The incentive spirometer is also issued to patients recovering from rib damage to help minimize the chance of fluid buildup in the lungs. It can be used as well by wind instrument players who want to improve their air flow.

The patient breathes in from the device as slowly and as deeply as possible, then holds his or her breath for 2–6 seconds. This provides back pressure which pops open the alveoli. It is the same maneuver in a yawn. An indicator provides a gauge of how well the patient's lung or lungs are functioning, by indicating sustained inhalation vacuum. The patient is generally asked to do many repetitions a day while measuring his or her progress by way of the gauge.

Chest Physiotherapy

- Chest physiotherapy (CPT) is a technique used to mobilize or loosen secretions in the lungs and respiratory tract.

- This is especially helpful for patients with large amount of secretions or ineffective cough.
- Chest physiotherapy consists of external mechanical maneuvers, such as chest percussion, postural drainage, vibration, to augment mobilization and clearance of airway secretions, diaphragmatic breathing with pursed lips, coughing, and controlled coughing.

Techniques in CPT
- A nurse or respiratory therapist may administer CPT, though the techniques can often be taught to patients' family members.
- The most common procedures used are postural drainage and chest percussion, in which the patient is rotated to facilitate drainage of secretions from a specific lobe or segment while being clapped with cupped hands to loosen and mobilize retained secretions that can then be expectorated or drained.
- The procedure is somewhat uncomfortable and tiring for the patient.

Percussion
- Chest percussion involves striking the chest wall over the area being drained.
- Percussing lung areas involves the use of cupped palm to loosen pulmonary secretions, so that they can be expectorated with ease.
- Percussing with the hand held in a rigid dome-shaped position, the area over the lung lobes to be drained in rhythmic pattern.
- Usually the patient will be positioned in supine or prone and should not experience any pain.
- Cupping is never done on bare skin or performed over surgical incisions, below the ribs, or over the spine or breasts, because of the danger of tissue damage.
- Typically, each area is percussed for 30–60 seconds several times a day.
- If the patient has tenacious secretions, the area must be percussed for 3–5 minutes several times per day. Patients may learn how to percuss the anterior chest as well.

Vibration
- In vibration, the nurse uses rhythmic contractions and relaxations using his or her arm and shoulder muscles while holding the patient flat on the patient's chest as the patient exhales.
- The purpose is to help loosen respiratory secretions, so that they can be expectorated with ease. Vibration (at a rate of 200 per minute) can be done for several times a day.
- To avoid patient causing discomfort, vibration is never done over the patient's breasts, spine, sternum, and rib cage.
- Vibration can also be taught to family members or accomplished with mechanical device.

Postural drainage
- Postural drainage is the positioning techniques that drain secretions from specific segments of the lungs and bronchi into the trachea.
- Because some patients do not require postural drainage for all lung segments, the procedure must be based on the clinical findings.
- In postural drainage, the person is tilted or propped at an angle to help drain secretions from the lungs.
- Also, the chest or back may be clapped with a cupped hand to help loosen secretions—the technique called chest percussion.
- Postural drainage cannot be used for people who are:
  - unable to tolerate the position required
  - are taking anticoagulation drugs
  - have recently vomited blood
  - have had a recent rib or vertebral fracture or
  - have severe osteoporosis

- Postural drainage also cannot be used for people who are unable to produce any secretions (because when this happens, further attempts at postural drainage may lower the level of oxygen in the blood).

Oxygen Therapy

Definition

To increase the fraction of inspired oxygen concentration (FiO_2) available to a patient, a variety of oxygen delivery devices are employed to administer medical oxygen. The oxygen may be administered with or without humidity.

Uses

- To improve breathing pattern
- To restore body functions
- To improve gases exchange

Devices used for Oxygen Administration

The devices used for oxygen administration are the following:

- **Nasal catheter:** The light rubber nasal catheter is inserted after lubricating its tip with liquid paraffin until the tip is visible behind the uvula in the oropharynx.
- **Nasal cannula (NC):** It is a thin tube with two small nozzles separated by 1.5 mm in diameter that protrude into the patient's nostrils. It can only comfortably provide oxygen at low flow rates, 2–6 L/minute, delivering a concentration of 24–40%.
- **Simple face mask:** It is often used at between 6 and 12 L/minute, with an oxygen concentration to the patient of between 28 and 50%. This is a plastic mask with several small vent holes on each side. It is attached to the oxygen supply using 7 mm oxygen tubing. No humidification is required or should be added.
- **Venturi masks:** A venturi is a simple design of valve that uses oxygen supplied through a port which allows room air to be drawn in. This generates a rate of flow that may in some situations approach the patient's peak inspiratory flow.

  Advantage: It delivers a precise percentage of oxygen at high rates. On the side of each rating of venturi valve is printed the flow rate that is required to maintain the stated oxygen concentration.

  The green 60% venturi valve is not recommended for use as humidification is inadequate for a venturi valve of this rating.
- **Reservoir bag mask:** This is a mask that is designed to provide high concentrations of oxygen for short periods. At 15 L/minute, the system will deliver about 90% oxygen; at 10 L/minute the system will deliver about 70% oxygen. In the immediate and acute situation, the flow of gas can be titrated over whatever range (up to 15 L) that is required to achieve a target saturation. This type of mask is a variable performance mask and should be used for no longer than 3 hours. Long-term use leads to complications associated with dry lung tissue (i.e., reduced ciliary action, sputum retention, mucus plugging, and desiccation of lung tissue).
- **Partial rebreathing mask:** It can be used, which is based on a simple mask, but featuring a reservoir bag, which increases the provided oxygen rate to 40–70% oxygen at 5–15 L/minute.
- **Non-rebreather masks:** Draw oxygen from an attached reservoir bags, with one-way valves that direct exhaled air out of the mask. When properly fitted and used at flow rates of 10–15 L/minute or higher, they deliver close to 100% oxygen. This type of mask is indicated for acute medical emergencies.

ARTIFICIAL AIRWAYS

Definition

A tube or tube-like device that is inserted through the nose, mouth, or into the trachea to provide an opening for ventilation.

Indications for Artificial Airways

- Relief of airway obstruction guarantees the patency of upper airway regardless of soft tissue obstruction
- Protecting or maintaining an airway
- Reflexes
  - Pharyngeal reflex
    - Ninth and tenth cranial nerves
    - Gag and swallowing
  - Laryngeal
    - Vagovagal reflex
    - Cause laryngospasm
  - Tracheal
    - Vagovagal reflex
    - Cough when a foreign body or irritation in trachea
  - Carinals cough with irritation of carina.
- **Facilitation of tracheobronchial clearance:** Mobilization of secretions from the trachea requires either an adequate cough or direct suctioning of the trachea.
- **Facilitation of artificial ventilation:** Ventilation with a mask should be used for short periods during gastric insufflation.

Hazards of Artificial Airways

- Infection during bypassing the normal defense mechanisms that prevent bacterial contamination
- Ineffective cough maneuver
- Impaired verbal communication
- Loss of personal dignity

Types of Artificial Airways

- Oropharyngeal airways (OPAs)
- Nasopharyngeal tubes
- Orotracheal tubes
- Nasotracheal tubes
- Tracheostomy tubes
- Esophageal obturator airway
- Cricothyroid tubes
- Laryngeal masks

Oropharyngeal Airway (Fig. A-7.2)

Introduction

The OPA is a medical device called an airway adjunct used to maintain a patent (open) airway. It does this by preventing the tongue from covering the epiglottis, which could prevent the person from breathing. When a person becomes unconscious, the muscles in their jaw relax and allow the tongue to obstruct the airway.

- Device designed for insertion along the tongue until the teeth and/or gingiva limit the insertion
- Lies between the posterior pharynx and the tongue and pushes the tongue forward
- Activates the gag reflex and used on unconscious patient
- Correct sizing of airway is imperative

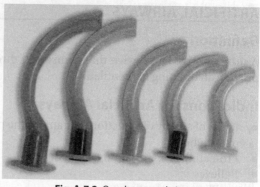

Fig. A-7.2: Oropharyngeal airways.

Purposes

Use of an OPA does not remove the need for the recovery position and ongoing assessment of the airway, and it does not prevent obstruction by liquids (blood, saliva, food, cerebrospinal fluid) or the closing of the glottis. But can facilitate ventilation during cardiopulmonary resuscitation (CPR) and for persons with a large tongue.

Indication

The OPAs are indicated only in unconscious people, because of the likelihood that the device would stimulate a gag reflex in conscious or semiconscious individuals. This could result in vomiting and potentially lead to an obstructed airway. Nasopharyngeal airways are mostly used instead as they do not stimulate a gag reflex.

In general OPAs need to be sized and inserted correctly to maximize effectiveness and minimize possible complications, such as oral trauma.

Sizes of Oropharyngeal Airways

The OPAs come in a variety of sizes, from infant to adult, and are used commonly in pre-hospital emergency care and for short-term airway management postanesthetic or when manual methods are inadequate to maintain an open airway.

The OPAs come in sizes ranging from 50, 60, and 70 mm (nos. 0, 1, and 2) for neonates and 80, 90, and 100 mm (nos. 3, 4, and 5) for adults.

Hazards of Oropharyngeal Airways

The hazards of OPAs are as follows:

- If too small, may not displace tongue or may cause tongue to obstruct airway or may aspirate.
- If too large, may cause epiglottis impaction.
- Roof of mouth may be lacerated upon insertion.
- Aspiration from intact gag reflex.

Nasopharyngeal Airway (Fig. A-7.3)

It is a tube that is designed to be inserted into the nasal passageway to secure an open airway. When a patient becomes unconscious, the muscles in the jaw commonly relax and can allow the tongue to slide back and obstruct the airway. The purpose of the flared end is to prevent the device from becoming lost inside the patient's nose.

- Located so that it can provide a clear path for gas flow into the pharynx
- Is a soft rubber catheter
- Can be tolerated by the conscious patient

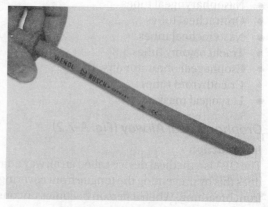

Fig. A-7.3: Nasopharyngeal airway.

- Useful for patients with a soft tissue obstruction who have jaw injury or spasm of jaw muscles
- Proper sizing and insertion.

Indications
Nasopharyngeal airways are sometimes used by people who have sleep apnea; however, these are only used in rare cases and are not a common form of treatment for sleep apnea.

Contraindications
The contraindications of nasopharyngeal airways are as follows:
- Patients with severe head or facial injuries
- Basilar skull fracture (Battle's sign, raccoon eyes, cerebrospinal fluid/blood from ears, etc.)

Insertion
Insertion of nasopharyngeal airways can be achieved as follows:
- The correct size airway is chosen by measuring the device on the patient.
- The device should reach from the patient's nostril to the earlobe or the angle of the jaw.
- The outside of the tube is lubricated with a water-based lubricant, so that it enters the nose more easily.
- The device is inserted until the flared end rests against the nostril.
- Some tubes contain a safety pin to prevent inserting the tube too deeply.
- Care must be taken to ensure the pin does not stick into the nostril.

Hazards of Nasopharyngeal Airways
- Using an airway that is too long may cause the tip to enter the esophagus.
- Injuring the nasal mucosa causes bleeding. This can lead to aspiration of blood or clots.
- If nasal airway does not have flange at the nasal end, the airway can be lost in nose and the airway.

Orotracheal Airway (Fig. A-7.4)
The orotracheal airway is used in the following conditions:
- Used in conditions of, or leading to, respiratory failure
- Usually the method of choice in emergencies that do not involve trauma to the mouth or mandible
- Oral route is usually the easiest
- Accomplished by using a laryngoscope to directly visualize the trachea

Endotracheal Tubes
The ET tubes are of the following:
- Size: (Age/4) + 4 mm internal diameter
- Tube of size calculated above, + tube 0.5 mm internal diameter
- 0.5 mm internal diameter larger, should above on the child's bed
- For example, 6-year-old child: (6/4) + 4 = 5.5 mm in diameter
- As such on the child's bed should be 5, 5.5, and 6 mm in diameter tubes.

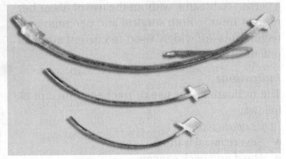

Fig. A-7.4: Orotracheal airway.

Drugs Used
The drugs used are as follows:

Thiopentone
- 3–5 mg/kg in a normovolemic child
- 0.5–1 mg/kg in a hypovolemic child

Midazolam
- 0.3 mg/kg in a child

Propofol
- 2.5 mg/kg in a normovolemic child
- 1 mg/kg in a hypovolemic child

Suxamethonium
- 1–2 mg/kg in a child

Rocuronium
- 1 mg/kg in a child

Saline flush: Ten milliliters intravenous (IV) cannula + 3-way tap on extension tubing: all patent and visible.

Nasotracheal Airway
The use of nasotracheal airway has the following features:
- More difficult route than oral
- Requires a longer and more flexible tracheal tube
- Insert through nose by touch and when in oropharynx use laryngoscope and forceps (can perform "blind")
- Usually nasotracheal tube is better tolerated by patient compared to oral.

Tracheostomy
Tracheostomy is performed as follows:
- Through the anterior tracheal wall either by the open method or by the percutaneous method.
- Performed usually to prevent or treat long-term respiratory failure.
- Decreases anatomic dead space by 50%.

Tracheostomy is defined as an incision on the anterior aspect of the neck and opening a direct airway through an incision in the trachea (windpipe). The resulting stoma (hole) can serve independently as an airway or as a site for a tracheostomy tube to be inserted; this tube allows a person to breathe without the use of his or her nose or mouth. Both surgical and percutaneous techniques are widely used in current surgical practice **(Fig. A-7.5)**.

Indications
The indications for use of tracheostomy are as follows:

In the acute setting:
- Severe facial trauma
- Head and neck cancers
- Large congenital tumors of the head and neck (e.g., bronchial cleft cyst)
- Acute angioedema and inflammation of the head and neck

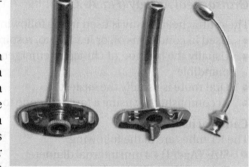
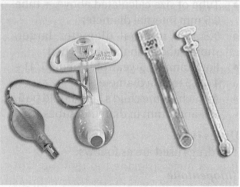

Fig. A-7.5: Tracheostomy airway.

In the chronic setting:
- Mechanical ventilation and tracheal toilet (e.g., comatose patients or extensive surgery involving the head and neck)
- Severe uvulopalatopharyngoplasty
- Maxillomandibular advancement surgeries

Other specialized ET tubes:
- Rae tube directs the airway connection away from the surgical field.
- Endotrol tube controls the distal tip for intubation.
- Hi-Lo Jet tube for high-frequency jet ventilation.
- Laser Flex tube reflects a diffused beam if it comes in contact with tube.
- Endobronchial tubes

Complications and Hazards of Tracheostomy
- Postsurgical bleeding
- Infection
- Mediastinal emphysema
- Pneumothorax
- Subcutaneous emphysema
- Stoma collapse (should not be moved or changed in the first 36 hours)

Esophageal Obturator Airway
The features of esophageal obturator airway (EOA) are as follows:
- Placed in the esophagus to prevent stomach contents from entering the lungs while the patient is being artificially ventilated.
- Cuff must be passed beyond carina before being inflated.
- Inflated cuff with 35 cc air
- Mask must fit tightly to ensure ventilation.

Pharyngeal Tracheal Lumen Airway
The features of pharyngeal tracheal lumen airway (PTL) are the following:
- Double-lumen airway combining an EOA and an ET tube
- Designed to be inserted blindly
- Has an oropharyngeal cuff and a cuff that can seal off either the trachea or the esophagus.

CRICOTHYROTOMY

Introduction
Also called thyrocricotomy, cricothyroidotomy, inferior laryngotomy, intercricothyrotomy, coniotomy, or emergency airway puncture.

This procedure provides a temporary emergency airway in situations where there is obstruction at or above the level of the larynx, such that oral/nasal ET intubation is impossible. Compared with an emergency tracheostomy, it is quicker and easier to perform and associated with fewer complications. It is a relatively quick procedure, taking up to about 2 minutes to complete. In an emergency, without access to medical equipment, cricothyroidotomy has even been improvised using a drinking straw and penknife.

Definition
It is an incision made through the skin and cricothyroid membrane to establish a patent airway during certain life-threatening situations, such as airway obstruction by a foreign body, angioedema, or massive facial trauma. Cricothyrotomy is nearly always performed as a last resort in cases where orotracheal and nasotracheal intubation are impossible or

contraindicated. Cricothyrotomy is easier and quicker to perform than tracheotomy, does not require manipulation of the cervical spine, and is associated with fewer complications. However, while cricothyrotomy may be lifesaving in extreme circumstances, this technique is only intended to be a temporizing measure until a definitive airway can be established.

Indications

Indications for cricothyrotomy are as follows:
- Cannot ventilate
- Severe facial or nasal injuries (that do not allow oral or nasal tracheal intubation)
- Massive midfacial trauma
- Possible cervical spine trauma preventing adequate ventilation
- Anaphylaxis
- Chemical inhalation injuries

Contraindications

- Inability to identify landmarks (cricothyroid membrane)
- Underlying anatomical abnormality (tumor)
- Tracheal transection
- Acute laryngeal disease due to infection or trauma
- Small children under 10 years old (a 12–14 gauge catheter over the needle may be safer)

Techniques

The three techniques used are as follows:
- Needle
- Intubation (with purpose-built kits)
- Surgical

Needle Cricothyroidotomy (Figs. A-7.6 and A-7.7)

Procedure

The procedures to use a needle cricothyroidotomy are the following:
- A needle or cannula (usually a large-bore IV cannula) is inserted through the cricothyroid membrane:
  - Place the patient supine and, assuming there is no cervical spine injury, extend the neck using a pillow under the shoulders.
  - Run a finger down the front of the neck in midline and find the notch in the upper border of the thyroid cartilage. Below this is a depression between the thyroid and cricoid cartilages—the cricothyroid membrane.
- Stabilize the cricothyroid membrane with one hand between finger and thumb.
- Pierce it with a large-bore cannula (14G) attached to a syringe aiming at 45° to the skin, caudally in the sagittal plain.

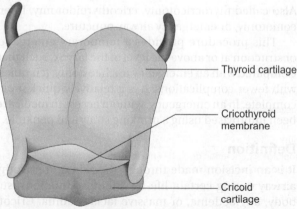

Thyroid cartilage

Cricothyroid membrane

Cricoid cartilage

Fig. A-7.6: Cricothyroidotomy.

- Aspirate as the needle is introduced and confirm position by withdrawal of air; slide the cannula over the needle into the airway.
- Connect to an O_2 supply via Y-connector, give 15 L/minute for an adult or, in a child, set the gas flow to the age of the child in years.
- Ventilate by covering the patent port of Y-connector with a thumb to allow O_2 to flow for 1 second (transtracheal insufflation). Remove thumb to allow expiration for 4 seconds via the upper airway. If no Y-connector is available, use a 2-mL syringe or IV giving set with a hole in the side that can be occluded by the thumb.

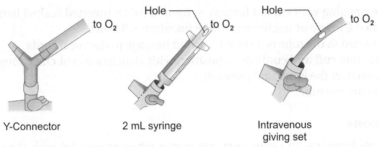

Fig. A-7.7: Needle cricothyroidotomy.

Cricothyroid Intubation with Purpose-Built Kits

Cricothyroidotomy may be achieved with a narrow tube using a pre-prepared kit, such as the Mini-Trach® II which contains a guarded blade, plastic introducer, 4 mm uncuffed tube to slide over introducer, ISO connection, tracheal suction tube, and neck fastenings. The patient can breathe spontaneously or be bagged using this form of airway, but they are usually only used as a temporary measure until a more permanent airway is secured. Retrograde intubation can be practiced with a Mini-Trach® II set by passing the introducer upward into the mouth and feeding an ET tube into place over it.

TABLE A-7.1: Complications and techniques to prevent complication.

Complications	Techniques to prevent complication
Thyrohyoid membrane incision	Attention to anatomy; vertical skin incision; confirm position of the cricothyroid membrane after skin incision
Intraoperative/postoperative bleeding	Incise directly over the cricothyroid membrane in the midline; vertical skin incision; horizontal incision in inferior half membrane; avoid the thyroid isthmus
Subglottic stenosis	Use a small-bore tube; avoid long-term use (>72 hours)
Dysphonia/hoarseness	Use a small tube; point inferiorly to avoid cords; avoid tracheal cartilage damage by not using force
Laryngeal damage	Avoid oversized tube and excessive traction on the thyroid cartilage during insertion
Tube misplaced in bronchus	Avoid insertion of too much of tube length so as not to enter the right main bronchus
Pulmonary aspiration	Protect the upper airway by suction and positioning
Tracheal stenosis	Use a low-pressure balloon cuff
Recurrent laryngeal nerve injury	Stay in midline and avoid the posterior subglottic wall by not inserting instruments too far
Esophageal perforation or tracheoesophageal fistula	Do not incise or insert the needle deeply after entering the subglottic space
Tracheo left brachiocephalic vein fistula	Use a low-pressure cuff
Fracture of thyroid cartilage	Avoid an oversized tube.

Surgical Cricothyroidotomy

This is usually not performed in children under 12.

- Delineate anatomy as above, clean the skin and instill a local anesthetic (if the patient is conscious).
- Make a small vertical skin incision in the midline, spread the wound edges laterally, and identify the cricothyroid membrane.
- Take care not to cut or remove the thyroid or cricoid cartilages.
- Make a horizontal incision through the membrane's inferior half and then extend gently through it.
- Dilate the opening with curved forceps or rotation of an inverted scalpel handle. Insert a small, cuffed ET tube or tracheotomy tube (maximum 8 mm).
- Aim downward as the tube is inserted to avoid damage to the vocal cords.
- Inflate the tube cuff and confirm its position with visualization of chest movements and auscultation over the lungs and stomach.
- Finally, secure the tube.

Complications

Although complications do occur, they are minor when compared with the catastrophic outcome normally associated with a failure to secure an airway. Complications can affect up to 40% in the emergency situation but, in experienced hands, the complication rate is usually much lower. Elective complication rate is ~ 6–8%.

Laryngeal Mask

Laryngeal mask enables anesthetists to channel oxygen or anesthesia gas to a patient's lungs during surgery. It has an airway tube that connects to an elliptical mask with a cuff. When the cuff is inflated, the mask conforms to the anatomy with the bowl of the mask (LMA) facing the space between the vocal cords. After correct insertion, the tip of the laryngeal mask sits in the throat against the muscular valve that is located at the upper portion of the esophagus.

- Ensure laryngeal mask airway has been previously sterilized.
- Check cuff and valve.
- Lubricate the LMA with KY jelly or other sterile surgical lubricant, specifically avoiding the bowl of the LMA, so that lubricant cannot get into the LMA aperture.
- Evacuate all air from cuff, preferably using the LMA deflator.

Laryngeal Mask Airway Sizes (Table A-7.2)

Size	Weight	Maximum air in cuff (mL)
TABLE A-7.2: Laryngeal mask airway sizes.		
1	Under 5 kg	4
1.5	5–10 kg	7
2	10–20 kg	10
2.5	20–30 kg	14
3	30 kg to small adult	20
4	Adult 50–70 kg	30
5	Big adult 70–100 kg	40
6	Adult over 100 kg	50

Preparation of the Laryngeal Mask Airway for Clinical Use

Procedure

The steps involved in laryngeal mask airway are as follows:

Step #1: Deflate the LMA using syringe and optional cuff deflation device	
Step #2: Press mask tip upward against the hard palate to flatten it out and advance the mask into the pharynx using the index finger. (CAUTION: Be sure to carefully "fit" the deflated LMA tip into the convexity of the hard palate as this is the KEY to successful insertion)	
Step #3: With neck flexed and head extended, press the laryngeal mask airway into the posterior pharyngeal wall using the index finger	
Step #4: Complete the insertion by exerting cephalad pressure by the nondominant hand prior to removing the index finger	

Contd...

Contd...

Step #5: Inflate laryngeal mask airway and secure in place with tape	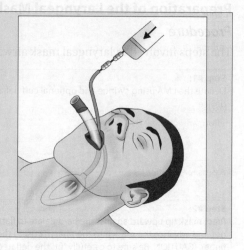

Prevention of Airway Obstruction

Many types of airway obstructions can be prevented. Reduce your risk by doing the following:
- Avoid drinking a lot of alcohol before eating.
- Eat small bites of food.
- Eat slowly.
- Supervise small children when eating.
- Chew thoroughly before swallowing.
- Make sure your dentures fit properly.
- Keep small objects away from children.
- Do not smoke.
- Visit your doctor regularly if you have a condition that can cause a chronic airway obstruction.

NURSING CARE PLAN

The nursing care plan to treat airway obstruction is listed below:

Nursing diagnosis: Ineffective airway clearance with regard to tracheobronchial obstruction

Long-term goal: Patient will maintain a patent airway

Short-term goals/outcomes: ➤ Patient's lung sounds will be clear to auscultate ➤ Patient will be free of dyspnea ➤ Patient will demonstrate correct coughing and deep breathing techniques

Intervention	Rationale	Evaluation
Assess airway for patency by asking the patient to state his or her name	Maintaining an airway is always top priority especially in patients who may have experienced trauma to the airway. If a patient can articulate an answer, their airway is patent	Patient is able to state their name without difficulty
Inspect the mouth, neck, and position of trachea for potential obstruction	Foreign materials or blood in the mouth, hematoma of the neck, or tracheal deviation can all mean airway obstruction	No foreign objects, blood in mouth noted. Neck is free of hematoma. Trachea is midline

Contd...

Contd...

Auscultate lungs for the presence of normal or adventitious lung sounds	Decreased or absent sounds may indicate the presence of a mucous plug or airway obstruction. Wheezing indicates airway resistance. Stridor indicates emergent airway obstruction	Patient's lung sounds are clear to auscultate throughout all lobes
Assess respiratory quality, rate, depth, effort, and pattern	Flaring of the nostrils, dyspnea, use of accessory muscles, tachypnea, and/or apnea are all signs of severe distress that require immediate intervention	Patient is free of signs of distress
Assess for mental status changes	Increasing lethargy, confusion, restlessness, and / or irritability can be early signs of cerebral hypoxia	Patient is awake, alert, and oriented X3
Assess changes in vital signs	Tachycardia and hypertension occur with increased work of breathing	Patient is normotensive with heart rate 60–100 bpm
Monitor arterial blood gases (ABGs)	Increasing $PaCO_2$ and decreasing PaO_2 are signs of respiratory failure	ABGs show $PaCO_2$ between 35 and 45 and PaO_2 between 80 and 100
Administer supplemental oxygen	Early supplemental oxygen is essential in all trauma patients since early mortality is associated with inadequate delivery of oxygenated blood to the brain and vital organs	Patient is receiving oxygen. SaO_2 via pulse oximetry is 90–100%
Position patient with head of bed 45° (if tolerated)	Promotes better lung expansion and improved gas exchange	Patient's rate and pattern are of normal depth and rate at 45° angle
Assist patient with coughing and deep breathing techniques (positioning, incentive spirometry, frequent position changes)	Assist patient to improve lung expansion, the productivity of the cough and mobilize secretions	Patient is able to cough and deep breathe effectively
Prepare for placement of endotracheal or surgical airway (i.e., cricothyroidectomy, tracheostomy)	If a patient is unable to maintain an adequate airway, an artificial airway will be required to promote oxygenation and ventilation and prevent aspiration	Artificial airway is placed and maintained without complications
Confirm placement of the artificial airway	Complications, such as esophageal and right main stem intubations can occur during insertion. Artificial airway placement should be confirmed by CO_2 detector, equal bilateral breath sounds and a chest X-ray	CO_2 detector changes color, bilateral breath sounds are audible equally and artificial airway is at the tip of the carina on X-ray
If maxillofacial trauma is present: 1. Position the patient for optimal airway clearance and constant assessment of airway patency	The patient with maxillofacial trauma is usually more comfortable sitting up. Any time of trauma to the maxillofacial area there is the possibility of a compromised airway	Patient exhibits normal respiratory rate and depth in sitting position. Patient is free of wheezing, stridor, and facial edema
2. Note the degree of swelling to the face and amount of blood loss	Noting swelling is important as a baseline for comparison later	
3. Prepare the patient for definitive treatment		

Contd...

Contd...

If neck trauma is present:		
1. Assess for potential hemorrhage and disruption of the larynx or trachea	Hemorrhage or disruption of the larynx and trachea can be seen as hoarseness in speech, palpable crepitus, pain with swallowing or coughing, or hemoptysis. The neck should also be assessed for ecchymosis, abrasions, or loss of thyroid prominence	Patient is free of signs of hemorrhage or disruption. CT scan reveals no injury to the larynx
2. Prepare the patient for computed tomography (CT) scan	Laryngeal injuries are most definitely diagnosed by CT scans as soft tissue neck films are not sensitive to these injuries	

- Teach patient correct coughing and deep breathing techniques.
- Weak, shallow breathing, and coughing is ineffective in removing secretions.
- Patient is able to demonstrate correct coughing and breathing techniques.

BIBLIOGRAPHY

1. Chandler T. Oxygen administration. 2001. [online]. Available from www.perinatal.nhs.uk. Accessed June 21, 2006.
2. Davies P, Cheng D, Fox A, et al. The efficacy of noncontact oxygen delivery methods. Pediatrics. 2002;110(5):964-7.

Oxygen Administration: Partial Breathing Bag, B-Pap, C-Pap Masks

INTRODUCTION

Noninvasive positive-pressure ventilation is a method of positive-pressure ventilation that can be given via mask that covers the nose and mouth, nasal masks or other oral or nasal devices, such as the nasal pillow (a small nasal cannula that seals around the nares to maintain the prescribed pressure). It eliminates the need for endotracheal intubation or tracheostomy and decreases the risk of nosocomial infections, such as pneumonia. The most comfortable mode for patient is pressure-controlled ventilation with pressure support. This eases the work of breathing and enhances gas exchange. The ventilator can be set with a minimum backup rate for patients with periods of apnea.

DEFINITION

The definitions of oxygen administration are the following:
- To increase the fraction of inspired oxygen concentration (FiO_2) available to a patient, a variety of oxygen delivery devices are employed to administer medical oxygen. The oxygen may be administered with/without humidity.
- It is the administration of oxygen as a medical intervention, which can be used for a variety of purposes in both chronic and acute patient care.

USES

Its uses are as listed below:
- To improve breathing pattern
- To restore body functions
- To improve gas exchange

INDICATIONS

Acute Conditions

Its use in acute conditions are as follows:
- Emergency medical services
- Advanced first aiders
- Resuscitation
- Major trauma
- Anaphylaxis
- Major hemorrhage, shock
- Active convulsions
- Hypothermia
- Increased work of breathing

- Increased myocardial work
- Pulmonary hypertension
- Peri- and postcardiac or respiratory arrest
- Hypoxia—diminished blood oxygen levels (oxygen saturation levels of <92%)
- Acute and chronic hypoxemia [Partial pressure of oxygen (PaO_2) <65 mm Hg, SaO_2 <92%]
- Signs and symptoms of shock
- Low cardiac output and metabolic acidosis (HCO_3 < 18 mmol).

In Chronic Conditions

Its use in chronic conditions are as follows:
- Chronic obstructive pulmonary disease (COPD)
- Smoking

CONTRAINDICATIONS

The contraindications of oxygen administration are the following:
- No absolute contraindications of oxygen therapy exist when indications are judged to be present.
- The relative contraindications of oxygen therapy relate to the dangers of hyperoxemia.

PRECAUTIONS/HAZARDS/COMPLICATIONS

The precautions to be observed and the complications involved in oxygen administration are the following:

Oxygen Toxicity

Oxygen toxicity is a condition resulting from the harmful effects of breathing molecular oxygen at elevated partial pressure known as oxygen toxicity.

Classification (Flowchart A-8.1)

Flowchart A-8.1: Classification of oxygen toxicity.

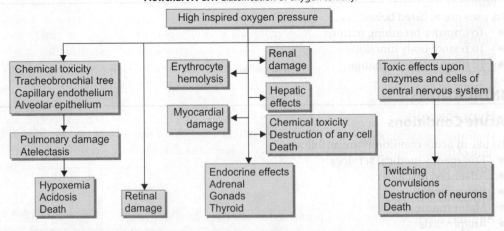

The effects of oxygen toxicity may be classified by the organs affected:
  I. Central nervous system (Bert effect)
 II. Pulmonary (Smith effect)
III. Ocular (Retinopathy conditions)

I. Central nervous system

- Unconsciousness
- Visual changes (especially tunnel vision)
- Ringing in the ears (tinnitus)
- Nausea
- Twitching (especially of the face)
- Irritability
- Personality change
- Anxiety
- Confusion
- Dizziness
- Tonic–clonic seizure

II. Pulmonary

- Chest pain
- Progresses to frequent coughing
- Shortness of breath
- Dyspnea
- Fever
- Pulmonary edema

III. Ocular

Increased ocular pressure

Exposure (minutes)	Symptoms
96	Prolonged dazzle; severe spasmodic vomiting
60–69	Severe lip twitching; euphoria; nausea and vertigo; arm twitching
50–55	Severe lip twitching; dazzle; blubbering of lips; fell asleep; dazed
31–35	Nausea, vertigo, lip twitching; convulsed
21–30	Convulsed; drowsiness; severe lip twitching; epigastric aura; twitch L arm; amnesia
16–20	Convulsed; vertigo and severe lip twitching; epigastric aura; spasmodic respiration
11–15	Inspiratory predominance; lip twitching and syncope; nausea, confusion
6–10	Dazed and lip twitching; paresthesia; vertigo, severe nausea

Nasal Irritation

Many patients get supplemental oxygen through a nasal cannula—flexible plastic tubing with prongs that fit into the nose. Over time, the cannula may irritate the lining of the nose, causing soreness or occasional bleeding. A nasal cannula of a different style or size, or changing to a face mask oxygen delivery system, alleviates this problem for most patients. A small amount of petroleum jelly placed just inside the nose may also help alleviate local irritation.

Hyperoxemia

High-dose oxygen therapy ($FO_2(I) > 50$ %) can cause $pO_2(a)$ to rise well in excess of the upper limit of the reference range, a condition called hyperoxemia, that potentially results in hyperoxia (increased oxygen in tissues).

Mucosal Damage

Appropriate flow rates are imperative for effective and safe oxygen delivery. Drying and dehydration of the nasal mucosa, respiratory epithelial degeneration, and impaired mucosal ciliary clearance increase the risk of infection in patients receiving supplemental oxygen. Humidification decreases the risk of mucosal damage exponentially.

- Absorption atelectasis
- Fire hazard
- Nasal obstruction, especially in infants and children
- Aspiration of vomitus

PARTIAL REBREATHING MASK

Introduction

Partial rebreathing mask has an inflammable bag to store 100% oxygen and a one-way valve between the bag and mask to prevent exhaled air from entering the bag.

a. Has one-way valve covering one or both exhalation ports to prevent entry of room air on inspiration.

b. Has a flap or spring-loaded valve to permit entry of room air, should the oxygen source fail or patient needs exceed the available oxygen flow.

c. All the patient's in spiratory volume will be provided by the mask/reservoir, allowing delivery of nearly 100% oxygen.

d. Consists of mask with exhalation ports and reservoir bag

e. Reservoir bag must remain inflated.

f. O_2 flow rate—6–10 L

g. $FiO_2 = 60\%–80\%$

Definition

The definitions of partial rebreathing mask are as follows:

- A face mask and a reservoir bag permitting a portion of exhaled gas to enter the bag for mixing with source gas.
- **Partial rebreather mask:** Conserves oxygen and can be administered in concentrations of 40–60% using flow rates of 6–10 L. This is useful when oxygen concentrations must be raised. It cannot be used with a high degree of humidity. Not recommended for COPD patients. It should NEVER be used with a nebulizer.

Equipment

The following equipment are used:

- Oxygen source
- Plastic face mask with reservoir bag and tubing
- Humidifier with distilled water
- Flow meter
- No smoking signs

Procedure

Steps	Rationale
Preparatory phase:	
1. Determine current vital signs and level of consciousness	Provides a baseline data for evaluating patient condition
2. Determine most recent saturation of oxygen (SaO_2) or arterial blood gases (ABGs)	Allow objective evaluation of patient response
Performance phase:	
1. Post no smoking signs on the patient's door and in view of the patient and visitors	Oxygen use increases the risk of fire hazard

Contd...

Contd...

Steps	Rationale
2. Attach tubing to flow meter	Bag serves as a reservoir, holding oxygen for patient inspiration
3. Show the mask to the patient and explain the procedure	Make sure mask fits snugly, because there must be an airtight seal between the mask and the patient's face
4. Flush the reservoir bag with oxygen to inflate the bag and adjust flow meter to 6–10 L/min	With a well-fitting rebreathing bag adjusted so the patient's inhalation does not deflate the bag, inspired oxygen concentration of 60–90% can be achieved. Some patient may require flow rate higher than 10 L/minute to ensure that the bag does not collapse on inspiration
5. Place the mask on the patient's face	
6. Adjust liter flow so the rebreathing bag will not collapse during inspiratory cycle, even during deep inspiratory	
Nursing alert:	
Adjust the flow to prevent collapse of the bag, even during inspiration.	
A partial rebreathing mask does not have a one-way valve between the mask and reservoir bag. If the bag is allowed to collapse on inspiration, more exhaled air can enter the reservoir and the patient can inhale high concentration of CO_2	
7. Stay with patient for a time to make the patient comfortable and observe reactions	These actions reduce moisture accumulation under the mask. Massage for the force stimulates circulation and reduce pressure over area
8. Remove mask periodically to dry the face around the mask. Apply water-based lotion to skin and massage force around the mask	
Follow-up phase:	
1. Record flow rate and immediate patient response. Note the patient's tolerance of treatment. Report if intolerance occurs	Assess the patient for change in mental status, diaphoresis, change in blood pressure, and respiratory rates
2. Observe the patient for change in condition. Assess equipment for malfunctioning and low water level in humidifier	
Nursing alert:	
Monitor functioning of mask to ensure that side ports of mask do not get blocked. This could be lead to patient inability to exhale and may lead to suffocation	

Postprocedure

The postprocedure process involved are as follows:
1. Monitor the effect of therapy with pulse oximetry and/or blood gas analysis.
2. Assess the patient for tolerance and appropriateness of therapy per the patient assessment policy at least once per 12-hour shift.
3. All "continuous" oxygen therapy must be verified for proper setup and function.
4. Change equipment as specified by changing of equipment policy.

Documentation

The documentation involved are as follows:
1. Document the initiation of oxygen therapy, changes in therapy, and the effect and tolerance of therapy.

2. **Documentation:**
   - Mode of delivery
   - Device
   - FiO_2 and/or liter flow
   - SpO_2
   - Indications

BILEVEL POSITIVE AIRWAY PRESSURE

Introduction

Bilevel positive airway pressure (BiPAP) is a mode used during noninvasive positive pressure ventilation (NPPV). First used in 1988 by Professor Benzer in Austria, it delivers a preset inspiratory positive airway pressure (IPAP) and expiratory positive airway pressure (EPAP). The BiPAP can be described as a continuous positive airway pressure (CPAP) system with a time-cycled change in the applied CPAP level. The CPAP, BiPAP, and other noninvasive ventilation modes have been shown to be effective management tools for COPD and acute respiratory failure.

Definition

The BiPAP is a CPAP mode used during NPPV. It delivers a preset IPAP and EPAP.
The BiPAP machine is a relatively small device that assists with a patient's breathing. It is connected by flexible tubing to a face mask worn by the patient. The BiPAP machine helps push air and oxygen into the lungs and then helps to hold the lungs inflated, thereby allowing more oxygen to enter the lungs.

When is a BiPAP Machine Used?

A BiPAP machine is used when a patient cannot breathe effectively enough to maximize the transport of oxygen into the lungs and then into the blood. It can at times be used instead of a ventilator (breathing machine). Patients can be given short breaks from the BiPAP mask which will normally then be replaced with an ordinary oxygen mask.

How Long is a BiPAP Machine Used?

The intensive care doctor determines how long the BiPAP machine is used. It has been used successfully for periods varying from several hours to several weeks in the intensive care unit. The BiPAP machines may also be used in specialized respiratory wards. Similar machines can be used at home for long periods.

Uses

The BiPAP is used when positive airway pressure is needed with the addition of pressure support.

Indication

It can be used for the following indications:
- Pneumonia
- Chronic obstructive pulmonary disease
- Asthma
- Status asthmaticus
- Cardiac failure
- Adult respiratory distress syndrome

Bilevel Pressure Devices

The "VPAP" or "BiPAP" (variable/BiPAP) provides two levels of pressure:
1. The IPAP
2. The EPAP

Modes

The three modes involved are as follows:
1. **Spontaneous (S):** In spontaneous mode, the device triggers IPAP when flow sensors detect spontaneous inspiratory effort and then cycles back to EPAP.
2. **Timed (T):** In timed mode, the IPAP/EPAP cycling is purely machine triggered, at a set rate, typically expressed in breaths per minute (BPM).
3. **Spontaneous/Timed (S/T):** Like spontaneous mode, the device triggers to IPAP on patient inspiratory effort. But in an S/T mode a "backup" rate is also set to ensure that patients still receive a minimum number of BPM if they fail to breathe spontaneously.

Contraindications

- Preexisting pneumothorax or pneumomediastinum
- Hypotension due to or associated with intravascular volume depletion
- Preexisting bullous lung disease may represent a contraindication
- Pneumocephalus has been reported in patients using nasal CPAP5
- Facial/skull fractures as well as patients with elevated intracranial pressure (ICP)
- Postoperative patients who have recently undergone abdominal surgery may not be appropriate candidates for BiPAP or nasal CPAP.

Operational Considerations

- Experience has shown that the best results occur when trial periods of 30 minutes or longer are attempted on two or three occasions prior to their first overnight trial. Patients who are gradually acclimated to this device in the above-mentioned fashion do considerably better than those whose initial exposure/trial is initiated at bedtime.
- Patients should refrain from eating 1–2 hours prior to the application of the BiPAP system.
- Heat moisture exchangers (HMEs) should not be used with the BiPAP system. Testing has shown that the HMEs may interfere with the ability of the BiPAP system to maintain the prescribed pressures.
- Supplemental humidification, if necessary, can be provided by a passover humidifier. Experience has shown that with adult patients, foregoing the addition of a humidifier for 2–3 days in most instances negates the need for such a device. The patient's mucociliary blanket appears to adapt to the new conditions. Pediatric patients, however, have all the required humidification.
- Oximetry should be performed prior to the initiation of this therapy as well as when the BiPAP system is in place. The oximetry will not only aid in the titration of the oxygen but will serve as tool to monitor the effectiveness of this therapy.
- Although no reports of gastric distension or aspiration have been reported, the most common complication has been abrasion of the bridge of the nose. Application of wound-care dressing appears to eliminate this problem.

Continuous Positive Airways Pressure

Introduction

The CPAP is an NPPV. The CPAP is simply a pressure applied at the end of exhalation to keep the alveoli open and not fully deflate. This mechanism for maintaining inflated alveoli helps increase the partial pressure of oxygen in arterial blood, an appropriate increase in CPAP increases the PaO_2.

It provides positive pressure to the airways throughout the respiratory cycle. It can be used as an adjunct to mechanical ventilation with a cuffed endotracheal tube or tracheostomy tube to open the alveoli, it is also used with a leak-proof mask to keep the alveoli open, thereby preventing respiratory failure.

Indications

The indications for CPAP use are the following:
- Sleep apnea
- Loud continuous snoring
- Alternative to intubation in severe respiratory illness (BiPAP)
- Adult respiratory distress syndrome (ARDS)
- Refractory hypoxemia

Contraindications

The only contraindications involved in this situation is central sleep apnea.

TYPES OF CONTINUOUS PRESSURE DEVICES

Fixed-Pressure CPAP

A CPAP machine was initially used mainly by patients for the treatment of sleep apnea at home, but now is in widespread use across intensive care units as a form of ventilation. Obstructive sleep apnea occurs when the upper airway becomes narrow as the muscles relax naturally during sleep. This reduces oxygen in the blood and causes arousal from sleep. The CPAP machine blows air at a prescribed pressure (also called the titrated pressure). The necessary pressure is usually determined by a sleep physician after review of a study supervised by a sleep technician during an overnight study (polysomnography) in a sleep laboratory. The titrated pressure is the pressure of air at which most (if not all) apneas and hypopneas have been prevented, and it is usually measured in cm of water (cmH_2O). The pressure required by most patients with sleep apnea ranges between 6 and 14 cmH_2O. A typical CPAP machine can deliver pressures between 4 and 20 cmH_2O. More specialized units can deliver pressures up to 25 or 30 cmH_2O.

Automatic Positive Airway Pressure

An automatic positive airway pressure (APAP) device automatically tunes the amount of pressure delivered to the patient to the minimum required to maintain an unobstructed airway on a breath-by-breath basis by measuring the resistance in the patient's breathing, thereby giving the patient the precise pressure required at a given moment and avoiding the compromise of fixed pressure.

Physiology

The physiology involved are as follows:
- Pressure above atmosphere maintained at airway opening
  - Maintained throughout respiratory cycle
  - Acts as airway splint to prevent collapse
  - Used during spontaneous breathing
- Same end-expiratory pressure as with positive end expiratory pressure (PEEP)

- Lower inspiratory pressure excursion than with PEEP
  - The CPAP requires less pressure to open
  - PEEP requires a greater work of breathing

Normal Range/Dosing

- Usual dose: 6–12 cmH$_2$O (range: 3–20 cm H$_2$O)
- Higher pressure (within range above) indications
  - Heavier weight
  - Short-thick necks
  - More severe sleep Apnea

Technique

- Requires especially designed, tightly fitting masks
- Mask should have pressure-limiting valves.

Adverse Effects

Relates to decreased mask tolerance
- Nasal dryness or congestion
- Mask air leakage
- Claustrophobia
- Skin irritation or abrasions
- Conjunctivitis

Precautions

- The CPAP will worsen central sleep apnea.
- Do not use CPAP empirically without sleep study
- Decreases respiratory drive

Weight Change Since CPAP Was Started

- Reassess CPAP if weight gain exceeds 10%
- Consider overnight oximetry
  - Calculate desaturation index = (4% desats)/hours
  - Desaturation index <5 is normal

CPAP Last Checked

- Mask should be changed every 6 months
- Check blower every 12 months

EQUIPMENT

The following equipment are required for CPAP:
- Oxygen blender
- Flow meter
- The CPAP mask
- Valve for prescribed PEEP (2, 5, 7.5, 10 cmH$_2$O)
- Nebulizer with distilled water
- Large bore tubing
- Nasogastric tube

Steps	Rationale
Preparatory phase	
1. Assess the patient's level of consciousness and gag reflex	CPAP mask may lead to aspiration unless the patient is breathing spontaneously and is able to protect the airway
2. Determine current arterial blood gases (ABGs)	Document that patient meets criteria for use of this mask
Nursing alert	
CPAP is used when patient has not responded to attempt to increase PaO$_2$ with other types of masks	
The patient will require frequent assessment to detect changes in respiratory status, cardiovascular status, and LOC	
If the patient's lack of conciseness (LOC) decrease or ABGs deteriorate, intubation may be necessary	
Performance phase	
1. Post no smoking signs on the patient's door and in view of the patient and visitors	O$_2$ use increases the risk of fire hazard
2. Show the mask to the patient and explain the procedure	With CPAP, the patient may swallow air, causing gastric dissention or emesis. Prophylactic NG suction diminishes this risk
3. Insert nasogastric tube (NG) if ordered	Use of adapter may decreases air leak around the mask
4. Attach NG tube adapter	
5. Set desired concentration of O$_2$ blender rate, so it is sufficient to meet the patient's inspiratory demand	O$_2$ blenders are devices that mix air and O$_2$ using a proportioning valve. Concentrations of 21–100% may be delivered, depending on the model. Because patient will be receiving all minutes, ventilation from this "closed system," it is essential that the flow rate be adequate to meet changes in the patient's breathing pattern
6. Place the mask on the patient's face, adjust the head strap, and inflate the mask cushion to ensure a tight seal	If the mask is removed (for coughing and suctioning), CPAP is not maintained and inspired O$_2$ concentration drop
7. Organize care to remove the mask as infrequently as possible	
Follow-up phase	
1. Assess ABGs, homodynamic status, and LOC frequently	Provides objective documentation of patient response. CPAP may increase the work of breathing
2. Immediately report any increase in PaCO$_2$	Resulting in patient tiring and inability to maintain ventilation without intubation
3. Assess patency of NG tube at frequent intervals	An increase in PaCO$_2$ suggests hypoventilation, resulting from tiring of the patient or inadequate alveolar ventilation. Need for intubation and mechanical ventilation should be evaluated
4. Assess patient comfort and functioning of the equipment frequently	May become obstructed, causing gastric distention
5. Record patient response. With improvement, O$_2$ therapy without positive airway pressure can be substituted. With deterioration, intubation and mechanical ventilation may be required. Note the patient's tolerance of treatment. Report if intolerance occurs	Tight fit of the mask may predispose to skin breakdown. System may develop leaks, resulting in air escaping between the patient's face and mask. Face mask CPAP is usually continued only for short periods because of patient tiring and the necessity to remove mask for suctioning and coughing

PROBLEMS WITH CPAP

The common problems associated with CPAP are the following:

Intolerance of Air Pressure

- Activate CPAP ramp up or increase ramp time (machine slowly builds to maximal pressure as the night progresses)
- Add a CPAP humidifier
- Consider a full CPAP face mask
- Consider specific devices (Auto-adjust, C-flex)
- Consider lowering CPAP pressure by 1–2 cmH$_2$O
- Sleep center to calibrate device pressure

Vasomotor Rhinitis or Congestion

- The CPAP heated humidifier
- Consider nasal steroid for congestion
- Consider intranasal ipratropium for rhinitis

Mask or Pillow Leaks

- Adjust the straps and pads
- Check that the device is not upside down
- Wash face at bedtime and wash device daily
- Sleep center to switch mask types

Claustrophobia

- Wear mask when reading or watching television
- Sleep center to resize mask

Patient Pulls Off Headgear While Asleep (Very Common)

- Add chin strap or adjust for better fit
- Use a disconnect alarm
- Contour pillows can comfortably support the mask with position changes in bed.

Difficulty Initiating Sleep

- See sleep hygiene
- Wear mask when reading or watching television
- Assess for other causes (e.g., restless legs)
- Newer sedative hypnotics, such as Ambien or Sonata are considered safe and will not significantly exacerbate obstructive sleep apnea.

Dry Mouth

- Start or increase heated humidification
- Consider a chin strap (e.g., PureSom Ruby)
- Consider full face mask (covers nose and mouth)
- Consider artificial saliva
- Avoid drinking water overnight as solution due to secondary nocturia

Pressure Sores or Skin Breakdown from Mask

- Consider topical skin protection (e.g., moleskin, comfort care pad, RemZzzs, sore spot).
- Consider topical ointment at pressure areas (e.g., aquaphor)
- Refer to CPAP vendor for different mask or nasal pillows.

WHAT ARE CONTINUOUS POSITIVE AIRWAY PRESSURE AND BILEVEL POSITIVE AIRWAY PRESSURE?

The CPAP machine gives a predetermined level of pressure. It releases a gust of compressed air through a hose which is connected to the nose mask. The continuous air pressure is what keeps the upper airway open. Thus, air pressure prevents obstructive sleep apnea, which occurs as a result of narrowing of the air passage due to the relaxation of upper respiratory tract muscles while the patient sleeps. It assists in increasing the flow of oxygen by keeping the airway open.

- The IPAP is a high level of pressure applied when the patient inhales.
- The EPAP is a low level of pressure exerted during exhalation.

BiPAP is used to treat central sleep apnea and severe obstructive sleep apnea. It is also prescribed for patients who suffer from respiratory and heart diseases.

DIFFERENCE BETWEEN CONTINUOUS AND BILEVEL POSITIVE AIRWAY PRESSURE

Uses

Their uses are as follows:

- The CPAP was originally designed to treat sleep apnea and it is also used to treat patients with neuromuscular diseases and respiratory problems.
- The BiPAP is used in cases of central sleep apnea along with respiratory and heart diseases.

Airway Pressure

Their airway pressures are the following:

- The CPAP delivers air pressure at a single level. The air pressure cannot be altered.
- The BiPAP has two levels of airway pressure—high, when the patient inhales, and low when the patient exhales. The air pressure in the BiPAP can be altered.

User-Friendliness

Their user-friendly aspects are listed below:

- Patients using the CPAP have to exert extra force against the air flow while exhaling, as the airway pressure remains constant. This, at times, may disrupt the patient's sleep.
- With the BiPAP, the airway pressure is set at high and low levels, making it more user-friendly.

Cost: The CPAP comes at a lower price tag, as compared to the BiPAP.

Other Differences

- Patients who have used both machines report that the BiPAP machine tends to be noisier than the CPAP machine, which can be an influencing factor.
- Usually, patients who cannot adapt to the CPAP machine are advised to use the BiPAP.
- Unlike the CPAP, the airway pressure settings of the BiPAP need to be monitored.
- Other differences

CLEANING OF EQUIPMENT

Continuous and Bilevel Positive Airway Pressure System/Machine Cleaning

- Wipe machine off twice monthly with damp cloth
- Replace disposable filters monthly or per manufacturer manual

- Clean nondisposable filters weekly and replace when needed
- Use warm soapy water and let air dry before inserting back into machine
- Both disposable and nondisposable filters can be purchased from your home-care provider.

Headgear (Strap)

- Wash as needed
- Hand wash in mild detergent (i.e., Woolite, Ivory) and air dry. DO NOT machine wash headgear and do not use dryer to dry. Let air dry only.

Masks and Nasal Pillows

- Wash daily with mild detergent (i.e., Ivory); rinse thoroughly with warm water to remove all detergent and residue; air dry. DO NOT place in dishwasher.
- Use detergent that is free of perfumes, dyes, and moisturizers. They can shorten the useful life of the mask or pillow.

Tubing

Wash bimonthly with mild detergent or white vinegar solution, rinse with warm water, and air dry between uses.

Humidifier (If Indicated by Physician)

- Change distilled water daily right before bed. It is best to put the distilled water in right before bed.
- Clean chamber weekly and let air dry
- Do not place in a dishwasher
- Soak all other humidifier chambers for 30 minutes in a solution of equal parts white vinegar and water. This solution can remain in refrigerator for one week (label container with contents and date).

Oxygen Administration

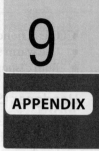

DEFINITION

To increase the fraction of inspired oxygen concentration (FiO_2) available to a patient, a variety of oxygen delivery devices are employed to administer medical oxygen. The oxygen may be administered with/without humidity.

Or

Oxygen therapy is the administration of oxygen as a medical intervention, which can be used for a variety of purposes in both chronic and acute patient care.

USES

The uses of oxygen are the following:
- To improve breathing pattern
- To restore body functions
- To improve gas exchange

INDICATIONS

Acute Conditions
- Emergency medical services
- Advanced first aiders
- Resuscitation
- Major trauma
- Anaphylaxis
- Major hemorrhage and shock
- Active convulsions
- Hypothermia
- Increased work of breathing
- Increased myocardial work
- Pulmonary hypertension
- Peri- and postcardiac or respiratory arrest
- Hypoxia—diminished blood oxygen levels (oxygen saturation levels of <92%)
- Acute and chronic hypoxemia (PaO_2 <65 mm Hg, SaO_2 <92%)
- Signs and symptoms of shock
- Low cardiac output and metabolic acidosis (HCO_3 <18 mmol).

Chronic Conditions
- Chronic obstructive pulmonary disease (COPD)
- Smoking

CONTRAINDICATIONS

No absolute contraindications of oxygen therapy exist when indications are judged to be present. The relative contraindications of oxygen therapy relate to the dangers of hyperoxemia.

MAIN SOURCES OF OXYGEN THERAPY

The main sources of oxygen therapy are the following:

Liquid Storage

Liquid oxygen is stored in chilled tanks until required and then allowed to boil [at a temperature of 90.188 K (−182.96°C)] to release oxygen as a gas. This is widely used at hospitals due to their high usage requirements but can also be used in other settings.

Compressed Gas Storage

The oxygen gas is compressed in a gas cylinder, which provides a convenient storage, without the requirement for refrigeration found with liquid storage. Large oxygen cylinders hold 6500 L and can last about 2 days at a flow rate of 2 L/minute.

MANUAL RESUSCITATION BAG

Artificial manual breathing unit (AMBU) also called Ambu bag, generically a manual resuscitator or "self-inflating bag," is a hand-held device commonly used to provide positive pressure ventilation to patients who are not breathing or not breathing adequately.

Or

A resuscitation bag is a hollow, football-shaped device used to manually push air into the lungs to assist children in taking breaths.

Indications

Indications for the use of resuscitation are as follows:
- During emergencies
- To give larger breaths than the child can take
- When disconnected from the ventilator during circuit changes or problems
- After suctioning
- A resuscitation bag and mask must accompany the child with a tracheotomy at all times
- Try to match the child's breathing efforts and rate
- Give a breath that is big enough to make the chest rise, but not too big.

Standard Components

The standard components of Ambu bag are the following:

Mask

Bag valve mask: Part 1 is the flexible mask to seal over the patient's face, part 2 has a filter and valve to prevent backflow into the bag itself (prevents patient deprivation and bag contamination), and part 3 is the soft bag element that is squeezed to expel air to the patient.

Bag and Valve (Fig. A-9.1)

Bag and valve combinations can also be attached to an alternate airway adjunct, instead of to the mask. For example, it can be attached to an endotracheal tube or laryngeal mask airway. Small heat and moisture exchangers, or humidifying/bacterial filters, can be used.

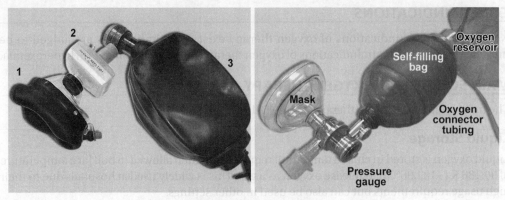

Fig. A-9.1: Bag and valve.

A bag–valve mask can be used without being attached to an oxygen tank to provide "room air" (21% oxygen) to the patient; however, manual resuscitator devices also can be connected to a separate bag reservoir that can be filled with pure oxygen from a compressed oxygen source—this can increase the amount of oxygen delivered to the patient to nearly 100%.

Bag valve masks come in different sizes to fit infants, children, and adults. The face mask size may be independent of the bag size; for example, a single pediatric-sized bag might be used with different masks for multiple face sizes, or a pediatric mask might be used with an adult bag for patients with small faces.

Most types of the device are disposable and therefore single use, while others are designed to be cleaned and reused.

Types of Manual Resuscitators

Self-inflating Bags

This type of manual resuscitator is the standard design most often used in both in-hospital and out-of-hospital settings. The material used for the bag portion of a self-inflating manual resuscitator has a "memory," meaning after it is manually compressed it will automatically re-expand on its own in-between breaths (drawing in air for the next breath). These devices can be used alone (thus delivering room air) or can be used in connection with an oxygen source to deliver nearly 100% oxygen. As a result of these features, this type of manual resuscitator is appropriate for in-hospital use and out-of-hospital settings (e.g., ambulances).

Flow-inflating Bags

Also termed "anesthesia bags," these are a specialized form of manual resuscitator with a bag portion that is flaccid and does not reinflate on its own. This necessitates an external flow source of pressurized inflation gas for the bag to inflate; once inflated, the provider can manually squeeze the bag or, if the patient is breathing on his/her own, the patient can inhale directly through the bag itself. These types of manual resuscitators are used extensively during anesthesia induction and recovery and are often attached to anesthesia consoles so anesthesia gases can be used to ventilate the patient. They are primarily utilized by anesthesiologists during most general surgery procedures but also during some in-hospital emergencies which may involve anesthesiologists or respiratory therapists. They are not typically used outside hospital settings.

Anesthesia

The requirement of anesthesia for oxygen administration is indicated below:
- Generally not required when indication exists
- Elective ventilation in the operating room may require a sedative agent (e.g., propofol).

Equipment

The equipment that are needed for oxygen administration are the following:
- Oxygen connector tubing
- Oxygen source suction
- Nasal pharyngeal airway (NPA)
- Oral pharyngeal airway (OPA)

Positioning

The positioning method to administer oxygen are as follows:
- Place towels under the patient's head to position the ear level with the sternal notch
- Extend the patient's head slightly

Technique

Open the Airway

The following techniques are performed while administering oxygen:
- Perform the head-tilt chin-lift maneuver or the jaw thrust. In patients with suspected cervical spine injury, do not perform a head-tilt; rather, only perform a chin-lift maneuver.
- Use an airway adjunct
- Place an OPA in unresponsive patients without a gag reflex
- If the patient is awake, place one or two NPA devices instead, as this may be better tolerated. However, because of the risk of intracranial placement, avoid the use of an NPA in patients with significant head and facial trauma.

Position the Mask

The list below provides as how to position the mask:
- Place the mask on the patient's face before attaching the bag.
- Cover the nose and the mouth with the mask without extending it over the chin
- Change the size of the mask, as appropriate, to create a good seal
- Hold the mask in place using the one-hand E-C technique, as shown in **Figure A-9.2**.
    - Use the nondominant hand

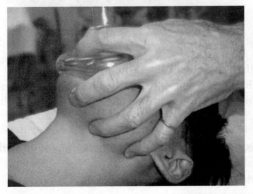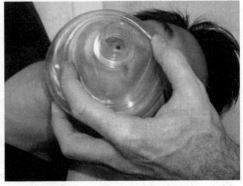

Fig. A-9.2: One-hand E-C technique.

- ■ Create a C-shape with the thumb and index finger over the top of the mask and apply gentle downward pressure.
- ■ Hook the remaining fingers around the mandible and lift it upward toward the mask, creating the E.
- The alternative one-hand technique shown in **Figure A-9.3** can also be used.
- If a second person is available to provide ventilations by compressing the bag, a two-hand technique can be used.
  - ■ Create two opposing semicircles with the thumb and index finger of each hand to form a ring around the mask connector and hold the mask on the patient's face. Then lift up on the mandible with the remaining digits, as shown **Figure A-9.4** two-hand technique.

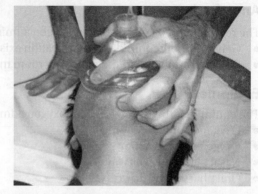

Fig. A-9.3: Alternate one-hand technique.

  - ■ Alternatively, place both thumbs opposing the mask connector, using the thenar eminence to hold the mask on the patient's face, while lifting up the mandible with the fingers, as shown in **Figure A-9.5**.
- No matter which technique is being used, avoid applying pressure on the soft tissues of the neck or on the eyes.

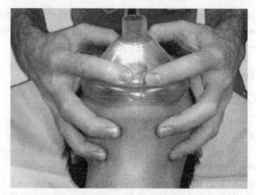

Fig. A-9.4: Two-hand technique.

- The two-hand technique is preferred to the one-hand technique and should be used whenever possible.
  - ■ Place the web space of the thumb and index finger against the mask connector
  - ■ Push downward with gentle pressure
  - ■ Wrap the remaining fingers around the mandible and lift it upward
  - ■ Ventilate the patient
- Provide a volume of 6–7 mL/kg per breath (approximately 500 mL for an average adult).

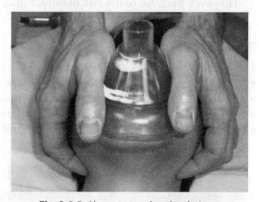

Fig. A-9.5: Alternate two-hand technique.

- For a patient with a perfusing rhythm, ventilate at a rate of 10–12 breaths per minute.
- During cardiopulmonary resuscitation (CPR), give two breaths after each series of 30 chest compressions until an advanced airway is placed. Then ventilate at a rate of 8–10 breaths per minute.
- Give each breath over 1 second.
- If the patient has intrinsic respiratory drive, assist the patient's breaths. In a patient with tachypnea, assist every few breaths.
- Ventilate with low pressure and low volume to decrease gastric distension.
- Maintain cricoid pressure consistently

■ This pressure is meant to compress the esophagus and reduce the risk of aspiration. However, it does not completely protect against regurgitation, especially in cases of prolonged ventilation or poor technique.

■ Care must be taken to avoid excessive pressure, which can result in compression of the trachea.

Assess the adequacy of ventilation.

● Observe for chest rise, improving color and oxygen saturation
● Monitor for air leak
● Be cognizant of the increasing gastric distention

Complications

The complications that can develop during oxygen administration are the following:

● Air to inflate the stomach (gastric insufflation)
● Lung injury from overstretching (volutrauma)
● Lung injury from overpressurization (barotrauma)

CLIENT WITH AN ARTIFICIAL AIRWAY

Airway management is the medical process of ensuring an open pathway between a patient's lungs and the outside world as well as reducing the risk of aspiration. Airway management is a primary consideration in CPR anesthesia, emergency medicine, intensive care medicine, and first aid.

Indications for an Artificial Airway

The following are the indications for the availability of an artificial airway:

● To facilitate mechanical ventilation
● To protect the airway, e.g., prevent aspiration
● To facilitate suctioning
● To relieve upper airway obstruction

AIRWAY MANEUVERS

Head-Tilt Chin-Lift

The head-tilt chin-lift is the most reliable method of opening the airway. The head-tilt chin-lift is the primary maneuver used in any patient in whom cervical spine injury is not a concern. The simplest way of ensuring an open airway in an unconscious patient is to use a head-tilt chin-lift technique, thereby lifting the tongue from the back of the throat. This is taught on most first-aid courses as the standard way of clearing an airway.

Jaw-Thrust Maneuver

The jaw-thrust maneuver is an effective airway technique, particularly in the patient in whom cervical spine injury is a concern. The jaw thrust is a technique used on patients with a suspected spinal injury and is used on a supine patient. The practitioner uses their index and middle fingers to physically push the posterior (back) aspects of the mandible upward, while their thumbs push down on the chin to open the mouth. When the mandible is displaced forward, it pulls the tongue forward and prevents it from occluding (blocking) the entrance to the trachea, helping to ensure a patent (secure) airway.

Cervical Spine Immobilization

Most airway maneuvers are associated with some movement of the cervical spine (c-spine). Even though collars for holding the head in-line can cause problems maintaining an airway and maintaining a blood pressure, it is not recommended to remove the collar without adequate personnel to manually hold the head in place.

Invasive Airway Management

Oropharyngeal Airway (Fig. A-9.6)

OPAs are rigid plastic curved devices used to maintain an open airway. It does this by preventing the tongue from covering the epiglottis, which could prevent the person from breathing. When a person becomes unconscious, the muscles in their jaw relax and allow the tongue to obstruct the airway. An OPA should only be used in a deeply unresponsive patient because in a responsive patient they can cause vomiting and aspiration by stimulating the gag reflex. A conscious patient cannot tolerate this airway.

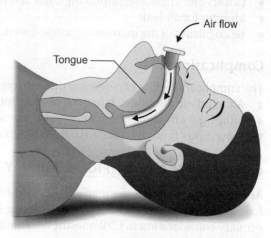

Fig. A-9.6: Oropharyngeal airway.

Oropharyngeal Airway Sizes

The optimal sizes of OPAs are as follows:

- 6 mm
- Most adults take between 3–5 mm
- Correct size by measuring from corner of mouth to bottom of earlobe.

Nasopharyngeal Airway

The NPA (also known as a nasal trumpet) is a soft rubber or plastic hollow tube that is passed through the nose into the posterior pharynx. Patients tolerate NPAs more easily than OPAs, so NPAs can be used when the use of an OPA is difficult, such as when the patient's jaw is clenched or the patient is semiconscious and cannot tolerate an OPA, NPAs are generally not recommended if there is suspicion of a fracture to the base of the skull, due to the possibility of the tube entering the cranium. However, the actual risks of this complication occurring compared to the risks of damage from hypoxia if an airway is not used are debatable.

Laryngeal Mask Airway

A laryngeal mask airway is an airway placed into the mouth and set over the glottis and inflated. This tube does not enter the trachea.

Tracheal intubation: Tracheal intubation, often simply referred to as intubation, is the placement of a flexible plastic or rubber tube into the trachea (windpipe) to maintain an open airway or to serve as a conduit through which to administer certain drugs. It is frequently performed in critically injured, ill, or anesthetized patients to facilitate ventilation of the lungs, including mechanical ventilation, and to prevent the possibility of asphyxiation or airway obstruction. The most widely used route is orotracheal, in which an endotracheal tube is passed through the mouth and vocal apparatus into the trachea. In a nasotracheal procedure, an endotracheal tube is passed through the nose and vocal apparatus into the trachea.

Role of Nurse During the Procedure

The role of nurse while performing the procedure is as follows:
- Monitor the patient
- Maintain adequate ventilation and oxygenation
- Assist physician as needed
- Suctioning obviously must be performed but as gently as possible

Intubation Complications

The complications involved while intubating the patient are the following:
- Trauma to oral cavity, pharynx, and vocal cords
- Bleeding
- Laryngospasm
- Perforation of trachea
- Improper tube placement
- Contamination/infection
- The pressure in the cuff should be checked often, e.g., each ventilator check.

AIRWAY MANAGEMENT

The following are the airway management options:
- **Humidification:** Heated cascade provides 100% humidification of inhaled gases. Ensure systemic hydration is monitored to help keep secretions thin.
- **Aerosol therapy:** Nebulizers delivering aerosols increase secretion clearance and liquefy mucus; nebulizers may become a source of bacterial contamination.
- **Cuff management:** Essential for the prevention of necrosis and aspiration.
- **Minimal leak (ML) technique:** Inject air into cuff until no leak is heard and then withdrawing the air until a small leak is heard on inspiration. (Problems are related to maintaining positive end-expiratory pressure (PEEP), aspiration around the cuff, and increased movement of the tube).
- **Minimal occlusive volume (MOV) technique:** Inject air into the cuff until no leak is heard, then withdrawing the air until a small leak is heard on inspiration, and then adding more air until no leak is heard on inspiration. (Problems are related to higher cuff pressures than an ML technique.) Use only if patient needs a seal to provide adequate ventilation and/or is at high risk of aspiration.
- Maintain pressure 18–22 mm Hg (25–30 cm H_2O). Greater pressures decrease capillary blood flow in tracheal wall and lesser pressures increase the risk of aspiration. Do not routinely deflate cuff.
- Postural drainage and positioning
- Key point: Pneumonia = "Good lung down position"
- **Adult respiratory distress syndrome (ARDS)** = prone positioning for improved oxygenation
- **Suctioning:** Performed as a sterile procedure only when patient needs it, not on a routine schedule. Observe for hypoxemia, atelectasis, bronchospasms, cardiac dysrhythmias, hemodynamic alterations, increased intracranial pressure, and airway trauma.

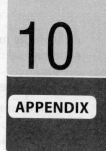

Pacemaker

INTRODUCTION

Pacemaker is that part of the heart that produces the electrical stimuli or provides the electrical stimuli to contract. When the natural pacemaker of the heart is unable to do so, there is need to insert an artificial pacemaker through the surgical procedure. The natural pacemaker of the heart is the sinoatrial node (SA).

DEFINITION

A cardiac pacemaker is an electronic device that provides electrical stimuli to the heart muscles or myocardium.

CLINICAL INDICATIONS

The clinical indications of requiring an artificial pacemaker are as follows:
- Bradydysrhythmias
- Secondary and tertiary heart block
- Tachydysrhythmias
- Atrioventricular (AV) block
- Decreased cardiac output
- Before and after cardiac surgery
- Before permanent pacing

Other Disorders

Artificial pacemakers are used under the following conditions:
- Myocardial infarction
- Myocardial ischemia
- Cardiac trauma

Pacemakers are of three major types **(Flowchart A-10.1)**, namely—permanent pacemaker, temporary pacemaker, and biventricular pacemaker. The permanent pacemaker is of three types, i.e., single chamber, dual chamber, and rate responsive. The temporary pacemaker are of four types, namely— transvenous, epicardial, transcutaneous, and transthoracic.

Permanent Pacemaker

Permanent pacemaker is used under the following conditions:
- It is used to treat chronic conditions of the heart.
- It is placed surgically utilizing a local anesthesia.
- The leads are placed transvenously in an appropriate chamber of the heart.

Flowchart A-10.1: Types of pacemaker.

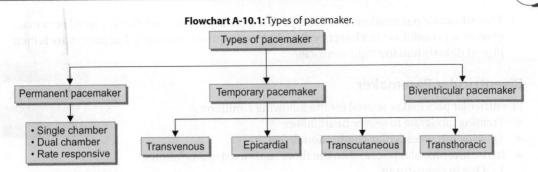

- The leads are attached to the small sealed battery-powered pulse generator inserted in the chest wall or abdominal cavity.

The three basic types of permanent pacemakers classified according to the number of chambers involved and their basic operating mechanism are as follows:

1. **Single-chamber pacemaker:** In this type, only one pacing lead is placed into a chamber of the heart, either the atrium or the ventricle. It is called unipolar lead.
2. **Dual-chamber pacemaker:** Here wires are placed in two chambers of the heart. One lead paces the atrium and one paces the ventricle. This type more closely resembles the natural pacing of the heart by assisting the heart in coordinating the function between the atria and ventricles. It is called as bipolar lead.
3. **Rate-responsive pacemaker:** This pacemaker has sensors that detect changes in the patient's physical activity and automatically adjust the pacing rate to fulfill the body's metabolic needs.

Temporary Pacemaker

Temporary pacemaker is used under the following conditions:
- It is commonly used during an emergency condition.
- Main indication of the temporary pacemaker is the following:
  - Atrioventricular block
  - Bradycardia
  - Low cardiac output

According to the site of placement, the temporary pacemakers are of four types:

1. **Transvenous pacemaker:** The pacemaker in which leads are inserted transvenously is known as transvenous pacemaker.
   The main veins used for insertion are the following:
   - Subclavian
   - Internal jugular
   - Femoral
   The leads are placed into the particular chamber of the heart under fluoroscopy and then attached to an external pulse generator.
2. **Epicardial pacemaker:** In this, the leads are attached to the endocardium of the heart. It is inserted through a surgical incision into the chest and then attached to an external pulse generator.
   This is commonly used when a patient is undergoing cardiac surgery.
3. **Transcutaneous pacemaker:** In this, the noninvasive electrodes are placed on posterior and anterior chest wall, i.e., right of the upper sternum below the clavicle and to the back of the patient. Or the procedure is performed by placing two pacing pads on the patient's chest, either in the anterior/lateral position or in the anterior/posterior position.

4. **Transthoracic pacemaker:** It is the type of temporary pacemaker that is placed only in an emergency condition via a long needle using a subxiphoid approach. The pacer wire is then placed directly into the right ventricle.

Biventricular Pacemaker

Biventricular pacemaker is used for the following conditions:

- Treating moderate to severe heart failure
- Treating intraventricular conduction defect
- In the biventricular pacemaker, the three leads used are as follows:
  1. One in right atrium
  2. One in right ventricle
  3. One in left ventricle to coordinate ventricular conduction and improve cardiac output

Leads are implanted through a vein into the right ventricle and into the coronary sinus vein to pace or regulate the left ventricle. Usually (but not always), a lead is also implanted into the right atrium. This helps the heart beat in a more balanced way.

Traditional pacemakers are used to treat slow heart rhythms. Pacemakers regulate the right atrium and right ventricle to maintain a good heart rate and keep the atrium and ventricle working together. This is called AV synchrony. Biventricular pacemakers add a third lead to help the left ventricle contract at the same time as the right ventricle.

PACEMAKER DESIGN

A pacemaker has the following parts:

- Pulse generator
- Pacemaker leads
- A tiny computer circuit

Pulse generator

In permanent pacing system	In temporary pacing system
➢ In the permanent pacing system, the pulse generator is encapsulated in a metal can, which protects the generator from electromagnetic interference	➢ A temporary pacing system generator is contained in a small box with a dial for programming
➢ In this, the lithium or nuclear batteries are used	➢ The external box is attached to the patient with velcro straps
➢ The life span of the lithium battery is 3–5 years and life span of nuclear battery is 5–20 years	➢ The battery used in temporary pacemaker is replaceable or rechargeable

Pacemaker leads are parts of the pacemaker through which the electrical signals are transmitted from the pulse generator to the heart.

A tiny computer circuit that converts energy from the battery into electrical impulses, which flow down the wires and stimulate the heart to contract.

MODES OF PACEMAKER

The major modes of a pacemaker are fixed and demand modes.

Fixed mode: In this, the pulses are generated at a fixed predetermined or preset rate, irrespective of what the intrinsic rhythm is.

Demand mode: The pacemaker generates the impulses intermittently only on demand, when it senses or receives the signal or information for slow intrinsic rhythm.

HOW PACEMAKER WORKS?

Pacemaker works in two phases i.e., sensing and pacing.

Sensing: In the first step, the information about the intrinsic heart rhythm goes to the pacemaker generator. The generator senses that information and responds accordingly.

Responding: In this, the electrical current flows through lead wire to a negative pole, i.e., at the tip of lead (electrode).

Then it stimulates the heart for contraction and electrical impulse travels back to the positive lead to complete the circuit.

FUNCTIONAL CODES

The functional codes are established by Intersociety Commission for Heart Disease (ICHD). The five letters explain normal functioning of the pacemaker/characteristics of the pacemaker.

1	2	3	4	5
Chamber paced	*Chamber sensed*	*Mode of response*	*Programmable function*	*Antitachycardia function*
V = Ventricle	V = Ventricle	T = Triggered	R = Rate modulated	O = None
A = Atrium	A = Atrium	I = Inhibited	R = Rate modulated	P = Paced
D = Dual (A & V)	D = Dual (A & V)	D = Dual (T & I)	C = Communicating	S = Shocks
O = None	O = None	O = None	M = Multiprogrammable	D = Dual (P & S)
			O= None	

PACEMAKER INSERTION

Equipment required for permanent pacemaker insertion includes the following:
- Fluoroscope
- Instrument tray
- Pacing system analyzer
- Introducer kit
- Lidocaine or bupivacaine 1–2%
- Antimicrobial flush and saline for pocket irrigation
- Emergency crash cart with medications
- Battery or electric cautery
- Suture material
- External pacemaker/defibrillator

PATIENT PREPARATION

Before the procedure, all blood tests are to be performed, including X-ray. Consent forms are signed by patients. Part preparation is done.

Anesthesia

Implantation of pacing systems usually involves a combination of local anesthesia and conscious sedation. Infiltration of skin and subcutaneous tissue at the implant site with 1–2% lidocaine or bupivacaine provides sufficient local anesthesia for the majority of implant procedures. Conscious sedation may be administered in the form of carefully titrated intravenous (IV) midazolam and fentanyl by trained and qualified personnel. On rare occasions, general anesthesia may be required in an extremely uncooperative or high-risk patient.

Positioning

The patient is usually positioned on his/her back, with the arms tucked.

IMPLANTATION OF PACEMAKER

Routinely, cefazolin 1 g is administered IV 1 hour before the procedure. If the patient is allergic to penicillins or cephalosporins, vancomycin 1 g IV or another appropriate antibiotic may be administered preoperatively.

Venous Access

Venous access is established as follows:
- A central vein (i.e., the subclavian, internal jugular, or axillary vein) is accessed via the percutaneous approach. In patients in whom this is technically difficult because skeletal landmarks are deviated, an initial brief fluoroscopic examination will greatly reduce the time and complications associated with obtaining the access.
- The subclavian vein is typically accessed at the junction of the first rib and the clavicle. Occasionally, phlebography may be required to visualize the vein adequately or to confirm its patency. Some centers employ the first-rib approach under fluoroscopy, with no or minimal incidence of pneumothorax.
- After venous access is obtained, a guidewire is advanced through the access needle, and the tip of the guidewire is positioned in the right atrium or the vena caval area under fluoroscopy. The needle is then withdrawn, leaving the guidewire in place. If indicated, a second access can be obtained in a similar fashion for positioning of a second guidewire.
- Sometimes a double-wire technique is used, whereby two guidewires are inserted through the first sheath and the sheath is then withdrawn, so that two separate sheaths can be advanced over the two guidewires. This technique can cause some resistance or friction during sheath or lead advancement.

Creation of Pocket

Pocket is created as follows:
A 1.5- to 2-inch incision is made in the infraclavicular area parallel to the middle third of the clavicle, and a subcutaneous pocket is created with sharp and blunt dissection where the pacemaker generator will be implanted. Some physicians prefer to make the pocket first and obtain access later through the pocket or via venous cut down; once the access is obtained, they position the guidewires as described above.

Placement of Leads

Leads are placed as follows:
- Over the guidewire, a special peel-away sheath and dilator are advanced. The guidewire and dilator are withdrawn, leaving the sheath in place. A stylet (a thin wire) is inserted inside the center channel of the pacemaker lead to make it more rigid, and the lead–stylet combination is then inserted into the sheath and advanced under fluoroscopy to the appropriate heart chamber. Usually, the ventricular lead is positioned before the atrial lead to prevent its dislodgment.
- Making a small curve at the tip of the stylet renders the ventricular lead tip more maneuverable, so that it can more easily be placed across the tricuspid valve and positioned at the right ventricular apex. Techniques for positioning the ventricular lead have been described.

- Once the correct lead positioning is confirmed, the lead is affixed to the endocardium either passively with tines (such as a grappling hook) or actively via a helical screw located at the tip. The screw at the tip of the pacemaker is extended or retracted by turning the outer end of the lead with the help of a torque device. Adequate extension of the screw is confirmed with fluoroscopy. Each manufacturer has its own proprietary identification marks for confirming adequate extension of the screw.
- Once the lead is secured in position, the introducing sheath is carefully peeled away, leaving the lead in place. After the pacing lead stylet is removed, pacing and sensing thresholds and lead impedances are measured with a pacing system analyzer, and pacing is performed at 10 V to ensure that it is not causing diaphragmatic stimulation. After confirmation of lead position and thresholds, the proximal end of the lead is secured to the underlying tissue (i.e., pectoralis) with a nonabsorbable suture that is sewn to a sleeve located on the lead.
- If a second lead is indicated, it is positioned in the right atrium via a second sheath, with the lead tip typically positioned in the right atrial appendage with the help of a J-shaped stylet.
- In a patient who is without an atrial appendage as a result of previous cardiac surgery, the lead can be positioned medially or in the lateral free wall of the right atrium. As with the ventricular lead, the atrial lead position is confirmed, impedance is assessed, the stylet is withdrawn, and the lead is secured to the underlying pectoralis with a nonabsorbable suture.

Positioning of Pulse Generator

The pulse generator is placed as follows:
- When the leads have been properly positioned and tested and sutured to the underlying tissue, the pacemaker pocket is irrigated with antimicrobial solution, and the pulse generator is connected securely to the leads. Many physicians secure the pulse generator to underlying tissue with a nonabsorbable suture to prevent migration or twiddlers syndrome.
- Typically, the pacemaker is positioned superficial to the pectoralis, but occasionally, a subpectoral or inframammary position is required. After hemostasis is confirmed, a final look under fluoroscopy before closure of the incision is recommended to confirm appropriate lead positioning.

Completion and Closure

The steps involved in completion and closure of the pacemaker placement are listed below:
- The incision is closed in layers with absorbable sutures and adhesive strips. Sterile dressing is applied to the incision surface. An arm restraint or immobilizer is applied to the unilateral arm for 12–24 hours to limit movement.
- A postoperative chest radiograph is usually obtained to confirm lead position and rule out pneumothorax. Before discharge on the following day, posteroanterior and lateral chest radiographs will be ordered again to confirm lead positions and exclude delayed pneumothorax.
- Pain levels are typically low after the procedure, and the patient can be given pain medication to manage breakthrough pain associated with the incision site.

Complications

The various complications associated with pacemaker placement are the following:
- Local infection at the entry site of leads
- Bleeding and hematoma

- Tachycardia
- Hemothorax from puncture of subclavian vein

POINTS TO BE KEPT IN MIND

Patients with an artificial pacemaker implanted in them should remember the following:

- Microwave ovens, electric blankets, remote controls for TV and other common household appliances would not affect pacemaker.
- Hold the phone to the ear on the side of body opposite from pacemaker.
- When phone is on, try to keep it at least six inches away from the pacemaker. For example, do not carry phone in breast pocket over pacemaker.

Postural Drainage

INTRODUCTION

Postural drainage is an airway clearance technique that, along with chest percussion and vibration, helps patients with respiratory illnesses, such as chronic obstructive pulmonary disease (COPD) clear mucus from their lungs.

- Postural drainage is the positioning techniques that drain secretions from specific segments of the lungs and bronchi into the trachea.
- In postural drainage, the person is tilted or propped at an angle to help drain secretions from the lungs.
- The chest or back may be clapped with a cupped hand to help loosen secretions—the technique called chest percussion.

CONTRAINDICATIONS

The contraindications involved in postural drainage are as follows:

- Unable to tolerate the position required
- Taking anticoagulation drugs
- Have recently vomited blood
- Have had a recent rib or vertebral fracture or
- Have severe osteoporosis

PROCEDURE

The following are the procedures performed during postural drainage:

- The patient's body is positioned in such a manner that the trachea is inclined downward and below the affected chest area.
- Postural drainage is essential in treating bronchiectasis and patients must receive physiotherapy to learn to tip themselves into a position in which the lobe to be drained is uppermost at least three times daily for 10 to 20 minutes.
- The treatment is often used in conjunction with the technique for loosening secretions in the chest cavity called chest percussion.

ARTICLES REQUIRED

The following articles are used for postural drainage:

- Pillows
- Tilt table
- Sputum cup
- Paper tissues

STEPS

The steps involved in postural drainage are the following:

- Use specific positions, so the force of gravity can assist in the removal of bronchial secretions from affected lung segments to central airways by means of coughing and suctioning.
- The patient is positioned, so that the diseased area is in a near vertical position, and gravity is used to assist the drainage of specific segment.
- The positions assumed are determined by the location, severity, and duration of mucous obstruction.
- The exercises are performed two to three times a day, before meals and bedtime. Each position is done for 3 to 15 minutes.
- The procedure should be discontinued if tachycardia, palpitations, dyspnea, and chest tightness occurs. These symptoms may indicate hypoxemia. Discontinue if hemoptysis occurs.
- Bronchodilators, mucolytic agents, water, or saline may be nebulized and inhaled before postural drainage and chest percussion to reduce bronchospasm, decrease thickness of mucus and sputum, and combat edema of the bronchial walls, thereby enhancing secretion removal.
- Perform secretion removal procedures before eating
- Ensure patient is comfortable before the procedure starts and as comfortable as possible he/she assumes each position.
- Auscultate the chest to determine the areas of needed drainage
- Encourage the patient to deep breathe and cough after spending the allotted time in each position.
- Encourage diaphragmatic breathing throughout postural drainage and this helps widen airways so secretions can be drained.

POSITIONS

The various positions that adult and pediatric patients can adopt during postural drainage are listed in **Table A-11.1**:

TABLE A-11.1: Positions for postural drainage.

Adult	Positions
Lung segment	Position recommended
Bilateral	High Fowler's
Apical right upper lobe anterior segment	Sitting on side of the bed, supine with head elevated
Left upper lobe anterior	Supine with head elevated
Right upper lobe posterior	Side lying with right side of the chest elevated on pillows
Left upper lobe posterior	Side lying with left side of the chest elevated on pillows
Right middle lobe anterior segment	Three-fourth supine position with dependent lung in Trendelenburg's position
Right middle lobe posterior segment	Prone with thorax and abdomen elevated
Both lower lobes anterior segments	Supine in Trendelenburg's position
Left lower lobe lateral position	Right side lying in Trendelenburg's position
Right lower lobe lateral segment	Left side lying in Trendelenburg's position
Right lower lobe posterior segment	Prone with right side of chest elevated in Trendelenburg's position
Both lower lobes posterior segment	Prone in Trendelenburg's position
Child	Positions
Bilateral apical segments	Sitting on nurse's lap, leaning slightly forward flexed over pillow
Bilateral middle anterior segments	Sitting on nurse's lap, leaning against nurse
Bilateral anterior segments	Lying supine on nurse's lap, back supported with pillow

Upper Lobe Apical Segments

The various positions for postural drainage involving the upper lobe apical segments are in **Figure A-11.1**.

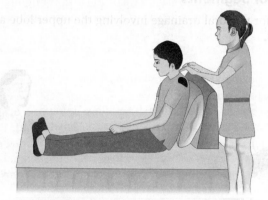

Fig. A-11.1: Upper lobe apical segments (Position 1).

- To drain mucus from the upper lobe apical segments, the patient sits in a comfortable position on a bed or flat surface and leans on a pillow against the headboard of the bed or the caregiver.
- The caregiver percusses and vibrates over the muscular area between the collar bone and the very top of the shoulder blades (shaded areas of the diagram) on both sides for 3–5 minutes.
- Encourage the patient to take a deep breath and cough during percussion to help clear the airways.
- Do not percuss over bare skin.

Upper Lobe Posterior Segments

The various positions for postural drainage involving the upper lobe posterior segments are depicted in **Figure A-11.2**:

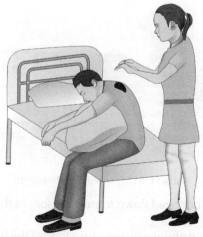

Fig. A-11.2: Upper Lobe posterior segments (Position 2).

- The patient sits comfortably in a chair or on the side of the bed and leans over, arms dangling, against a pillow.

- The caregiver percusses and vibrates with both hands over upper back on both the right and left sides.

Upper Lobe Anterior Segments

The various positions for postural drainage involving the upper lobe anterior segments are depicted **Figure A-11.3.**

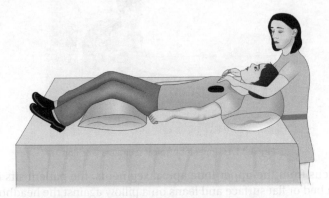

Fig. A-11.3: Upper lobe anterior segments (Position 3).

- The patient lies flat on the bed or table with a pillow for comfort under his/her head and legs.
- The caregiver percusses and vibrates the right and left sides of the front of the chest, between the collar bone and nipple.

Lingula

The various positions for postural drainage involving the lingula are depicted in **Figure A-11.4:**

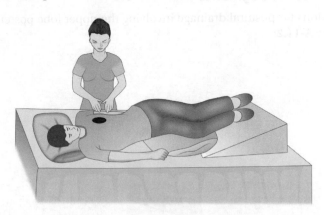

Fig. A-11.4: Lingula position (Position 4).

- The patient lies with his/her head down toward the foot of the bed on the right side, hips and legs up on pillows.
- The body should be rotated about a quarter-turn toward the back.
- A pillow can also be placed behind the patient and his/her legs slightly bent with another pillow between the knees.
- The caregiver percusses and vibrates just outside the nipple area.

Postural Drainage of the Middle Lobe

The various positions for postural drainage involving the middle lobe are depicted in **Figure A-11.5**.

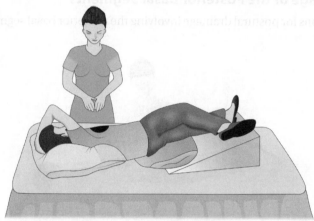

Fig. A-11.5: Middle lobe (Position 5).

- The patient lies head down on his/her left side.
- A quarter-turn toward the back with the right arm up and out of the way.
- The legs and hips should be elevated as high as possible.
- A pillow may be placed in back of the patient and between slightly bent legs.
- The caregiver percusses and vibrates just outside the right nipple area.

Postural Drainage of the Anterior Basal Segments

The various positions for postural drainage involving the anterior basal segments are depicted in **Figure A-11.6**.

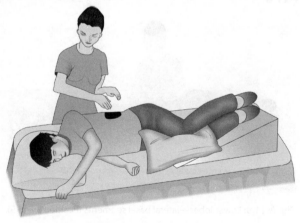

Fig. A-11.6: Lower lobes—anterior basal segments (Position 6).

- The patient lies on his/her right side with his/her head facing the foot of the bed and a pillow behind his/her back.
- The hips and legs should be elevated as high as possible on pillows.
- The knees should be slightly bent and a pillow should be placed between them for comfort.
- The caregiver percusses and vibrates over the lower ribs on the left side.

- This should then be repeated on the opposite side, with percussion and vibration over the lower ribs on the right side of the chest.

Postural Drainage of the Posterior Basal Segments

The various positions for postural drainage involving the posterior basal segments are depicted in **Figure A-11.7**.

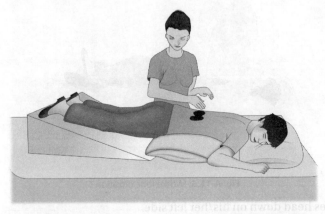

Fig. A-11.7: Lower lobes—posterior basal segments (Position 7).

- The patients lies on his/her stomach, with the hips and legs elevated by pillows.
- The caregiver percusses and vibrates at the lower part of the back, over the left and right sides of the spine, careful to avoid the spine and lower ribs.

Postural Drainage of the Lower Lobes Lateral Basal Segments

The various positions for postural drainage involving the lower lobes lateral basal segments are depicted in **Figure A-11.8**.

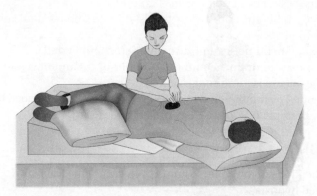

Fig. A-11.8: Lower lobes—lateral basal segments (Position 8 and 9).

- The patient lies on his/her right side, leaning forward about one quarter of a turn with hips and legs elevated on pillows.
- The top leg may be flexed over a pillow for support and comfort.
- The caregiver percusses and vibrates over the uppermost portion of the lower part of the left ribs.
- This should then be repeated on the opposite side, with percussion and vibration over the uppermost portion of the right side of the lower ribs.

Postural Drainage of the Lower Lobes Superior Segments

The various positions for postural drainage involving the lower lobes superior segments are depicted in **Figure A-11.9**:

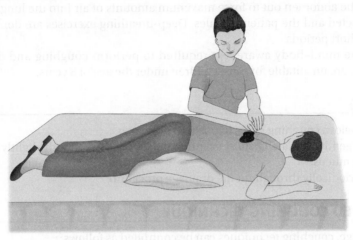

Fig. A-11.9: Lower lobes—superior segments (Position 10).

- For this position, the patient lies on his/her stomach on a flat bed or table.
- Two pillows should be placed under the hips.
- The caregiver percusses and vibrates over the bottom part of the shoulder blades, on both the right and left sides of the spine.
- Avoiding direct percussion or vibration over the spine itself.

TIMING OF POSTURAL DRAINAGE

It is necessary to strictly follow the timing for postural drainage:
- Each treatment session can last for 20 to 40 minutes.
- Postural drainage is best be done before meals or 1½ to 2 hours after eating to minimize the chance of vomiting.
- Early morning and bedtime sessions usually are recommended.
- The length of postural drainage and the number of treatment sessions may need to be increased if the person is more congested.
- The recommended positions and durations of treatment are prescribed by the cystic fibrosis (CF) doctor or therapist.

COMPLICATIONS

The major complications involved in postural drainage are the following:
- Position-related hypoxia
- Aspiration of secretions in other lung regions
- Hypotension

TURNING

Turning from side-to-side permits lung expansion. The child may turn on his/her own or be turned by a caregiver. Turning should be done at a minimum of every 2 hours if the child is bedridden. The head of the bed can also be elevated in order to promote drainage.

DEEP-BREATHING EXERCISES

Deep breathing helps expand the lungs and forces an improved distribution of the air into all sections of the lungs. The patient either sits in a chair or sits upright in bed and inhales and then pushes the abdomen out to force maximum amounts of air into the lung. The abdomen is then contracted and the patient exhales. Deep-breathing exercises are done several times each day for short periods.

Because of the mind–body awareness required to perform coughing and deep-breathing exercises, they are unsuitable for most children under the age of 8 years.

COUGHING

As indicated below, coughing helps in postural drainage:
- Coughing gently or making short grunting noises with the mouth slightly open will help loosen the mucus.
- Do this periodically throughout the drainage procedure.

CONTROLLED COUGHING TECHNIQUE

During drainage, coughing techniques can be controlled as follows:
- Controlled coughing is one of the essential techniques in good respiratory care.
- Patient performs this maneuver after each drainage position and often throughout the day.

HUFFING

At the end of each drainage position, the person can take a deep breath and then expel it quickly in a "huff." This huff forces the air and mucus out, making the cough more effective.

AFTERCARE

Many children may wish to perform **oral hygiene** measures after therapy to lessen the poor taste of the secretions they have expectorated.

Suctioning

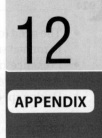

INTRODUCTION

The patient with an artificial airway is not capable of effectively coughing, and the mobilization of secretions from the trachea must be facilitated by aspiration. This is called as suctioning.

DEFINITION

It is the process of removing secretions from the airways.

PURPOSE

The main purposes of suctioning are the following:
- To maintain a patent airway
- To help in maintaining airway of the patient who cannot clear his/her airway effectively with coughing.

METHODS OF SUCTIONING

The three major suctioning methods are the following:
1. Oropharyngeal
2. Nasopharyngeal
3. Tracheostomy and end tracheal tubes

INDICATION

Therapeutic

Therapeutic indications for suctioning are as follows:
- Coarse breath sounds
- Noisy breathing
- Visible secretions in the airway
- Decreased SpO_2 in the pulse oximeter and deterioration of arterial blood gas values
- Clinically increased work of breathing
- Suspected aspiration of gastric or upper airway secretions
- Patient's inability to generate an effective spontaneous cough
- Changes in monitored flow/pressure graphics
- Increased peak inspiratory pressure (PIP) and decreased tidal volume (Vt) during ventilation
- X-ray changes consistent with retained secretions
- The need to maintain the patency and integrity of the artificial airway

- The need to stimulate a cough in patient's unable to cough effectively secondary to changes in mental status or the influence of medication
- Presence of pulmonary atelectasis or consolidation presumed to be associated with secretion retention
- During special procedures, such as bronchoscopy and endoscopy.

Diagnostic

The following are the diagnostic aspects of suctioning:

- The need to obtain a sputum specimen/endotracheal aspiration (ETA) for bacteriological or microbiological or cytological investigations.
- This is the picture that shows us about the ETA sampling.

HAZARDS AND COMPLICATIONS

The hazards and complications of suctioning are as follows:

- Hypoxia/hypoxemia
- Tracheal and/or bronchial mucosal trauma
- Cardiac or respiratory arrest
- Pulmonary hemorrhage/bleeding
- Cardiac dysrhythmias
- Pulmonary atelectasis
- Bronchoconstriction/bronchospasm
- Hypotension/hypertension
- Elevated intracranial pressure (ICP)
- Interruption of mechanical ventilation

ASSESSMENT OF NEED

Qualified personnel should assess the need for tracheal suctioning as a routine part of a patient/ventilator system check.

NECESSARY EQUIPMENT

The equipment necessary for suctioning are the following:

- Vacuum source or portable suction apparatus with adjustable regulator suction jar, collection bottle, and connection tubing.
- Stethoscope
- Sterile gloves for open suctioning method.
- Clean gloves for closed suctioning method.
- Clear protective goggles, apron and mask.
- Sterile normal saline
- Bain's circuit or Ambu bag to preoxygenate the patient.
- Suction tray with hot water for flushing.
- Nasopharyngeal or oropharyngeal airway.
- Water-soluble lubricant
- Sterile catheter

For an adult, 12–14 French catheters; for a child, 8–10 French catheters; and for an infant, pediatric feeding tubes are used.

TYPES OF SUCTIONING

The types of suctioning are as listed below:
- Open suction system: Regularly using system in the intubated patients
- Closed suction system:
  - This is used to facilitate continuous mechanical ventilation and oxygenation during suctioning.
  - Closed suctioning is also indicated when PEEP level is above 10 cm H_2O.

POINTS TO BE KEPT IN MIND

While performing the suctioning procedure, the following points are to be remembered:
- Never suction for more than 10–15 seconds at a time to prevent hypoxia.
- Do not apply suction pressure during insertion catheter.
- Preoxygenate the patient.
- Provide 3-minute interval before each suction followed by hypotension related to the stimulation of vagus nerve.
- Use genital insertion and manipulation of catheter.
- Lubricate catheter before inserting.
- Monitor patient's pulse.
- Follow strict aseptic technique.
- Suction patient only when need arises.

It is also necessary to record the following:
1. Date and time
2. Amount, color, consistency, and odor.

MONITORING

The following should be monitored prior to, during, and after the procedure:
- Breath sounds
- Oxygen saturation
- Respiratory rate (RR) and pattern
- Hemodynamic parameters (pulse rate, blood pressure)
- Cough effort
- Intracranial pressure (ICP) (if indicated and available)
- Sputum characteristics (color, volume, consistency, and odor)
- Ventilator parameters (PIP, Vt, and FiO_2).

PATIENT PREPARATION

For preparing patients undergoing suction, the following aspects are to be remembered:
- Explain the procedure to the patient (if patient is conscious).
- The patient should receive hyperoxygenation by the delivery of 100% oxygen for >30 seconds prior to the suctioning (either with Bain's circuit or by increasing the FiO2 by mechanical ventilator).
- Position the patient in supine position.
- Auscultate the breath sounds.

PROCEDURE

The procedures involved are as follows:
- Perform hand hygiene, i.e., wash hands. It reduces transmission of microorganisms.

- Turn on suction apparatus and set vacuum regulator to appropriate negative pressure. For adult, a pressure of 100–120 mm Hg, for children 80–100 mm Hg, and for infants it is 60–80 mm Hg.
- Goggles, mask, and apron should be worn to prevent splash from secretions.
- Preoxygenate with 100% O_2.
- Wear sterile gloves with sterile technique.
- With the help of an assistant, open suction catheter package and connect it to suction tubing (if you are alone, then open the end of the suction catheter package and connect it to suction tubing).
- With the help of an assistant, disconnect the ventilator.
- Kink the suction tube and insert the catheter into the endotracheal (ET) tube until resistance is felt.
- Resistance is felt when the catheter impacts the carina or bronchial mucosa, and the suction catheter should be withdrawn by 1 cm before applying suction.
- Apply continuous suction while rotating the suction catheter during removal.
- The duration of each suctioning should be <15 seconds.
- Instill 3–5 mL of sterile normal saline into the artificial airway, if required.
- Assistant resumes the ventilator.
- Give four to five manual breaths with bag or ventilator.
- Continue making suction passes, bagging patient between passes, until clear of secretions, but no more than four passes.
- Return patient to ventilator.
- Flush the catheter with hot water in the suction tray.
- Suction nares and oropharynx above the artificial airway.
- Discard used equipment.
- Flush the suction tube with hot water.
- Auscultate the chest
- Wash hands
- Document including indications for suctioning and any changes in vitals and patient's tolerance.

If nurse is alone then:
- Explain the procedure to the patient even if patient is unresponsive.
- Inform patient that suctioning may stimulate transient coughing or gagging (but tell patient that coughing helps to mobilize secretions).
- Reassure patient throughout the procedure to minimize anxiety and fear which can increase oxygen consumption.
- Wash your hands
- Place the patient in semi-Fowler's or high Fowler's position, to promote lung expansion and effective coughing (if patient is responsive).
- Turn on the suction from the portable unit.
- Set the pressure according to your facility's policy (the pressure is usually set between 80 and 120 mm Hg (higher pressure causes excessive trauma without enhancing secretion removal).
- Occlude the end of the connection tubing to check suction pressure.
- Using strict aseptic technique, open the suction catheter kit.
- Disposable container and gloves are to be used.
- Consider your dominant hand sterile and your nondominant hand nonsterile.
- Using your nondominate hand, pour the sterile water or saline into the sterile container.
- With your nondominant hand, place a small amount of water-soluble lubricant on the sterile area (the lubricant is used to facilitate passage of the catheter during nasopharyngeal suctioning).
- Pick-up the catheter with your dominant (sterile) hand and attach it to the connecting tube.

- Use your nondominant hand to control the suction valve, while your dominant hand manipulates the catheter.
- Instruct the patient to cough and breathe slowly and deeply several times before beginning suction. Coughing helps loosen secretions and may decrease the amount of suctioning necessary.

Closed Suctioning Procedure

The following are to be followed for closed suctioning procedure:
- Wash hands
- Wear clean gloves
- Connect tube to closed suction port.
- Preoxygenate the patient with 100% O_2.
- Gently insert catheter tip into artificial airway without applying suction, stop if you meet resistance or when patient starts coughing and pull back by 1 cm.
- Place the dominant thumb over the control vent of the suction port, applying continuous or intermittent suction for no more than 10 seconds as you withdraw the catheter into the sterile sleeve of the closed suction device.
- Repeat steps above if needed.
- Clean the suction catheter with sterile saline until clear; being careful not to instill solution into the ET tube.
- Suction oropharynx above the artificial airway.
- Wash hands

ASSESSMENT OF OUTCOME

The outcome of the procedure is assessed using the following:
- Improvement in breath sounds
- Decreased peak inspiratory pressure and increased tidal volume delivery during ventilation
- Improvement in arterial blood gas values or saturation as reflected by pulse oximetry (SpO_2)
- Removal of pulmonary secretions.

CONTRAINDICATIONS

- Most contraindications are relative to the patient's risk of developing adverse reactions or worsening clinical condition as result of the procedure.
- Suctioning is contraindicated when there is fresh bleeding.
- When indicated, there is no absolute contraindication to endotracheal suctioning because the decision to abstain from suctioning in order to avoid a possible adverse reaction may, in fact, be lethal.

LIMITATIONS OF METHOD

- Suctioning is potentially a harmful procedure if carried out improperly.
- Suctioning should be done when clinically necessary (not routinely).
- The need for suctioning should be assessed at least every 2 hours or more frequently as need arises.

Nasopharyngeal suctioning should be used with caution in patients who have the following problems:
- Nasopharyngeal bleeding
- Spinal fluid leakage into the nasopharyngeal area.
- Receiving anticoagulant therapy because these conditions increase the risk of bleeding.

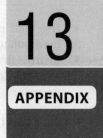

Thoracic Surgeries

APPENDIX

13

INTRODUCTION

Assessment and management are frequently important in the patient undergoing thoracic surgery. Patient undergoing such surgery also have obstructive pulmonary disease with compromised breathing. The objectives of preoperative care for the patient undergoing thoracic surgery are to ascertain the patient's functional reserve to determine if the patient can survive the surgery and to ensure that the patient is in optimal condition for surgery.

Various types of thoracic surgical procedures are performed to relieve the disease condition, such as lung abscesses, lung cancer, cysts, and benign tumor. An exploratory thoracotomy may be performed to diagnose lung or chest disease. A biopsy may be performed in this procedure with a small amount of lung tissue removed for analysis; the chest incision is then closed.

RISK FACTORS FOR SURGERY-RELATED ATELECTASIS AND PNEUMONIA

Preoperative Risk Factors

The risk factors of undergoing a surgery are the following:
- Increased age
- Obesity
- Poor nutritional status
- Smoking history
- History of aspiration

Interoperative Risk Factors

The risk factors involved while undergoing a surgery are the following:
- Thoracic incision
- Prolonged anesthesia

Postoperative Risk Factors

- Supine position
- Decreased level of consciousness
- Inadequate pain management
- Presence of nasogastric tube
- Immobilization
- Prolonged intubation/mechanical intubation

TYPES OF THORACIC SURGERY

Thoracic surgeries are operative procedure performed to aid in the diagnosis and treatment of certain pulmonary conditions and procedures include the following:

- Pneumonectomy
- Lobectomy
- Sleeve lobectomy
- Resection
  - Wedge resection
  - Segment resection or segmentectomy
- Laser surgery
- Video-assisted thoracoscopic surgery (VATS)
- Lung volume reduction
- Advances in thoracic surgeries

Pneumonectomy

Pneumonectomy is of the following two types:
1. **Simple pneumonectomy:** Removal of only the affected lung
2. **Extrapleural pneumonectomy (EPP):** Removal of the affected lung, plus part of the diaphragm, the parietal pleura (lining of the chest), and the pericardium (lining of the heart) on that side.

Extrapleural Pneumonectomy

Introduction: Extrapleural pneumonectomy is a surgical treatment of malignant pleural mesothelioma (MPM). In an EPP, the surgeon removes the diseased lung, part of the pericardium (membrane covering the heart), part of the diaphragm (muscle between the lungs and the abdomen), and part of the parietal pleura (membrane lining the chest).

An EPP is an invasive and complex operation and performed only on patients with early stage localized disease that has not spread to the lymph nodes or invaded surrounding tissues and organs. Candidates for surgery must be otherwise in good health with adequate heart and lung function since removal of an entire lung will increase the load on the heart and remaining lung. Because the EPP is a technically complex operation, it is generally only performed at large medical centers by surgeons with extensive experience in treating mesothelioma.

Procedure: For EPP, general anesthesia is required and the surgeon opens the patient's chest cavity, at either the front, a sternotomy, or the side, a thoracotomy, and makes an incision of approximately 9 inches. The surgeon visually inspects the chest cavity and removes any visible cancer including the entire diseased lung, the pleural lining of the chest and heart, and the diaphragm.

Recovery is extensive often requiring up to a 2-week hospital stay. After discharge, an additional 6–8 weeks is required for a full recovery.

Risks and Benefits:
- An EPP is the most effective method for disease control of malignant mesothelioma.
- It can slow disease progression.
- It improves quality of life, especially breathing.
- When combined with radiation and chemotherapy, EPP can have a significant impact on life expectancy.

Techniques of Pneumonectomy
- **Drainage after pneumonectomy:** After most pneumonectomies, the pleural space can be safely closed without drainage. If a chest tube must be used, a balanced drainage system is recommended. It also describes the indications, advantages, and disadvantages of drainage and the methods commonly used for this purpose. Balanced drainage system will prevent mediastinal shift following pneumonectomy.

- **Pneumonectomy through an empyema:** The practical management of the patient with a destroyed lung in association with a pre-existing empyema. Control of infection before proceeding with pneumonectomy by adequate drainage of the empyema and control of tuberculosis and pneumonia, particularly on the opposite side, are stressed. Pneumonectomy is undertaken through the empyema and usually in the intrapleural plane.
- **Completion pneumonectomy:** Completion pneumonectomy refers to an operation intended to remove what is left of a lung partially resected during previous surgery. Completion pneumonectomy is a technically demanding procedure, which carries an increased operative mortality and morbidity. If the planning and the surgical technique are done meticulously, the good prospect for long-term survival justifies the higher risk.

Lobectomy

Also called a pulmonary lobectomy, it is a common surgical procedure that removes one lobe of the lung that contains cancerous cells. Removal of two lobes is called bilobectomy.

Sleeve Lobectomy

A surgical procedure that removes a cancerous lobe of the lung along with part of the bronchus (air passage) that is attached to it. The remaining lobes are then reconnected to the remaining segment of the bronchus. This procedure preserves part of a lung and is an alternative to removing the lung as a whole (pneumonectomy).

Resection

Resection refers to the removal of a smaller amount of lung tissue, that is, less than one lobe. It is of two types.

1. **Wedge resection:** In a wedge resection, a small, localized area of tumor near the surface of the lung is removed using special stapling devices. This operation can be performed either through a thoracotomy or by VATS. Because the resected area is small, the pulmonary structure and function are relatively not changed. It is performed for random lung biopsy and small peripheral nodules.
2. **Segmental resection:** It is removal of one or more lung segments (a bronchiole and its alveoli). The remaining lung tissue overexpands to fill the previously occupied space. A segment resection removes a larger portion of the lung lobe than a wedge resection but does not remove the whole lobe.

Laser Surgery

Laser therapy is used as a palliative measure for relief of endobronchial obstructions that are not surgically resectable. However, the tumor must be accessible by bronchoscopy. Therefore, tumors pressing on bronchial tissue from outside the bronchus are not amenable to laser therapy. Laser procedures do not produce systemic or cumulative toxic effects and are well tolerated. Laser therapy may be provided in an outpatient setting.

Video-assisted Thoracoscopic Surgery

Video-assisted thoracoscopic surgery is minimally invasive thoracic surgery that does not use a formal thoracotomy incision. It provides adequate visualization despite limited access to the thorax, allowing the procedure to be performed in a state of debilitation and for patients who have marginal pulmonary reserve.

Video-assisted thoracoscopic surgery is principally employed in the management of pulmonary, mediastinal, and pleural pathology. Its main benefit has been the avoidance of a thoracotomy incision, which allows a shorter operative time, less postoperative morbidity, and earlier return to normal activity.

Indications

Video-assisted thoracoscopic surgery is used in both diagnostic and therapeutic pleural, lung, and mediastinal surgery. Specific indications include the following:

- Stapled lung biopsy
- Pericardial window
- Sympathectomy
- Pleural biopsy
- Bullectomy
- Lobectomy
- Pneumonectomy
- Resection of peripheral pulmonary nodule
- Evaluation of mediastinal tumors or adenopathy
- Treatment of recurrent pneumothorax
- Management of loculated empyema
- Pleurodesis of malignant effusions
- Repair of a bronchopleural fistula
- Chest trauma (mainly diaphragmatic injuries)

Contraindications

- Markedly unstable or shocked patient
- Extensive adhesions obliterating the pleural space

Relative contraindications

The relative contraindications are the following:

- Inability to tolerate single lung ventilation
- Previous thoracotomies
- Extensive pleural diseases

Procedure

General anesthesia is used on the patient for a pneumonectomy. The surgery requires an incision that is 7–9 inches in length. After the incision is made, part of the rib may be taken out, so that the lungs can be easily viewed. It will collapse the lung to be removed and then any blood vessels that are attached, as well as the air tube (main bronchus) that goes into the cancerous lung are clamped, cut, and tied off.

At this point, the lung is taken out through the incision. To ensure that no fluid leaks into the chest cavity, all of the tubes and vessels that were tied off are closely inspected. If an EPP procedure is done, at the same time that the lung is removed, the pleural lining for the chest, diaphragm, and heart are also taken out.

Recovery

For several days after the surgery, the patient's breathing will be assisted by a respirator. Tubes for drainage will remove any fluid that may build up. Two weeks is the normal hospital stay duration for a pneumonectomy patient.

Lung Transplantation

Lung transplant can benefit patients with a variety of serious pulmonary disorders, including pulmonary hypertension, emphysema, cystic fibrosis, and bronchiectasis. A single lung, both lungs or heart and lungs have been successfully transplanted. Better criteria for selecting patients and donors as well as advancements in surgical techniques have improved outcomes for these patients.

Advances in Thoracic Surgeries

Advanced minimally invasive thoracic surgical procedure include the following:
- Video-assisted thoracoscopic surgery lobectomy
- Video-assisted thoracoscopic surgery segmentecomy
- Minimally invasive esophagectomy
- Thymectomy
- Endobronchial ultrasound
- Electromagnetic navigation bronchoscopy
- Lung resection after chemoradiation
- Pleurectomy

VIDEO-ASSISTED ENDOBRONCHIAL SURGERY

It was rigid bronchoscopy that first provided direct access to the tracheobronchial tree. With the adaptation of new technologic advances, endoscopic evaluation and management of disorders of the trachea and bronchi have attained full circle, enabling surgeons and pulmonologists to perform a wide range of minimally invasive endobronchial procedures.

Indications

Simple diagnostic and therapeutic procedures such as biopsy and foreign body or tumor removal were possible with rigid bronchoscopy performed under general anesthesia.

The subsequent development of fiberoptic technology and refinements in instrumentation made it possible to evaluate the tracheobronchial tree with the flexible fiberoptic bronchoscope, thus alleviating the requirement for general anesthesia. However, therapeutic limitations existed with flexible fiberoptic bronchoscopy in the management of large airway maladies, including tumor or foreign body obstruction, tracheoesophageal fistula, bronchopleural fistula, and anastomotic stricture or dehiscence. An ingenious combination of the "older" rigid bronchoscope, modified to incorporate "newer" fiberoptic lenses, video cameras, and television monitors broadened the horizon of minimally invasive endobronchial surgery. This concomitant development of instrumentation and devices, keeping pace with advances in endoscopy, has made it possible to treat many conditions that could formerly be managed only by open surgical operations.

Preoperative Management

The goal is to maximize respiratory function to improve outcome postoperatively and reduce risk of complications.
- Encourage the patient to stop smoking to restore bronchial ciliary action and to reduce the amount of sputum and likelihood of postoperative atelectasis.
- Teach an effective coughing technique.
  - Sit upright with knees flexed and body bending slightly forward.
  - Splint the incision with hands or folded towel.
  - Take three short breaths, followed by a deep inspiration, inhaling slowly and evenly through the nose.
  - Contract abdominal muscles and cough twice forcefully with mouth open and tongue out.
  - Alternate technique—huffing and coughing—is less painful. Take a deep diaphragmatic breath and exhale forcefully against hand; exhale in a quick distinct pant or huff.

- Humidify the air to loosen secretions
- Administer bronchodilators to reduce bronchospasm
- Administer antimicrobials for infection
- Encourage deep breathing using incentive spirometer to prevent atelectasis postoperatively.
- Teach diaphragmatic breathing.
- Carry out chest physical therapy and postural drainage to reduce pooling of the lung secretions.
- Evaluate cardiovascular status for risk and prevention of complications.
- Encourage activity to improve exercise tolerance.
- Administer medications and limit sodium and fluid to improve congestive heart failure, if indicated.
- Correct anemia, dehydration, and hypoproteinemia with intravenous infusions, tube feedings, and blood transfusions as indicated.
- Give prophylactic anticoagulant as prescribed to reduce perioperative incidence of DVT and pulmonary embolism.
- Provide teaching and counseling.
- Orient the patient to events that will occur in the postoperative period—coughing and deep breathing, suctioning, chest tube and drainage bottles, oxygen therapy, ventilator therapy, pain control, leg exercises, and range-of-motion (ROM) exercises for affected shoulder.
- Ensure that the patient fully understands the surgery and is emotionally prepared for it; verify that informed consent has been obtained.

Postoperative Management

The postoperative management involves the following steps:
1. Use mechanical ventilator until respiratory function and cardiovascular status stabilize. Assist with weaning and extubating.
2. Auscultate chest, monitor vital signs, monitor ECG, and assess respiratory rate and depth frequently. Arterial line, central venous pressure (CVP), and pulmonary artery catheter are usually used.
3. Frequently monitor arterial blood gases (ABGs) and/or SaO_2.
4. Monitor and manage chest drainage system to drain fluid, blood, clots, and air from the pleura after surgery. Chest drainage is usually not used after pneumonectomy; however, because it is desirable that the pleural space is filled with an effusion that eventually obliterates the space.

Complications

- Hypoxia: Watch for restlessness, tachycardia, tachypnea, and elevated blood pressure.
- Postoperative bleeding: Monitor for restlessness and anxiety, pallor, tachycardia, and hypotension.
- Pneumonia, atelectasis.
- Bronchopleural fistula from disruption of a bronchial suture or staple, and bronchial stump leak.
  - Observe for sudden onset of respiratory distress or cough productive of serosanguineous fluid.
  - Position with the operative side down.
  - Prepare for immediate chest tube insertion and/or surgical intervention.
- Cardiac dysrhythmias; myocardial infarction (MI) or heart failure.

Nursing Assessment

- Monitor for manifestations of acute pulmonary edema: Dyspnea, crackles, persistent cough, frothy sputum, and cyanosis.
- Monitor chest tube drainage system: Amount and color, water seal chamber for tidaling and bubbling, suction control chamber filled to appropriate level.
- Monitor for manifestations of tension pneumothorax: Severe dyspnea, tachypnea and tachycardia, extreme restlessness and agitation, cyanosis, laryngeal and tracheal deviation to unaffected side.
- Observe for subcutaneous emphysema around incision and in the chest and neck.
- Monitor for manifestations of pulmonary embolus: Chest pain, dyspnea and tachypnea, fever, hemoptysis, and indications of right-sided heart failure.
- Assess for cardiac dysrhythmias, particularly atrial fibrillation, atrial flutter and paroxysmal atrial tachycardia.
- Monitor intravenous fluid rate.
- Assess dressing and incisional area every 4 hours for evidence of bleeding.
- Monitor for the signs of hypovolemic shock.
- Monitor for thrombophlebitis

Nursing Diagnosis

- Ineffective airway clearance related to increased secretions and to decreased coughing effectiveness due to pain
- Ineffective breathing pattern related to hypoventilation
- Acute pain related to surgical procedure
- Impaired physical mobility related to pain, muscle dissection, restricted positioning, and chest tubes
- Activity intolerance related to difficulty in maintaining oxygenation secondary to reduced lung volume
- Risk for ineffective coping related to temporary dependence and loss of full respiratory function
- Knowledge deficit related to self-care after discharge.

Nursing Interventions

The seven major steps involved in nursing interventions are the following:

I. **Maintaining airway clearance**
   - Once vital signs are stable, place the client in semi or high Fowler's position.
   - Help the client cough and deep breathe every 1 or 2 hours during the first 24–48 hours.
   - Instruct the client to take deep breath slowly and to hold it for 3–5 seconds, then exhale; to take a second breath and then, while exhaling, to cough forcefully twice.
   - When possible, schedule coughing and deep breathing sessions at times when pain medication is maximally effective.
   - Assess the breath sounds before and after coughing.

II. **Maintain respiratory status**
   - Monitor for manifestations of ineffective breathing pattern: Tachypnea, tachycardia, dyspnea, use of accessory muscles, cyanosis, restlessness, and decreased level of consciousness.
   - Monitor for and report significant decrease in SaO_2 and PaO_2 levels.
   - Provide interventions to reduce chest pain.
   - Maintain semi to high Fowler's positioning unless contraindicated.
   - Implement measures to reduce client anxiety and fear.

- Provide calm and supportive environment, answer each question, and instruct the relaxation techniques.

III. Maintain the comfort level

- Assess pain intensity using a self-report measure tool.
- Administer pain medication as ordered.
- Observe for side effects of medication used.
- Offer and instruct the clients to ask for pain medication before pain becomes severe.
- Assess medication effectiveness and avoid overmedication.
- Relaxation techniques are taught to the client and also provided with diversional therapy.

IV. Encouraging mobility in the patient

- Position client as indicated by phase of recovery and surgical procedure.
  - ♦ Nonoperative side lying position may be used until consciousness is regained.
  - ♦ Semi Fowler's position is recommended as the vital signs are stable.
  - ♦ Avoid positioning client on operative side.
  - ♦ Avoid complete lateral position after pneumonectomy.
  - ♦ Avoid traction on chest tubes while changing client position; check for kinking or compression of tubing.
- Gently turn the client every 1–2 hours, unless contraindicated.
- Encourage regular ambulation, once the client's condition is stable. Maintain supplemental oxygen, if ordered.
- Begin passive ROM exercises of arm and shoulder on the affected side 4 hours after recovery from anesthesia.
- Encourage the client to use the affected side arm for daily living activities.

V. Ensure activity tolerance

- Carefully assess the client's response to activity and exercise. Observe for manifestations of dyspnea, fatigue, tachycardia, and tachypnea that do not subside in 3 minutes.
- Allow adequate rest periods between activities.

VI. Help the client and family members to cope with the situation

- Provide opportunity to the client to express feelings.
- Encourage the use of positive coping strategies.
- Allow the client to have as much control over daily activities and decision-making as is possible.
- Support and praise all independent activities that promote recovery.

VII. Enhancing the knowledge of the patient: It involves providing thorough instruction and preparation for hospital discharge:

- Surgical wound and chest tube insertion site care
- Continuation of exercise program
- Precautions regarding activity and environmental irritants
- Clinical manifestations to be reported to health-care professionals.
- Community agencies that can provide resources, as needed.

Exercise Stress Test

ERGOMETER

Ergometer comes from the Greek words *ergon*, meaning "work" and *metron*, meaning "measure."

An apparatus which measures work or energy expended during a period of physical exercise.

Types of Ergometer
- Treadmill
- Cycle
- Arm ergometer

EXERCISE TESTING PROTOCOLS

A variety of exercise testing protocols are available, whether the test is conducted using treadmill, cycle, or arm ergometer.
- Amputee patients use arm ergometer.
- Treadmill testing provides a more common form of physiologic stress (i.e., walking).
- The cycle ergometer has the advantage of requiring less space and generally is less costly than the treadmill. Minimized movements of the arm and thorax facilitates better quality electrocardiogram (ECG) recording and blood pressure (BP) monitoring.
- To perform a stress test in an above-knee amputee, an upper extremity ergometer is used.

TREADMILL

A stress test in which the patient walks on a moving treadmill while the heart and breathing rates are monitored.

Exercise stress test allows us to assess the response of heart to the increased workload and demand for blood during exercise. This is done by recording the ECG of heart while walking on a treadmill machine. It is useful in diagnosing ischemic heart disease (reduced blood supply to the heart muscles due to coronary artery disease).

INDICATIONS AND CONTRAINDICATIONS

Treadmill stress testing is indicated for diagnosis and prognosis of cardiovascular disease, specifically coronary artery disease (CAD).
- Evaluate for myocardial ischemia.
- Evaluate for exercise-induced arrhythmia.
- Evaluate exercise tolerance.

Absolute contraindications include the following:
- Acute myocardial infarction (MI; within 2 days)
- Unstable angina not previously stabilized by medical therapy
- Uncontrolled cardiac arrhythmias causing symptoms or hemodynamic compromise
- Symptomatic severe aortic stenosis
- Uncontrolled symptomatic heart failure
- Acute pulmonary embolus or pulmonary infarction
- Acute myocarditis or pericarditis
- Acute aortic dissection

Relative contraindications can be superseded if the benefits of exercise outweigh the risks. They include the following:
- Left main coronary stenosis
- Moderate stenotic valvular heart disease
- Electrolyte abnormalities
- Severe arterial hypertension, i.e., systolic BP (SBP) higher than 200 mm Hg and diastolic BP (DBP) higher than 110 mm Hg or both
- Tachyarrhythmia or bradyarrhythmias
- Hypertrophic cardiomyopathy and any other forms of outflow tract obstruction
- Mental or physical impairment leading to an inability to exercise adequately
- High-degree atrioventricular (AV) block

EQUIPMENT

- Treadmill
- The ECG machine and the BP monitor
- Oxygen delivery nasal cannula and wall oxygen on hand
- Resuscitation capability: Crash cart/defibrillator with emergency pharmaceuticals

PLACEMENT OF THE ECG ELECTRODES

It is important to be familiar with proper placement of ECG electrodes for exercise treadmill test (ETT). Four limb leads are placed either on the patient's limbs or on the torso near the patient's limbs. A standardized color scheme is used to designate limb leads:
- **White:** Right upper extremity or right upper torso (shoulder)
- **Green:** Right lower extremity or right lower torso (hip)
- **Black:** Left upper extremity or left upper torso (shoulder)
- **Red:** Left lower extremity or left lower torso (hip)
  Precordial leads (standard ECG includes six leads, termed V1 through V6) are placed across the chest wall.
- V1: Right sternal margin, fourth intercostal space
- V2: Left sternal margin, fourth intercostal space
- V3: Midway between V2 and V4
- V4: Left midclavicular line, fifth intercostal space
- V5: Left anterior axillary line, same horizontal plane as V4
- V6: Left midaxillary line, same horizontal plane as V4.

PREPROCEDURE

- Requisition form is reviewed by nurse or physician.
- Provide patients instruction and determine appropriateness of study on the basis of clinical history and current status.

- Instruct patients to hold beta-blockers, calcium channel blockers, and long-acting nitrates 24 hours before the test.
- Instruct patients to wear comfortable clothing and comfortable, stable shoes for treadmill use.
- Instruct patients to not eat or drink for 3 hours before the test.
- Do not apply lotion, oil, or powder to the chest.
- For men, please shave the chest before the test, so that the ECG electrodes can be placed on the chest.
- Calculate the targeted heart rate (THR), i.e., calculated by formula of 85% of 220 − age = THR.

How is the Test Done?

- The medical technologist will place some ECG electrodes on chest and a BP cuff around arm for continuous monitoring throughout the test.
- Thereafter, the doctor will assess the condition.
- Blood pressure will be taken and an ECG of heart at rest will then be recorded.
- The medical technologist will show the patient how to walk on the treadmill.
- The treadmill will start off at a slow speed.
- Thereafter, the speed and gradient of the treadmill will increase gradually at a regular interval of 3 minutes.
- Blood pressure, heart rate, ECG, and general condition will be monitored closely during the test.
- As the stages of the test progress, it can get quite strenuous.
- Ask the patient to tell the doctor or medical technologist to stop the treadmill at any time should the patient feel tired, unwell, or unable to continue.
- Please note that once the patient discontinues the test, he or she will not be able to redo or continue with the test.

After Procedure (Recovery Period)

- When the exercise test ends, the patient will be asked to rest on the bed for approximately 5 minutes while the ECG and BP are being monitored and recorded.
- The ECG, heart rate, BP response, and symptoms recorded during the test will be analyzed and the report will be given to the doctor.

INDICATIONS FOR STOPPING AN EXERCISE TEST

Symptom-limited Maximal Test

1. Progressive angina
2. Ventricular tachycardia
3. Any significant drop (20 mm Hg) in systolic BP or a failure of the systolic BP to rise with an increase in exercise load
4. Light-headedness, confusion, pallor, cyanosis, nausea, or signs of severe peripheral circulatory insufficiency
5. The 3-mm horizontal or downsloping ST depression or elevation (in the absence of other indicators of ischemia)
6. Excessive rise in BP: systolic >250 mm Hg; diastolic pressure >120 mm Hg.

Urinary Catheterization

DEFINITION

Urinary catheterization is the insertion of a especially designed tube into the bladder using an aseptic technique, for the purpose of draining urine, removal of clots/debris, and the instillation of medication.

Catheters are sized in units called French, where one French (FR) equals 1/3 of 1 mm. Catheters vary from 12 (small) FR to 48 (large) FR (3–16 mm) in size.

Age	Weight	Catheter Size
0–6 months	3.5–7 kg	6
1 year	10 kg	6–8
2 years	12 kg	8
3 years	14 kg	8–10
5 years	18 kg	10
6 years	21 kg	10
8 years	27 kg	10–12
12 years	Varies	12–14

INDICATIONS FOR CATHETERIZATION

Investigations (Diagnostic Purposes)

- To determine residual urine
- To enable bladder function test to be performed

Drainage

Pre- or postoperatively:
- To drain blood clots and debris
- To obtain an accurate measurement of urine output
- To empty the bladder before childbirth if necessary

Retention of urine

Acute or chronic caused by:
- Outflow obstruction, e.g., prostate hyperplasia or urethral stricture
- Neurological diseases, e.g., multiple sclerosis
- Trauma to brain or spinal cord
- Spina bifida

Drug Instillation

- Catheter maintenance solution
- Chemotherapy

Management of Incontinence

Contraindications

- Foley catheters are contraindicated in the presence of urethral trauma
- Urethral injuries
- Patients with multisystem injuries and pelvic fractures

Equipment

A tray containing the following:
- A pair of sterile gloves
- A pair of clean gloves
- Sterile drapes
- Cleansing solution—betadine
- A bowl with soapy swabs
- Sterile water (usually 10 cc)
- Foley catheter (usually 16–18 French)
- Syringe (usually 10 cc)
- Lubricant (water-based jelly or xylocaine jelly)
- Collection bag and tubing
- Kidney tray and paper bag
- Mackintosh and towel/paper
- Specimen bottle if sample is required
- A sterile tray containing bowl with sterile swabs, thumb forceps, and artery forceps
- Recording and reporting chart

PRELIMINARY ASSESSMENT

- The nurse should assess the patient's fluid intake and urinary output in the previous 12 hours.
- Palpate bladder to assess the level of distension.
- Identify the purpose of catheterization.
- Check patient's level of consciousness and ability to follow instructions.

PROCEDURE

The steps of procedure are as follows:
- Gather equipment
- Explain procedure to the patient
- Maintain privacy
- Wash hands and wear clean gloves
- Remove patient's cloth and place a Mackintosh with towel under patient's buttocks
- Assist patient into supine position with legs spread and feet together
- Drape the patient
- Clean perineal area with soapy swabs
- Remove gloves and wash hands

- Prepare sterile field
- Put on sterile gloves
- Open catheterization kit and catheter
- Tell assistant to put betadine solution in sterile bowl with sterile swabs
- Clean the perineal area with betadine-soaked sterile swabs from inner to outer, one swipe per swab, discard swab away from the sterile field
- Tell assistant to remove the covering of catheter 3–4 inches only
- Hold catheter in one hand and part the labia/foreskin with other hand
- Tell assistant to generously coat the distal portion (2–5 cm) of the catheter with lubricant
- Gently insert catheter 2–4 inches in female or 7–9 inches in male
- Collect a urine specimen, if needed, by placing the open end of catheter into specimen bottle or otherwise attach the catheter with tubing and urobag
- Inflate balloon, using correct amount of sterile liquid (usually 10 cc)
- Gently pull catheter until inflation balloon is snug against bladder neck
- Secure catheter to abdomen (in male) or thigh (in females), without tension on tubing
- Place drainage bag below the bladder level
- Evaluate catheter function and amount, color, odor, and quality of urine
- Remove gloves, dispose of equipment appropriately, and wash hands
- Document the size of catheter inserted, amount of water in balloon, patient's response to procedure, and assessment of urine.

AFTERCARE

- Remove the drape sheet and replace the bed linen
- Make the patient comfortable with proper body alignment
- Wash articles and replace in the utility room
- Send urine specimen to laboratory

Complications

- Tissue trauma and infection. After 48 hours of catheterization, most catheters are colonized with bacteria, thus leading to possible bacteriuria and its complications.
- Renal inflammation
- Cystitis, urethritis
- Pyelonephritis if left in for prolonged periods

Points to Remember for Preventing Infection

- Follow good hand washing techniques
- Do not open the drainage bag
- If the drainage tube is disconnected, then clean the end of catheter with antiseptic solution and then reconnect it.
- Empty the bag at least 8 hourly
- Perform routine perineal hygiene
- Catheter should be changed before 14 days.

INDEX

Page numbers followed by *f* refer to figure, *fc* refer to flowchart, and *t* refer to table.

D